Urogenital Trauma: A Practical Guide

Said Abdallah AL-Mamari

Urogenital Trauma: A Practical Guide

Springer

Said Abdallah AL-Mamari
Department of Urology
The Royal Hospital
Muscat, Oman

ISBN 978-981-99-6170-2 ISBN 978-981-99-6171-9 (eBook)
https://doi.org/10.1007/978-981-99-6171-9

This Springer imprint is published by the registered company Springer Nature Singapore Pte Ltd.
The registered company address is: 152 Beach Road, #21-01/04 Gateway East, Singapore 189721, Singapore

Foreword

It gives me pleasure to introduce the book written by Said Abdallah Al-Mamari from Muscat, Oman.

Urogenital trauma is a complex topic and Dr. Said Al-Mamari has assembled its latest management. We always learn from the experience of others and the guidelines-based approach. He has effortfully compiled various chapters on all genito-urinary organs in a book that brings out practical points in the management options for complex situations.

The book is handy to the ones treating trauma and to the ones in education.

I wish you all a good reading and congratulate Said Abdallah Al-Mamari for this book.

Sanjay B. Kulkarni
Kulkarni Reconstructive Urology Center
Pune, India

Preface

While conceiving, writing, completing, and publishing a book is always a daunting task, questions on the very interest of the present work were constantly troubling my mind during its preparation. However, when remembering some confusing scenarios in urogenital trauma in my personal practice whose management was not clearly predicted by the current guidelines, it became obvious that a thorough look at **the most relevant and most recent publications** was necessary to learn more and deeper about other centers' experiences and to share my efforts with as many practitioners and researchers as possible.

While carrying out a broad review of the literature treating this subject, a delicate approach was undertaken to summarize the most practical knowledge and present it in a didactical and easily digestible way to the readers.

Abundant illustrations were added to this book to enhance the learning and memorizing process.

An account of life-saving minimally invasive interventions and invasive surgical procedures was given as well as a detailed review of reconstructive operations of the urinary tract and genital organs. **Nevertheless, these are by no means intended to be substituted for more comprehensive manuals of operative techniques and will never replace attendance to workshops and assiduous observation and participation in real-life situations in the operating theaters.**

Apart from being useful in daily practice, I believe this book will also be a good vade mecum for the students and residents, serving them as a last-day-revision material before their Board or fellowship examinations.

It is my pleasure to acknowledge **Professor Sanjay B. Kulkarni (Pune, India)** who kindly and promptly accepted to review the content of this manuscript and to write his expert foreword that will surely add value to this manual and raise the interest of the readers.

Said Abdallah Al-Mamari
Urology Department, The Royal Hospital
Muscat, Oman

Acknowledgment

1. To Professor Sanjay Balwant Kulkarni, Kulkarni Reconstructive Urology Center, Pune, India, President of the Urology Society of India, for reviewing this manual and for his expert foreword.
2. To Dr. Ayman Mohamed Abozekry and Dr. Hamidreza Shemsheki, Urology Department, The Royal Hospital, for their help in images collection and their technical advices.
3. To all my colleagues who kindly shared relevant images (pictures, X-rays) from their personal collection to illustrate this book.
4. To Mr. Naren Aggarwal, Mrs. Raman Shukla, Mrs. Neeraja Padmanabhan, and Ms. Momoko Asawa, Editors and Executives for Springer Nature, for their expert technical assistance in the production, finalization, and publication of this book.

Introduction

Along with the improvement of trauma management, safety measures have been implemented with appreciable efficacy as evidenced by a 31% decrease in the global age-standardized injury-related disability-adjusted life year (DALY) rate between 1990 and 2013 [1]. Yet trauma remains unpredictable. It occurs anywhere, at any time of the day, at any period of the year, and each medical practitioner must be prepared for its occurrence in his/her daily practice.

With the development of modern transport technology, the increased dependence on machinery in human daily activities, the intensive construction of higher buildings and highways, the widespread sports practice, the easy procurement of weapons, the development of urban criminality, and the multiplication of conflicts in the world, the magnitude of trauma and its consequences have become greater than ever. In 2013, approximately 973 million people in the world sustained injuries of various grades that required medical attention [1]. Global estimation of mortality suggests that between 14,000 and 16,000 people lose their lives every day, i.e., 5.8 million each year, as a result of trauma, accounting for 10–11% of mortalities, and being currently the sixth leading cause of death in the world [2, 3]. Projections made by WHO suggest that by 2030, **road traffic accidents (RTA)** are likely to become the fifth leading cause of death and the third leading cause of disability in the world [2]. In the USA, trauma is reported to be the leading cause of death among people aged 1–44 years old and to be the third leading cause of death in all age groups. Statistically, 214,000 people die in the USA from traumatic injuries every year, which equals 586 persons every day [4]. In the UK, trauma is also the leading cause of death in children and young adults (≤44 years) according to the Trauma Audit and Research Network (TARN), and approximately 16,000 people die every year after injury, or 44 daily, in England and Wales [5].

Contrary to malignancies, heart and renal diseases, hypertension, diabetes mellitus, and other degenerative disorders which mostly affect older people, the higher likelihood of trauma affecting the young population in the productive age provokes grim economic consequences that cannot be overlooked. Indeed, in addition to direct medical costs, five other components should be considered in the estimation of the total socio-economic costs of any serious injury: production loss, human costs (quality of life and life-years lost), administrative costs (police, fire service, insurance, legal costs), material damage (vehicles, infrastructure, freight, etc.), and others (traffic congestion, vehicle unavailability, funeral costs) [6]. Statistics have shown that over 2.8 million people are hospitalized in the USA every year because of trauma, with estimated annual costs of $406 billion including medical management and lost productivity [7]. Moreover, when this calculation was revisited by a recent study including the human costs, the estimated total burden steeply rose to $4.2 trillion per year, comprising $327 billion for medical management, $69 billion for productivity loss, and $3.8 trillion for the losses of statistical life and quality of life [8]. There is a wide disparity in the serious injuries cost, and a European study has shown that this may vary from €28,205 to €975,074, and the estimated total burden might represent between 0.04% and 2.7% of a country's gross domestic product (GDP) [6].

Regrettably, there is a disparity in the budget allocated for trauma research compared to other health problems. Thus in 2018, the American National Institute of Health (NIH) funded an estimated $639 million to traumatic injury research projects, representing less than 2% of its budget and only a tenth of the estimated amount allocated to cancer research ($6.3 billion). The great paradox is that trauma accounts for more years of potential life lost (YPLL) before 75 years than cancer with 24.1% and 21.3%, respectively [4], and the greater negative impact of this financial disparity is observed in lower socio-economic status victims who have higher recorded mortality than the richer population following minor trauma [9].

Specifically, **urogenital trauma (UGT)** of various anatomopathology and grade is a common condition presenting to the hospital. Its causes and circumstances are multiform and comprise a broad spectrum that includes RTAs (renal trauma, pelvic trauma with membranous urethra injury, bladder rupture, external genital injuries), home, recreational, or sports accidents where the external genitals are mostly involved, assaults, work accidents (falling astride with bulbar urethral injury), iatrogenic injuries occurring either during gyneco-obstetrical interventions (bladder or ureteral injury in cesarean section or hysterectomy), colorectal operations (ureteric injury), endourological interventions (urethral, bladder, or ureteral injury of various degrees) or percutaneous nephrolithotomy (PCNL). Rarely do patients present with self-inflicted genital trauma, and this entity will be dealt with in a special section.

The management of UGT has been addressed by many retrospective research articles (meta-analyses, systematic reviews, series, national databases, population-based studies, and case reports). However, due to a lack of funding in the field of trauma on the one hand [4], and the stressful patient's presentation potentially requiring urgent life-saving management; on the other hand, there is not enough room left for prospective randomized controlled trials. This paucity of high-quality research causes a lack of high level of evidence to support authoritative guidelines; therefore, recommendations from expert panels are seldom strong [10]. Nonetheless, there are robust retrospective research and strong clinical experience pleading for many consensuses in this field that are published by experts' panels. Because of the complexity of the UGT, each injury has got its special approach guided by the mechanism of the trauma, the anatomopathology of the lesion, the organ involved, and the patient's condition at presentation.

In this book, a systematic approach will be adopted, summarizing all available data and progressing from proximal to distal throughout the urogenital system.

However, female genital trauma will not be discussed in this manual since it would better be addressed by gynecological experts. At the same time, efforts were made to avoid oversaturating the didactic material and to provide the readers with pieces of useful and practical knowledge about the management of this entity.

References

1. Haagsma JA, Graetz N, Bolliger I, et al. The global burden of injury: incidence, mortality, disability-adjusted life years and time trends from the Global Burden of Disease study 2013. Inj Prev. 2016;22(1):3–18. https://doi.org/10.1136/injuryprev-2015-041616. Epub 2015 Dec 3.
2. World Health Organization. Global status report on road safety: time for action. Geneva: WHO; 2009.
3. Greaves I, Porter K, Garner J, editors. Trauma care manual. 3rd ed. CRC Press. 2021. https://doi.org/10.1201/9781003197560.
4. Dowd B, McKenney M, Boneva D, Elkbuli A. Disparities in National Institute of Health trauma research funding: the search for sufficient funding opportunities. Medicine (Baltimore). 2020;99(6):e19027. https://doi.org/10.1097/MD.0000000000019027.
5. The Trauma Audit and Research Network (TARN). Trauma care in England and Wales. https://tarndev.exchdev.man.ac.uk/#:~:text=Welcome,left%20severely%20disabled%20for%20life.
6. Schoeters A, Wijnen W, Carnis L, et al. Costs related to serious road injuries: a European perspective. Eur Transp Res Rev 2020;12:58. https://doi.org/10.1186/s12544-020-00448-0.
7. Haider AH, Saleem T, Leow JJ. Influence of the National Trauma Data Bank on the study of trauma outcomes: is it time to set research best practices to further enhance its impact? J Am Coll Surg. 2012;214(5):756–68.
8. Peterson C, Miller GF, Barnett SB, Florence C. Economic cost of injury—United States, 2019. MMWR Morb Mortal Wkly Rep. 2021;70:1655–6.
9. McHale P, Hungerford D, Taylor-Robinson D, Lawrence T, Astles T, Morton B. Socioeconomic status and 30-day mortality after minor and major trauma: a retrospective analysis of the Trauma Audit and Research Network (TARN) dataset for England. PLoS One. 2018;13(12):e0210226. https://doi.org/10.1371/journal.pone.0210226.
10. Sharma DM, Serafetinidis E, Sujenthiran A, Elshout PJ, Djakovic N, Gonsalves M, Kuehhas FE, Lumen N, Kitrey ND, Summerton DJ, EAU Guidelines Panel on Urological Trauma. Grey areas: challenges of developing guidelines in adult urological trauma. Eur Urol Focus. 2016;2(1):109–10. https://doi.org/10.1016/j.euf.2015.11.005. Epub 2015 Dec 8.

Contents

Abbreviations

AAST	American Association for the Surgery of Trauma
AIS	Abbreviated Injury Scale
AKI	Acute renal injury
AMH	Anti-Mullerian hormone
AUA	American Urological Association
AUF	Arterio-ureteral fistula
AVF	Arteriovenous fistula
BAUS	British Association of Urological Surgeons
BMG	Buccal mucosa graft
BPD	Berlin polytrauma definition
CECT	Contrast-enhanced computed tomography
CPAs	Congenital penile anomalies
CTE	Crossed testicular ectopia
CTU	Computerized-tomography urography
DJ (stent)	Double J stent
DVIU	Direct vision internal urethrotomy
EAU	European Association of Urology
EBRT	External beam radiation therapy
EPA	Excision and primary anastomosis
ESWL	Extracorporeal shock wave lithotripsy
G/U Index	Gapometry-urethrometry index
GCS	Glasgow Coma score
GSM	Genital self-mutilation
GSW	Gunshot wound
HSK	Horseshoe kidney
ISS	Injury severity score
IVU/IVP	Intravenous urography/pyelography
MRI	Magnetic resonance imaging
MVA	Motor vehicle accidents
MVC	Motor vehicle collisions
NTDB	National Trauma Data Bank
OIS	Organ injury scale
PBS	Prune belly syndrome
PCN	Percutaneous nephrostomy

PCNL	Percutaneous nephrolithotomy
PF	Penile fracture
PFUDD	Pelvic fracture urethral distraction defects
PFUI	Pelvic fracture urethral injury
PSA	Pseudoaneurysm
PTFE	Polytetrafluoroethylene
PUV	Posterior urethral valves
RAFF	Radial artery free flap phalloplasty
RFFF	Radial forearm free flap
RGU/RGP	Retrograde urography/pyelography
RIRS	Retrograde intrarenal surgery
RTA	Road traffic accidents
RTS	Revised trauma score
RUG	Retrograde urethrography
SIU	Societé Internationale d'Urologie
SIU-ICUD	Sociétè Internationale d'Urologie—International Consultation on Urological Diseases
SNVB	Subcutaneous nephron-vesical bypass
SPC	Suprapubic catheter
SSCs	Spermatogonial stem cells
TAE	Transcatheter angiographic embolization
TARN	Trauma Audit and Research Network
TDT	Traumatic dislocation of the testis
TESE	Testicular sperm extraction
TURBT	Transuretheral resection of bladder tumour
TURP	Transuretheral resection of prostate
UGT	Urogenital trauma
US	Ultrasound (ultrasonography)
USI	Urological Society of India
UTI	Urinary tract infection
WHO	World Health Organization
WSES	World Society of Emergency Surgery
WSES-AAST	World Society of Emergency Surgery and the American Association for the Surgery of Trauma
ZIRPI	Zipper-related penis injuries

Part I

Renal Trauma

Kidneys are double-edged swords. They are indispensable for your life by removing waste and excess water. But they are also blood bombs that might explode when hit and jeopardize your life.

Introduction to Renal Trauma

Although ancient humans did not know the exact function of the kidneys, they suspected very early their vital importance in the body. Thus, when mummifying important personalities, old Egyptians used to remove all organs, except the heart and the kidneys [1]. The biblical conception of kidneys also placed them as the seat of conscience and impetus for ethical yearning [2].

Nowadays, thanks to tremendous progress in the anatomy, anatomical pathology, physiology, and physiopathology of the kidney, the spiritual part of these old thoughts has completely faded while the vital role of this organ has been confirmed. However, this role doesn't provide any shield to the kidney against internal or external insults, since this organ is frequently the target of various infections, malignancies, congenital abnormalities, and other pathologies that interfere with its noble function: stones, diabetes, hypertension, atherosclerosis, systemic lupus erythematosus, drugs, etc. As if that weren't enough, the kidneys are also the most vulnerable urogenital organs in trauma, being involved in 41% of cases [3].

In the majority of cases, the kidneys are subjected to **blunt trauma** as a result of **motor vehicle accidents (MVA)** [4, 5]. Less frequently, they are injured in **penetrating trauma** by projectiles (bullets), i.e., gunshot wounds (GSW) or by stubbing instruments (knives). A minority of cases are iatrogenic resulting from minimally invasive treatment such as extracorporeal shock wave lithotripsy (ESWL), endourological procedures, percutaneous nephrolithotomies (PCNL), percutaneous kidney biopsy, and angiographic procedures. More rarely the kidneys can suffer deceleration injuries during falls from height.

In almost all cases, the specific cause of the trauma is obvious, and the patient is present with loin pain associated or not with hematuria. Depending on the severity of the injury, he/she might be stable or in a state of cardiovascular shock caused by massive bleeding and hypovolemia. Fever can be observed in late presentations associated with a hematoma or urinoma.

Nowadays, the cornerstone of the diagnosis and grading of renal trauma is **contrast-enhanced computed tomography (CECT)**. The current trend is toward **conservative treatment**, and interventions are seldom required being triggered either by the patient's cardiovascular instability or when his condition deteriorates, and minimally invasive procedures are the preferred approach here, while open surgical interventions are exceptionally performed [6–8].

References

1. Greydanus DE, Kadochi M. Reflections on the medical history of the kidney: from Alcmaeon of Croton to Richard Bright—standing on the shoulders of giants. J Integr Nephrol Androl. 2016;3:101–8.
2. Kopple JD. The biblical view of the kidney. Am J Nephrol. 1994;14(4–6):279–81. https://doi.org/10.1159/000168735.
3. Terrier J-E, Paparel P, Gadegbeku B, Ruffion A, Jenkins LC, N'Diaye A. Genitourinary injuries after traffic accidents. J Trauma Acute Care Surg. 2017;82(6):1087–93. https://doi.org/10.1097/ta.0000000000001448.
4. McGeady JB, Breyer BN. Current epidemiology of genitourinary trauma. Urol Clin North Am. 2013;40(3):323–34. https://doi.org/10.1016/j.ucl.2013.04.001.
5. Voelzke BB, Leddy L. The epidemiology of renal trauma. Transl Androl Urol. 2014;3(2):143–9. https://doi.org/10.3978/j.issn.2223-4683.2014.04.11.
6. EAU Guidelines. Edn. presented at the EAU annual congress Amsterdam, Mar 2022. ISBN: 978-94-92671-16-5. https://d56bochluxqnz.cloudfront.net/documents/full-guideline/EAU-Guidelines-on-Urological-Trauma-2022_2022-03-24-104100_fwda.pdf.
7. Morey AF, Brandes S, Dugi DD 3rd, Armstrong JH, Breyer BN, Broghammer JA, Erickson BA, Holzbeierlein J, Hudak SJ, Pruitt JH, Reston JT, Santucci RA, Smith TG 3rd, Wessells H, American Urological Association. Urotrauma: AUA guideline. J Urol. 2014;192(2):327–35. https://doi.org/10.1016/j.juro.2014.05.004. Epub 2014 May 20.
8. Coccolini F, Moore EE, Kluger Y, et al. Kidney and uro-trauma: WSES-AAST guidelines. World J Emerg Surg. 2019;14:54. https://doi.org/10.1186/s13017-019-0274-x.

Anatomy of the Kidney

1

Animal and human cadaveric dissection has been performed since antiquity, and the oldest available illustration of the kidney is said to be a bronze figure found in the Kition temples in Cyprus and dated to the thirteenth century BC [1]. The Italian artist Michelangelo (1475–1564) is reported to have had a strong interest in anatomy, particularly in the kidneys, having participated in many dissections and having suffered from chronic nephrolithiasis. His portrayal of "*God Separating the Earth from Waters*," painted on the Sistine Chapel ceiling in Vatican City in 1511 and showing the story of Genesis, is considered by analysts to represent kidney anatomy [2].

However, modern anatomy was born a few decades later, in the middle of the sixteenth century AD, thanks to great anatomists and anatomopathologists such as the Belgian Andreas Vesalius (1514–64) with his publication of "De Humani Corporis Fabrica" (1543) and the Roman Bartolomeo Eustachio (1500 or 1510–1574) with his posthumous publication "Tabulae anatomicae Bartholomaci Eustachii" [3, 4]. Eustachio was the first to describe the adrenal glands and is also credited for a great contribution to the modern knowledge of kidney anatomy: the lower position of the right kidney compared with the left, the intrarenal kidney vasculature, the renal calyceal system and its relation to the renal papillae, and the renal collecting ducts [1]. From the seventeenth century onward, many other contributors did their bits for the development of kidney anatomy science: The Dutch Frederik Ruysch (1638–1731), the Italian Lorenzo Bellini (1643–1704), the Dutch Govard Bidloo (1649–1713), the Italian Giovanni Battista Morgagni (1682–1771), the English William Cheselden (1688–1752), the Italian Marcello Malpighi (1628–1694/8), and so on. [1]. The French anatomist Exupère Joseph Bertin (1712–1781) is credited for the description of intra-renal septa in 1744 which evolved later into the concept of "Columns of Bertin" and is also regarded by some authors as the first discoverer of the "Tubes of Henle" which he described as "petits siphons recourbés" (small curved siphons) a century before the German anatomist Friedrich Gustav Jakob Henle (1809–1885) [5, 6].

S. A. AL-Mamari, *Urogenital Trauma: A Practical Guide*,
https://doi.org/10.1007/978-981-99-6171-9_1

Because of the determination and sacrifices of all these old anatomists and to the continuous efforts of modern researchers, more detailed and precise knowledge is available nowadays about the kidney. Hereafter, a practical summary is given to help understand the basis of trauma management of this organ.

1.1 Embryology

The **mesoderm** which gives rise to the urinary tract appears on the 15th day of development. Then the **metanephros** starts its growth during the fifth week of embryogenesis and starts its cranial migration in the following weeks to ultimately form the definitive kidneys that have a dual mesodermal origin: **The glomeruli and tubules develop from metanephric blastema and the excretory segments (pelvicalyceal system) from the ureteric bud** [7–9] (Figs. 1.1 and 1.2).

During its ascent, the arterial supply of the metanephros also migrates cranially with the following adaptation:

- At the most caudal initial stage: from the pelvic branches of the umbilical (iliac) arteries
- Then from the sequential branches of the dorsal aorta
- At the most cranial final stage: from a persistent lateral intersegmental artery of the mesonephros, supplying also adrenal glands and gonads [7–10]

The embryological origin of accessory arteries is therefore considered the result of persistent primordial arteries arising from more caudal sources during the ascent (Fig. 1.3a–d), but some authors considered them as the result of an early or precocious division of the renal artery [11, 12].

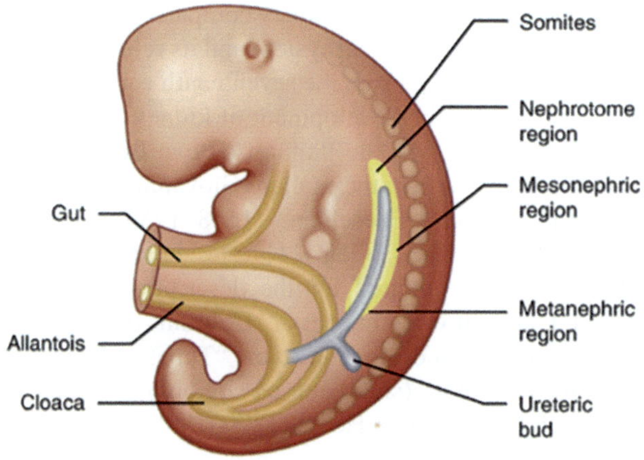

Fig. 1.1 Diagram of the embryo depicting the nephrotome, mesonephric, and metanephric regions from which the pronephros, mesonephros, and metanephros will, respectively, arise. The pronephros and mesonephros will regress, while the metanephros develops into the permanent kidney. (From Kassab G.H. et al. [8], with permission from Springer Nature)

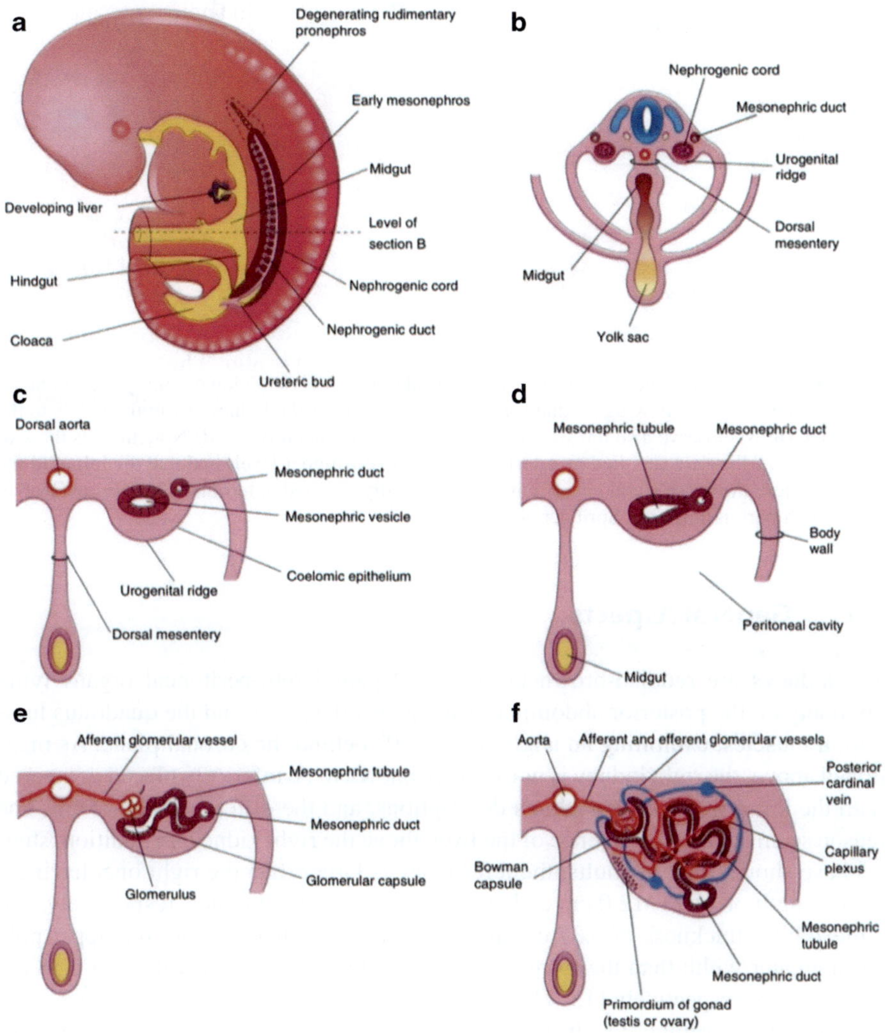

Fig. 1.2 (**a**) Sketch of a lateral view of a 5-week embryo showing the extent of the mesonephros and the primordium of the metanephros or permanent kidney. (**b**) Transverse section of the embryo showing the nephrogenic cords from which the mesonephric tubules develop. Observe the position of the urogenital ridges and nephrogenic cords. (**c–f**) Sketches of transverse sections showing successive stages in the development of a mesonephric tubule between the 5th and 11th weeks. Note that the mesenchymal cell cluster in the nephrogenic cord develops a lumen, thereby forming a mesonephric vesicle. The vesicle soon becomes an S-shaped mesonephric tubule and extends laterally to join the pronephric duct, now renamed the mesonephric duct. The expanded medial end of the mesonephric tubule is invaginated by blood vessels to form a glomerular capsule (Bowman capsule). The cluster of capillaries projecting into this capsule is the glomerulus. (From Zweyer M [9], with permission from Springer Nature)

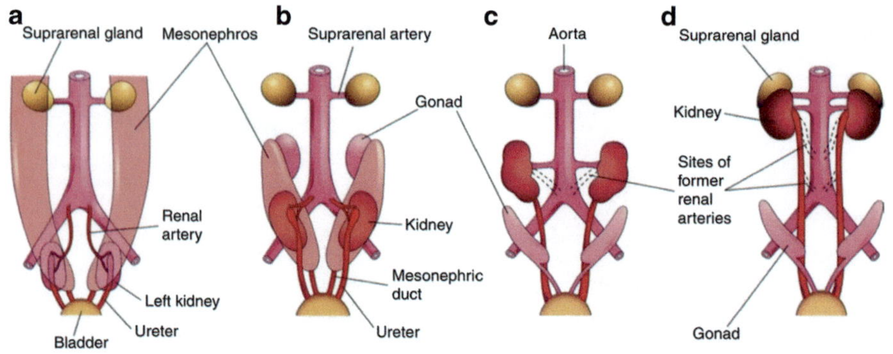

Fig. 1.3 (**a–d**) Diagrammatic ventral views of the abdominopelvic region of embryos and fetuses (sixth to ninth weeks) showing medial rotation and "ascent" of the kidneys from the pelvis to the abdomen. (**a, b**) Observe also the size regression of the mesonephroi. (**c, d**) Note that, as the kidneys "ascend," they are supplied by arteries at successively higher levels and that the hilum of the kidney (where the vessels and nerves enter) is eventually directed anteromedially. (From Zweyer M [9], with permission from Springer Nature)

1.2 General Aspects

The kidneys are reddish-brown bean-shaped paired retroperitoneal organs lying obliquely on the posterior abdominal wall against the psoas and the quadratus lumborum muscles, exhibiting an angle of 30°–50° behind the coronal plane. As mentioned above, the right kidney is notoriously known to be inferiorly placed compared with the left one since Eustachio's descriptions, and the difference is 1–2 cm. The reason seems to be the presence of the liver above the right kidney. In addition, studies have shown that, in adults, the left kidney is larger than the right one, having a mean length of 11.21–12.0 cm and 10.97–11.4 cm in adult males, respectively, and a mean hilar thickness of 3.37 cm and 3.21 cm, respectively. Also, the upper pole has a greater width than the lower pole in the same kidney, with values of 6.48 cm and 5.39 cm, respectively [13–16].

The kidney weight steeply increases until the age of 20 years, then continues slowly to increase, reaching its maximum at the age of 30–40 years with an average of 318 g for males and 255 g for females, and then maintains a plateau until the age of 50 years before declining progressively [13].

1.3 General Structure and Coverings

The kidney is composed of a **cortex**, a **medulla**, and a **pelvicalyceal system**. The cortex is the outer layer containing the **glomeruli** and **convoluted tubules** of the functional units, namely, the **nephrons**, and the medulla is formed by **pyramids**

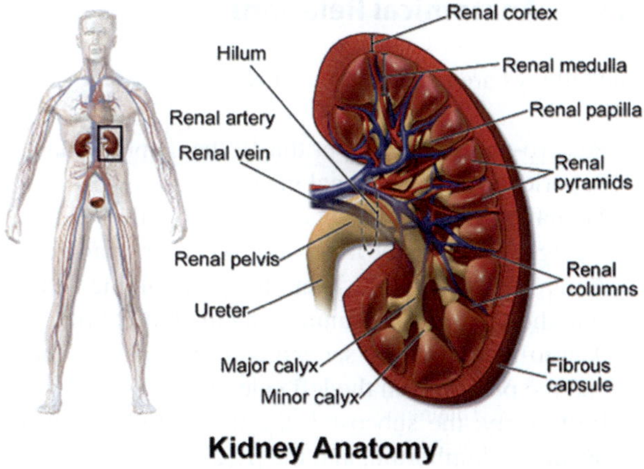

Fig. 1.4 Kidney anatomy. (From Blausen.com [18]—CC BY 3.0 Creative Commons Attribution License)

containing the remaining parts of the nephrons: the **loops of Henle** and the **collecting tubules**. The cortex has projections that divide and limit the pyramids called **columns of Bertin**. In some cases, the columns of Bertin increase in thickness and form a mass that is made of glomerular tissues. These so-called cortical **pseudotumors** have sometimes been mistaken for vascular tumors [16–18] (Fig. 1.4). Another classical renal pseudotumor consists of a focal protrusion in the lateral border of the midportion of the left kidney where the renal cortex is indented by the adjacent spleen, the so-called **dromedary hump** [8].

More internally is the excretory system formed by the **minor and major calyces**, which merge toward the **hilum** to form the **renal pelvis** in close contact with the renal vessels. The topography of these structures at the renal hilum is well known by the mnemonic **VAP** from anterior to posterior: the renal vein, the renal artery, and the renal pelvis.

The kidney surface is covered with a **renal capsule**, surrounded by the perirenal fat, which is enclosed by the fibrous **Gerota's fascia**. The Gerota's fascia, also simply called renal fascia, is surrounded anteriorly and posteriorly by the **pararenal fat** [14]. The Gerota's fascia comprises two layers: a strong posterior layer and a delicate anterior layer. The two layers fuse superiorly above the adrenals, laterally behind the ascending and descending colons, and medially to adjacent fascia and vessels, but they only touch each other inferiorly with no fusion [14, 15]. The posterior leaves of the diaphragm arch as a dome above the superior pole of the kidneys. The pleura lines the thoracic side of this dome and extends posteriorly and inferiorly up to the 12th rib, being therefore exposed to punctures during nephrostomy or injuries during the lumbar approach to nephrectomy [14, 15].

1.4 Anatomical Relations

The kidneys are in close contact with [15–17]:

- Postero-superiorly (upper third): the diaphragm.
- Superiorly: the suprarenal gland.
- Medially: the inferior vena cava (IVC), the head of the pancreas (hilar level) on the right side, and the aorta and body of the pancreas (hilar level) (on the left side).
- Antero-superiorly: the liver, the right colonic flexure on the right side, the stomach, the spleen, the jejunum, and the left colonic flexure on the left side.
- Antero-medially: the second and third part of the duodenum on the right side, and the pancreas on the left side.
- Posteriorly: the subcostal, the ilioinguinal, and the iliohypogastric nerves, the quadratus lumborum, and the psoas muscles.
- Lateral to the psoas muscle: The abdominal wall is built of the transversal, internal, and external oblique muscles.
- Posterior to the 12th rib: the latissimus dorsi and slips of the serratus posterior inferior muscle.

The kidneys are situated at an average depth of 4–5 cm from the skin of the back. When approaching it through a lumbar incision, the following structures will be encountered in progressive order from posterior to anterior: **skin**, **subcutaneous tissue**, subcutaneous latissimus dorsi, serratus posterior inferior (often difficult to detect), the lateral border of the erector spinae (iliocostalis, longissimus, and spinalis), the **external oblique**, the **internal oblique**, and the **transversus abdominis muscles**, whose posterior aponeurosis contributes to the thoracolumbar fascia, the quadratus lumborum muscle (located between the iliac crest and the 12th rib, immediately lateral to the transverse processes of lumbar vertebrae), and the **pararenal fat** that covers the kidneys [16, 19] (Fig. 1.5).

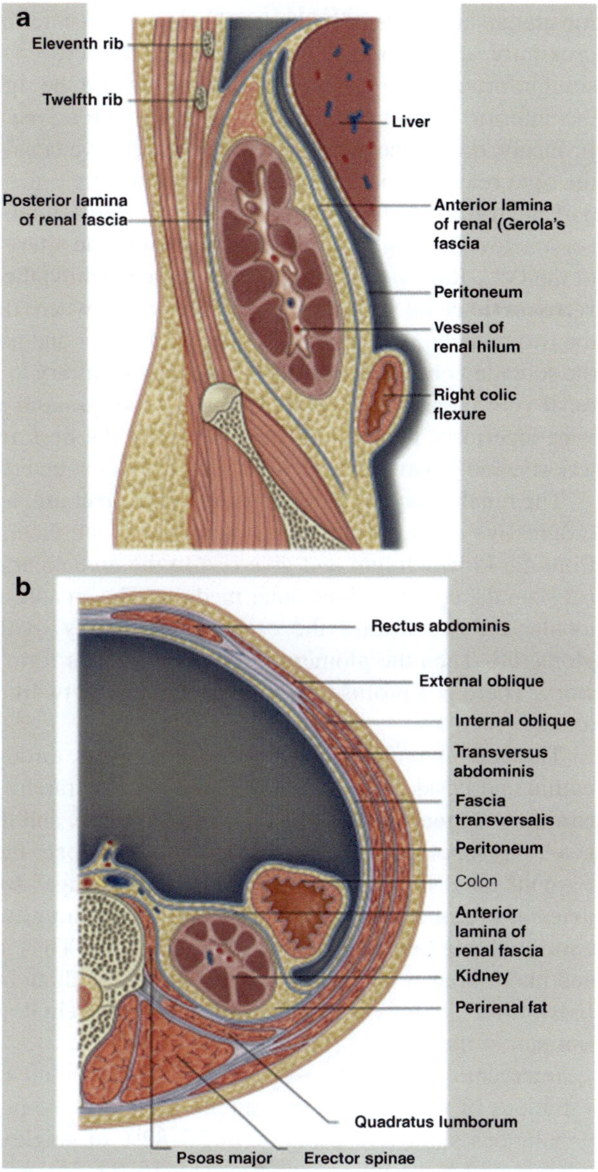

Fig. 1.5 Schematic sagittal and transverse sections of the right kidney showing the renal fascia and its relationship to the peritoneum and posterior abdominal wall. (From Mahadevan, V. [16] 2019, with permission from Elsevier)

1.5 Arterial Supply and Venous Drainage

Together the two kidneys receive more than 1.2 L of blood per minute, representing more than 20% of the total cardiac output. The renal arteries arise from the lateral sides of the abdominal aorta at the L1–L2 level, more precisely at the lower third of L1, immediately caudal to the origin of the superior mesenteric artery, and usually run cranial and anterior to the renal pelvis when entering the hilum [15]. Due to the proximity of the aorta to the left kidney, the left renal artery is short and travels straightforwardly to its respective kidney, while the right artery is long and crosses the inferior vena cava (IVC) posteriorly before reaching its respective kidney. Inversely, due to the proximity of the inferior vena cava (IVC) to the right kidney, the right renal vein is approximately two to three times shorter than its left counterpart and travels straight to the IVC [15, 20]. The left renal vein travels anterior to the aorta below the origin of the superior mesenteric artery before entering the left side of the IVC. Rarely the left renal vein travels behind the aorta, being referred to as a **retroaortic renal vein**. In the very rare cases where the left renal vein duplicates, the two branches can separate and travel anterior and posterior to the aorta, forming the so-called **circumaortic left renal vein**. Contrary to its right counterpart, the left renal vein has many tributaries, namely the **gonadal vein** inferiorly, the **adrenal vein** superiorly, the **inferior phrenic veins**, the **first or second lumbar veins** posteriorly, and **paravertebral veins** which are encountered in one-third of cases [15].

The renal artery divides into **interlobar**, **arcuate**, and **interlobular arteries**, in progressive order. With no anastomosis between them, the interlobar arteries arise from the kidney hilum and give rise to the arcuate arteries that lie at the junction between the cortex and the outer medulla. The arcuate arteries give rise to the interlobular arteries toward the capsule and finally to the **afferent vessels** of the glomeruli. Then the glomerular **efferent vessels** form a peritubular capillary network. There is a profuse peritubular vascular network surrounding the convoluted tubules.

The venous return from the medulla occurs through numerous vessels rising within and beside the vascular bundles. The hierarchy starts with the **peritubular capillary venous plexus**, then the **venae rectae,** and the **arcuate veins**. From this level, the venous system resembles the arterial one: the interlobular veins unite to form the renal vein anterior to the renal pelvis (Fig. 1.6). **However, contrary to the arterial organization, there are anastomotic longitudinal venous arcades that communicate between the interlobular veins.** Thus, these veins are not terminal, and major branches can be surgically ligated without risking a venous obstruction. In two-thirds of the cases, there is a **retrocolic vein** draining a portion of the posterior part of the kidney [15, 16, 21, 22].

Interventional radiologists and urologists should be aware of the anatomical variations of the renal arterial supply. Roughly, the published series from various populations show a distribution of 70–82% of single arteries, 17–20% of double arteries, and 1–2% of triple arteries [14, 15, 23, 24]. After an analysis of 266 cadaveric kidneys performed in Brazil, Sampaio, and Passos provided more details on these variations: **53.3%** had one hilar artery, **14.3%** had one hilar artery with one superior pole extra-hilar branch, 7.9% had two hilar arteries, 6.8% had a superior polar artery, 5.3% had an inferior polar artery, 3.4% had two hilar arteries with one superior pole extra-hilar branch, **2.6%** had one hilar artery with early bifurcation, 1.9% had three hilar arteries, and other variations in 2.5% [25, 26] (Fig. 1.7).

Note: The numbers in bold represent cases of single arteries for a total of 70.2%.

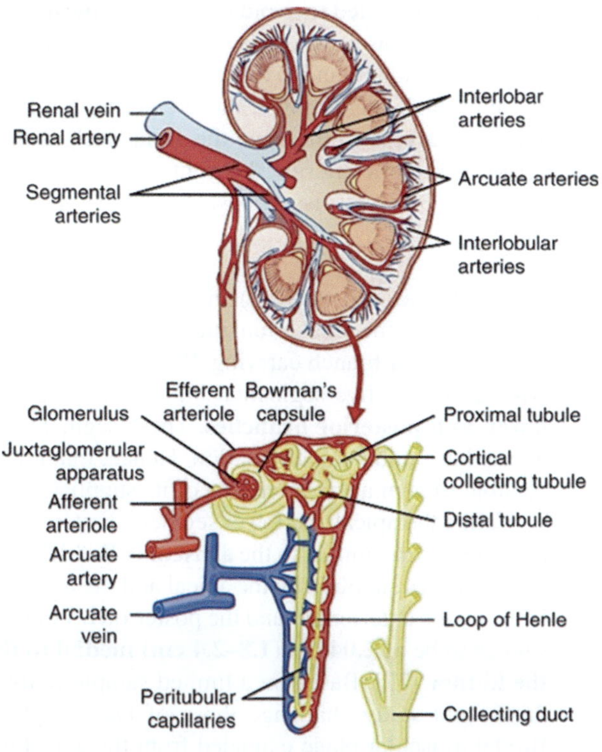

Fig. 1.6 Section of the human kidney showing the major vessels that supply the blood flow to the kidney and schematic of the microcirculation of each nephron. (From Guyton and Hall [21], with permission from Elsevier)

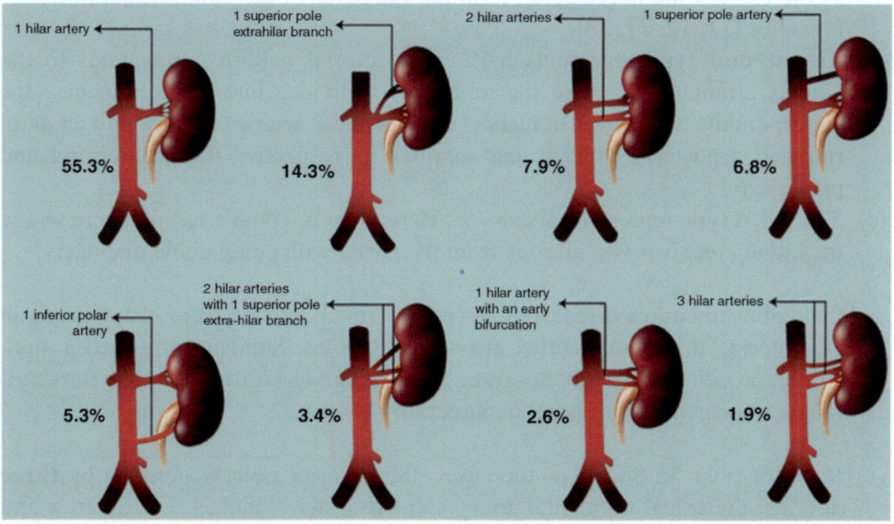

Fig. 1.7 Graphic illustration of variant renal anatomy. (From Lopez-Gonzalez et al. [26], with permission from Georg Thieme Verlag KG)

It has been suggested to avoid the term "**supernumerary**" when referring to the accessory arteries, as no artery is superfluous, each being essential for one or more segments in the kidney, and to reserve the term "**aberrant**" for vessels whose course is truly abnormal, for example, those entering the kidney by the poles, or whose origin is from a vessel other than the aorta, such as the hepatic artery, the superior or inferior mesenteric arteries, the right colic artery, or the lumbar arteries [11, 15].

Based on 153 kidney dissections, David Sykes proposed to divide the renal artery into three types [12]:

(a) **The first type** ("the typical") represents 83.1%. The artery is unique and divides near or within the renal hilum into an anterior branch carrying 75% of the blood and a posterior branch carrying 25% of the blood [14]. From the two divisions arise a total of five segmental branches, namely, the **apical, upper, middle, lower, and posterior branches**. These segmental arteries are end arteries and do not have collateral circulation. Hence, ligation of each of them causes irreversible ischemia and infarction of its supplied territory [15, 16].

Unlike the apical and lower segmental arteries, the upper, middle, and posterior arteries are limited to the **avascular Brödel's line** which only runs between the territories supplied by the apical and the lower segmental arteries, in a plane between the anterior 2/3 and the posterior 1/3 of the kidney, measured by recent studies to be **at 2.04 cm (1.8–2.4 cm) medial to the lateral convex border of the kidney** [27]. Based on a limited sample (only 15 kidneys), the findings of this recent study challenge those of David Sykes, as they mention that the Brödel avascular plane extended from the apical to the inferior segment in six cases (40%). Anyway, it is important to know that this line is not truly avascular as there are some overlapping terminal branches of the anterior and posterior branches [11, 12, 27, 28].

(b) **The second type** represents 8.4%: The arterial pattern corresponds to the venous arrangement. Here the renal artery divides into three branches: the upper, middle, and lower branches. Each of these arteries divides into an anterior and a posterior branch and supplies its respective third, anteriorly and posteriorly.

(c) **The third type** represents also 8.4%: Here there is a dual arterial pattern where the kidney receives two arteries from the aorta, with comparable diameters.

In the abovementioned research, accessory renal arteries were encountered in 25.8%, entering the kidney cortex at one of its poles. Sampaio proposed a more practical approach that demarcates three arterial regions worthy of notice for surgical trauma management or partial nephrectomy [14]:

(a) Superior pole: In 86.6% of the cases, the superior pole is supplied by **three** arteries: the apical segmental artery and two other branches (i.e., anterior and posterior).

(b) Inferior pole: In 62.2% of the cases, the inferior pole is supplied **only by the inferior segmental artery**, anteriorly and posteriorly, and its bleeding control is less complicated than for the upper pole.
(c) Mid- or hilar zone: Its anatomy is **very complex**. Mid-kidney resection is also technically more challenging to perform than a polar one, as it must not only control a complex vascular network but also maintain adequate vascularization and a patent collecting system for the superior and inferior poles.

1.6 Congenital Abnormalities

Nowadays, due to generalized antenatal ultrasonography, many abnormalities have become detectable. A German study including over 30,000 infants and fetuses showed major malformations in 6.9% and mild errors of morphogenesis in 35.9% of all infants. Among major malformations, the most frequent were musculoskeletal, internal urogenital, and cardiovascular malformations, which collectively accounted for more than 60%, with the incidence of 239, 162, and 113 per 10,000 infants, respectively [29].

Kidney anomalies are reported to account for 20–30% of all detectable anomalies [30]. The congenital kidney malformations include the following phenotypes [8, 9, 30, 31] (Fig. 1.8):

- **Horseshoe kidney (HSK) or renal fusion**: This is the most frequent abnormality with an incidence of 1 in every 400–500 live births.
- **Malrotation**: The result of the malrotation is the hilum facing anteriorly, and the incidence is 1/500.
- **Duplex kidney**.
- **Polycystic kidney disease**.
- **Multicystic dysplastic kidney (MCDK):** 1 in 3640 births.
- **Ectopic kidney**: Often in pelvic location, can be unilateral or bilateral. The incidence of simple ectopia is 1/10,000. Bilateral pelvic kidneys can fuse in a so-called **pancake kidney**. The ectopic kidney can cross and fuse with the contralateral one with an incidence of 1/2000. Very rarely, a three-in-one anomaly consisting of a **solitary crossed renal ectopia** has been described with only about 35 cases reported in the literature and an estimated incidence of 1/1,500,000. **However, in all crossed kidneys, the ureters retain the embryological memory, crossing back the midline and inserting into the normal bladder site**.
- **Renal dysplasia**: Can be unilateral with an incidence of 1/4300 for multicystic dysplastic kidneys and 1/1000 for dysplastic kidneys, or rarely bilateral with an incidence of 1/7500.
- **Renal hypoplasia**: Can be unilateral (1/1000) or bilateral (1/4000).
- **Supernumerary or accessory kidney**.
- **Renal agenesis**: Unilateral (1/1000) or bilateral (1/10,000). The latter is more common in males and is incompatible with life.

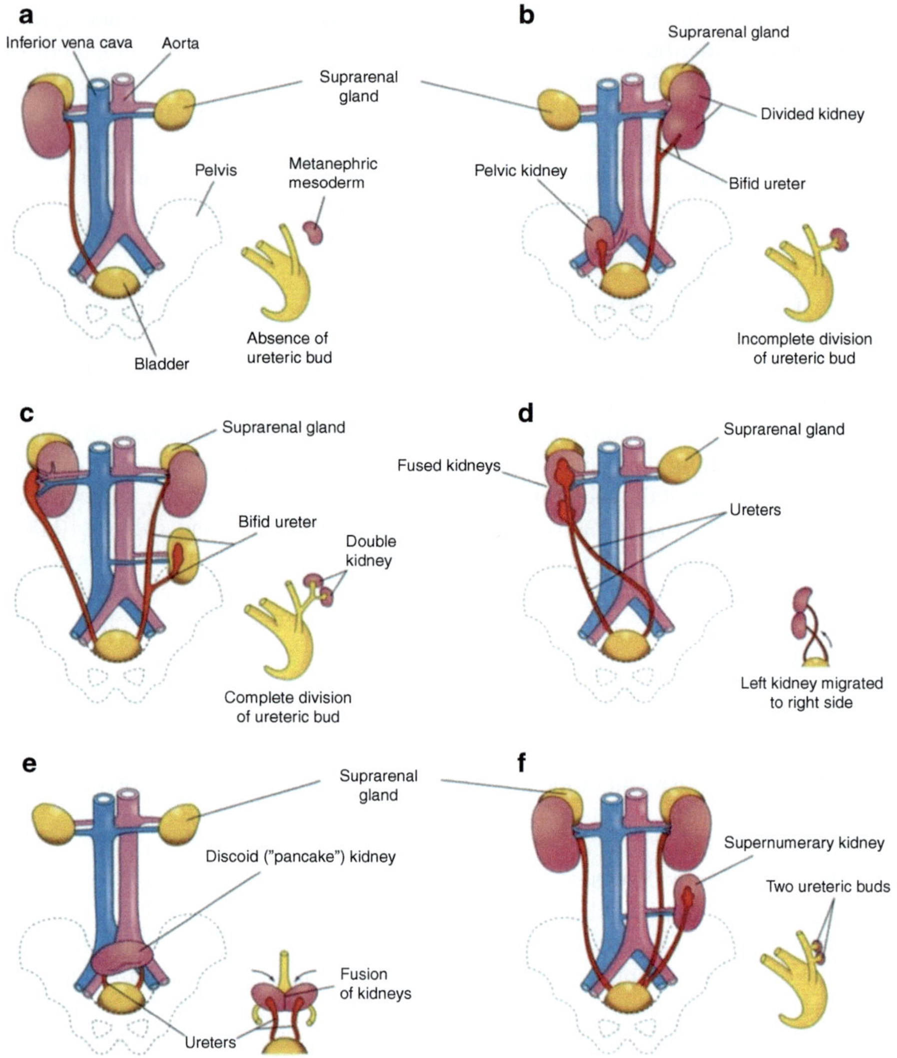

Fig. 1.8 Drawings illustrating various anomalies of the urinary system. The small sketch to the lower right of each drawing illustrates the probable embryological basis of the anomaly. (**a**) Unilateral renal agenesis. (**b**) Right side, pelvic kidney; left side, divided kidney with a bifid ureter. (**c**) Right side, malrotation of the kidney; left side, bifid ureter and supernumerary kidney. (**d**) Crossed renal ectopia. The left kidney crossed to the right side and fused with the right kidney. (**e**) Discoid (also pancake kidney) resulting from the fusion of the kidneys while they are in the pelvis. (**f**) Supernumerary left kidney resulting from the development of two ureteric buds. (From Zweyer M [9], with permission from Springer Nature)

References

1. Purkerson ML, Wechsler L. Depictions of the kidney through the ages. Am J Nephrol. 1997;17(3–4):340–6. https://doi.org/10.1159/000169121.
2. Eknoyan G. Michelangelo: art, anatomy, and the kidney. Kidney Int. 2000;57(3):1190–201. https://doi.org/10.1046/j.1523-1755.2000.00947.x.
3. Vesalius A. De Humani Corporis Fabrica. Basel: Oporinus; 1543.
4. Eustachio B. Tabulae anatomicae Bartholomaci Eustachii. Amsterdam: Wetsten; 1722.
5. Bertin M. Mémoire pour servir à l'histoire des reins. Mémoires de l'Académie Royale des Sciences; 1744.
6. Mezzogiorno A, De Santo NG, Bisaccia C, Di Iorio B, Cirillo M, Savica V, Ricciardi B, Menditti D, Richet G. Exupère-Joseph Bertin (1712-1781) and his description of the "petits siphons recourbez" (Henle's loops, a century earlier). J Nephrol. 2013;26(Suppl. 22):93–8. https://doi.org/10.5301/jn.5000374. Epub ahead of print.
7. Ntoulia A, Papadopoulou F, Benz-Bohm G. Urinary tract embryology, anatomy, and anatomical variants. In: Riccabona M, editor. Pediatric urogenital radiology, Medical radiology. Cham: Springer; 2018. https://doi.org/10.1007/978-3-319-39202-8_7.
8. Kassab GH, et al. Urinary tract. In: Paltiel HJ, Lee EY, editors. Pediatric ultrasound. Cham: Springer; 2021. https://doi.org/10.1007/978-3-030-56802-3_17.
9. Zweyer M. Embryology of the kidney. In: Quaia E, editor. Radiological imaging of the kidney, Medical radiology. Berlin: Springer; 2010. https://doi.org/10.1007/978-3-540-87597-0_1.
10. White RD, Moore KS, Salahia MG, Thomas WR, Gordon AC, Williams IM, Wood AM, Zealley IA. Renal arteries revisited: anatomy, pathologic entities, and implications for endovascular management. Radiographics. 2021;41(3):909–28. https://doi.org/10.1148/rg.2021200162.
11. Vordermark JS 2nd. Segmental anatomy of the kidney. Urology. 1981;17(6):521–31. https://doi.org/10.1016/0090-4295(81)90067-4.
12. Sykes D. The arterial supply of the human kidney with special reference to accessory renal arteries. Br J Surg. 1963;50:368.
13. Part I: Size of normal kidneys in adults. Acta Radiol. 1961;os-56(206_Suppl):7–31. https://doi.org/10.1177/0284185161056S20602.
14. Sampaio FJ. Renal anatomy. Endourologic considerations. Urol Clin N Am. 2000;27(4):585–607, vii. https://doi.org/10.1016/s0094-0143(05)70109-9.
15. Klatte T, Ficarra V, Gratzke C, Kaouk J, Kutikov A, Macchi V, Mottrie A, Porpiglia F, Porter J, Rogers CG, Russo P, Thompson RH, Uzzo RG, Wood CG, Gill IS. A literature review of renal surgical anatomy and surgical strategies for partial nephrectomy. Eur Urol. 2015;68(6):980–92. https://doi.org/10.1016/j.eururo.2015.04.010.
16. Mahadevan V. Anatomy of the kidney and ureter. Surgery (Oxford). 2019;37(7):359–64. https://doi.org/10.1016/j.mpsur.2019.04.005.ISSN: 0263-9319.
17. Hodson J. The lobar structure of the kidney. Br J Urol. 1972;44(2):246–61. https://doi.org/10.1111/j.1464-410x.1972.tb10072.x.
18. Blausen.com Staff. Medical gallery of Blausen Medical 2014. WikiJournal Med. 2014;1(2) https://doi.org/10.15347/wjm/2014.010. ISSN: 2002-4436.
19. Daly FJ, Bolender DL, Jain D, Uyeda S, Hoagland TM. Posterior approach to kidney dissection: an old surgical approach for integrated medical curricula. Anat Sci Educ. 2015;8(6):555–63. https://doi.org/10.1002/ase.1520. Epub 2015 Feb 16.
20. Ishii H, Aboumarzouk OM, Van Poppel H. Kidney and ureter anatomy. In: Aboumarzouk OM, editor. Blandy's urology. 3rd ed. John Wiley & Sons Ltd.; 2019. p. 91–106.
21. Chap. 26: Urine formation by the kidneys: I. Glomerular filtration, renal blood flow, and their control. In: Guyton and Hall textbook of medical physiology. 12th ed. Philadelphia, PA: Elsevier; 2011. p. 305.
22. Beeuwkes R 3rd. The vascular organization of the kidney. Annu Rev Physiol. 1980;42:531–42. https://doi.org/10.1146/annurev.ph.42.030180.002531.

23. Khamanarong K, Prachaney P, Utraravichien A, Tong-Un T, Sripaoraya K. Anatomy of renal arterial supply. Clin Anat. 2004;17:334–6. https://doi.org/10.1002/ca.10236.
24. Pradhay G, Gopidas GS, Karumathil Pullara S, Mathew G, Mathew AJ, Sukumaran TT, Pavikuttan N, Sudhakaran R Sr. Prevalence and relevance of multiple renal arteries: a Radioanatomical perspective. Cureus. 2021;13(10):e18957. https://doi.org/10.7759/cureus.18957.
25. Sampaio FJ, Passos MA. Renal arteries: anatomic study for surgical and radiological practice. Surg Radiol Anat. 1992;14(2):113–7. https://doi.org/10.1007/BF01794885.
26. Lopez-Gonzalez DB, Zurkiya O. Interventional radiology in renal trauma. Semin Intervent Radiol. 2021;38(1):113–22. https://doi.org/10.1055/s-0041-1726006.
27. Macchi V, Picardi E, Inferrera A, Porzionato A, Crestani A, Novara G, De Caro R, Ficarra V. Anatomic and radiologic study of renal avascular plane (Brödel's line) and its potential relevance on percutaneous and surgical approaches to the kidney. J Endourol. 2018;32(2):154–9. https://doi.org/10.1089/end.2017.0689.
28. Brödel M. The intrinsic blood-vessels of the kidney and their significance in nephrotomy. Johns Hopkins Hosp Bull. 1961;118:10.
29. Queisser-Luft A, Stolz G, Wiesel A, Schlaefer K, Spranger J. Malformations in newborn: results based on 30,940 infants and fetuses from the Mainz congenital birth defect monitoring system (1990-1998). Arch Gynecol Obstet. 2002;266(3):163–7. https://doi.org/10.1007/s00404-001-0265-4.
30. Stonebrook E, Hoff M, Spencer JD. Congenital anomalies of the kidney and urinary tract: a clinical review. Curr Treat Options Pediatr. 2019;5(3):223–35. https://doi.org/10.1007/s40746-019-00166-3.
31. Jain S, Chen F. Developmental pathology of congenital kidney and urinary tract anomalies. Clin Kidney J. 2019;12(3):382–99. https://doi.org/10.1093/ckj/sfy112.

2 Epidemiology of Renal Trauma

The kidney is the third most injured organ in abdominal trauma after the spleen and liver [1, 2] (Fig. 2.1).

By the end of the last century (1997–1998), a population-based study showed an incidence of renal trauma in the USA of 4.9 per 100,000 population, comprising 1.2% of all trauma cases [3]. However, more recent estimations based on the American **National Trauma Data Bank (NTDB)** suggest a lower rate of 0.3–0.5% [4, 5]. The same proportion has been found elsewhere in Europe in general and in France in particular [6, 7]. A systematic review of 15 adult renal trauma articles including nearly 11,000 patients showed an overall male predominance of 72% and a mean age of 30.8 years [8]. A more recent and larger review of 46 articles including 48,660 patients confirmed the above data showing 75.3% of males and a mean age of 33 years [9], and a Japanese retrospective study conducted during the same period and including 3550 patients showed a nearly equal male predominance (74.2%) but a higher median age of 43 years, which probably correlated to the age distribution in this country [10]. In the Middle East, higher male predominance and younger age of the victims might prevail in urogenital trauma (UGT) as suggested by an Iranian study that found a male rate of 91% and an average age of 25 years [11].

The majority of renal injuries are caused by blunt trauma accounting for 80.5% versus only 19.5% for penetrating trauma, and the overall mortality rate is 6.4% (4.8–8.4%) [9]. However, penetrating injuries are reported to predominate in underdeveloped countries and areas of social insecurity and civil unrest. This fact was suggested by a retrospective study in a Turkish region subjected to increased sociopolitical tensions, which showed that 59% of the encountered renal injuries were secondary to gunshot wounds [12], and by a South African study that showed three-quarters of renal injuries being caused by penetrating agents and half by gunshots only [13]. In penetrating renal injuries, the median age of patients is lower (28 years), and the male predominance of the victims is strikingly higher, reaching 93% [14].

When specifying UGT after road traffic accidents (RTA), the male predominance increases to 76% and the mean age remains almost the same (30.3 years) [6]. When

S. A. AL-Mamari, *Urogenital Trauma: A Practical Guide*,
https://doi.org/10.1007/978-981-99-6171-9_2

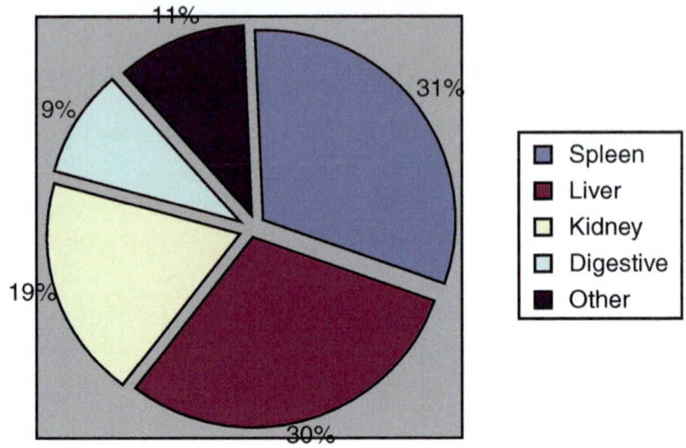

Fig. 2.1 Distribution of the four most frequent abdominal injuries in the combined data set for the years 1993–1998. (From Yoganandan N et al. [2], with permission from the Association for the Advancement of Automotive Medicine)

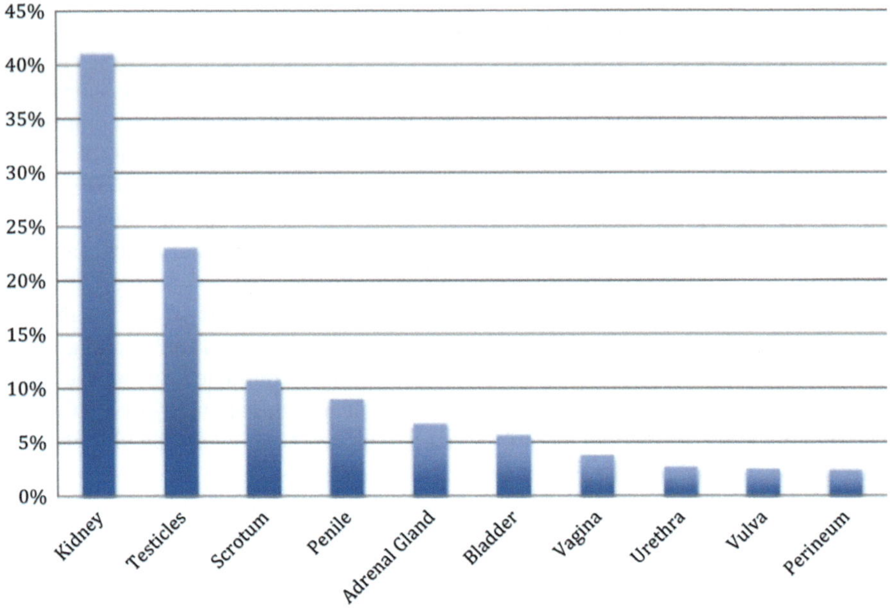

Fig. 2.2 Overall distribution of GUI after traffic accidents ($n = 963$ victims). (From Terrier et al. [7], with permission from Wolters Kluwer Health, Inc.)

especially addressing penetrating renal trauma, the male predominance even deepens to 88% and the mean age falls to 28 years. For the pediatric group, there is a lesser male predominance, 67%, and the mean age is 9.3 years [8].

Among urogenital organs, the most frequently injured ones after motor vehicle accidents (MVA) are the kidneys and the testicles with 41–43% and 23–24%, respectively, and ureteric trauma is almost not observed [6, 7] (Fig. 2.2). However, when considering only motorcyclists, 62% of injuries involved the external genitalia, and the testes were the most injured organs (38–41%). The penis was the most involved organ among cyclists (23–41%), while the pedestrians showed a nearly equal frequency for all organs [6, 7].

Minor renal trauma grades are fortunately more frequently encountered than major ones, and data show the following distribution: grade I, 22–28%; grade II, 28–30%; grade III, 20–26%; grade IV, 15–19%; and grade V, 6–7%. Details of this grading will be discussed later in this section [8, 15, 16].

Notably, 85% of children sustaining renal trauma are older than 6 years with a mean age of 9.3 years. The distribution parallels that of the adults with the majority of blunt injuries occurring in males (67–77%) [8, 17]. However, there is a discrepancy with regard to the injury grade distribution in the pediatric group due to a lack of large reviews; some studies show a great proportion of high-grade injuries [8], while others present a predominance of low-grade ones [17].

References

1. Syarif, Palinrungi AM, Kholis K, et al. Renal trauma: a 5-year retrospective review in single institution. Afr J Urol. 2020;26:61. https://doi.org/10.1186/s12301-020-00073-2.
2. Yoganandan N, Pintar FA, Gennarelli TA, Maltese MR. Patterns of abdominal injuries in frontal and side impacts. Annu Proc Assoc Adv Automot Med. 2000;44:17–36.
3. Wessells H, Suh D, Porter JR, Rivara F, MacKenzie EJ, Jurkovich GJ, Nathens AB. Renal injury and operative management in the United States: results of a population-based study. J Trauma. 2003;54(3):423–30. https://doi.org/10.1097/01.TA.0000051932.28456.F4.
4. Bjurlin MA, Fantus RJ, Fantus RJ, Villines D. Comparison of nonoperative and surgical management of renal trauma. J Trauma Acute Care Surg. 2017;82(2):356–61. https://doi.org/10.1097/ta.0000000000001316.
5. Ho P, Hellenthal NJ. Independent predictors of mortality for patients with traumatic renal injury. World J Urol. 2021;39:3685. https://doi.org/10.1007/s00345-020-03552-x. Epub ahead of print.
6. Paparel P, N'Diaye A, Laumon B, Caillot J-L, Perrin P, Ruffion A. The epidemiology of trauma of the genitourinary system after traffic accidents: analysis of a register of over 43000 victims. BJU Int. 2006;97(2):338–41. https://doi.org/10.1111/j.1464-410x.2006.05900.x.
7. Terrier JE, Paparel P, Gadegbeku B, Ruffion A, Jenkins LC, N'Diaye A. Genitourinary injuries after traffic accidents: analysis of a registry of 162,690 victims. J Trauma Acute Care Surg. 2017;82(6):1087–93. https://doi.org/10.1097/TA.0000000000001448.
8. Voelzke BB, Leddy L. The epidemiology of renal trauma. Transl Androl Urol. 2014;3(2):143–9. https://doi.org/10.3978/j.issn.2223-4683.2014.04.11.
9. Petrone P, Perez-Calvo J, Brathwaite CEM, Islam S, Joseph DK. Traumatic kidney injuries: a systematic review and meta-analysis. Int J Surg. 2020;74:13–21. ISSN: 1743-9191. https://doi.org/10.1016/j.ijsu.2019.12.013.
10. Nakao S, Katayama Y, Hirayama A, et al. Trends and outcomes of blunt renal trauma management: a nationwide cohort study in Japan. World J Emerg Surg. 2020;15:50. https://doi.org/10.1186/s13017-020-00329-w.
11. Salimi J, Nikoobakht MR, Zareei MR. Epidemiologic study of 284 patients with urogenital trauma in three trauma center in Tehran. Urol J. 2004;1(2):117–20.
12. Ersay A, Akgün Y. Experience with renal gunshot injuries in a rural setting. Urology. 1999;54(6):972–5.
13. Madiba TE, Haffejee AA, John J. Renal trauma secondary to stab, blunt and firearm injuries: a 5-year study. S Afr J Surg. 2002;40(1):5–9; discussion 9–10.

14. Kansas BT, Eddy MJ, Mydlo JH, Uzzo RG. Incidence and management of penetrating renal trauma in patients with multiorgan injury: extended experience at an inner city trauma center. J Urol. 2004;172(4 Pt 1):1355–60. https://doi.org/10.1097/01.ju.0000138532.40285.44.
15. Hotaling JM, Wang J, Sorensen MD, et al. A national study of trauma level designation and renal trauma outcomes. J Urol. 2012;187(2):536–41. https://doi.org/10.1016/j.juro.2011.09.155.
16. Erlich T, Kitrey ND. Renal trauma: the current best practice. Ther Adv Urol. 2018;10:295–303. https://doi.org/10.1177/1756287218785828.
17. Dangle PP, Fuller TW, Gaines B, Cannon GM, Schneck FX, Stephany HA, Ost MC. Evolving mechanisms of injury and management of pediatric blunt renal trauma—20 years of experience. Urology. 2016;90:159–63. https://doi.org/10.1016/j.urology.2016.01.017. Epub 2016 Jan 26.

3 Etiology and Anatomopathology of Kidney Trauma

The causes of renal trauma strongly correlate with the anatomopathology of the injury and can be divided into two major groups: blunt and penetrating trauma. However, two more groups will be added in the following discussion as they require special attention: pediatric and iatrogenic renal trauma.

3.1 Blunt Trauma

Motor vehicle collisions (MVC) are the main causes of blunt renal injury in the adult population being encountered in 63–70% of the cases, followed by falls, sports trauma, and pedestrian accidents representing 43%, 11%, and 4%, respectively [1–3].

3.2 Penetrating trauma

A systematic literature review recruiting a total of 1793 penetrating renal injuries showed that firearms were more common than stab wounds in a proportion of 65% and 35%, respectively [2]. However, these proportions vary considerably among countries. Due to the permissive laws and the easy procurement of firearms, the USA has a very high record of gunshot injuries, accounting for 72.2% of all penetrating renal injuries, while other countries such as the United Kingdom and Canada have a higher rate of stabbing wound representing 87.3% and 88% of penetrating renal traumas, respectively [4–6].

From an anatomopathological point of view, an American population-based study showed 64% of patients with contusions/hematoma, while 26.3% had lacerations, 5.3% had parenchymal disruption, and 4% had vascular injuries. However, when considering penetrating injuries alone, 74% had lacerations, 15% had parenchymal disruption, and 11% had vascular injuries [7].

S. A. AL-Mamari, *Urogenital Trauma: A Practical Guide*,
https://doi.org/10.1007/978-981-99-6171-9_3

3.3 Pediatric Population

If subjected to an equal force of trauma, children are hypothetically more susceptible to kidney injury than adults due to the lack of perirenal fat cushion, the relatively larger size of the pediatric kidney in relation to the body, and the decreased protection from the abdominal wall muscles and the less ossified pediatric thoracic cage [8]. A systematic review recruiting a total of 458 blunt pediatric renal traumas showed that, while motor vehicle collisions (MVC) are still the most frequent cause in this age category, their proportion is lower than in the adult group (30% vs 63%), and the proportions of falls and pedestrian accidents are much higher being 27% and 13%, respectively [2].

Some studies are even clearly showing the predominance of falls as the first cause of trauma in children. Indeed, the Pennsylvania Trauma System Foundation has recorded over two decades (1993–2013) a total of 354 children who suffered blunt renal trauma, of whom 228 cases were sufficiently imaged and graded. This study showed that falls comprised 20.6% of all cases, followed by all-terrain vehicles (ATV) (18.9%), bikes (17.1%), MVC (12.7%), sport (11.4%), Ski-Sled (6.6%), pedestrian accidents (6.1%), and others (6.6%) [9]. This research sounded the alarm about the widespread use of recreational motor vehicles (RMV) by children despite the restrictive recommendations in this age category.

3.4 Iatrogenic Causes

Iatrogenic causes of kidney trauma include many procedures: extracorporeal shockwave lithotripsy (ESWL), percutaneous nephrolithotomy (PCNL), percutaneous nephrostomy (PCN), renal biopsy, nephron-sparing surgery (partial nephrectomy), ureterorenoscopy, renal angiography or renal artery stenting with guidewire-induced arterial perforation, endopyelotomy, or pyeloplasty. Hereinafter, the most frequent of them are developed, and a brief account of their management is given.

3.4.1 Extracorporeal Shockwave Lithotripsy (ESWL)

Most of the time ESWL is safe. However, complications have been described such as symptomatic subcapsular or perirenal hematoma (0.7%) with decreased hemoglobin [10, 11] (Fig. 3.1a, b). While clinically significant or symptomatic hematomas are rare after ESWL, it is important to remember that, strictly speaking, the incidence of hematomas would rise up to 4.1% if one proceeds to systematic imaging after the treatment (ultrasound and CT scan) [11].

Pre-existing hypertension appears to be a significant risk factor as it was found in 57% of patients who developed post-ESWL perirenal hematoma [10]. The patient's age is another risk factor with each 10-year increase in age carrying a 1.67 times greater probability of hematoma [11]. Other associated factors were urinary tract infections (UTI) and simultaneous bilateral treatment [10]. On the

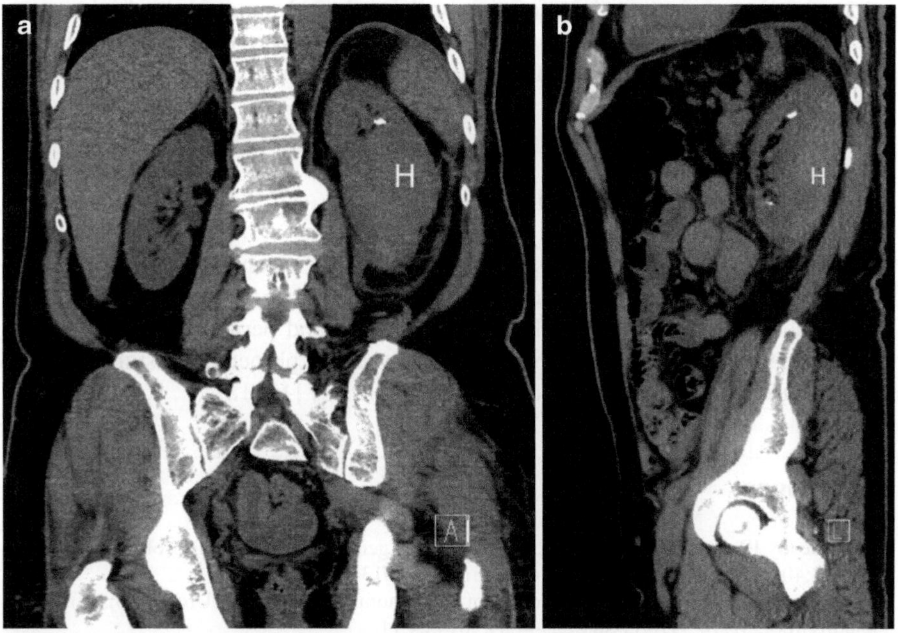

Fig. 3.1 (**a**, **b**) Coronal and sagittal views of a plain CT abdomen showing a large post-ESWL subcapsular hematoma (H) of the left kidney

contrary, no correlation was found between the occurrence of post-ESWL subcapsular or perinephric hematoma and the stones' number, size, or location, the history of renal surgery, the presence of kidney malformations, the patient body habitus (size and weight), the number of shock waves, and the level of energy applied [10, 11].

In general, these hematomas are managed conservatively and resolve rapidly within weeks. Rarely, however, the hemorrhage may be severe necessitating embolization [12, 13], or sometimes percutaneous drainage [14].

3.4.2 Percutaneous Nephrolithotomy (PCNL)

Bleeding is a worrisome complication of PCNL. Its incidence is decreasing with the introduction of miniaturized techniques, evolving from standard PCNL to MiniPerc and MicroPerc. Depending on the published series, it occurs in a wide range of frequency from 0.5% to 2.4% for severe bleeding requiring intervention (embolization) and from 3.4% to 24% for those only requiring blood transfusion, and many contributing factors have been incriminated: stone complexity (Guy's stone score Grades 3 and 4) and high Hounsfield Unit (HU) value, high body mass index (BMI), prolonged operating time, the thickness of the renal parenchyma and absence of hydronephrosis, history of ipsilateral renal stone surgery, occurrence of intraoperative pelvicalyceal perforation, upper calyceal puncture, multiple access tracts, method of tract dilatation (balloon dilatation decreases bleeding), presence of diabetes mellitus (DM), preoperative urinary infection, surgeon's inexperience, and so on. [15].

3.4.3 Flexible and Rigid Ureteroscopy

Ureteroscopy carries potential risks for the ureters but is generally safe for the kidneys [16]. Rarely, however, especially when a ureteral access sheath is not used in retrograde intrarenal surgery (RIRS), extravasation and peri-renal collection may occur. Exceptional cases of peri-renal hematoma and nephroenteric fistula have also been reported following ureteroscopic laser lithotripsy [17, 18].

References

1. McGeady JB, Breyer BN. Current epidemiology of genitourinary trauma. Urol Clin North Am. 2013;40(3):323–34. https://doi.org/10.1016/j.ucl.2013.04.001.
2. Voelzke BB, Leddy L. The epidemiology of renal trauma. Transl Androl Urol. 2014;3(2):143–9. https://doi.org/10.3978/j.issn.2223-4683.2014.04.11.
3. Nance ML. National Trauma Data Bank 2012 annual report. 2012. Available: https://www.facs.org/media/ebgfrtdn/ntdb-annual-report-2012.pdf.
4. Bjurlin MA, Fantus RJ, Fantus RJ, et al. Comparison of nonoperative and surgical management of renal trauma: can we predict when nonoperative management fails? J Trauma Acute Care Surg. 2017;82:356–61.
5. Hadjipavlou M, Grouse E, Gray R, et al. Managing penetrating renal trauma: experience from two major trauma centres in the UK. BJU Int. 2018;121:928–34.
6. Mann U, Zemp L, Rourke KF. Contemporary management of renal trauma in Canada: a 10-year experience at a level 1 trauma Centre. Can Urol Assoc J. 2019;13:E177–82.
7. Wessells H, Suh D, Porter JR, Rivara F, MacKenzie EJ, Jurkovich GJ, Nathens AB. Renal injury and operative management in the United States: results of a population-based study. J Trauma. 2003;54(3):423–30. https://doi.org/10.1097/01.ta.0000051932.28456.f4.
8. Buckley JC, McAninch JW. The diagnosis, management, and outcomes of pediatric renal injuries. Urol Clin North Am. 2006;33(1):33–40.
9. Dangle PP, Fuller TW, Gaines B, Cannon GM, Schneck FX, Stephany HA, Ost MC. Evolving mechanisms of injury and management of pediatric blunt renal trauma—20 years of experience. Urology. 2016;90:159–63. https://doi.org/10.1016/j.urology.2016.01.017. Epub 2016 Jan 26.
10. Knapp PM, Kulb TB, Lingeman JE, Newman DM, Mertz JHO, Mosbaugh PG, Steele RE. Extracorporeal shock wave lithotripsy-induced perirenal hematomas. J Urol. 1988;139(4):700–3. https://doi.org/10.1016/s0022-5347(17)42604-8.
11. Dhar N, Thornton J, Karafa M, Streem S. A multivariate analysis of risk factors associated with subcapsular hematoma formation following electromagnetic shock wave lithotripsy. J Urol. 2004;172(6):2271–4. https://doi.org/10.1097/01.ju.0000143459.03836.2d.
12. Silberstein J, Lakin CM, Kellogg PJ. Shock wave lithotripsy and renal hemorrhage. Rev Urol. 2008;10(3):236–41.
13. Assaf E, Abou Zahr R, Ghabi E, Ghantous I. Perinephric hematoma with active arterial hemorrhage following extracorporeal shockwave lithotripsy. Case Rep Urol. 2019;2019:1–3. https://doi.org/10.1155/2019/1547437.

14. Jang YB, Kang KP, Lee S, Kim W, Kim MK, Kim YG, Park SK. Treatment of subcapsular haematoma, a complication of extracorporeal shock wave lithotripsy (ESWL), by percutaneous drainage. Nephrol Dial Transplant. 2006;21(4):1117–8. https://doi.org/10.1093/ndt/gfk002.
15. Poudyal S. Current insights on haemorrhagic complications in percutaneous nephrolithotomy. Asian J Urol. 2021;9:81. https://doi.org/10.1016/j.ajur.2021.05.007.
16. Alenezi H, Denstedt JD. Flexible ureteroscopy: technological advancements, current indications and outcomes in the treatment of urolithiasis. Asian J Urol. 2015;2(3):133–41. https://doi.org/10.1016/j.ajur.2015.06.002.
17. Zhang P, Hu W. Sudden onset of a huge subcapsular renal hematoma following minimally invasive ureteroscopic holmium laser lithotripsy: a case report. Exp Ther Med. 2015;10(1):335–7.
18. Correia DC, Antunes RM, Ferreira P. Nephroenteric fistula after lithotripsy: a rare complication. Int J Radiol Imaging Technol. 2019;5:048. https://doi.org/10.23937/2572-3235.1510048.

4 Mechanism and Physiopathology of Kidney Trauma

4.1 Blunt Trauma

The kidneys are anatomically protected by the 10th, 11th, and 12th ribs and the strong lumbar muscles posteriorly and laterally, namely, the erector spinae, quadratus lumborum, and psoas major, the transverse and oblique muscles. Anteriorly, they are cushioned by the abdominal viscera. However, despite this anatomical shield, they are the most often traumatized genitourinary organs, in deceleration (MVA, fall from a height) or acceleration injuries (pedestrian, kick at the lumbar area during sports or assaults) because they are held in place only by the renal pedicle and the pelviureteric junction (PUJ) [1].

Moreover, pathologically enlarged or abnormally located kidneys such as hydronephrotic kidney, polycystic kidney, cystic kidney, ectopic kidney, duplication, horseshoe kidneys, angiomyolipoma, and malignancies make them vulnerable even to minor trauma, and their association with renal trauma was found to be 19% [2]. An attempt to explain the high vulnerability of these pathological kidneys, especially those with fluid-filled lesions, to blunt trauma was provided by a computerized simulation where the force of the trauma impact was amplified by the presence of a liquid-filled incompressible compartment. It has been observed that maximum stress concentrations were found at the periphery of the kidney model and corresponded to the clinically observed injury sites [3].

Studies addressing the biochemical response of pig kidneys to pendulum impacts identified an energy-based injury threshold: **A strain energy density of 21 kJ/m^3 corresponded to a 50% risk of renal injury level AIS 3 (AAST grade III) or higher**. [1]

[1] Details of AAST and AIS grading are available in Chap. 5.

S. A. AL-Mamari, *Urogenital Trauma: A Practical Guide*,
https://doi.org/10.1007/978-981-99-6171-9_4

Further experimental results confirmed the prediction of renal capsule rupture and underlying parenchyma viscoelastic failure from a finite element model of the human kidney at a **threshold of an impact energy level of 4.0 J,** which is therefore considered a threshold of AAST grade III renal injury [4] (Fig. 4.1). Furthermore, in blunt lateral abdominal impact, the kidney is squeezed between the fractured ribcage and the lumbar spine, and **impact velocities between 5.2 and 6.5 m/s** were predicted to cause tearing or contusion of the renal parenchyma (AAST grade I or II injury), but not renal capsule rupture, and the threshold speed for kidney rupture was predicted to be **6.7 m/s** (AAST grade III or higher) (Fig. 4.2). This model

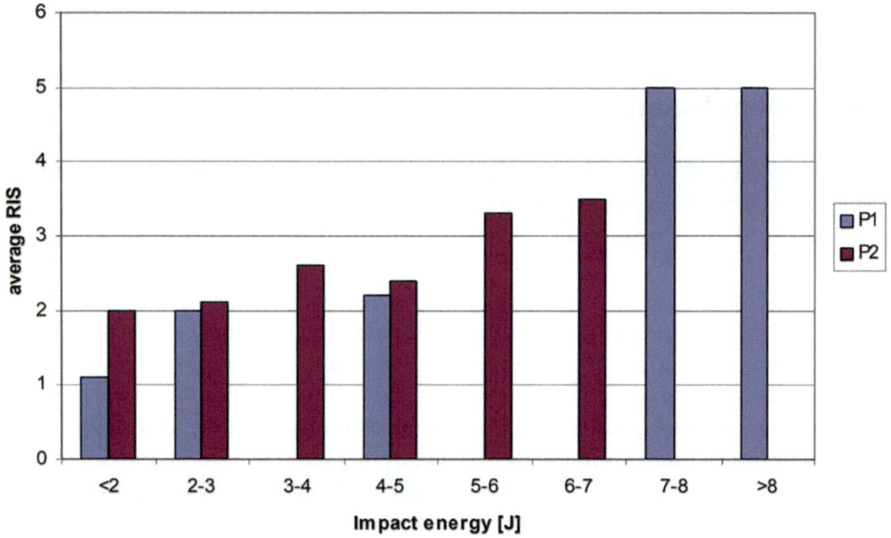

Fig. 4.1 Average grade on the AAST renal injury scale for different impact energy intervals and different pendulum masses. (From K.-U. Schmitt and J. G. Snedeker [4], with permission from the authors)

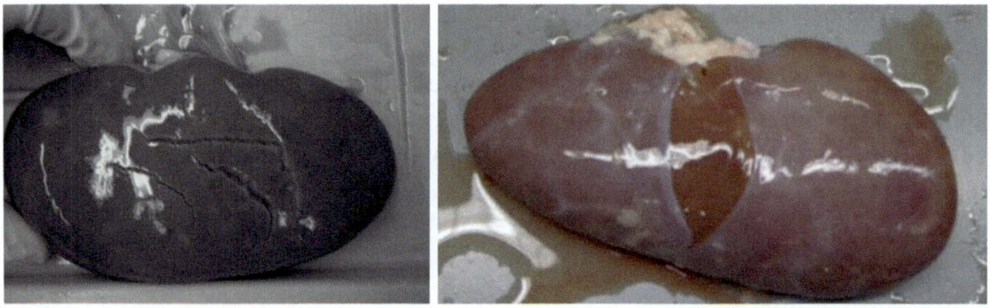

Fig. 4.2 Typical injuries observed include rupture of the renal membrane (right) and the parenchyma (left). (From K.-U. Schmitt and J. G. Snedeker [4], with permission from the authors and from Taylor & Francis)

permits a hypothetical prediction of the grade of injury from the impact severity and impact geometry [4, 5].

Four components have been proposed in the mechanism of collision in a motor vehicle crash: collision between the vehicle and the external object (another car, tree, wall, rock, etc.), collision of the unrestrained occupant (driver or passenger) and the interior of the vehicle, collision between the occupant organs and the body walls (skull, chest wall, abdominal wall), and the collision between the occupants and loose objects within the vehicle [6]. Logically, another component can be added for some victims of a high-speed car accident: a collision of the ejected unrestrained occupant with an object outside the vehicle.

The medical literature contains a handful of cases of diaphragmatic rupture after blunt abdominal trauma, with intrathoracic herniation of the kidney. This occurs mostly on the left side as the right side is protected by liver interposition. Very scanty reports mention a renal injury in association with this migration. By now, we can only hypothesize that the "give way" of the diaphragm acts as a safety valve in addition to the role of the internal airbag played by the lungs. One can understand that this mechanism might logically protect the renal parenchyma from being shattered but would not prevent avulsion of the herniated kidney vessels in high-speed blunt trauma which calls for urgent life-saving surgical intervention [7, 8].

The body damages are caused not only by deceleration but also by a direct hit. The deceleration magnitude may be reduced by the deformability of the vehicle. This is the reason why new vehicles are designed to have a higher deforming ability during crashes, absorbing partially the effect of the impact on the occupants [6].

Seat belts were designed in 1885, and the front lap belt use became widely distributed in 1964 and was upgraded into a three-point harness in 1973 [9]. Their use was shown to reduce head injury by a third (from 46.0% to 30.6%) and the mortality rate by half (from 12% to 6%) [10]. However, no statistical difference was observed for abdominal organs in general or genito-urinary tract trauma in particular, and controversies arose with regard to their possible harmfulness being incriminated in provoking increased deceleration injury to intraabdominal organs [11]. Nevertheless, seat belt compliance, and especially the correct use of three-point restraints, has been shown to be inversely proportionate to the rate of fatal accidents [12] (Fig. 4.3).

The same controversy has been raised for airbags; however, more advantages were again demonstrated than detrimental effects [6]. The risks also vary with the individual role and position inside the car. Being a passenger, especially in the right outboard position, increases the odds of serious abdominal injury by 2.67. These odds are reduced by front airbag deployment. A frontal impact is associated with decreased odds of severe abdominal injury than a side impact [13]. Moreover, when seatbelt restraints are combined with an airbag, there is statistically better protection including for intra-abdominal organs. A study of the Crash Injury Research and Engineering Network (CIREN) database for a period of over a decade (1996–2008) showed that frontal airbags and side airbags were associated with a 45.3% and 52.8% reduction in renal injury, respectively, after adjusting for the change in velocity [14] (Tables 4.1 and 4.2).

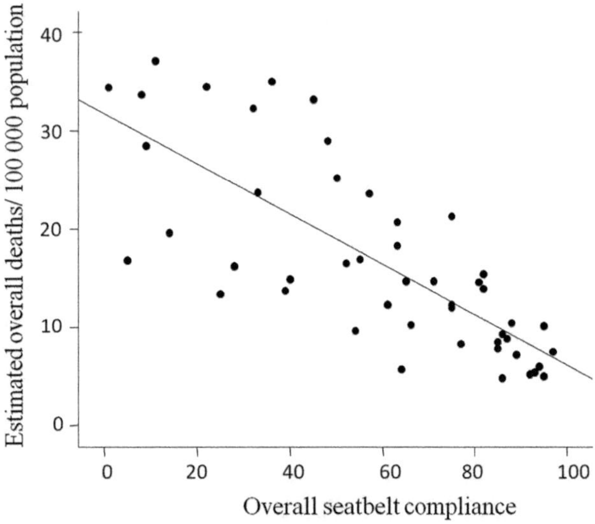

Fig. 4.3 Linear regression between seatbelt compliance and road traffic death rates in 46 high-income countries. (From Abbas et al. [12]. Creative Commons Attribution License)

Table 4.1 Front impact renal injury stratified by a change in velocity

	Δv < 40 kph						Δv > 40 kph				
	Air bag: front						Air bag: front				
	No		Yes				No		Yes		
Renal injury	n	Frequency	n	Frequency	Total, n	Renal injury	n	Frequency	n	Frequency	Total, n
No	66	86.8	624	97.4	690	No	64	94.1	679	96.2	743
Yes	10	13.2	17	2.7	27	Yes	4	5.9	27	3.8	31
Total	76		641		717	Total	68		706		774

Δv, change in velocity.

From Thomas G. Smith III et al. [14], with permission from Wolters Kluwer Health

Table 4.2 Side impact renal injury stratified by change in velocity

	Δv < 40 kph						Δv > 40 kph				
	Air bag: side						Air bag: side				
	No		Yes				No		Yes		
Renal injury	n	Frequency	n	Frequency	Total, n	Renal injury	n	Frequency	n	Frequency	Total, n
No	356	92.7	84	95.5	440	No	165	92.2	22	95.65	187
Yes	28	7.3	4	4.6	32	Yes	14	7.8	1	4.35	15
Total	384		88		472	Total	179		23		202

Δv, change in velocity.

From Thomas G. Smith III et al. [14], with permission from Wolters Kluwer Health

Scarce articles have studied the specific protection of these devices against urogenital trauma. A review of the NTDB research data for a 3-year period (2010, 2011, and 2012) recruited 3846 renal injuries and demonstrated that those without a protective device had a higher rate of high-grade renal injuries (45.1%) than those with seat belts, airbags, and combined seatbelts with airbags with 39.9%, 42.3%, and 34.7%, respectively [15].

Among patients with high-grade renal injury, those who used no protective device had a higher nephrectomy rate (56.2%) compared with those who used seat belts, airbags, and combined seatbelts with airbags who lost their kidneys in 20.0%, 10.5%, and 13.3%, respectively. Also, the combination of seatbelts and airbags was associated with a significant reduction in the total hospital length of stay and ICU days [15].

Falls are generally associated with a higher proportion of lower grades in patients who survived the accident deceleration impact. Notably, 94% of the injuries were grade I, and no grade V injury was observed in a retrospective study of 372 cases [16]. The mean height of free fall was 23.1 ft, or 7 m (range, 10–60 ft or 3–18 m), and the mean ISS was 20.6. There was no statistical correlation between the height of free fall with the grade of renal injury or with the Injury Severity Score (ISS) [16]. This statement must, however, be taken with caution as the study excluded patients who did not survive their injuries.

Regarding injuries sustained during team sports, statistics show that renal and testis injuries occur at a much lower rate than from other causes (MVA). Therefore, recommendations against team sport participation for people with solitary kidney or testis seem to be less justified than advising them to avoid motor vehicle transport [17–19].

4.2 Penetrating Injuries

As opposed to blunt trauma, penetrating trauma has a higher occurrence of intermediate- and high-grade injuries than low-grade injuries with proportions of 44%, 37%, and 19%, respectively, and nearly all patients have associated multiorgan injury (94.6%), involving the liver, the small bowel, and the vertebrae on the right side, and the stomach, the colon, and spleen on the left side [20].

4.2.1 Gunshot Injuries

According to a global estimate, 251,000 deaths were caused by firearms injuries in the world in 2016 outside the context of wars [21]. In the USA, the number of daily gunshot injury-related deaths is estimated to be 46–90 and is the second leading cause of mortality in children and adolescents, representing 15.4% of all deaths [22]. It is important for the readers to have some information about the basics of guns and ammunition, as well as the anatomopathology of a gunshot wound. However, by no means, the following notes should be substituted for comprehensive forensic studies or wound ballistics, and interested readers are referred to specialized publications for deeper and more complete information.

The muzzle velocity is defined as the initial velocity of the bullet when it exits the gun barrel after the ignition of the gunpowder. It depends on the quantity of the propellant (i.e., the explosive powder contained in the cartridge case) and the length of the gun barrel. Therefore, as rifles are long-barreled and contain larger cartridges, their bullets are considered high-velocity projectiles and they travel three times faster than conventional handgun bullets (pistols), whose velocity range is from 250 to 370 m/s [23, 24]. Roughly handgun projectiles are considered low-velocity ones, and rifles missiles are considered high-velocity ones. Low-velocity bullets are also called subsonic being less than 350 m/s, while high-velocity ones are considered to travel approximately at 600–700 m/s, carrying a high potential of explosive effects. The term "medium or intermediate velocities" is seldom used and applies to projectiles traveling at 350–600 m/s such as Magnum bullets [24].

The bullet also exhibits a high-frequency rotational motion (spin) due to the spiral grooves of the bore, but the head-on orientation is maintained through gyroscopic stabilization. However, due to the effects of the surrounding medium (air), there is a yawing of the bullet, which increases the projectile–tissue interface, hence the devastating effect of the bullet. In this context, the yaw can simply be defined as the angle between the path of flight of the bullet and its long axis [23, 25].

As mentioned above, the yawing or deformation causes enlargement of the presenting area of the bullet, thus logically aggravating the damage, and is accentuated by the tissues (muscles) in long wound tracts traversing the abdomen. The bullet may tumble in around 90° (greater damage and larger exit wound) or even at 180° yaw making the projectile base exit first (greater damage, but with a smaller exit wound) (Fig. 4.4) [23, 24]. A 90° yaw makes the entire long axis of the bullet to strike the tissue, and its amount of crush has been estimated to be three times greater than at 0° yaw [25].

The damage produced by bullets also depends on the intensity of their impact energy on the tissues, and the characteristics (elasticity, density, and anatomic relationships) of the area subjected to cavitation from high-energy projectiles [24, 25]. Also, the conception of the bullet tips is dictated by the intended effects on the targets: The bullets may be either soft-point tipped or hollow-point tipped (Fig. 4.4). The tip can also be fully covered by a metal jacket or only partially jacketed. Upon impact, when the tip is not fully covered with a metal jacket, the bullets become flattened or deformed into a mushroom and create more tissue destruction. This is the characteristic of most civilian handguns' ammunitions. On the contrary, military ammunitions have full-metal-jacket bullets and do not deform in mushroom tips aiming at producing less lethal but still debilitating injuries. The rationale is that a wounded and weakened enemy soldier who is still alive uses more resources than a killed one. The requirement for fully jacketed tips does not apply to civilian bullets that may therefore be more tissue-devastating [25, 26]. Hollow-point rifle bullets have also an increased tendency to mushroom deformation and produce excessive tissue destruction. They are mandatory by law for hunting purposes for their instant "humane" killing of the animal, avoiding prolonged suffering of the prey from a disabling but nonlethal wound. Hollow-point handgun bullets are also used by some police units to avoid over-penetration and perforation of their targets and accidental collateral injury of bystanders beyond their targets [24, 25].

Another factor that increases the devastating potential of bullets is their tendency to fragment which increases their surface area. Striking a bone with a rifle or large handgun bullet increases the potential of bullet fragmentation and ricochet in addition to the fact that bone fragments themselves become secondary missiles [25, 26] (Fig. 4.5).

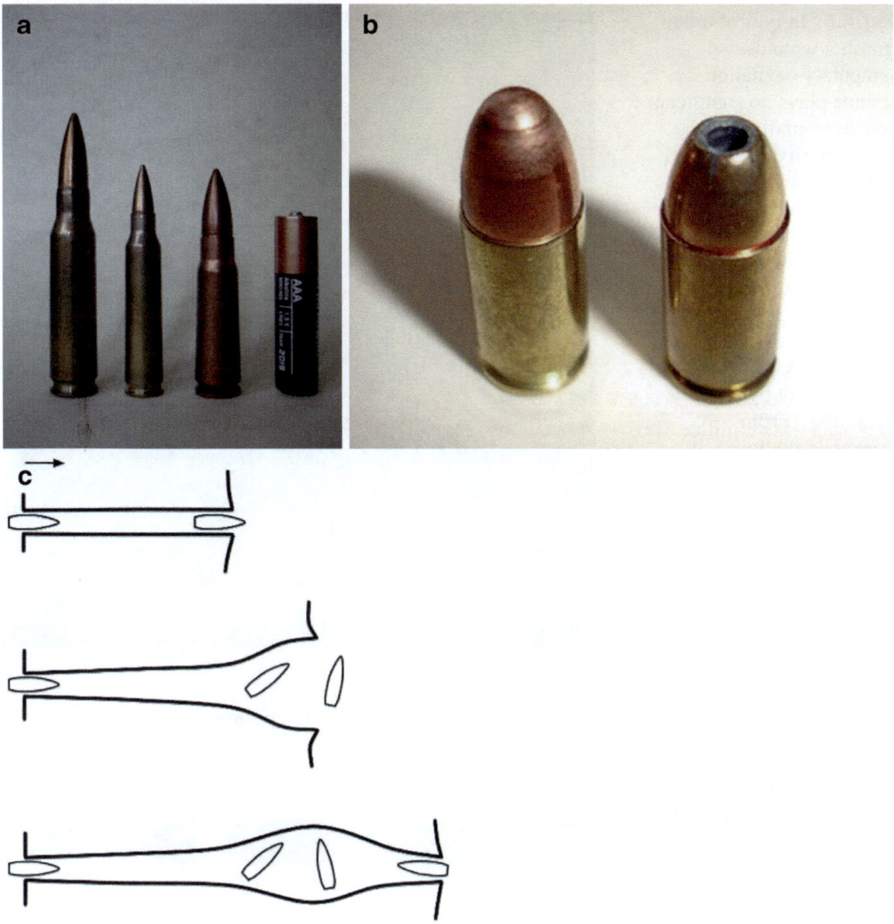

Fig. 4.4 (**a**) Common military rifle cartridges, compared with AAA battery. From left to right, with muzzle velocities in parentheses: 7.62 mm NATO (830 m/s); 5.56 mm NATO (920 m/s) used in the M16 assault rifle; and 7.62 × 39 mm Kalashnikov (700 m/s) used in the AK-47 assault rifle. The designation is according to military ammunition terminology, with the first number indicating bullet diameter and the second number (where present) indicating the cartridge case length, both in millimeters. (**b**) Hollow-point handgun bullet (right) compared with a full metal-jacketed one (left). Both cartridges are 9 mm Luger. The manufacturer's scoring of the semi-jacketed hollow-point bullet serves to facilitate the expansion of the hollowed tip upon impact. (**c**) Ballistic behavior of a military rifle bullet in tissue and the resultant perforating wounding effects. Top: the bullet traverses a limited width of tissue in stable flight without significant cavitation producing a wound similar to that from a non-deforming handgun bullet. Middle: the bullet yaw results in a gaping exit wound because of marked cavitation, a so-called "explosive" effect. Bottom: bullet tumbling and the resultant cavitation beneath the fascia. The movement of the bullet is indicated by the arrow. (From Stefanopoulos PK et al. [23], with permission from Springer)

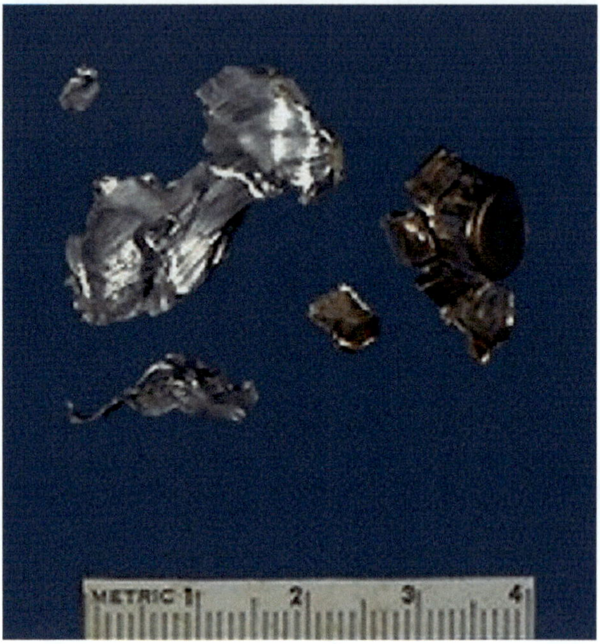

Fig. 4.5 In typical urban gunshot wounds, temporary cavitation trauma plays no significant role in wounding. In the vast majority of gunshot wounds, all significantly injured tissues have been crushed either by the intact bullet, or by its fragments (if the bullet breaks up like in this case), or by secondary missiles created by the breaking up of structures hit by the projectile. (From Alexandropoulou et al. [26], Health Science Journal. Creative Commons Attribution)

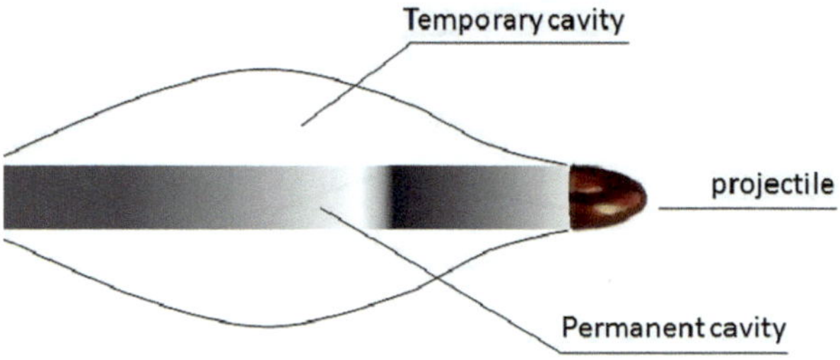

Fig. 4.6 The mechanism of cavitation can cause tissue destruction along the bullet diameter. (From Lichte P et al. [27]. Creative Commons Attribution License)

Two major mechanisms of wounding occur, namely, the crushing of the tissue struck by the projectile (forming the permanent cavity) and the radial stretching of the projectile path walls (forming the temporary cavity) [26]. When a bullet penetrates tissues, its path directly creates a crush or a central area of irreversible tissue disruption, while there is a radial stretching or temporary cavitation in the surrounding area developing in milliseconds. The crushing of tissues by a high-velocity missile results from the overpressure which is estimated to reach thousands of atmospheres. The resulting wound channel left by the bullet, filled with blood clots, fragmented tissues, and eventual foreign material, is referred to as the "permanent cavity" and roughly corresponds to the initial direct bullet crush [23–25]. The temporary cavitation can be 10–40-fold larger than the bullet diameter, and if developing from elastic tissues, such as skeletal muscle, blood vessels, and skin, these can rebound after their stretching like an accordion. However, if the tissues are inelastic such as bone and liver, more damage will occur consisting of fractures and tissue destruction [27] (Fig. 4.6).

The severity of tissue trauma is related to the degree of energy transfer which is governed by several factors including the projectile velocity (low vs. high), the entrance profile, the caliber of the projectile, the distance traveled within the body, particularities of the impacted tissue, and the mechanisms of tissue disruption (e.g. stretching, tearing, crushing) [27].

It is also important to get rid of the misconception of bullets being sterilized by the firing heat. Indeed, they can carry microorganisms (bacteria) from the body surface (skin, mucosa) into deeper tissues or spread them from perforated hollow viscus (colon) along their path [26].

Isolated penetrating renal injury is rare and the great majority (94.6%) present in the context of multiorgan [20]. These are caused either by gunshot or by stabbing, in a proportion of 81–86% and 14–16%, respectively [20]. Firearms cause more damage than stabbing injuries, and high-velocity bullets are more destructive than low-velocity ones [27, 28] (Figs. 4.7a, b and 4.8).

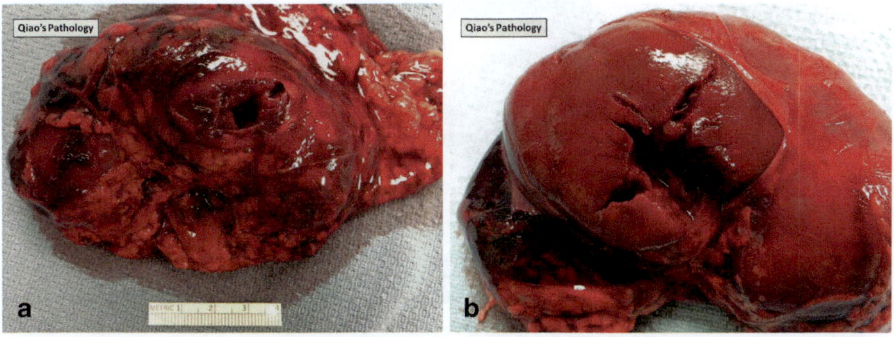

Fig. 4.7 (**a**) Gross photo of a nephrectomy with focal entrance gunshot wound. (**b**) Gross photo of a nephrectomy specimen with focal exit gunshot wound. (Jian-Hua Qiao, MD, FCAP, Los Angeles, CA, USA)

Fig. 4.8 A complex renal injury produced by an M-16A2; this wound resulted in nephrectomy. (From Hudak SJ et al. [28], with permission from Elsevier)

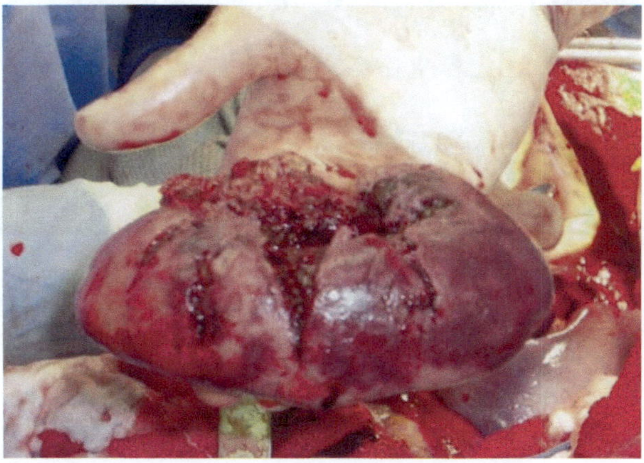

4.2.2 Stab Injuries

Instruments or objects with tissue-impaling ability comprise a wide range of heterogeneous items which are typically narrow-tipped and sharp. They include knives, scissors, animal horns, vegetable thorns, wooden sticks, glace pieces, concrete iron rods, metal pins, nails, antennas, screw-drivers [29, 30], and so on (Figs. 4.9, 4.10, and 4.11a, b). They can traverse anatomic tissues, penetrating through the skin, the fascia, the skeletal muscles, the nerves, the solid organs, and the hollow viscus, the blood vessels. When pushed with enough force, some of them may even fracture bones. Obviously, the outcome of their damage depends on the crossed organs.

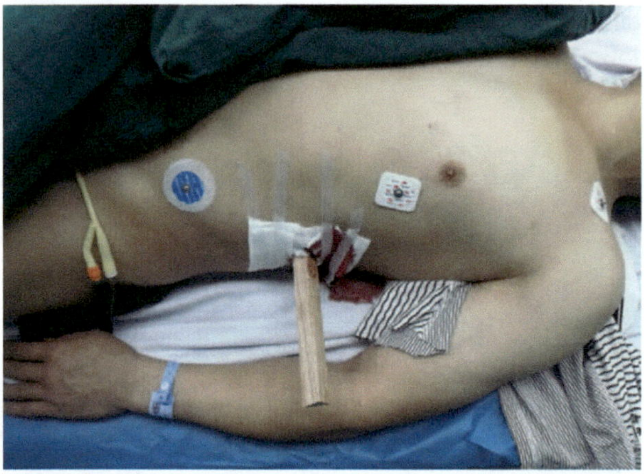

Fig. 4.9 A case of bilateral renal injury by a penetrating wooden stick. Above: Picture of the wooden stick penetrating the patient's left flank. (From Jing X et al. [29], with permission from Wolters Kluwer Health)

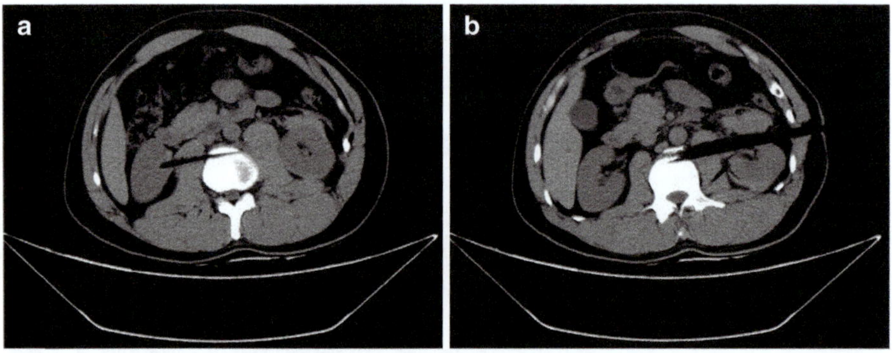

Fig. 4.10 A case of bilateral renal injury by a penetrating wooden stick. Preoperative CT scan (**a**: End course of the stick which went through the right psoas muscle and terminated in the right renal parenchyma. **b**: The stick went through the left kidney, the left psoas muscle, and the anterior body of the second lumbar vertebra). (From Jing X et al. [29], with permission from Wolters Kluwer Health)

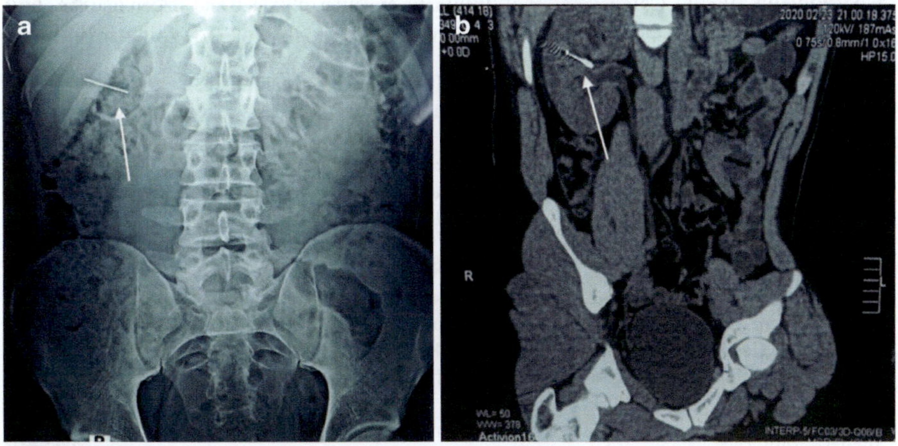

Fig. 4.11 (**a**) Plain abdomen X-ray: A metallic nail is seen in the right renal area. (**b**) Abdominal CT without contrast: The 2-in. nail is seen within the right kidney. (From Alothman AS et al. [30], Creative Commons Attribution License)

Studies have shown that stab renal injury had associated organ injuries in 61% of cases, and the wounds were mostly present in the flanks, followed by the abdomen, chest, and back in 52%, 35%, 22%, and 19%, respectively, considering that some patients had multiple wound sites with a mean of 1.27 stab per patient. The associated organ injury included the liver, the pleura (hemothorax or pneumothorax), the spleen, the Colon, and the small bowel in 42%, 37%, 20%, 19%, and 17%, respectively. Less involved organs were the lungs, the stomach, the great vessels and the heart, the diaphragm, the mesentery, the renal pelvis, the ureter, and the adrenal in decreasing order [31].

References

1. Schmidlin F, Farshad M, Bidaut L, et al. Biomechanical analysis and clinical treatment of blunt renal trauma. Swiss Surg. 1998;5:237–43.
2. Schmidlin FR, Iselin CE, Naimi A, et al. The higher injury risk of abnormal kidneys in blunt renal trauma. Scand J Urol Nephrol. 1998;32:388–92.
3. Schmidlin FR, Schmid P, Kurtyka T, et al. Force transmission and stress distribution in a computer-simulated model of the kidney: an analysis of the injury mechanisms in renal trauma. J Trauma. 1996;40:791–6.
4. Schmitt KU, Snedeker JG. Analysis of the biomechanical response of kidneys under blunt impact. Traffic Inj Prev. 2006;7(2):171–81. https://doi.org/10.1080/15389580500482021.
5. Snedeker JG, Barnstuble BB, Iaizzo PA, Farshad M, Niederer P, Schmidlin FR. A comprehensive renal injury concept based on a validated finite element model of the human abdomen. J Trauma. 2007;62(5):1240–9. https://doi.org/10.1097/01.ta.0000215531.05677.19.
6. Wallis LA, Greaves I. Injuries associated with airbag deployment. Emerg Med J. 2002;19:490–3.
7. Yoo DG, Kim CW, Park CB, Ahn JH. Traumatic right diaphragmatic rupture combined with avulsion of the right kidney and herniation of the liver into the thorax. Korean J Thorac Cardiovasc Surg. 2011;44(1):76–9. https://doi.org/10.5090/kjtcs.2011.44.1.76.

8. Stamatiou K, Ilias G, Chlopsios C, et al. Traumatic avulsion of kidney and spleen into the chest through a ruptured diaphragm in a young worker: a case report. J Med Case Rep. 2007;1:178. https://doi.org/10.1186/1752-1947-1-178.
9. Huecker MR, Chapman J. Seat belt injuries [updated 2022 Mar 7]. In: StatPearls. Treasure Island, FL: StatPearls Publishing; 2022. Available from: https://www.ncbi.nlm.nih.gov/books/NBK470262/.
10. Porter RS, Zhao N. Patterns of injury in belted and unbelted individuals presenting to a trauma center after motor vehicle crash: seat belt syndrome revisited. Ann Emerg Med. 1998;32(4):418–24. https://doi.org/10.1016/s0196-0644(98)70169-6.
11. Chandler CF, Lane JS, Waxman KS. Seatbelt sign following blunt trauma is associated with increased incidence of abdominal injury. Am Surg. 1997;63:885–8.
12. Abbas AK, Hefny AF, Abu-Zidan FM. Seatbelts and road traffic collision injuries. World J Emerg Surg. 2011;6(1):18. Published 2011 May 28. https://doi.org/10.1186/1749-7922-6-18.
13. Bansal V, Conroy C, Tominaga GT, Coimbra R. The utility of seat belt signs to predict intra-abdominal injury following motor vehicle crashes. Traffic Inj Prev. 2009;10(6):567–72. https://doi.org/10.1080/15389580903191450.
14. Smith TG III, Wessells HB, Mack CD, Kaufman R, Bulger EM, Voelzke BB. Examination of the impact of airbags on renal injury using a national database. J Am Coll Surg. 2010;211(3):355. https://doi.org/10.1016/j.jamcollsurg.2010.05.009.
15. Bjurlin MA, Fantus RJ, Fantus RJ, Mellett MM, Villines D. The impact of seat belts and airbags on high grade renal injuries and nephrectomy rate in motor vehicle collisions. J Urol. 2014;192(4):1131–6. https://doi.org/10.1016/j.juro.2014.04.093.
16. Brandes SB, McAninch JW. Urban free falls and patterns of renal injury: a 20-year experience with 396 cases. J Trauma. 1999;47(4):643–9; discussion 649–50. https://doi.org/10.1097/00005373-199910000-00007.
17. McAleer IM, Kaplan GW, LoSasso BE. Renal and testis injuries in team sports. J Urol. 2002;168(4 Pt 2):1805–7. https://doi.org/10.1097/01.ju.0000028021.97382.bc.
18. Bernard JJ. Renal trauma: evaluation, management, and return to play. Curr Sports Med Rep. 2009;8(2):98–103. https://doi.org/10.1249/JSR.0b013e31819e2e52.
19. Johnson B, Christensen C, Dirusso S, Choudhury M, Franco I. A need for reevaluation of sports participation recommendations for children with a solitary kidney. J Urol. 2005;174(2):686–9; discussion 689. https://doi.org/10.1097/01.ju.0000164719.91332.42.
20. Kansas BT, Eddy MJ, Mydlo JH, Uzzo RG. Incidence and management of penetrating renal trauma in patients with multiorgan injury: extended experience at an inner city trauma center. J Urol. 2004;172(4 Pt 1):1355–60. https://doi.org/10.1097/01.ju.0000138532.40285.44.
21. Rivara FP, Studdert DM, Wintemute GJ. Firearm-related mortality: a global public health problem. JAMA. 2018;320(8):764–5. https://doi.org/10.1001/jama.2018.9942.
22. Shrestha R, Kanchan T, Krishan K. Gunshot wounds forensic pathology (2022 May 15). In: StatPearls. Treasure Island, FL: StatPearls Publishing; 2022.
23. Stefanopoulos PK, Pinialidis DE, Hadjigeorgiou GF, Filippakis KN. Wound ballistics 101: the mechanisms of soft tissue wounding by bullets. Eur J Trauma Emerg Surg. 2017;43(5):579–86. https://doi.org/10.1007/s00068-015-0581-1. Epub 2015 Oct 15.
24. Stefanopoulos P, Hadjigeorgiou G, Filippakis K, Gyftokostas D. Gunshot wounds: a review of ballistics related to penetrating trauma. J Acute Dis. 2014;3:178. https://doi.org/10.1016/S2221-6189(14)60041-X.
25. Hollerman JJ, Fackler ML, Coldwell DM, Ben-Menachem Y. Gunshot wounds: 1. Bullets, ballistics, and mechanisms of injury. AJR Am J Roentgenol. 1990;155(4):685–90.
26. Alexandropoulou C-A, Panagiotopoulos EE. Wound ballistics: analysis of blunt and penetrating trauma mechanisms. Health Sci J. 2010;4:225–36.

27. Lichte P, Oberbeck R, Binnebösel M, et al. A civilian perspective on ballistic trauma and gunshot injuries. Scand J Trauma Resusc Emerg Med. 2010;18:35. https://doi.org/10.1186/1757-7241-18-35.
28. Hudak SJ, Morey AF, Rozanski TA, Fox CW Jr. Battlefield urogenital injuries: changing patterns during the past century. Urology. 2005;65(6):1041–6. https://doi.org/10.1016/j.urology.2004.11.031.
29. Xie J, Liu Y, Chen T, Xiao K-F. Case report of bilateral penetrating renal trauma caused by a wooden stick. Medicine. 2020;99(16):e19853. https://doi.org/10.1097/MD.0000000000019853.
30. Alothman AS, Alhajress GI, Elshaer A, Hamri SB. Nail gun penetrating renal injury: a case report. Cureus. 2022;14(2):e22697. Published 2022 Feb 28. https://doi.org/10.7759/cureus.22697.
31. Armenakas NA, Duckett CP, McAninch JW. Indications for nonoperative management of renal stab wounds. J Urol. 1999;161(3):768–71.

Grading of Renal Trauma

5

Before considering the kidney trauma grade itself, it is important to remember some vital principles.

Renal trauma is likely to occur in the context of a polytrauma, and other organs might have precedence over the kidneys in terms of emergency and treatment priority, calling for urgent life-saving interventions (e.g., massive intrathoracic or abdominal bleeding control, chest, and brain decompression) [1]. Using empirical data on outcome, namely, a mortality of 30% or greater, the Berlin Polytrauma Definition (BPD) was introduced in 2014 through an international consensus. Its criteria include significant injuries in two or more anatomical regions greater or equal to 3 on the Abbreviated Injury Scale (AIS [1]), in conjunction with one or more of the following additional diagnoses (pathologic condition): hypotension (systolic blood pressure ≤90 mmHg), unconsciousness

The original version of this chapter was revised. A correction to this chapter can be found at https://doi.org/10.1007/978-981-99-6171-9_57

[1] The Abbreviated Injury Scale (AIS) is an anatomical-based, consensus-derived, global severity scoring system created by the Association for the Advancement of Automotive Medicine. Its first version was published in 1969 and has undergone major updates since then. It classifies an individual injury by body region according to its relative severity on a 6-point scale [3, 4]:

AIS 1—Minor
AIS 2—Moderate
AIS 3—Severe but not life-threatening
AIS 4—Severe and life-threatening (survival probable)
AIS 5—Critical (survival uncertain)
AIS 6—Fatal (currently untreatable)

S. A. AL-Mamari, *Urogenital Trauma: A Practical Guide*,
https://doi.org/10.1007/978-981-99-6171-9_5

(Glasgow Coma Scale score[2] ≤8), acidosis (base deficit ≤−6.0), coagulopathy (PTT ≥40 s or INR ≥1.4), and age (≥70 years) [2].

The BPD was subsequently validated by many studies including a recent Dutch observational study [7]. Well before a consensus was reached to define polytrauma, its physiopathology was intensively studied, and Gebhard and Huber-Lang proposed the following critical events [1]:

- Danger-sensing molecules phase: coagulation cascade, kallikrein-kinin system, complement system, acute phase reaction
- Trauma-induced complementopathy
- Trauma-induced intravascular coagulopathy (TIC)
- Trauma-induced neuroinflammation

In 1974, Baker et al. introduced a method for describing patients presenting with multiple injuries to evaluate their prognosis and emergency priorities: The **Injury Severity Score (ISS)**, which was developed from the **Abbreviated Injury Scale (AIS)** [8]. They defined the ISS as the sum of the squares of the highest AIS grade in each of the three most severely injured areas, with the purpose of dramatically increasing the correlation between the severity of the injury and the mortality, compared with the AIS.

---

[2] Glasgow Coma Score (GCS) [5, 6]:
Parameters:

- Best eye response (4 points)
  - No eye opening: 1
  - Eye opening to pain: 2
  - Eye opening to sound: 3
  - Eyes open spontaneously: 4
- Best verbal response (5 points)
  - No verbal response: 1
  - Incomprehensible sounds: 2
  - Inappropriate words: 3
  - Confused: 4
  - Orientated: 5
- Best motor response (6 points)
  - No motor response: 1
  - Abnormal extension to pain: 2
  - Abnormal flexion to pain: 3
  - Withdrawal from pain: 4
  - Localizing pain: 5
  - Obeys commands: 6

Total score:

GCS 3–8: severe
GCS 9–12: moderate
GCS 13–15: mild

The ISS is allocated a marking from 0 to 75 and correlates linearly with mortality, morbidity, and hospital stay. The ISS has been validated and categorized as follows [9]:

- <9 = Mild
- 9–15 = Moderate
- 16–24 = Severe
- ≥25 = Profound

Therefore, major trauma is defined by ISS >15.

Progressing further in our discussion, it is important to avoid confusing kidney trauma with **acute renal injury (AKI),** and a bracket is opened in the following paragraphs to elucidate this concept. AKI is defined as a sudden loss of kidney function arising from multiple causes such as sepsis, hypovolemic shock, drugs, and so on. AKI may develop in a polytrauma patient with or without a direct physical hit to the kidneys. According to the Kidney Disease Improving Global Guidelines (KDIGO), AKI has three stages and is defined by any of the following: an increase in serum creatinine (SCr) by ≥0.3 mg/dL (≥26.5 μmol/L) within 48 h; or an increase in SCr to ≥1.5 times baseline, which is known or presumed to have occurred within the prior 7 days; urine volume ≤0.5 mL/kg/h for 6 h [10]. The duration of AKI is limited to 7 days. Beyond this limit, the pathology will be called acute kidney disease or disorder, and if persisting for more than 3 months, the term will change to chronic kidney disease [11].

Following polytrauma, AKI is triggered by massive hemorrhage, systemic inflammatory response syndrome (SIRS), and multiple-organ dysfunction syndrome (MODS). Two or more criteria have to be fulfilled to define a SIRS: Temperature >38.8 or <36 °C, tachycardia >90 beats/min, tachypnea >20 breaths/min or $PaCO_2$ <32 mmHg, leukocytes >12,000/mm^3 or leukopenia <4000/mm^3, or >10% immature neutrophils [12].

AKI associated with trauma has a high mortality rate (28.08%) [13]. Severe AKI was found in 2.3% of 64,059 civilians with gunshot wounds and 0.9% required dialysis. It was associated with older age, male sex, history of diabetes or hypertension, hypotension at presentation (systolic blood pressure <90 mmHg), coagulopathy, lower Glasgow Coma Scale score, sepsis, hollow viscus injury, and higher injury severity score. The likelihood for patients with severe AKI to die was twice as high as that of patients without severe AKI, and it was even higher for those requiring dialysis as 28.4% of the latter group died [13, 14].

AKI might also develop in the context of isolated brain injury, as shown by a study recruiting 37,851 patients with isolated severe traumatic brain injuries, of whom 2.1% experienced severe (stage 3 or greater) AKI [15].

In developing countries, the risk of mortality for motor traffic accidents is far higher than in developed countries [16], and the polytrauma victims are younger, with a higher male predominance (92.3%) and a higher percentage (38.5%) of AKI [17].

Table 5.1 Kidney injury scale (from Moore et al. [18], with permission from Elsevier)

Grade[a]	Type	Injury description	AIS-90
I	Contusion	Microscopic or gross hematoma, urologic studies normal	2
	Hematoma	Subcapsular, nonexpanding without parenchymal laceration	2
II	Hematoma	Nonexpanding perineal hematoma confined to renal retroperitoneum	2
	Laceration	<1.0 cm parenchymal depth of renal cortex without urinary extravasation	2
III	Laceration	>1.0 cm parenchymal depth of renal cortex without collecting system rupture or urinary extravasation	3
IV	Laceration	Parenchymal laceration extending through the renal cortex, medulla, and collecting system	4
	Vascular	Main renal artery or vein injury with contained hemorrhage	4
V	Laceration	Completed shattered kidney	5
	Vascular	Avulsion of renal hilum which devascularizes the kidney	5

[a] Advance one grade for bilateral injuries up to grade III

In summary, AKI is far more frequent than direct kidney trauma and its presence portends a more serious prognosis. It can be associated or not with gross kidney trauma. It is important to remember that AKI per se is not a surgical pathology and is better managed by nephrologists and acute medicine specialists in a high dependency or an Intensive Care Unit, and the management is based on the treatment of the primary insult and control of systemic disorders and also short-term hemodialysis if required until the acute episode is over, and the kidneys recover.

After clarifying this potential source of confusion, let us close the bracket and get back to the grading of the kidney trauma.

The American Association for the Surgery of Trauma (AAST) grading score of kidney trauma was introduced by Moore et al. in 1989 (Table 5.1) [18].

This grading system has been validated by many studies: After a review of 54,148 entries containing the AIS-coded injuries in the National Trauma Data Bank (NTDB), Tinkoff et al. found that, in the 35,897 isolated abdominal solid organ injuries (including spleen, liver, and kidney), the outcome corresponded to the increase of injury grade [19]. And a monocentric retrospective review of 2467 patients with renal trauma showed a linear correlation between the AAST grades and the need for surgical exploration in general and for nephrectomy in particular [20] (Fig. 5.1).

In a large proportion of patients with blunt as well as penetrating renal injury, the need for nephrectomy and the overall outcome can be reliably predicted by a combination of the AAST grade of renal injury, the overall injury severity score, and the requirement of blood transfusion [21]. However, concerns were raised about the lack of clarification of certain subtypes of injuries within grades IV and V [22], and proposals were made in 2011 concerning segmental vascular injuries and ureteral pelvic injuries [23]. In 2018, the AAST Patient Assessment Committee revised the kidney AAST grading system to include vascular thrombosis, segmental renal artery or vein injury, and all collecting system injuries as grade IV injuries, and a devascularized kidney with active bleeding as grade V kidney injury [24]. In 2019, the American Society of Emergency Radiology adapted the description of CT findings in accordance with the above updated AAST revision and highlighted important differences from the prior grading scheme [25] (Table 5.2).

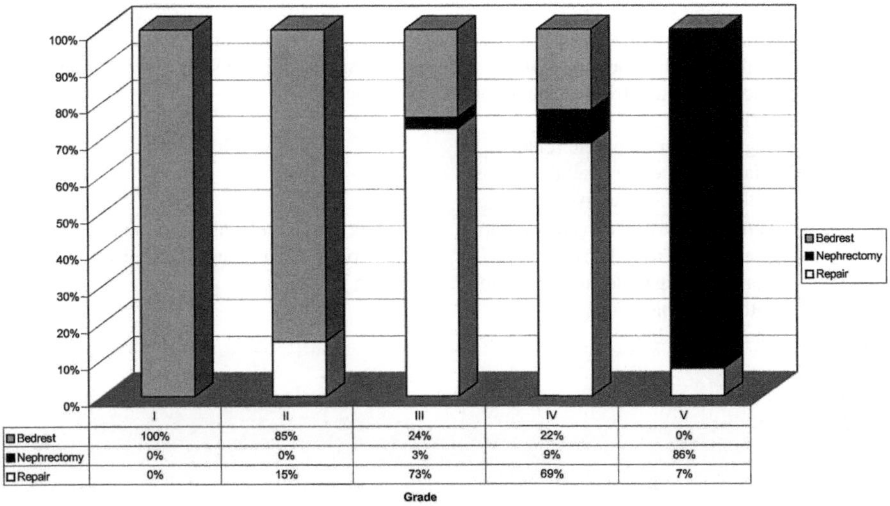

Fig. 5.1 Correlation between treatment and AAST grade. (From Santucci RA, et al. [20], with permission from Wolters Kluwer Health)

Table 5.2 Description of CT features associated with each AAST OIS grade in the 2018 revision. The last column emphasizes the new elements in the revised grading scheme (from Chien LC et al. [25], with permission from Springer Nature)

AAST grade	CT criteria in the revised grading system	New features in the revised grading system
I	– Isolated parenchymal contusion – Subcapsular hematoma	– Removes microscopic or macroscopic hematuria without imaging abnormality – Removes term nonexpanding from subcapsular hematoma
II	– Renal parenchymal laceration ≤1 cm in depth without extension to the collecting system – Perirenal hematoma contained by Gerota fascia	– Removes term nonexpanding from perirenal hematoma
III	– Renal parenchymal laceration >1 cm without extension to the collecting system – Any low-grade injury with associated vascular injury or active bleeding contained by Gerota fascia	– Adds vascular injury, defined as AVF or pseudoaneurysm – Includes active bleeding within Gerota fascia

(continued)

Table 5.2 (continued)

AAST grade	CT criteria in the revised grading system	New features in the revised grading system
IV	– Parenchymal laceration extending to the collecting system – Renal pelvis laceration or complete ureteropelvic laceration – Segmental renal artery or vein intimal injury/thrombus – Active bleeding beyond Gerota fascia into the retroperitoneum or peritoneum – Segmental or complete renal infarction due to vessel thrombosis in the absence of active bleeding	– Incorporates isolated renal collecting system injury – Includes active bleeding beyond Gerota fascia – Removes bleeding injuries to the main renal artery and vein (laceration or avulsion of hilar vessels now included in grade V)
V	– Main renal artery or vein laceration or avulsion from the renal hilum – Complete organ devascularization with active bleeding – Shattered kidney	– Adds active bleeding in setting of complete renal infarction in distinction from grade IV

Content excluded

Content excluded

Patients who are victims of gunshot kidney injury have higher grades than those assaulted by stabbing, and the latter group sustains higher injury grades than those who suffer blunt trauma [26]. The AAST grade has a statistically significant correlation with the need for surgery and for the risk of nephrectomy; 86–91% of patients undergoing exploration for grade V ultimately have nephrectomy vs only 9% for grade IV [22, 25, 27] (Fig. 5.3). These results are sufficient to emphasize the importance of a careful distinction between grades IV and V before venturing into a surgical exploration.

The World Society of Emergency Surgery (WSES) has adapted the AAST grading to the patient's hemodynamical condition and proposed four grades grouped into three categories: minor, moderate, and severe [28] (Table 5.3).

A different grading system (the Chatelain Classification) has been used in the French medical literature since 1981 but is almost abandoned now. It comprised four grades only and was based on intravenous urography (IVU) findings, hence its weakness. To date, the original AAST classification still holds the lion's share among trauma doctors, clinicians, and researchers.

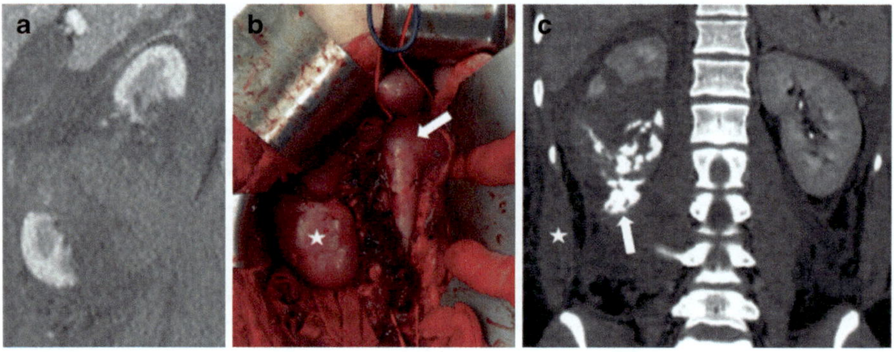

Fig. 5.3 AAST grade V injury in two separate patients. (**a**) Sagittal CECT of a patient with transected kidney demonstrates complete devascularization of the interpolar region of the right kidney. (**b**) Intraoperative photograph of the same patient as (**a**) demonstrating transection of the kidney, with a small superior pole attached to the IVC (arrow), which was subsequently repaired. The inferior pole is in the lower-left corner (star). No distinct arterial supply to the inferior pole could be identified. Superior pole parenchyma was well-vascularized but was avulsed from the entire collecting system. Nephrectomy was performed. (**c**) Coronal CECT in a separate patient. (From Chien LC et al. [25], with permission from Springer Nature)

Table 5.3 WSES kidney trauma classification (from Coccolini, F. et al. [28]. Creative Commons Attribution 4.0 International License)

	WSES grade	AAST	Hemodynamic
Minor	WSES grade I	I–II	Stable
Moderate	WSES grade II	III or segmental vascular injuries	Stable
Severe	WSES grade III	IV–V or any grade parenchymal lesion with main vessel dissection/occlusion	Stable
	WSES grade IV	Any	Unstable

References

1. Gebhard F, Huber-Lang M. Polytrauma—pathophysiology and management principles. Langenbeck's Arch Surg. 2008;393:825.
2. Pape HC, Lefering R, Butcher N, Peitzman A, Leenen L, Marzi I, Lichte P, Josten C, Bouillon B, Schmucker U, Stahel P, Giannoudis P, Balogh Z. The definition of polytrauma revisited: an international consensus process and proposal of the new 'Berlin definition'. J Trauma Acute Care Surg. 2014;77(5):780–6. https://doi.org/10.1097/TA.0000000000000453.
3. States J. The abbreviated and the comprehensive research injury scales. SAE Technical Paper 690810, 1969. https://doi.org/10.4271/690810.
4. Abbreviated Injury Scale (AIS). Overview. Association for the Advancement of Automotive Medicine. 2019 [cited 7 Aug 2019]. Available from: https://www.aaam.org/abbreviated-injury-scale-ais/.
5. Teasdale G, Jennett B. Assessment of coma and impaired consciousness. Lancet. 1974;304(7872):81–4. https://doi.org/10.1016/s0140-6736(74)91639-0.
6. Jain S, Iverson LM. Glasgow Coma scale. 2021. In: StatPearls. Treasure Island, FL: StatPearls Publishing; 2022.
7. Driessen MLS, Sturms LM, van Zwet EW, Bloemers FW, Ten Duis HJ, Edwards MJR, den Hartog D, de Jongh MAC, Leenhouts PA, Poeze M, Schipper IB, Spanjersberg R, Wendt KW, de Wit RJ, van Zutphen SWAM, Leenen LPH. Evaluation of the Berlin polytrauma definition: a Dutch nationwide observational study. J Trauma Acute Care Surg. 2021;90(4):694–9. https://doi.org/10.1097/TA.0000000000003071.
8. Baker SP, O'Neill B, Haddon W Jr, Long WB. The injury severity score: a method for describing patients with multiple injuries and evaluating emergency care. J Trauma. 1974;14(3):187–96.
9. Bolorunduro OB, Villegas C, Oyetunji TA, Haut ER, Stevens KA, Chang DC, Cornwell EE 3rd, Efron DT, Haider AH. Validating the Injury Severity Score (ISS) in different populations: ISS predicts mortality better among Hispanics and females. J Surg Res. 2011;166(1):40–4. https://doi.org/10.1016/j.jss.2010.04.012. Epub 2010 May 6.
10. KDIGO AKI Work Group. KDIGO clinical practice guideline for acute kidney injury. Kidney Int Suppl. 2012;2:1–138.
11. Kellum JA, Romagnani P, Ashuntantang G, et al. Acute kidney injury. Nat Rev Dis Primers. 2021;7:52. https://doi.org/10.1038/s41572-021-00284-z.
12. Ertel W, Friedl H, Trentz O. Multiple organ dysfunction syndrome (MODS) following multiple trauma: rationale and concept of therapeutic approach. Eur J Pediatr Surg. 1994;4(4):243–8. https://doi.org/10.1055/s-2008-1066112.
13. Ahmed N, Mathew RO, Kuo Y, et al. Risk of in-hospital mortality in severe acute kidney injury after traumatic injuries: a national trauma quality program study. Trauma Surg Acute Care Open. 2021;6:e000635. https://doi.org/10.1136/tsaco-2020-000635.
14. Athavale AM, Fu CY, Bokhari F, Bajani F, Hart P. Incidence of, risk factors for, and mortality associated with severe acute kidney injury after gunshot wound. JAMA Netw Open. 2019;2(12):e1917254. https://doi.org/10.1001/jamanetworkopen.2019.17254.
15. Luu D, Komisarow J, Mills BM, Vavilala MS, Laskowitz DT, Mathew J, James ML, Hernandez A, Sampson J, Fuller M, Ohnuma T, Raghunathan K, Privratsky J, Bartz R, Krishnamoorthy V. Association of severe acute kidney injury with mortality and healthcare utilization following isolated traumatic brain injury. Neurocrit Care. 2021;35:434. https://doi.org/10.1007/s12028-020-01183-z.
16. Museru LM, Mcharo CNLMT. Road traffic accidents in Tanzania: a ten year epidemiological appraisal. East Cent African J Surg. 2002;7:23–6. https://doi.org/10.1017/CBO9781107415324.004.
17. Muhamedhussein MS, Manji M, Nungu KS, Ruggajo P, Khalid K. Prevalence and risk factors of acute kidney injury in polytrauma patients at Muhimbili Orthopedic Institute, Tanzania. Afr J Emerg Med. 2021;11(1):74–8. https://doi.org/10.1016/j.afjem.2020.08.004.

18. Moore EE, Shackford SR, Pachter HL, McAninch JW, Browner BD, Champion HR, Flint LM, Gennarelli TA, Malangoni MA, Ramenofsky ML, et al. Organ injury scaling: spleen, liver, and kidney. J Trauma. 1989;29(12):1664–6. https://doi.org/10.1016/S0039-6109(16)46589-8.
19. Tinkoff G, Esposito TJ, Reed J, Kilgo P, Fildes J, Pasquale M, Meredith JW. American Association for the Surgery of Trauma Organ Injury Scale I: spleen, liver, and kidney, validation based on the national trauma data bank. J Am Coll Surg. 2008;207(5):646–55. https://doi.org/10.1016/j.jamcollsurg.2008.06.342.
20. Santucci RA, McAninch JW, Safir M, Mario LA, Service S, Segal MR. Validation of the American Association for the Surgery of Trauma organ injury severity scale for the kidney. J Trauma. 2001;50(2):195–200. https://doi.org/10.1097/00005373-200102000-00002.
21. Erlich T, Kitrey ND. Renal trauma: the current best practice. Ther Adv Urol. 2018;10:295–303. https://doi.org/10.1177/1756287218785828.
22. Costa IA, Amend B, Stenzl A, Bedke J. Contemporary management of acute kidney trauma. J Acute Dis. 2016;5:29–36.
23. Buckley JC, McAninch JW. Revision of current American Association for the Surgery of Trauma Renal Injury grading system. J Trauma. 2011;70(1):35–7. https://doi.org/10.1097/TA.0b013e318207ad5a.
24. Kozar RA, Crandall M, Shanmuganathan K, Zarzaur BL, Coburn M, Cribari C, Kaups K, Schuster K, Tominaga GT, AAST Patient Assessment Committee. Organ injury scaling 2018 update: spleen, liver, and kidney. J Trauma Acute Care Surg. 2018;85(6):1119–22. https://doi.org/10.1097/TA.0000000000002058. Erratum in: J Trauma Acute Care Surg. 2019;87(2):512.
25. Chien LC, Vakil M, Nguyen J, et al. The American Association for the Surgery of Trauma Organ Injury Scale 2018 update for computed tomography-based grading of renal trauma: a primer for the emergency radiologist. Emerg Radiol. 2020;27:63–73. https://doi.org/10.1007/s10140-019-01721-z.
26. Shariat SF, Roehrborn CG, Karakiewicz PI, Dhami G, Stage KH. Evidence-based validation of the predictive value of the American Association for the Surgery of Trauma Kidney Injury Scale. J Trauma. 2007;62(4):933–9. https://doi.org/10.1097/ta.0b013e318031ccf9.
27. Santucci RA, McAninch JM. Grade IV renal injuries: evaluation, treatment, and outcome. World J Surg. 2001;25:1565–72.
28. Coccolini F, Moore EE, Kluger Y, et al. Kidney and uro-trauma: WSES-AAST guidelines. World J Emerg Surg. 2019;14:54. https://doi.org/10.1186/s13017-019-0274-x.

Symptoms, Signs, and Diagnostic Means of Renal Trauma

6

6.1 Presentation and Physical Examination

Generally, the patient is brought to the hospital by relatives or by an ambulance from the accident (RTA, sports trauma, and fall) or the aggression scene, and history is readily provided by the patient himself if fully conscious, the rescuers, the relatives, or the bystanders. Usually, the mechanism of the injury is obvious. The first step is to assess his consciousness and hemodynamic status. Vital signs must be taken immediately, and the patient kept under monitoring (BP, pulse, RR, and O_2 saturation) and instructed on strict bed rest until definitely labeled as stable with minor trauma. Patients might present with anemia and hemodynamic instability (i.e., systolic blood pressure <90 mmHg). Patients who sustained penetrating renal injury are more likely to present with hemodynamic instability than those with blunt trauma in a proportion of 14.2% vs. 8.36%, respectively [1].

The patient can also present with loin or flank pain with or without hematuria. The presence of hematuria is an important positive finding, but its absence does not exclude renal trauma, and its importance does not correlate with the grade of the trauma. The physical examination will show bruising, ecchymosis, swelling, and tenderness at the loin, flank, or abdominal region. In penetrating injuries, the wound caused by the stabbing instrument will be obvious, and the entry and possibly the exit site of the bullet in a gunshot injury should also be determined. Signs of peritonitis might be observed if a hollow viscus has been perforated.

As renal trauma might present in the context of multiorgan injury, a general physical examination is of paramount importance to avoid missing injuries of other organs: in addition to the urgent consciousness and hemodynamical status assessment already mentioned above, the examination should rule out rib fracture or spine injury, hemoperitoneum (spleen or liver rupture), hemo- or pneumothorax (pleural or broncho-pulmonary injury), and peritonitis (injury of hollow abdominal viscera: colon, small bowel, stomach, etc.).

S. A. AL-Mamari, *Urogenital Trauma: A Practical Guide*,
https://doi.org/10.1007/978-981-99-6171-9_6

6.2 Laboratory Tests

The clinician should rapidly request a complete blood count (CBC) (hemoglobin and hematocrit), blood crossmatching, renal function tests, coagulation profile, as well as urine analysis to detect microscopic hematuria. Depending on the presentation, other blood tests might also be useful (amylase, troponin, D-dimer, C-RP, etc.).

6.3 Imaging

6.3.1 Contrast-Enhanced Computerized Tomography (CECT)

For more than two decades, intravenous urography (IVU) has been supplanted by **CECT which is now the gold standard imaging means** to define and grade the renal injury either for blunt or penetrating renal trauma. However, being time-consuming, CECT should be performed only in a stable patient as recommended by Experts' panel guidelines [2, 3].

Because of the poor correlation between hematuria and the injury grade, radiological investigations are recommended in all patients with penetrating injuries. For those with blunt trauma, due to the absence of prospective randomized trials, there is a consensus that hemodynamically stable patients with suspected renal trauma should undergo imaging examinations, the suspicion being built upon history and the presence of gross hematuria or microhematuria [4].

In this setting, it has been shown that patients with blunt trauma, microscopic hematuria, and systolic blood pressure >90 mmHg have a very low incidence of major renal injury (0.2%) and do not require imaging investigations. On the contrary, those who have BP <90 mmHg have 12.5% of major renal injury [5].

In addition, despite the total absence of hematuria, radiological investigations should be performed in patients with a suggestive history of deceleration injuries or those with multiple associated injuries: high-speed motor vehicle accident (MVA) and falls from height [4–6].

As the patient's hemodynamic stability status is a key factor in deciding on the management, it is important to refresh the readers' mind with some definitions [7]:

In adult patients, hemodynamic instability is defined by:

- Systolic blood pressure <90 mmHg + signs of skin vasoconstriction (cool, decreased capillary refill), altered level of consciousness, and/or shortness of breath or
- BP >90 mmHg but requiring bolus infusions or transfusions and/or inotropic support, and/or base excess (BE) >−5 mmol/L, and/or shock index [1] >1, and/or transfusion requirement of at least 4–6 units of packed red blood cells within the first 24 h

[1] The shock index (SI) is the ratio between heart rate and systolic blood pressure in mmHg (HR/SBP). It helps to detect early hemorrhagic shock and to determine the severity of the trauma.

In pediatric patients, hemodynamic stability is considered as:

- A systolic blood pressure of 90 mmHg plus twice the child's age in years (the lower limit is inferior to 70 mmHg plus twice the child's age in years or inferior to 50 mmHg in some studies)

As a rule of thumb, based on general consensus, experts' panels [2, 3, 8, 9] recommend performing diagnostic imaging with CECT in hemodynamically stable patients presenting with the following:

- Blunt trauma with visible (gross, macroscopic) haematuria
- Blunt trauma with non-visible (microscopic) haematuria + one episode of hypotension (syst BP <90 mmHg)
- History of rapid deceleration injury and/or significant associated injuries
- Penetrating trauma
- Clinical signs suggestive of renal trauma (flank pain, abrasions, fractured ribs, abdominal distension, and/or mass or tenderness elicited on palpation)

A complete CT study should include four phases [9]:

- Precontrast: help identifying renal calculi or intraparenchymal hematoma.
- Postcontrast arterial (35 s postintravenous injection): identify parenchymal and vascular damage, eventual presence of active extravasation, and another solid organ injury.
- Postcontrast nephrogenic/portal venous (75 s postintravenous injection): identify active extravasation and optimally demonstrate parenchymal contusions and lacerations.
- Delayed (5–10 min postintravenous injection): identify eventual collecting system and ureteral injury and urinoma.

After an initial imaging, general consensus also prevails that reimaging with a repeat CECT should be obtained for high-grade renal injuries after 2–4 days to reevaluate the progress or be requested whenever there are signs of complications such as fever, abdominal distension, unexplained decrease Hb and Hct, or significant flank pain [2, 3, 9].

6.3.2 Ultrasonography (U/S)

U/S is inferior to CECT and has limited use. However, it may help detect renal lacerations and hematoma but is unable to define the nature of a collecting fluid (urine or blood). It is useful in the follow-up of hydronephrosis and fluid resorption, with the advantage of being radiation-free, especially in the pediatric population [9].

6.3.3 Intravenous Urography (IVU) or Intravenous Pyelography (IVP)

IVP has become obsolete nowadays due to the widespread distribution of cross-sectional imaging (CT scan). Nonetheless, the European Association of Urology (EAU) recommends proceeding to a rapid one-shot intra-operative IVP to confirm the presence of the contralateral kidney before engaging in a surgical exploration in unstable patients who cannot undergo a CT scan beforehand: Practically, a bolus of 2 mL/kg of contrast is given followed by a single plain X-ray film after 10 min [2].

6.3.4 Other Imaging Modalities

Magnetic resonance imaging (MRI) is impracticable in the setting of a trauma as it requires a tedious arrangement and is not superior to CECT. However, MRI may be useful in a stable pregnant woman or in patients who are allergic to iodine [7].

Radionuclide studies have a role in the follow-up to evaluate scarring and loss of kidney or secondary obstruction.

References

1. McClung CD, Hotaling JM, Wang J, Wessells H, Voelzke BB. Contemporary trends in the immediate surgical management of renal trauma using a national database. J Trauma Acute Care Surg. 2013;75(4):602–6. https://doi.org/10.1097/TA.0b013e3182a53ac2.
2. EAU Guidelines. Edn. presented at the EAU annual congress Amsterdam, Mar 2022. ISBN: 978-94-92671-16-5. https://d56bochluxqnz.cloudfront.net/documents/full-guideline/EAU-Guidelines-on-Urological-Trauma-2022_2022-03-24-104100_fwda.pdf.
3. Morey AF, Brandes S, Dugi DD 3rd, Armstrong JH, Breyer BN, Broghammer JA, Erickson BA, Holzbeierlein J, Hudak SJ, Pruitt JH, Reston JT, Santucci RA, Smith TG 3rd, Wessells H, American Urological Assocation. Urotrauma: AUA guideline. J Urol. 2014;192(2):327–35. https://doi.org/10.1016/j.juro.2014.05.004. Epub 2014 May 20.
4. Santucci RA, Wessells H, Bartsch G, Descotes J, Heyns CF, McAninch JW, Nash P, Schmidlin F. Evaluation and management of renal injuries: consensus statement of the renal trauma subcommittee. BJU Int. 2004;93(7):937–54. https://doi.org/10.1111/j.1464-4096.2004.04820.x.
5. Mee SL, McAninch JW, Robinson AL, Auerbach PS, Carroll PR. Radiographic assessment of renal trauma: a 10-year prospective study of patient selection. J Urol. 1989;141:1095–8.
6. Ramchandani P, Buckler PM. Imaging of genitourinary trauma. AJR Am J Roentgenol. 2009;192(6):1514–23. https://doi.org/10.2214/AJR.09.2470.
7. Coccolini F, Moore EE, Kluger Y, et al. Kidney and uro-trauma: WSES-AAST guidelines. World J Emerg Surg. 2019;14:54. https://doi.org/10.1186/s13017-019-0274-x.
8. Serafetinides E, Kitrey ND, Djakovic N, et al. Review of the current management of upper urinary tract injuries by the EAU Trauma Guidelines Panel. Eur Urol. 2015;67:930–6.
9. Erlich T, Kitrey ND. Renal trauma: the current best practice. Ther Adv Urol. 2018;10(10):295–303. https://doi.org/10.1177/1756287218785828.

Treatment of Renal Trauma. I. Conservative and Mini-Invasive Management

7

Following a long period of lethargy with scarce publications about the conservative management of renal trauma in the post-World War II period, a new era of explosive interest in this subject arose in the mid-2000s [1].

Success was once considered when a patient survived a renal trauma and nephrectomy was frequently performed for any severe trauma to reach this goal. Then emotional progress was made in the management of renal trauma over the last 20 years. Nowadays, while still aiming at the patient's survival, true success is increasingly considered as salvaging the injured kidney. More and more researchers and clinicians rightly consider the unnecessary removal of a kidney during the treatment of renal trauma as "an avoidable disaster second only to death or extreme debility" and preconize preserving renal function while minimizing morbidity and eliminating kidney-related mortality [2].

Moreover, analysis of high-grade renal trauma patients in the National Trauma Data Bank (NTDB) for a 10-year period from 2007 to 2016 showed that nephrectomy is an independent factor associated with increased risk of mortality after adjusting for injury characteristics, overall injury severity, and patient demographics. In this study, nephrectomy was associated with 82% increased odds of death in multivariable logistic regression [3].

With the exception of critical scenarios where the patient is unstable and expectative management is obviously deemed dangerous, the great fear of the treating team in the approach of a renal trauma should be to do more harm than good. A meta-analysis has shown that nonoperative approaches result in lower mortality compared with operating management even when considering solely high-grade blunt as well as penetrating injuries [4] (Fig. 7.1a–d).

The conservative management or minimally invasive approaches for grades IV and V blunt renal trauma have also been supported in the pediatric population by systemic reviews which demonstrated short- and long-term favorable outcomes [5] and a lower rate of kidney loss with angioembolization than with surgical intervention [6].

S. A. AL-Mamari, *Urogenital Trauma: A Practical Guide*,
https://doi.org/10.1007/978-981-99-6171-9_7

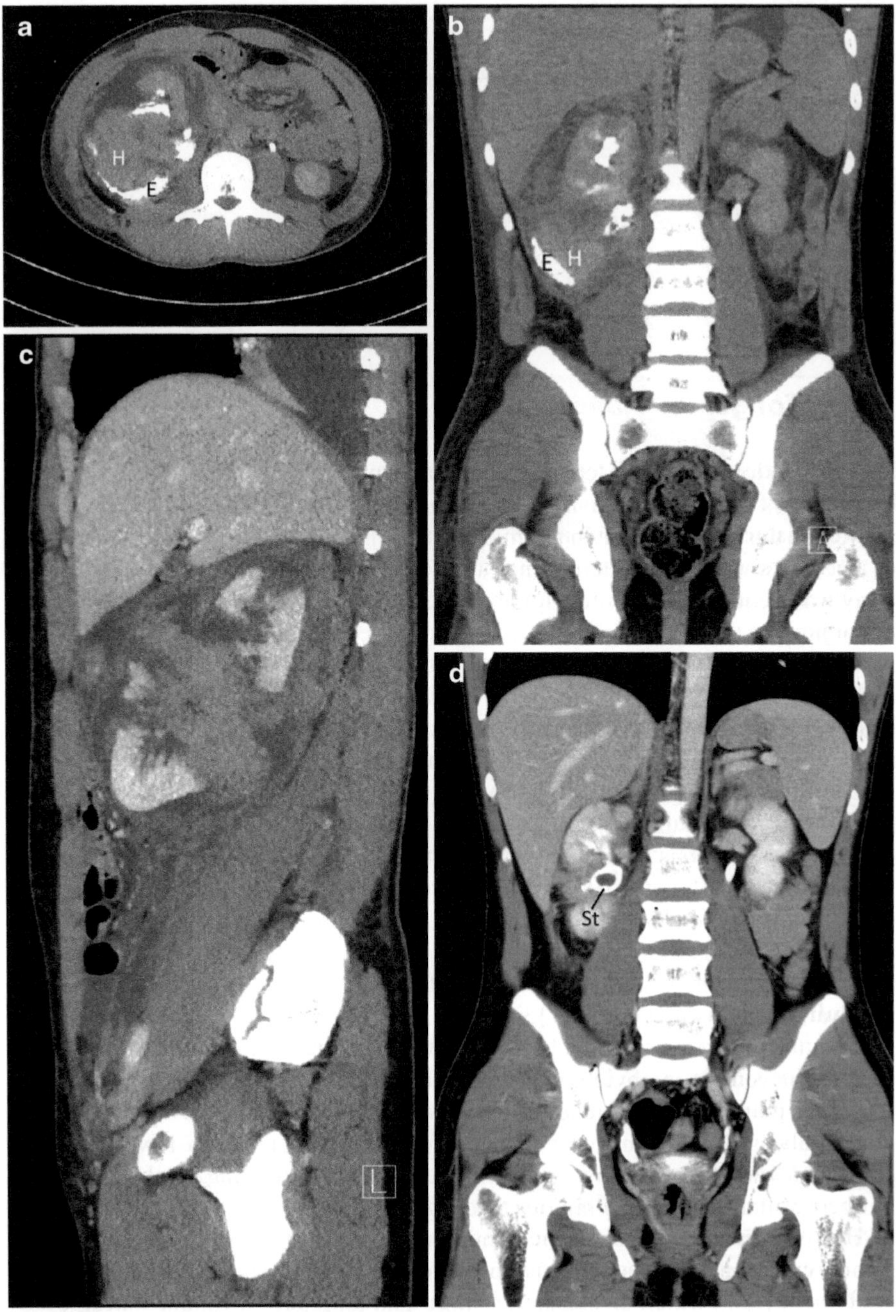

Fig. 7.1 (**a**–**d**) An 18-year-old fisherman who fell and sustained abdominal trauma resulting in a shattered right kidney (AAST grade V) and largely associated intra and perinephric hematoma (127 × 115 × 85 mm) (H) and extravasation (E): (**a**–**c**) Axial, coronal and sagittal image of the right kidney and hematoma. (**d**) The patient was stable, only a DJ stent (St) was inserted and the rest of management was conservative. (**e**) Follow-up repeat CT showed nearly complete healing at 8 months

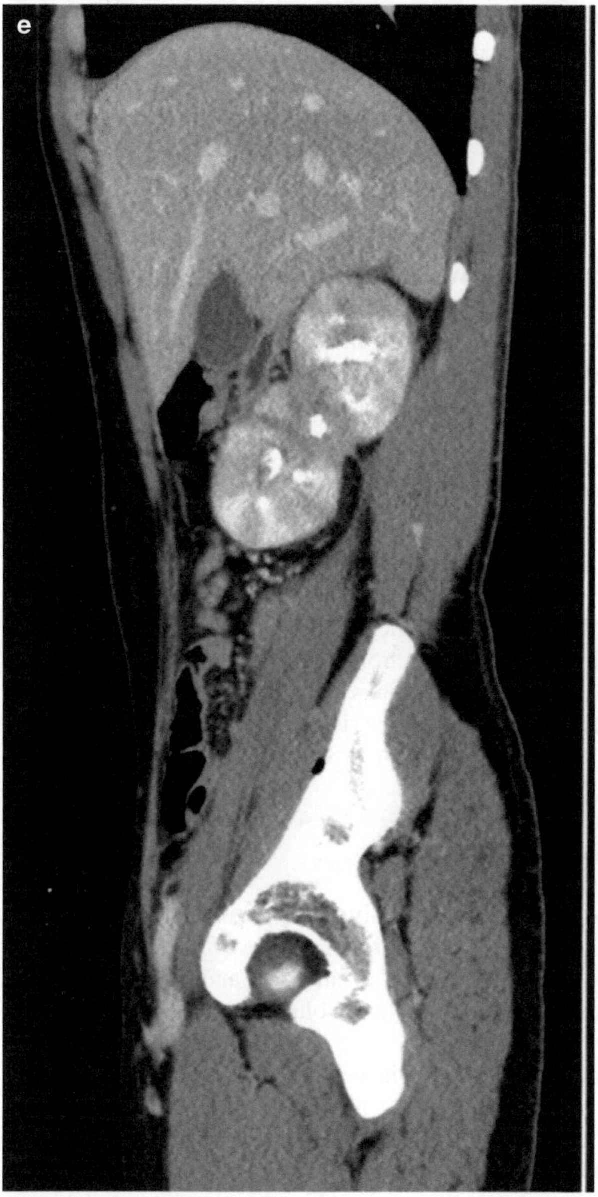

Fig. 7.1 (continued)

The National Trauma Data Bank (NTDB) research in the USA shows that 83.4% of renal traumata were managed nonoperatively, and only 16.6% were treated with interventional therapy for the period 2010–2014 [7].

Even when specifying high-grade injuries only (AAST grade III–V) for the period 2014–2017, data still show that 70% were managed nonoperatively, 11% underwent minimally invasive management, 19% were operated on, and 67% of the operated patients underwent nephrectomy. Thus, the overall nephrectomy rate for all patients with high-grade injury was 13%, and more specifically 0.4%, 15%, and 62% for grades III, IV, and V, respectively [8].

7.1 Supportive and Adjunctive Treatments

The critically sick and shocked patient is better resuscitated in a high dependency or intensive care unit with continuous monitoring, intravenous crystalloid infusion, blood transfusions, inotropic support if required, oxygen supplement if required, central venous pressure line, urine output monitoring, intubation, and so on. The details are outside the scope of this book. For most of the patients, there is no clear recommendation on DVT thromboprophylaxis, antibiotic prophylaxis, and mobilization due to a lack of evidence [9].

Consensus pleads, however, for antibiotic prophylaxis with a single dose, with the possibility to continue the antibiotic therapy in cases of urinary extravasation or high-grade injury. Also, putting into balance the ongoing or possible sudden occurrence of bleeding weighed against the risk of thrombosis in a traumatized bedridden patient with kidney trauma, compression stockings are advised while low molecular heparin can be given in selected cases only after risk balancing. Catheterization is advised in patients with high-grade trauma or in those with heavy hematuria.

7.2 Minimally Invasive Approach

7.2.1 The Rationale of Minimally Invasive Approach

Prioritizing less invasive management applies to all ages, and pediatric patients should be treated in the same way as adults, either in blunt or penetrating urogenital injuries [10].

However, experts' opinion states that non-invasive management in severe injuries should be supported by the availability of close clinical observation and hemodynamic monitoring facilities (ideally in high dependency/intensive care units), proper laboratory tests, and immediate procurement of whole blood, packed cells, and other blood products. Also, diagnostic means should be readily available, as well as immediate access to interventional radiology (angioembolization) and surgery [10].

While still considering the hemodynamical status of the patient as the key factor to decide on either nonoperative or operative management, the second factor that should be considered is the **AAST grade**, not because this will directly and immediately dictate the management option, but because it has a correlation with the hemodynamical status and will keep the clinician on alert:

- Grade I: Nonoperative management. These patients rarely require any intervention, and no nephrectomy has been associated with this grade.
- Grade II: Nonoperative management. Rarely require any intervention. However, due to small parenchymal laceration (<1 cm), persistent moderate pain might be present due to a larger subcapsular hematoma than in grade I. No nephrectomy has been associated with this grade.
- Grade III*:* Again, nonoperative management must be considered for any stable patient. However, as there is a deeper laceration of the cortex (>1 cm), a larger subcapsular hematoma is expected with subsequent increased pain requiring more analgesia and also the need for blood transfusion, percutaneous drainage if the hematoma is expanding, and even selective arterial embolization if the patient's Hb drops requiring repeated blood transfusion.
- Rarely, if embolization is ineffective, exploration might be needed to remove the hematoma and proceed to hemostatic renorrhaphy of the laceration. Failure to control the bleeding might lead to nephrectomy. Old studies showed higher rates of nephrectomy (3–9%) in grade III renal injury [11], which significantly decreased with the introduction of angioembolization to almost completely disappear [12].
- Grade IV: Conservative management has still a large place in grade IV blunt renal injury [13].
- However, when remembering the definition of this grade with deeper parenchymal laceration up to the collecting system and main renal artery or vein injury, one can expect the presence of a larger possibly pulsating hematoma, with a drop of hemoglobin requiring frequent blood transfusion and the presence of urinoma.
- Therefore, the need for interventional management must be permanently kept in mind consisting of percutaneous urinoma drainage, placement of a DJ stent, an angioembolization in the presence of continuous bleeding with expansive hematoma, and even surgical exploration in case of failed embolization, or severe pain, or sepsis from an infected hematoma or abscess.
- The chances of nephrectomy are higher in grade IV than in grade III, even if the trend is going down due to the development of angioembolization. A study showed that angioembolization and ureteral stent placement were necessary in 22 patients out of 124 (18%) patients with grade IV injury [14], and a 25-year retrospective study of 153 cases of grade IV kidney injury concluded in 2006 showed 67% (two-thirds) of cases treated operatively and 33% (one-third) treated nonoperatively [15]. Nephrectomy was performed in 15 patients from this cohort (9.8%).
- More recent research showed a higher rate of successful nonoperative management of grade IV renal injury (82%) and only 2 patients out of 124 underwent partial nephrectomy (1.6%) and 2 others total nephrectomy [14].
- Grade V injury: Again, a stable patient can still be managed conservatively.
- Indeed, in our practice, we have successfully managed conservatively cases of grade V trauma with shattered kidney, some of them without even a minimally invasive procedure (Fig. 7.1). More frequently, however, these patients require either a DJ stent insertion or angioembolization. Nonetheless, due to the higher

possibility of a rapidly expansive hematoma or the presence of a completely shattered kidney, a higher rate (52%) of grade V injuries requires operative exploration (half of the patients) with a rate of nephrectomy 23% of cases [14].
- Angioembolization is of great interest in avulsed main renal vessels when one is planning to proceed to exploration and removal of the kidney as it will minimize the bleeding during mobilization of the kidney and removal of the hematoma. It can also be considered for segmental arteries in shattered kidney with no main vessels' avulsion. It has a decreased rate of renal unit loss compared with surgical intervention in stable patients with persistent or delayed bleeding [6].

In the pediatric population also, there are robust data supporting conservative management protocols for high-grade (III, IV, and V) blunt renal trauma as these have favorable short- and long-term outcomes [5].

A European systematic review found a significant heterogeneity in the outcomes of high-grade renal trauma management according to the published series. However, when comparing the nonoperative with the operative approaches, it found that the overall mortality, renal preservation, and complication rates are significantly better in the nonoperative management group than in the operative one, with values of 0–3% vs. 0–29%, 84–100% vs. 0–82%, and 5–32% vs. 10–76%, respectively [16].

A great change has occurred in the last decade with the majority of isolated blunt renal artery injuries being also treated conservatively leaving only a minority of cases for nephrectomy, endovascular stenting, or open renal artery repair [17].

Another important factor to keep in mind after considering the patient's hemodynamic status and the AAST injury grade is the **mechanism of injury.** As for the AAST grade, the importance of the mechanism lies in its correlation with the patient's hemodynamic status. **Penetrating injuries have shown a higher rate of interventions than blunt trauma despite still being managed nonoperatively in the majority of cases**: 40% nonoperative, 38% renorrhaphy, and 22% nephrectomy. And among penetrating injuries, renal gunshot wounds were mostly managed surgically with 26% and 42% requiring nephrectomy and renorrhaphy, respectively, while only 32% were successfully managed nonoperatively [18] (Fig. 7.2).

7.2.2 Minimally Invasive Procedures

7.2.2.1 Angioembolization

Angiography in a patient after a renal trauma may reveal actively bleeding vessels, pseudoaneurysms, arteriovenous fistulas, or arterio-calyceal fistula or may show no abnormality or bleeding.

The technique of angioembolization is performed under **local anesthesia,** and the **common femoral artery** is the preferred approach. The patient's vital signs are monitored. The kidney side of interest is selected, and when the area of bleeding is visualized, a super-selective approach is undertaken so that distal embolization is limited to the site to avoid the devascularization of unaffected parenchyma. For this reason, the embolizing material should be positioned at, or beyond, the interlobar

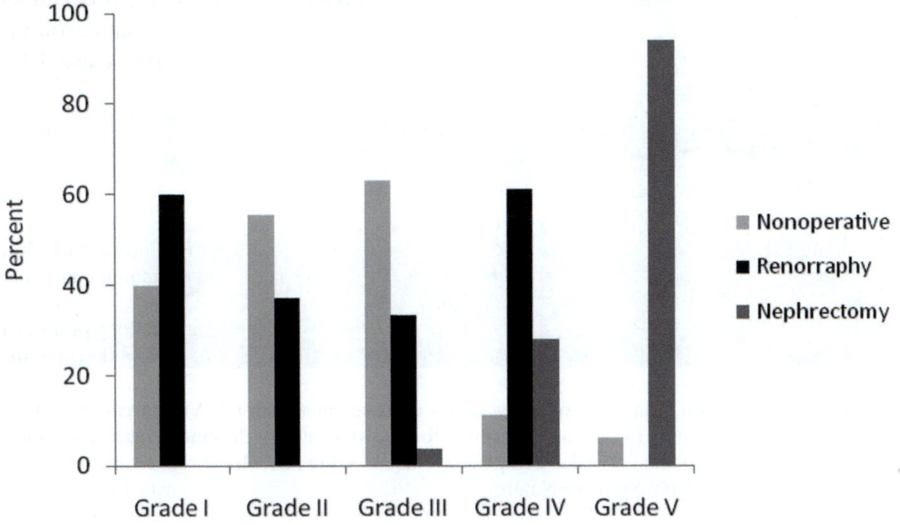

Fig. 7.2 Incidence of nonoperative management, renorrhaphy, and nephrectomy of penetrating renal injury grades I–V. (From Bjurlin MA et al. [18], with permission from Lippincott Williams and Wilkins (Wolters Kluwer Health))

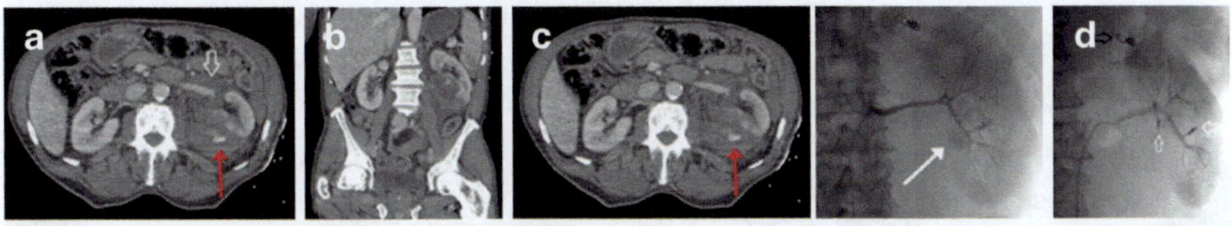

Fig. 7.3 Grade 4 left renal laceration after fall. Axial (**a**) and coronal (**b**) CT images showing laceration of the left kidney with hyperdense material (red arrow) showing active hemorrhage. Angiography (**c**) shows the area of bleeding in the inferior pole (white arrow). After coil embolization (**d**), the bleeding is controlled. The lack of parenchymal contrast peripheral to the coils in the medial inferior pole represents devascularized tissue. (From Lopez-Gonzalez DB et al. [19], with permission from Georg Thieme Verlag KG)

artery. Various materials may be utilized for an effective embolization: microcoils, gelfoam, polyvinyl-alcohol (PVA) particles, and vascular plug (Amplatzer) [19, 20] (Figs. 7.3, 7.4, and 7.5).

The combination of these materials might be used to potentiate their effects.

A review of angioembolization for iatrogenic kidney injury showed a 100% technical success rate and a 95% clinical success rate.

After the failure of the initial angioembolization, a repeat procedure should be considered in hemodynamically stable patients who have a continuous active bleeding with no other indications for surgical intervention [10].

Resuscitative endovascular balloon occlusion of the aorta (i.e., REBOA) may be used in hemodynamically unstable patients as a bridge for hemorrhage control until a more definitive procedure is performed [10].

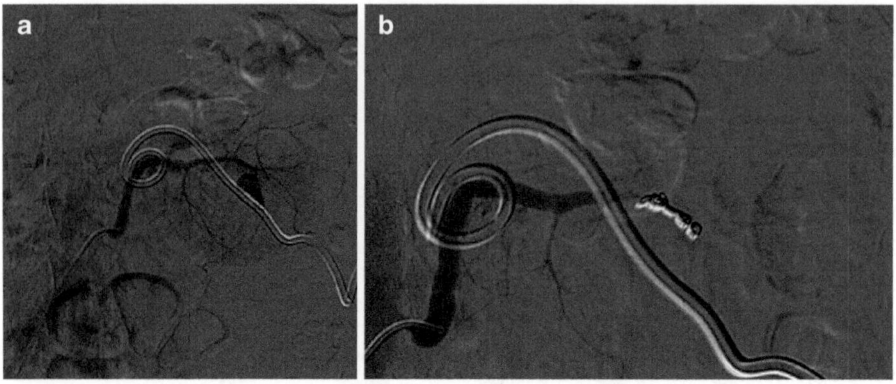

Fig. 7.4 Selective left renal arteriography shows a pseudoaneurysm (PSA) in a patient with a percutaneous nephrostomy (**a**); the angiogram performed at the end of the embolization procedure (carried out with microcoils) revealed complete exclusion of the PSA (**b**). (From Ierardi AM et al. [20], with permission from Springer Nature)

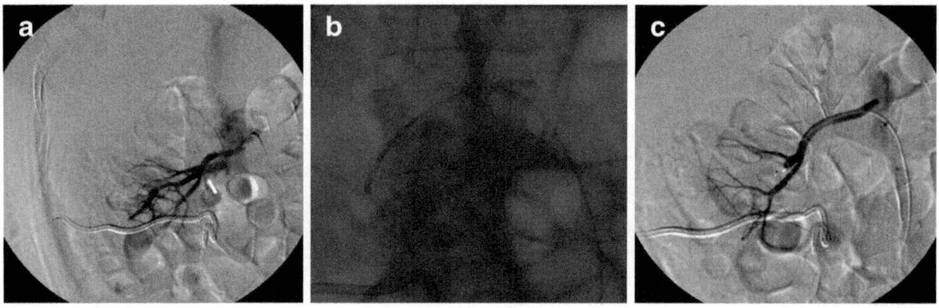

Fig. 7.5 Selective right renal arteriography shows early opacification of draining veins (white arrow) during the arterial phase due to postnephrostomy iatrogenic arteriovenous fistula (**a**); an 8 mm Amplatzer plug inside the delivery catheter (**b**); the angiogram performed at the end of the procedure revealed closure of the arteriovenous fistula (**c**). (From Ierardi AM et al. [20], with permission from Springer Nature)

REBOA might be associated with decreased mortality. However, like most of the procedures performed in life-saving situations, it suffers the lack of randomized trials to support its use, and its complications should be kept in mind (air emboli, lower limbs ischemia, aortic dissection, hematoma, rupture, perforation, pseudoaneurysm, etc.) [21, 22].

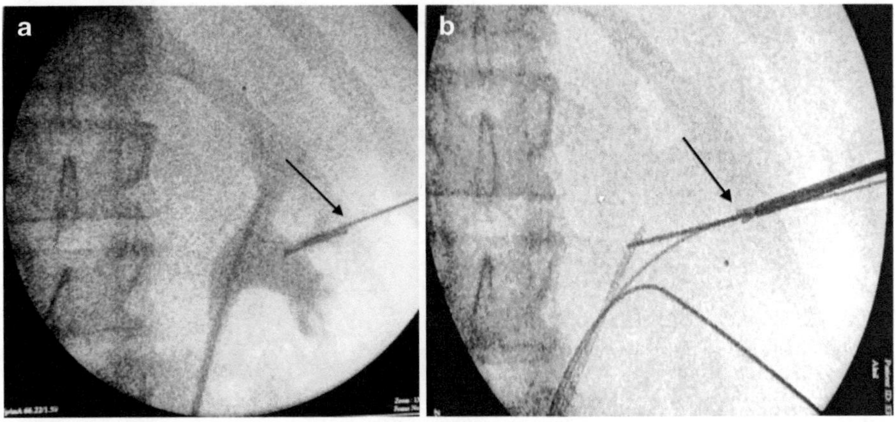

Fig. 7.6 (**a**) Intraoperative fluoroscopy. (**b**) Extraction of the nail by the ureteroscopy forceps with fluoroscopic guidance. (From Alothman AS et al. [23]. Creative Commons Attribution License)

7.2.2.2 Other Minimally Invasive Procedures

These may merely consist of a percutaneous drainage of urinoma and abscess, a percutaneous nephrostomy (PCN), an antegrade or retrograde DJ stent insertion, a percutaneous extraction of a nail under fluoroscopy guidance, and so on [23] (Fig. 7.6a, b).

In very rare cases, CECT may show a traumatic occlusion of the main renal artery which mandates an endovascular stent placement. Only short series are available in the literature, and one of them showed a high rate of kidney atrophy or recanalization failure with extravasation prompting embolization [24].

7.3 Special Management for Post-PCNL Renal Injury

As a urologist, you are expected to be able to manage iatrogenic kidney damages caused by yourself. The best example is a post-PCNL renal injury.

The following algorithm has been proposed for the management of post-PCNL bleeding (Figs. 7.7 and 7.8) [25, 26].

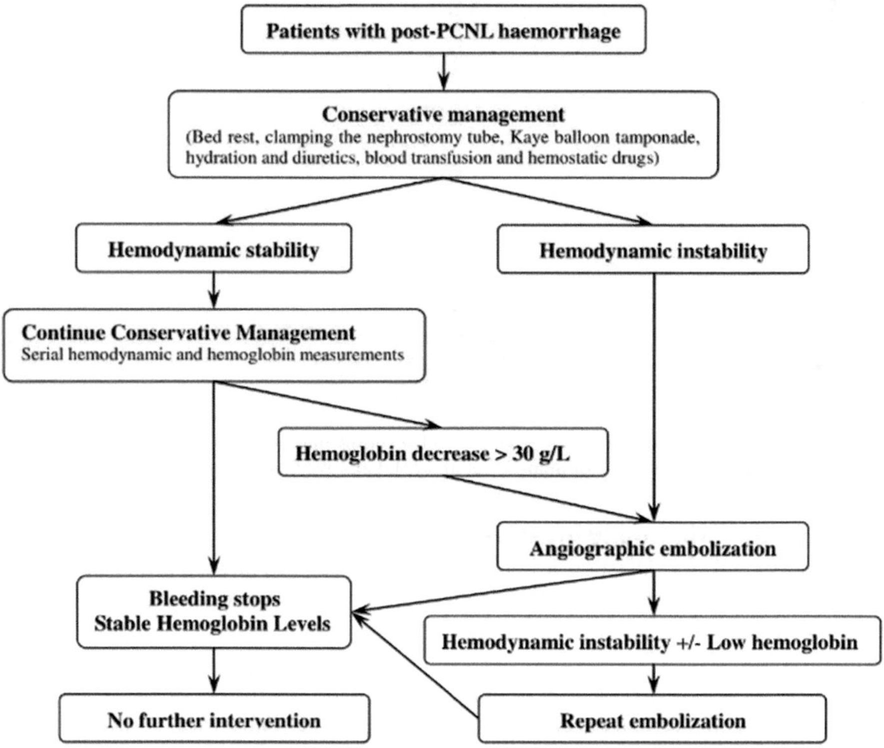

Fig. 7.7 Treatment algorithm for the management of post-PCNL hemorrhage. (From Long Li et al. [25], with permission from Springer Nature)

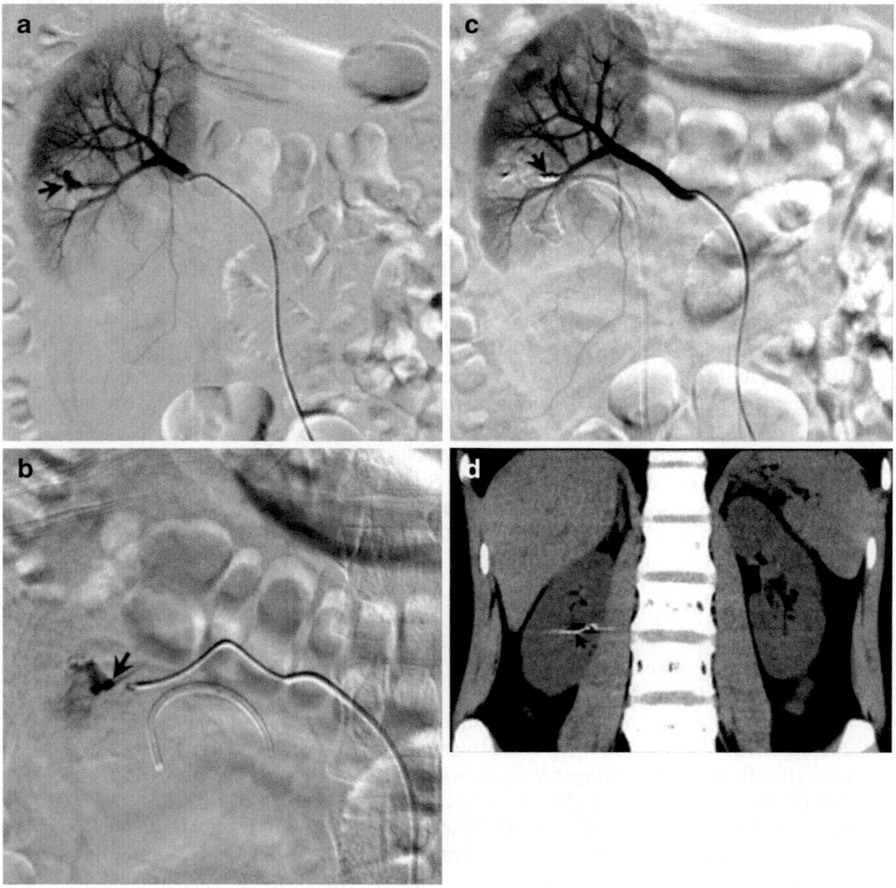

Fig. 7.8 Superselective TAE of a renal artery branch pseudoaneurysm resulting in delayed post-PCNL hemorrhage. (**a**) The right renal artery angiography revealed a pseudoaneurysm originated from the anterior inferior segmental branch. (**b**) The parent arterial branch of the pseudoaneurysm was catheterized superselectively using the microcatheter. (**c**) The right renal arteriography showed that the parent arterial branch of the pseudoaneurysm was completely occluded by a microcoil. (**d**) CT scan at 12-month follow-up showed the normal homogeneous density throughout the right renal parenchyma and the parapelvic metal artifact resulting from the microcoil. *TAE* transcatheter angiographic embolization. (From Long Li et al., with permission from Springer Nature)

References

1. Santucci RA. 2015 William Hunter Harridge lecture: how did we go from operating on nearly all injured kidneys to operating on almost none of them? Am J Surg. 2016;211(3):501–5. https://doi.org/10.1016/j.amjsurg.2016.01.001. Epub 2016 Jan 6.
2. Al-Qudah HS, Santucci RA. Complications of renal trauma. Urol Clin North Am. 2006;33(1):41–53, vi. https://doi.org/10.1016/j.ucl.2005.10.005.

3. Anderson RE, Keihani S, Das R, Hanson HA, McCrum ML, Hotaling JM, Myers JB. Nephrectomy is associated with increased mortality after renal trauma: an analysis of the National Trauma Data Bank from 2007-2016. J Urol. 2021;205(3):841–7. https://doi.org/10.1097/JU.0000000000001366. Epub 2020 Oct 6.
4. Mingoli A, La Torre M, Migliori E, et al. Operative and nonoperative management for renal trauma: comparison of outcomes. A systematic review and meta-analysis. Ther Clin Risk Manag. 2017;13:1127–38. Published 2017 Aug 31. https://doi.org/10.2147/TCRM.S139194.
5. LeeVan E, Zmora O, Cazzulino F, Burke RV, Zagory J, Upperman JS. Management of pediatric blunt renal trauma: a systematic review. J Trauma Acute Care Surg. 2016;80(3):519–28. https://doi.org/10.1097/TA.0000000000000950.
6. Hagedorn JC, Fox N, Ellison JS, Russell R, Witt CE, Zeller K, Ferrada P, Draus JM Jr. Pediatric blunt renal trauma practice management guidelines: collaboration between the Eastern Association for the Surgery of Trauma and the Pediatric Trauma Society. J Trauma Acute Care Surg. 2019;86(5):916–25. https://doi.org/10.1097/TA.0000000000002209.
7. Bjurlin MA, Fantus RJ, Fantus RJ, Villines D. Comparison of nonoperative and surgical management of renal trauma. J Trauma Acute Care Surg. 2017;82(2):356–61. https://doi.org/10.1097/ta.0000000000001316.
8. Keihani S, Xu Y, Presson AP, Hotaling JM, Nirula R, Piotrowski J, Dodgion CM, Black CM, Mukherjee K, Morris BJ, Majercik S, Smith BP, Schwartz I, Elliott SP, DeSoucy ES, Zakaluzny S, Thomsen PB, Erickson BA, Baradaran N, Breyer BN, Miller B, Santucci RA, Carrick MM, Hewitt T, Burks FN, Kocik JF, Askari R, Myers JB, Genito-Urinary Trauma Study Group, Contemporary management of high-grade renal trauma: results from the American Association for the Surgery of Trauma Genitourinary Trauma study. J Trauma Acute Care Surg. 2018;84(3):418–25. https://doi.org/10.1097/TA.0000000000001796. Erratum in: J Trauma Acute Care Surg. 2018 May;84(5):826.
9. Sharma DM, Serafetinidis E, Sujenthiran A, Elshout PJ, Djakovic N, Gonsalves M, Kuehhas FE, Lumen N, Kitrey ND, Summerton DJ, EAU Guidelines Panel on Urological Trauma. Grey areas: challenges of developing guidelines in adult urological trauma. Eur Urol Focus. 2016;2(1):109–10. https://doi.org/10.1016/j.euf.2015.11.005. Epub 2015 Dec 8.
10. Coccolini F, Moore EE, Kluger Y, et al. Kidney and uro-trauma: WSES-AAST guidelines. World J Emerg Surg. 2019;14:54. https://doi.org/10.1186/s13017-019-0274-x.
11. Santucci RA, McAninch JW, Safir M, Mario LA, Service S, Segal MR. Validation of the American Association for the Surgery of Trauma organ injury severity scale for the kidney. J Trauma. 2001;50(2):195–200. https://doi.org/10.1097/00005373-200102000-00002.
12. Aragona F, Pepe P, Patanè D, Malfa P, D'Arrigo L, Pennisi M. Management of severe blunt renal trauma in adult patients: a 10-year retrospective review from an emergency hospital. BJU Int. 2012;110(5):744–8. https://doi.org/10.1111/j.1464-410X.2011.10901.x. Epub 2012 Feb 7.
13. Erlich T, Kitrey ND. Renal trauma: the current best practice. Ther Adv Urol. 2018;10(10):295–303. Published 2018 Jul 10. https://doi.org/10.1177/1756287218785828.
14. Lanchon C, Fiard G, Arnoux V, Descotes JL, Rambeaud JJ, Terrier N, Boillot B, Thuillier C, Poncet D, Long JA. High grade blunt renal trauma: predictors of surgery and long-term outcomes of conservative management. A prospective single center study. J Urol. 2016;195(1):106–11. https://doi.org/10.1016/j.juro.2015.07.100. Epub 2015 Aug 6.
15. Buckley JC, McAninch JW. Selective management of isolated and nonisolated grade IV renal injuries. J Urol. 2006;176(6 Pt 1):2498–502; discussion 2502. https://doi.org/10.1016/j.juro.2006.07.141.
16. Sujenthiran A, Elshout PJ, Veskimae E, MacLennan S, Yuan Y, Serafetinidis E, Sharma DM, Kitrey ND, Djakovic N, Lumen N, Kuehhas FE, Summerton DJ. Is nonoperative management the best first-line option for high-grade renal trauma? A systematic review. Eur Urol Focus. 2019;5(2):290–300. https://doi.org/10.1016/j.euf.2017.04.011.
17. Owattanapanich N, Benjamin E, Lewis M, Cai J, Demetriades D. Epidemiology and management of isolated blunt renal artery injuries. J Trauma Acute Care Surg. 2021;90(6):1003–8. https://doi.org/10.1097/TA.0000000000003153.

18. Bjurlin MA, Jeng EI, Goble SM, Doherty JC, Merlotti GJ. Comparison of nonoperative management with renorrhaphy and nephrectomy in penetrating renal injuries. J Trauma. 2011;71(3):554–8. https://doi.org/10.1097/TA.0b013e318203321a.
19. Lopez-Gonzalez DB, Zurkiya O. Interventional radiology in renal trauma. Semin Intervent Radiol. 2021;38(1):113–22. https://doi.org/10.1055/s-0041-1726006.
20. Ierardi AM, Floridi C, Fontana F, Duka E, Pinto A, Petrillo M, Kehagias E, Tsetis D, Brunese L, Carrafiello G. Transcatheter embolisation of iatrogenic renal vascular injuries. Radiol Med. 2014;119(4):261–8. https://doi.org/10.1007/s11547-013-0343-2. Epub 2013 Dec 3.
21. Castellini G, Gianola S, Biffi A, et al. Resuscitative endovascular balloon occlusion of the aorta (REBOA) in patients with major trauma and uncontrolled haemorrhagic shock: a systematic review with meta-analysis. World J Emerg Surg. 2021;16:41. https://doi.org/10.1186/s13017-021-00386-9.
22. Ribeiro Junior MAF, Feng CYD, Nguyen ATM, et al. The complications associated with resuscitative endovascular balloon occlusion of the aorta (REBOA). World J Emerg Surg. 2018;13:20. https://doi.org/10.1186/s13017-018-0181-6.
23. Alothman AS, Alhajress GI, Elshaer A, Bin HS. Nail gun penetrating renal injury: a case report. Cureus. 2022;14(2):e22697. Published 2022 Feb 28. https://doi.org/10.7759/cureus.22697.
24. Lopera JE, Suri R, Kroma G, Gadani S, Dolmatch B. Traumatic occlusion and dissection of the main renal artery: endovascular treatment. J Vasc Interv Radiol. 2011;22(11):1570–4. https://doi.org/10.1016/j.jvir.2011.08.002. Epub 2011 Sep 19.
25. Li L, Zhang Y, Chen Y, et al. A multicentre retrospective study of transcatheter angiographic embolization in the treatment of delayed haemorrhage after percutaneous nephrolithotomy. Eur Radiol. 2015;25:1140–7.
26. Poudyal S. Current insights on haemorrhagic complications in percutaneous nephrolithotomy. Asian J Urol. 2021;9:81. https://doi.org/10.1016/j.ajur.2021.05.007.

Treatment of Renal Trauma. II: Operative Approaches

8

Repetition is the mother of learning, the father of action, which makes it the architect of accomplishment (Zig Ziglar, American Author (1926–2012)).

Before discussing the operative approaches, it is important to reemphasize that the patient's hemodynamical status is considered the key criterion for adopting either a non-invasive or an invasive approach.

It is never superfluous to highlight once more that, when facing a stable patient, expectant management prevails, and this applies for all grades, either minor (I–II), intermediate (III), or severe (IV–V). However, if the patient is unstable, with no or transient response to resuscitation, an immediate intervention must be performed, consisting of surgery or angio-embolization [1–3].

With the strict use of the AAST grading system and the increasing place of conservative management, the overall rate of nephrectomy in kidney trauma has shown a progressive decrease over decades, being 13% in 1995 [4] and decreasing to 7% in 1997–1998, as shown by a population-based study that also revealed that roughly 11% or renal trauma victims required surgical management [5]. In this study, nephrectomy was performed in 61% of operated patients.

Nowadays, the rate of nephrectomy is lower as suggested by the US National Trauma Data Bank research data for the period 2010–2014 showing a failure rate of 2.7% for the nonoperative management in the first 24 h [6]. The same trend was observed in the pediatric population where the rate of nephrectomy decreased from decade to decade to reach 1.4% in some institutions [7]. By 2016, the decrease was noteworthy with a rate reaching 7.5% for high-grade injury (III–V) [8]. However, when specifying the study to penetrating renal injuries only, studies suggest that the rate of nephrectomy is 22–27% and is mostly the consequence of gunshot wounds rather than renal stab wounds [9, 10].

Predictors of failure of nonoperative management are injury severity score (ISS) ≥25, highest renal injury grade, the need for transfusion within 24 h, penetrating

S. A. AL-Mamari, *Urogenital Trauma: A Practical Guide*,
https://doi.org/10.1007/978-981-99-6171-9_8

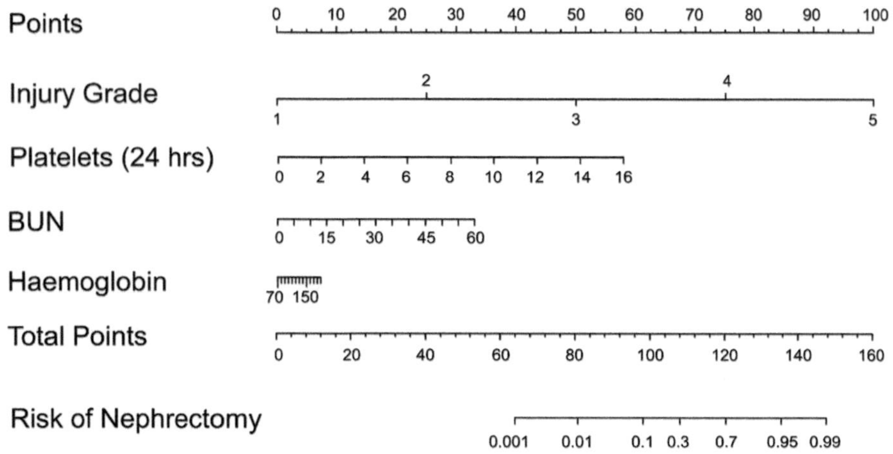

Fig. 8.1 Proposed nomogram to predict the need for nephrectomy in renal trauma. (From Shoobridge JJ et al. [13], with permission from Wolters Kluwer Health)

injury (Gunshot > Stabbing) with laceration, complete disruption, and vascular injury, highest abdominal injury grade for nonrenal organs (low RTS = Revised Trauma Score), low Glasgow Coma Scale (GCS score), and the presence of shock on presentation [5, 6, 11]. In contrast, age, gender, and institutional characteristics were not independent factors associated with nephrectomy [5, 12].

Shoobridge et al. proposed a nomogram to predict the odds of nephrectomy after high-grade renal injury in 2013, based on the injury grade, the number of platelet units transfused, the blood urea nitrogen (BUN) value, and the hemoglobin value on presentation [13] (Fig. 8.1).

More recently, the American Association for the Surgery of Trauma Multi-institutional Genito-Urinary Trauma Study (MiGUTS) proposed a nomogram to predict the need for bleeding interventions, namely, angio-embolization and nephrectomy, after high-grade renal trauma [14] (Fig. 8.2).

This nomogram successfully passed an external validation study through a CT-scan study of 569 cases, after high-grade renal trauma: this showed that **the presence of vascular contrast extravasation was associated with a threefold increase in the need for bleeding interventions and that every centimeter increase in the hematoma rim distance carries a 66% increase in odds of interventions aiming at controlling the bleeding** [15]. It is equally important to notice that the odds of nephrectomy decrease with the time elapsed since admission as shown by a multicentric review: 69% of nephrectomies were performed within 4 h and 89% were performed within 24 h [9]. In the pediatric population also, higher AAST grade and ISS were correlated with the odds of surgical intervention and nephrectomy [16]. In general, cases of RTA with GUT are not directly referred to or admitted under a urology department due to concerns about associated injuries, being managed first in emergency and trauma units [17]. However, this apparent delay does not negatively impact the urology management itself, as the trauma level

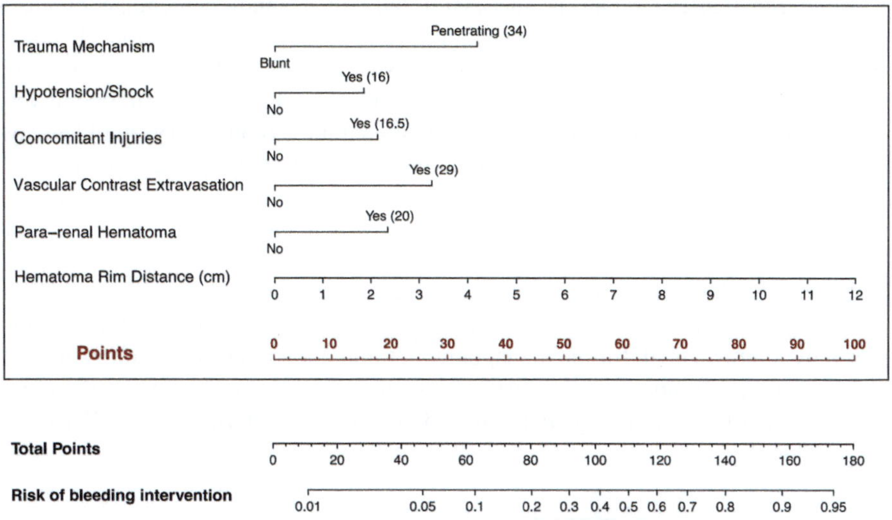

Fig. 8.2 Nomogram for the regression model predicting bleeding interventions after HGRT. (From Keihani S et al. [14], with permission from Wolters Kluwer Health)

designation (level I and nonlevel I) was not shown to be a predictive factor in the likelihood of more aggressive approaches [16].

Whatever the importance of all the factors discussed above, the strict indication for surgical exploration remains the non-responding hemodynamical instability. Other indications are severe renal vascular injuries (grade V vascular or penetrating injury) with ongoing bleeding showing no self-limiting tendency with expanding or pulsatile peri-renal hematoma. However, a shattered kidney per se is not an indication for urgent surgical intervention as long as the patient is stable, nor is a devascularized but non-bleeding kidney. Avulsion of the pyeloureteral junction or pelvis rupture not amenable to antegrade or retrograde stenting should not prompt an urgent repair [1, 3]. These patients are better managed conservatively with percutaneous drainage of the urinoma, and surgery might be considered later on if no tendency for self-repair. When the decision to operate is taken, the preferred approach is transperitoneal, and the early control of hilar vessels for nephrectomy, in general, has been advocated for more than half a century [18]. In the context of trauma, this maxim is even vital, and the surgeon must aim at controlling the renal artery and vein before manipulating the hematoma or starting any parenchymal repair (renorrhaphy) [19]. The strict observance of vessel control has shown a reduction in the rate of nephrectomy from 56% to 18% when two metachronous series were compared in a single institution [20].

As a rule of thumb, if a stable hematoma is found during exploration, it should not be disturbed and the surgery should be terminated without further manipulation, as opposed to a central or expanding hematoma, which is correlated to major vessels injuries (e.g., renal vessels, aorta, and vena cava), calling for surgical exploration [21].

Main renal artery repair is successful only in a small percentage of cases (10–26%) depending on the ischemia duration and the degree of the lesion. However, repair of isolated renal veins carries a larger success rate (51%) [22–24]. To date, most cases of arterial or severe parenchymal injuries discovered intraoperatively end in nephrectomy. However, efforts to repair an injured renal artery should always be made and the expertise of a vascular surgeon be requested in patients with a solitary kidney or bilateral renal injuries, or a minimal arterial tear, as the success depends on the incomplete nature of the injury which leaves some hope for a non-ischemic kidney [3, 21].

In view of the lack of high-grade evidence and strong guidelines, especially in intermingled scenarios, it is useful to follow some algorithms such as the one proposed by Santucci et al. for the management of unilateral renal artery injury, as well as blunt and penetrating renal injuries in general, based on a consensus of experts from the World Health Organization and the Societé Internationale d'Urologie (Fig. 8.3a–c).

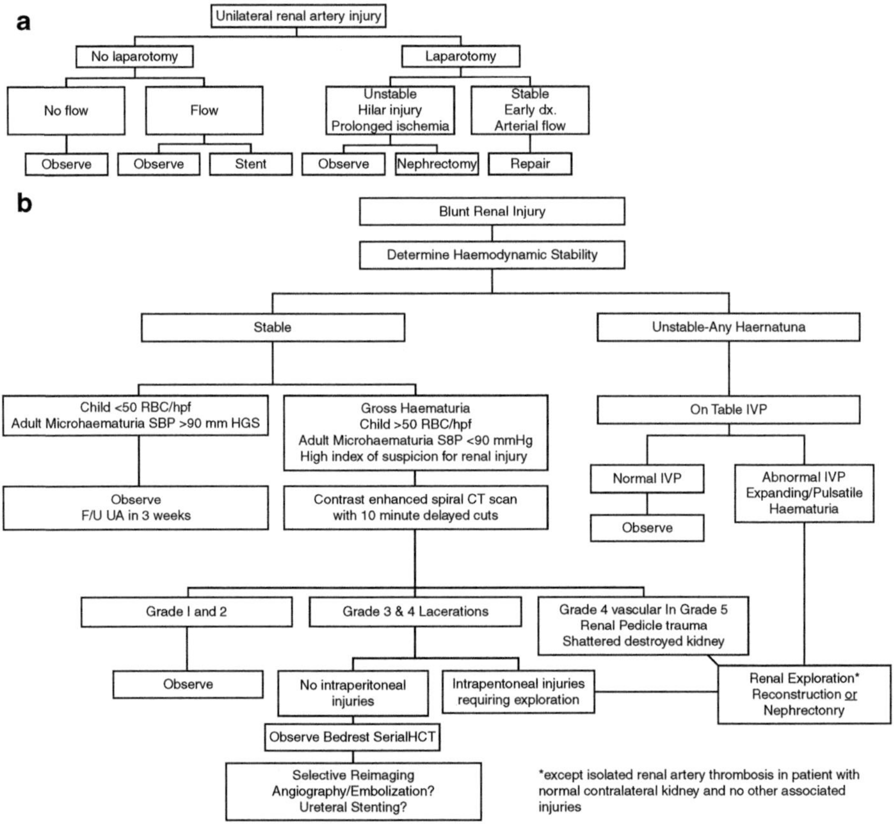

Fig. 8.3 Algorithms for managing: (**a**) renal arterial injury; (**b**) blunt renal injury; and (**c**) penetrating renal injury. (From Santucci et al. [21], with permission from John Wiley and Sons)

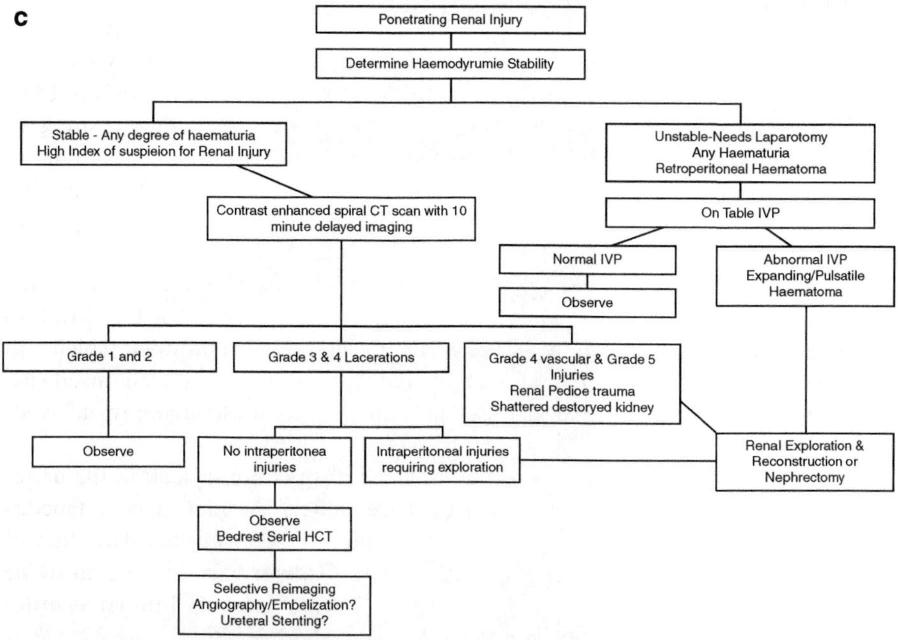

Fig. 8.3 (continued)

8.1 Surgical Technique

As mentioned above, intraperitoneal access is the preferred approach. Once the Gerota's fascia is opened and the kidney is exposed, the parenchymal tear must be identified. When the kidney is deemed salvageable and there is **diffuse bleeding**, a renal packing might be all that is needed, and if there is **focal bleeding** from a parenchymal tear, **renorrhaphy** can be undertaken after control of the main vessels and debridement of necrotic tissues. While proceeding to identify the main vessels, manual compression of the kidney should be started to temporarily control the bleeding. The technique of **renorrhaphy** is more or less the same as for partial nephrectomy. Any eventual breach in the collecting system must be closed with 4/0 absorbable suture material. To ensure watertightness of the PCS closure, the eventual leak may be identified by clamping the proximal ureter with a bulldog and injecting 2–3 mL of methylene blue into the renal pelvis using a 22-gauge or smaller butterfly [19, 25] (Fig. 8.4).

The renal parenchyma and capsule should be closed using tension-free 4-0 polypropylene sutures through protective pledgets (Surgicel, etc.) (Fig. 8.5). If the defect is very large, it should be filled by autologous or exogenous materials such as an omental pedicle flap, fibrin sealant, or thrombin-soaked Gelfoam bolsters, and the capsule should be closed above the interposed material using the same technique described above [25] (Fig. 8.6).

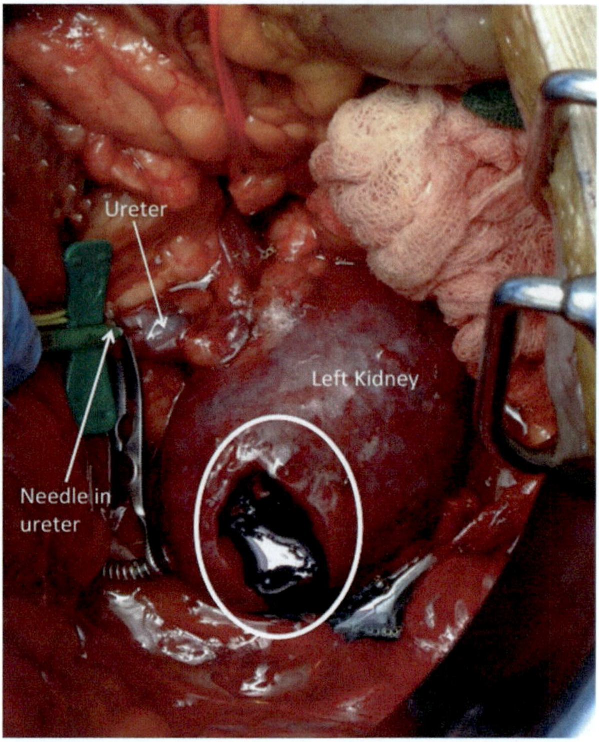

Fig. 8.4 Intraoperative evaluation of the integrity of the collecting system. Insertion of a 22-gauge needle into the proximal ureter, with bulldog clamp applied distally, and injection of 2–3 mL of methylene blue into the renal pelvis. Extravasation of the methylene blue (circle) confirms injury to the collective system. (From Doumanian et al. [25], with permission from Cambridge University Press)

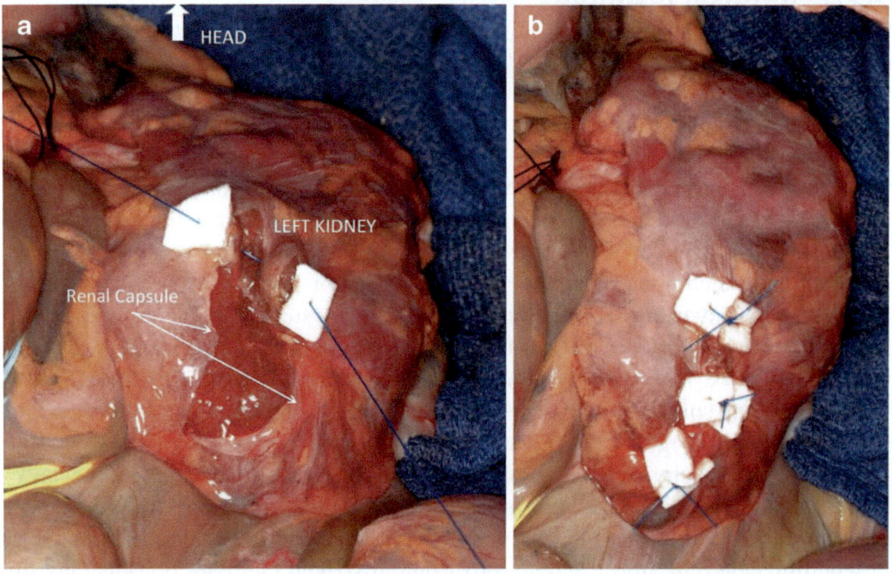

Fig. 8.5 (**a**) Suturing of pledgets on intact renal capsule edges, for primary repair of injury. (**b**) Definitive, tension-free repair of left kidney injury using pledgets. (From Doumanian et al. [25], with permission from Cambridge University Press)

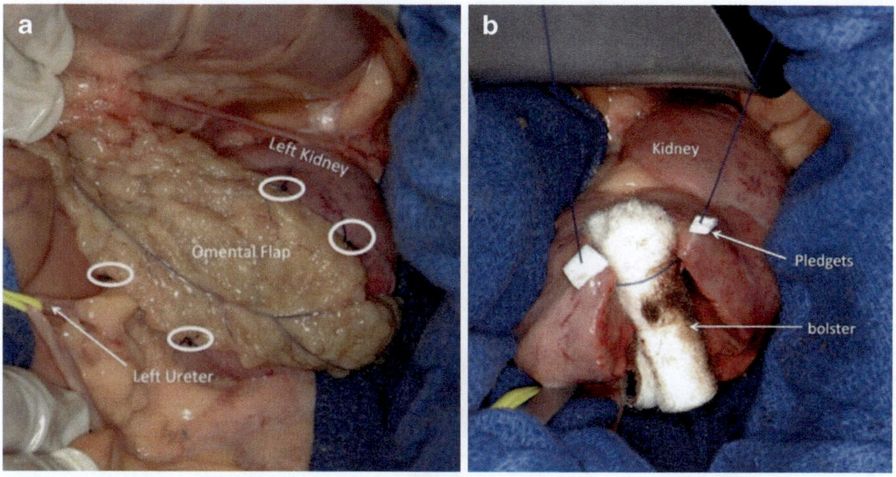

Fig. 8.6 (**a**) Omental pedicle flap may be used to fill in large parenchymal defects, not amenable to primary repair. The flap is anchored to the capsule with sutures (circles). (**b**) Hemostatic bolster used to repair a large defect that cannot be closed primarily without tension, with closure of the capsule over the bolster. (From Doumanian et al. [25], with permission from Cambridge University Press)

Sometimes, a partial nephrectomy is required when there is a significant loss of viability either at the upper or the lower pole. Here maximal exposure of the kidney is required, as complete removal of nonviable tissue, bleeding control with sutures, and again watertightness of the PCS and hemostasis have to be ensured [19, 25] (Fig. 8.7). In all cases, peri-renal drainage has to be maintained for at least 48 h.

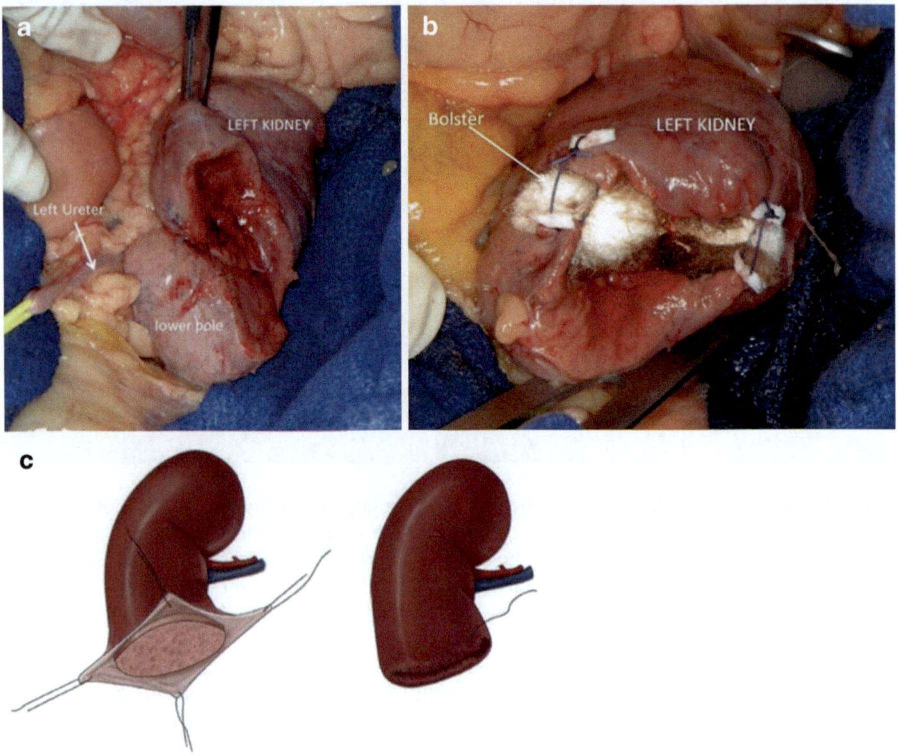

Fig. 8.7 (**a**) Extensive damage to the lower pole of the kidney is best managed with partial nephrectomy. (**b**) Partial lower pole nephrectomy with the raw surface covered with absorbable materials such as Gelfoam, which can be sutured to the remaining renal capsule. (**c**) Partial lower pole nephrectomy with preservation of the capsule. The capsule can be closed over the raw surface of the kidney. (From Doumanian et al. [25], with permission from Cambridge University Press)

References

1. EAU Guidelines. Edn. presented at the EAU annual congress Amsterdam, Mar 2022. ISBN: 978-94-92671-16-5. https://d56bochluxqnz.cloudfront.net/documents/full-guideline/EAU-Guidelines-on-Urological-Trauma-2022_2022-03-24-104100_fwda.pdf.
2. Morey AF, Brandes S, Dugi DD 3rd, Armstrong JH, Breyer BN, Broghammer JA, Erickson BA, Holzbeierlein J, Hudak SJ, Pruitt JH, Reston JT, Santucci RA, Smith TG 3rd, Wessells H, American Urological Assocation. Urotrauma: AUA guideline. J Urol. 2014;192(2):327–35. https://doi.org/10.1016/j.juro.2014.05.004. Epub 2014 May 20
3. Coccolini F, Moore EE, Kluger Y, et al. Kidney and uro-trauma: WSES-AAST guidelines. World J Emerg Surg. 2019;14:54. https://doi.org/10.1186/s13017-019-0274-x.
4. Nash PA, Bruce JE, McAninch JW. Nephrectomy for traumatic renal injuries. J Urol. 1995;153(3 Pt 1):609–11. https://doi.org/10.1097/00005392-199503000-00012.
5. Wessells H, Suh D, Porter JR, Rivara F, MacKenzie EJ, Jurkovich GJ, Nathens AB. Renal injury and operative management in the United States: results of a population-based study. J Trauma. 2003;54(3):423–30. https://doi.org/10.1097/01.TA.0000051932.28456.F4.

6. Bjurlin MA, Fantus RJ, Fantus RJ, Villines D. Comparison of nonoperative and surgical management of renal trauma: can we predict when nonoperative management fails? J Trauma Acute Care Surg. 2017;82(2):356–61. https://doi.org/10.1097/TA.0000000000001316.
7. Dangle PP, Fuller TW, Gaines B, Cannon GM, Schneck FX, Stephany HA, Ost MC. Evolving mechanisms of injury and management of pediatric blunt renal trauma—20 years of experience. Urology. 2016;90:159–63. https://doi.org/10.1016/j.urology.2016.01.017. Epub 2016 Jan 26.
8. Anderson RE, Keihani S, Das R, Hanson HA, McCrum ML, Hotaling JM, Myers JB. Nephrectomy is associated with increased mortality after renal trauma: an analysis of the National Trauma Data Bank from 2007-2016. J Urol. 2021;205(3):841–7. https://doi.org/10.1097/JU.0000000000001366. Epub 2020 Oct 6.
9. Keihani S, Xu Y, Presson AP, Hotaling JM, Nirula R, Piotrowski J, Dodgion CM, Black CM, Mukherjee K, Morris BJ, Majercik S, Smith BP, Schwartz I, Elliott SP, DeSoucy ES, Zakaluzny S, Thomsen PB, Erickson BA, Baradaran N, Breyer BN, Miller B, Santucci RA, Carrick MM, Hewitt T, Burks FN, Kocik JF, Askari R, Myers JB, Genito-Urinary Trauma Study Group. Contemporary management of high-grade renal trauma: results from the American Association for the Surgery of Trauma Genitourinary Trauma study. J Trauma Acute Care Surg. 2018;84(3):418–25. https://doi.org/10.1097/TA.0000000000001796. Erratum in: J Trauma Acute Care Surg. 2018 May;84(5):826.
10. Bjurlin MA, Jeng EI, Goble SM, et al. Comparison of nonoperative management with renorrhaphy and nephrectomy in penetrating renal injuries. J Trauma. 2011;71:554–8.
11. Davis KA, Reed RL, Santaniello J, Abodeely A, Esposito TJ, Poulakidas SJ, Luchette FA. Predictors of the need for nephrectomy after renal trauma. J Trauma. 2006;60(1):164170. https://doi.org/10.1097/01.ta.0000199924.3973.
12. McClung CD, Hotaling JM, Wang J, Wessells H, Voelzke BB. Contemporary trends in the immediate surgical management of renal trauma using a national database. J Trauma Acute Care Surg. 2013;75(4):602–6. https://doi.org/10.1097/TA.0b013e3182a53ac2.
13. Shoobridge JJ, Bultitude MF, Koukounaras J, Royce PL, Corcoran NM. Predicting surgical exploration in renal trauma: assessment and modification of an established nomogram. J Trauma Acute Care Surg. 2013;75(5):819–23. https://doi.org/10.1097/TA.0b013e3182a8fff5.
14. Keihani S, Rogers DM, Putbrese BE, Moses RA, Zhang C, Presson AP, Hotaling JM, Nirula R, Luo-Owen X, Mukherjee K, et al. A nomogram predicting the need for bleeding interventions after high-grade renal trauma: results from the American Association for the Surgery of Trauma Multi-institutional Genito-Urinary Trauma Study (MiGUTS). J Trauma Acute Care Surg. 2019;86(5):774–82.
15. Keihani S, Wang SS, Joyce RP, Rogers DM, Gross JA, Nocera AP, Selph JP, Fang E, Hagedorn JC, Voelzke BB, Rezaee ME, Moses RA, Arya CS, Sensenig RL, Glavin K, Broghammer JA, Higgins MM, Gupta S, Castillejo Becerra CM, Baradaran N, Zhang C, Presson AP, Nirula R, Myers JB, in Conjunction with the Trauma and Urologic Reconstruction Network of Surgeons. External validation of a nomogram predicting risk of bleeding control interventions after high-grade renal trauma: the Multi-institutional Genito-Urinary Trauma Study. J Trauma Acute Care Surg. 2021;90(2):249–56. https://doi.org/10.1097/TA.0000000000002987.
16. Mahran A, Fernstrum A, Swindle M, Mishra K, Bukavina L, Raina R, Narayanamurthy V, Ross J, Woo L. Impact of trauma center designation in pediatric renal trauma: National Trauma Data Bank analysis. J Pediatr Urol. 2020;16(5):658.e1–9. https://doi.org/10.1016/j.jpurol.2020.07.019.
17. Paparel P, N'Diaye A, Laumon B, Caillot J-L, Perrin P, Ruffion A. The epidemiology of trauma of the genitourinary system after traffic accidents: analysis of a register of over 43 000 victims. BJU Int. 2006;97(2):338–41. https://doi.org/10.1111/j.1464-410x.2006.05900.x.
18. Scott RF, Selzman HM. Coimplications of nephrectomy: review of 450 patients and a description of a modification of the transperitoneal approach. J Urol. 1966;95(3):307–12. https://doi.org/10.1016/s0022-5347(17)63452-9.
19. Erlich T, Kitrey ND. Renal trauma: the current best practice. Ther Adv Urol. 2018;10(10):295–303. Published 2018 Jul 10. https://doi.org/10.1177/1756287218785828.

20. McAninch JW, Carroll PR. Renal trauma: kidney preservation through improved vascular control-a refined approach. J Trauma. 1982;22(4):285–90.
21. Santucci RA, Wessells H, Bartsch G, Descotes J, Heyns CF, McAninch JW, Nash P, Schmidlin F. Evaluation and management of renal injuries: consensus statement of the renal trauma subcommittee. BJU Int. 2004;93(7):937–54. https://doi.org/10.1111/j.1464-4096.2004.04820.x.
22. Haas CA, Spirnak JP. Traumatic renal artery occlusion: a review of the literature. Tech Urol. 1998;4(1):1–11.
23. Turner WW, Snyder WH, Fry WJ. Mortality and renal salvage after renovascular trauma: a review of 94 patients treated in a 20 year period. Am J Surg. 1983;146(6):848–51. ISSN: 0002-9610. https://doi.org/10.1016/0002-9610(83)90357-4.
24. McAninch JW, Carroll PR, Klosterman PW, Dixon CM, Greenblatt MN. Renal reconstruction after injury. J Urol. 1991;145(5):932–7. ISSN: 0022-5347. https://doi.org/10.1016/S0022-5347(17)38494-X.
25. Doumanian L, Best C, Keeley J, Varga S. Urological trauma. In: Demetriades D, Velhamos G, editors. Atlas of surgical techniques in trauma. Cambridge University Press; 2019. p. 253–67. https://doi.org/10.1017/9781108698665.032.

Prognosis, Complications, and Follow-Up of Kidney Trauma

9

Analysis of over 40,000 high-grade renal injury victims from the NTDB showed that mortality was associated with the following factors: nephrectomy, lower Glasgow Coma Scale (GCS) score, higher Injury Severity Score (ISS), lower Revised Trauma Score, [1] hypotension, blood transfusion, penetrating mechanism of the trauma, age, and non-White race [1].

A meta-analysis confirmed the better outcome of nonoperative management compared with interventional approaches with mortality rates of 5.5% and 13.4%, respectively [3]. However, a study including nearly 5000 cases of renal trauma failed to find an increased likelihood of mortality with angioembolization and open renal surgery but confirmed the association with black race, age >45 years, penetrating trauma, and ISS >15 with mortality [4]. Anyway, the contradiction between these studies is only apparent because the latter study included all renal trauma injuries and not only the high grades. And rather than creating confusion in our mind, this should teach us that surgical exploration and nephrectomy must be avoided as much as possible and be performed only under strict indications as already discussed.

Not surprisingly, mortality after penetrating injury is higher than after blunt trauma and ranges from 6% to 7.5%, being highest after gunshot injury [5, 6]. It should be borne in mind that sole renal injuries account for a low rate of mortality and associated injuries play a large part in this grim outcome. Therefore, efforts made by researchers to differentiate between the specific cause of mortality helped

[1] The Revised Trauma Score (RTS) was introduced in 1989 by Champion et al. [2]. It aimed at including the Glasgow Coma Scale (GCS) score, the systolic blood pressure (SBP), and the respiratory rate (RR), while excluding capillary refill and respiratory expansion, as the last two are difficult to assess in the accident field. It is calculated by adding the scores of GCS (0–4 points), SBP (0–4 points), and RR (0–4 points) after multiplying them by a weighted coefficient: Thus, RTS = 0.9368 (GCS score) + 0.7326 (SBP score) + 0.2908 (RR score). In a post-trauma triage, RTS score of 12 is labeled delayed, 11 is urgent, and 3–10 is immediate. Below 3, the patient is declared dead or dying. The scores of GCS, SBP, and RR are given in Table 9.1.

S. A. AL-Mamari, *Urogenital Trauma: A Practical Guide*,
https://doi.org/10.1007/978-981-99-6171-9_9

elicit an overall mortality of 6.5% and a specific renal injury mortality of as low as 0.6% [3].

After throwing so many stones at the operative management, it is important to also mention that nonoperative management is not devoid of complications, and pneumonia (7.3%), urinary tract infection (UTI) (3.0%), deep vein thrombosis (DVT) (2.75%), acute respiratory distress syndrome (ARDS) (1.6%), unplanned intubation (1.4%), bleeding (0.4%), and urinoma (<0.1%) have been described [7, 8] (Fig. 9.1).

Al-Qudah and Santucci reported widely varying post-renal trauma complication rates of 3–33%, where urinary extravasation was the most frequently encountered with an occurrence of 10–30% in penetrating injury and 2–18% in blunt trauma [9].

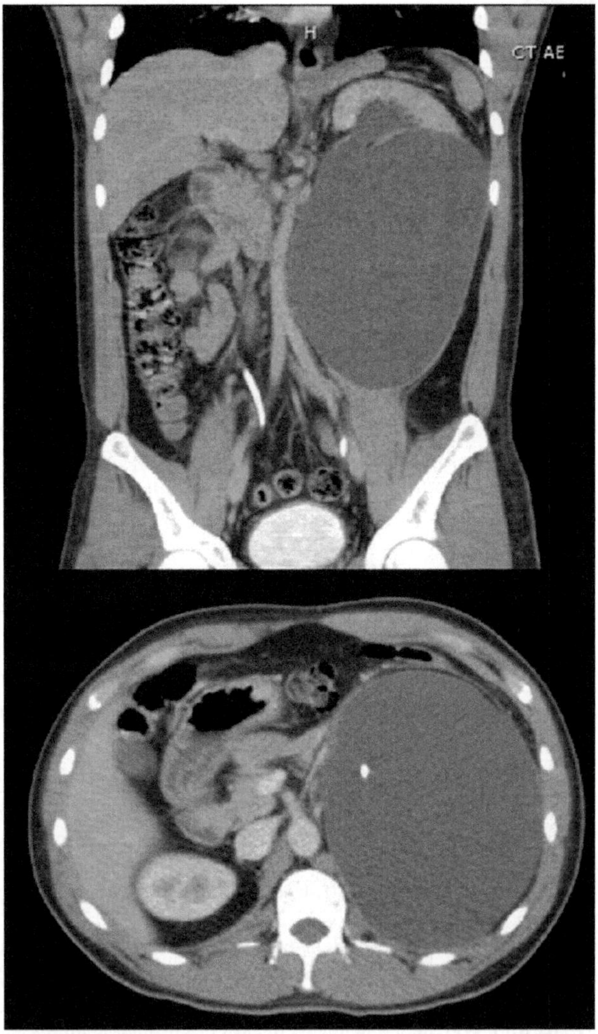

Fig. 9.1 Urinoma seen on repeat CT abdomen and pelvis with contrast after placement of ureteral stent. (From Shah PK, et al. [8]. Creative Commons Attribution License)

Other complications are urinoma (1–7% overall, 7–30% after penetrating injury), perinephric abscess (<1% overall, 5% after penetrating injury), unnecessary nephrectomy,, hypertension (5%), page kidney, UTI or pyelonephritis (2.3%), chronic flank pain (2%), impaired kidney function and renal insufficiency (1.3%), persistent or secondary bleeding (1.2%), vascular thrombosis (0.5%), pseudoaneurysm (0.3%), post-injury hydronephrosis (0–3%), reno-cutaneous fistula (mostly after partial nephrectomy, renorrhaphy, open drainage of collection), infarct and parenchymal loss (0.2%), arteriovenous fistula (0.1%) (Figs. 9.2 and 9.3), pulmonary complications (e.g., pneumonia, bronchitis, atelectasis, and iatrogenic pneumothorax), chylous ascites, and so on [10, 11].

It is recommended to observe a regular follow-up of post-renal trauma patients for early detection and management of these complications. The follow-up includes physical examination, urinalysis, diagnostic imaging (CT scan, ultrasonography, or radionuclides), regular measurement of blood pressure measurement, and serum creatinine. Ultrasonography is the preferred imaging modality for the pediatric population. However, by consensus, imaging follow-up for minor (AAST I–II) injuries might not be necessary according to experts' panels [12, 13].

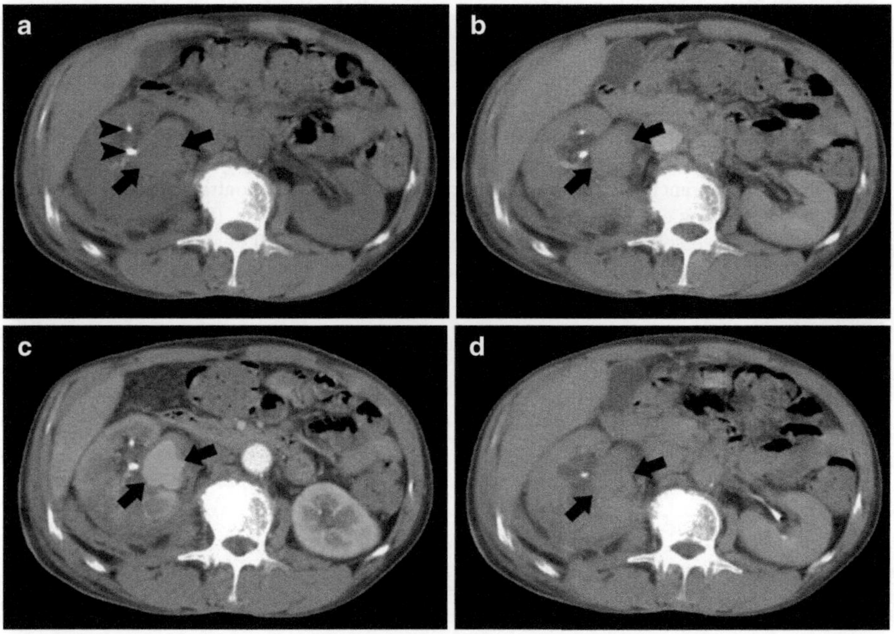

Fig. 9.2 Computed tomography images of unenhanced phase (**a**) and contrast-enhanced phases with the arterial (**b**), venous (**c**), and delayed (**d**). Arteriovenous fistula mimicking tumor in the right pelvis renal. Manifesting as a mass, enhancement in the arterial phase, and washout in the venous and delayed phase. They seemed to match the blood pool in every single phase of contrast enhancement (arrows). Note that there were several stones in the lower renal calyx (arrowheads). (From Hoang VT et al. [10], with permission from SAGE Publishing)

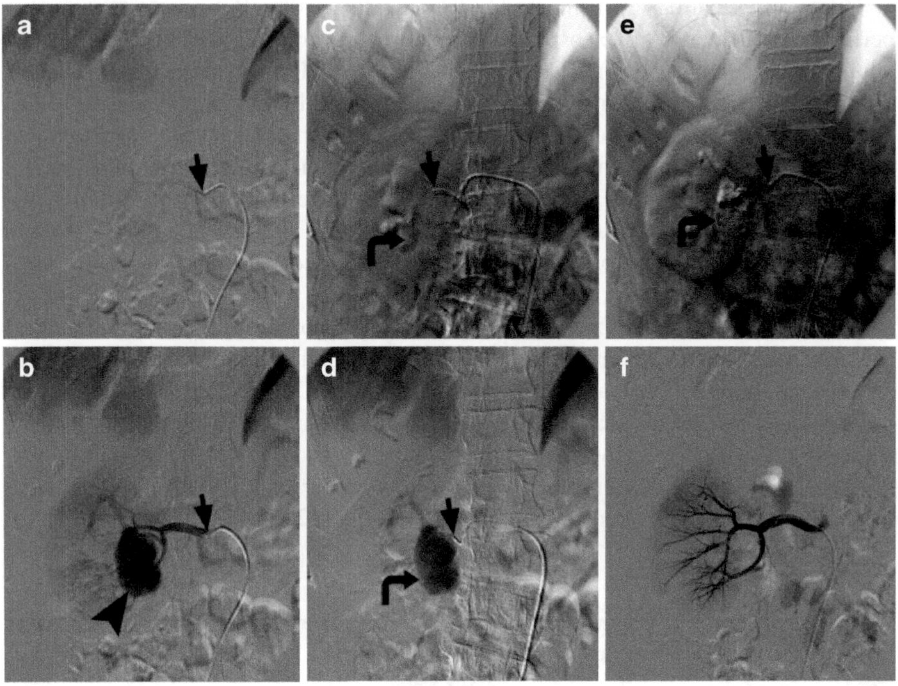

Fig. 9.3 Interventional therapy for right renal arteriovenous fistula (AVF) with digital subtraction angiography. (**a**) The catheter tip image in the right main renal artery (arrow). (**b**) After the injection of contrast, the AVF bulge was detected (arrowhead). (**c**) Push the tip of the catheter into the middle renal artery branch adjacent to AVF (arrow). (**d**) Inject more contrast material to identify the lesion. (**e**) Injecting embolization material to cause AVF obstruction. (**f**) The lesion was gone, and the renal blood vessels were circulated normally. (From Hoang VT et al. [10], with permission from SAGE Publishing)

Table 9.1 Revised Trauma Score variable breakpoints (from Champion HR et al. [2], with permission from Wolters Kluwer Health)

Glasgow Coma Scale	Systolic blood pressure (mmHg)	Respiratory rate	Coded value
13–15	>89	10–29	4
9–12	76–89	>29	3
6–8	50–75	6–9	2
4–5	1–49	1–5	1
3	0	0	0

There is no clearly defined timing for the return to normal activity after a renal trauma. However, as a rule, bed rest and reduced activity are to be observed as long as gross hematuria is present, and sports activities are suspended until microscopic hematuria is resolved. It is hypothesized that sports activities might be resumed 2–6 weeks after a minor or moderate renal injury or 6–12 months after a severe one [13].

References

1. Anderson RE, Keihani S, Das R, Hanson HA, McCrum ML, Hotaling JM, Myers JB. Nephrectomy is associated with increased mortality after renal trauma: an analysis of the National Trauma Data Bank from 2007-2016. J Urol. 2021;205(3):841–7. https://doi.org/10.1097/JU.0000000000001366. Epub 2020 Oct 6.
2. Champion HR, Sacco WJ, Copes WS, Gann DS, Gennarelli TA, Flanagan ME. A revision of the trauma score. J Trauma. 1989;29(5):623–9. https://doi.org/10.1097/00005373-198905000-00017.
3. Petrone P, Perez-Calvo J, Brathwaite CEM, Islam S, Joseph DK. Traumatic kidney injuries: a systematic review and meta-analysis. Int J Surg. 2020;74:13–21. https://doi.org/10.1016/j.ijsu.2019.12.013. Epub 2019 Dec 21.
4. Ho P, Hellenthal NJ. Independent predictors of mortality for patients with traumatic renal injury. World J Urol. 2021;39(9):3685–90. https://doi.org/10.1007/s00345-020-03552-x. Epub 2021 Jan 5.
5. McAninch JW, Carroll PR, Armenakas NA. Renal gunshot wounds: methods of salvage and reconstruction. J Trauma. 1993;35:279–83; discussion: 283–4.
6. Carroll PR, McAninch JW. Operative indications in penetrating renal trauma. J Trauma. 1985;25:587–93.
7. Bjurlin MA, Fantus RJ, Fantus RJ, Villines D. Comparison of nonoperative and surgical management of renal trauma: can we predict when nonoperative management fails? J Trauma Acute Care Surg. 2017;82(2):356–61. https://doi.org/10.1097/TA.0000000000001316.
8. Shah PK, Frieben RW, Desouza RA. Delayed nephron sparing surgery for grade IV renal injury. Case Rep Urol. 2013;2013:482320. https://doi.org/10.1155/2013/482320. Epub 2013 May 15.
9. Al-Qudah HS, Santucci RA. Complications of renal trauma. Urol Clin North Am. 2006;33(1):41–53, vi. https://doi.org/10.1016/j.ucl.2005.10.005.
10. Hoang VT, Pham NTT, Nguyen HQ, Van HAT, Vo MTT, Nguyen TTT, Chansomphou V, Trinh CT. A case of arteriovenous fistula after kidney trauma mimicking tumor. J Investig Med High Impact Case Rep. 2020;8:2324709620967877. https://doi.org/10.1177/2324709620967877.
11. Starnes M, Demetriades D, Hadjizacharia P, Inaba K, Best C, Chan L. Complications following renal trauma. Arch Surg. 2010;145(4):377–81. https://doi.org/10.1001/archsurg.2010.30.
12. EAU Guidelines. Edn. presented at the EAU annual congress Amsterdam, Mar 2022. ISBN: 978-94-92671-16-5. https://d56bochluxqnz.cloudfront.net/documents/full-guideline/EAU-Guidelines-on-Urological-Trauma-2022_2022-03-24-104100_fwda.pdf.
13. Coccolini F, Moore EE, Kluger Y, et al. Kidney and uro-trauma: WSES-AAST guidelines. World J Emerg Surg. 2019;14:54. https://doi.org/10.1186/s13017-019-0274-x.

Special Cases in Renal Trauma 10

The occurrence of trauma in ectopic kidneys, horseshoe kidneys (HSK), renal angiomyolipomas (AMLs), and kidney allografts is very rare, although they are more prone to damage than normal kidneys when hit. A simple explanation is the extreme rarity of these abnormal kidneys compared with normal kidneys.

10.1 Trauma in Simple Ectopic, Crossed Ectopic, and Crossed-Fused Ectopic Kidneys

Only a dozen of cases of ectopic kidneys injuries have been reported in the literature, including pelvic, thoracic, and crossed-fused ectopic kidneys. Studies have shown that these kidneys are likely to be injured by low-velocity impacts due to their poor anatomical protection; thus, they have a lower rate of associated trauma with other abdominal organs and a lower ISS [1]. The scantiness of cases does not plead for any reliable guideline to be formulated, and the traumatized ectopic kidney should be treated in the same way as the orthotopic one, i.e., conservatively even for high grades (IV–V), as long as the patients are hemodynamically stable [2–4]. And when there is a post-traumatic pseudoaneurysm of the ectopic kidney artery, this can be excluded through endovascular approach in the same way as for normal kidneys [5] (Fig. 10.1a–e).

There are also reports about trauma on crossed ectopic kidneys, either fused or not who were successfully managed conservatively or with minimally invasive procedures [6–8].

S. A. AL-Mamari, *Urogenital Trauma: A Practical Guide*, https://doi.org/10.1007/978-981-99-6171-9_10

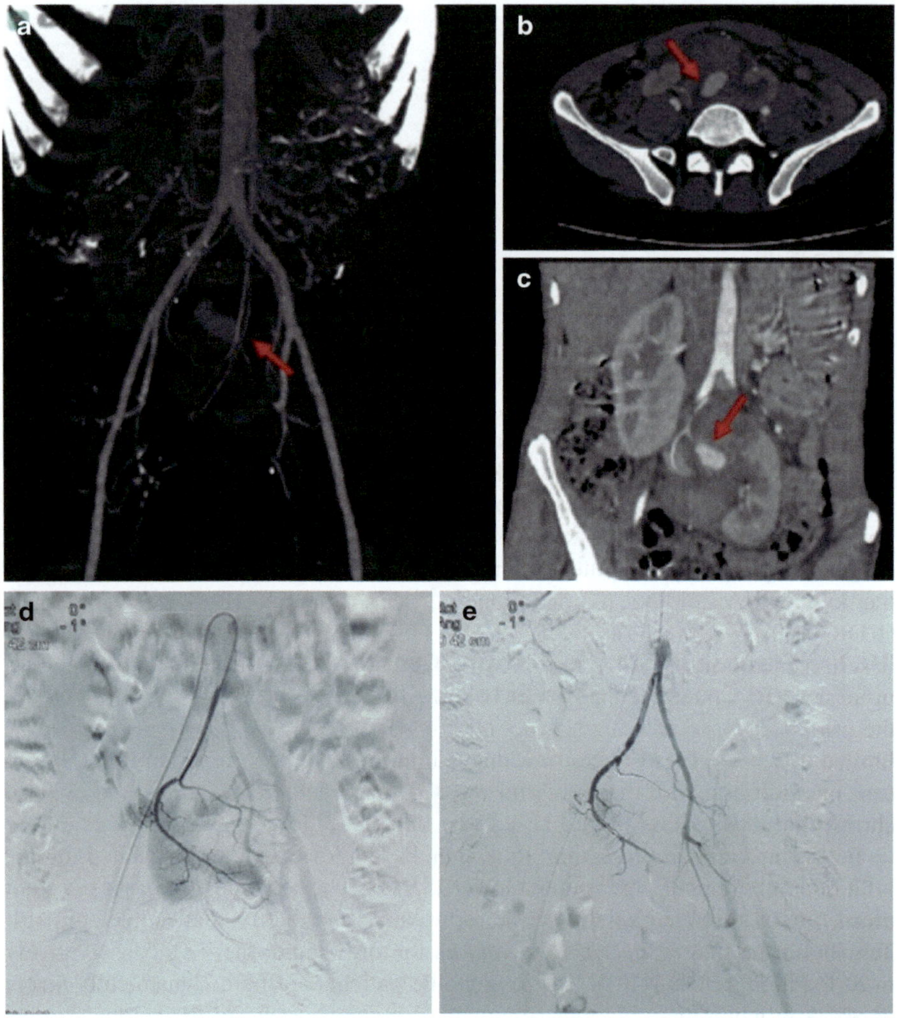

Fig. 10.1 (**a**–**c**) CT scan showing left pelvic kidney and distal pseudoaneurysm of one of the renal artery branches. (**d**) Selective arteriography of the left renal artery showing a pseudoaneurysm. (**e**) Angiography control: pseudoaneurysm exclusion and permeability of other branches of the renal artery. (Reproduced from Ibrahimi A et al. [5], with permission from Elsevier Masson SAS)

10.2 Trauma on Horseshoe Kidneys (HSK)

There are roughly a dozen cases of trauma on HSK reported in the literature, the oldest having been written as far back as 1964 [9].

HSK is vulnerable even to speeds lower than 15 km/h, and its injury is managed in the same manner as normal kidneys with conservative management being the first choice, followed by endovascular management, and surgery being reserved for exceptional situations with severe bleeding and hemodynamically unstable patients [10–12] (Figs. 10.2a, b and 10.3a, b).

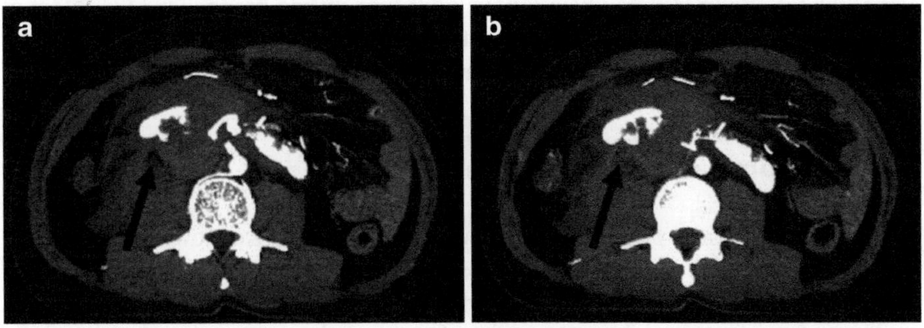

Fig. 10.2 CT angiography in axial view, showing an active contrast extravasation from accessory right renal artery and retroperitoneal hematoma (**a**, **b**) (black arrow). (From Krutsri et al. [11]. Creative Commons Attribution License)

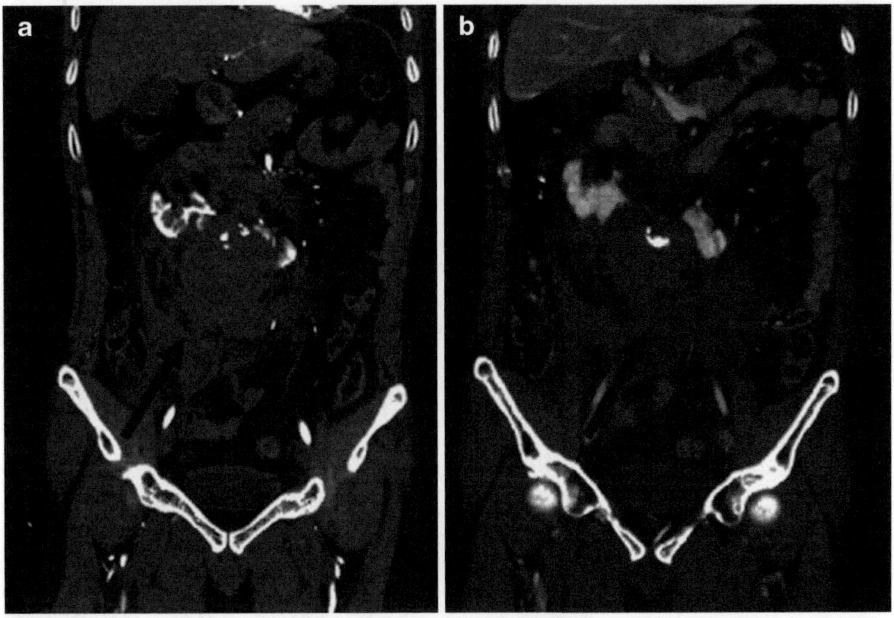

Fig. 10.3 CT angiography in coronal view, showing an active contrast extravasation from accessory right renal artery and retroperitoneal hematoma (**a**, **b**) (black arrow). (From Krutsri et al. [11]. Creative Commons Attribution License)

10.3 Trauma on Renal Angiomyolipoma (AML)

AML is known to have a propensity to rupture, especially if larger than 4 cm. This rupture can occur spontaneously in a so-called Wunderlich syndrome (up to 50% of cases), or following trauma (even low velocity), or during pregnancy [13]. Most of the modern reported cases were successfully managed with angioembolization or, rarely, surgery with nephrectomy for hemodynamically unstable patients [13–15].

10.4 Trauma and Kidney Allograft

The transplanted kidney is exposed to trauma in the iliac fossa. However, here again reported cases can be counted on the fingers of both hands. The rare cases are generally low-grade injuries happening after mild blunt trauma.

The trauma factor might just consist of a seat belt compression during a low-speed vehicle accident [16, 17] or a cat jumping on the patient's abdomen [18]. Most of the cases have been managed conservatively, even for high-grade injuries [19]. Some required superselective embolization considering the necessity of maximum preservation of the renal function in this situation (solitary functioning kidney) [20] (Figs. 10.4 and 10.5a, b).

Because of continuous bleeding with expanding and compressive hematoma, other patients required surgical exploration and renorrhaphy [21].

The same complications occurring in normal kidneys can be encountered in kidney allograft trauma, including urinomas, delayed hemorrhage, infections, pseudoaneurysm, arteriovenous fistula formation, and renal insufficiency.

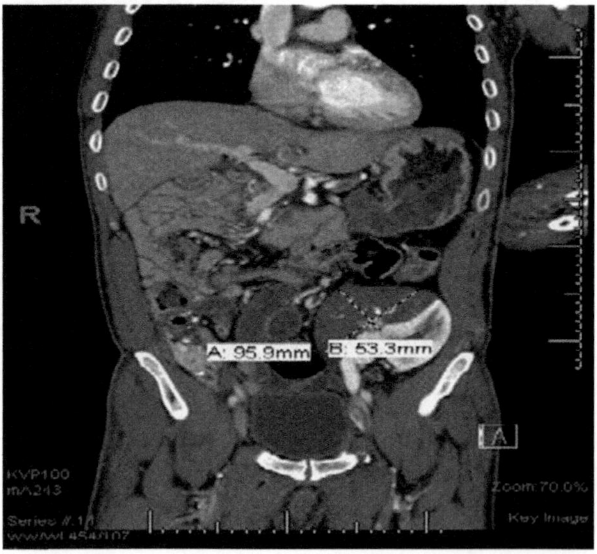

Fig. 10.4 Large peri-graft hematoma with grade III laceration (the patient had combined pancreas and kidney transplantation). (From Rajagopal P [20]. Creative Commons Attribution License)

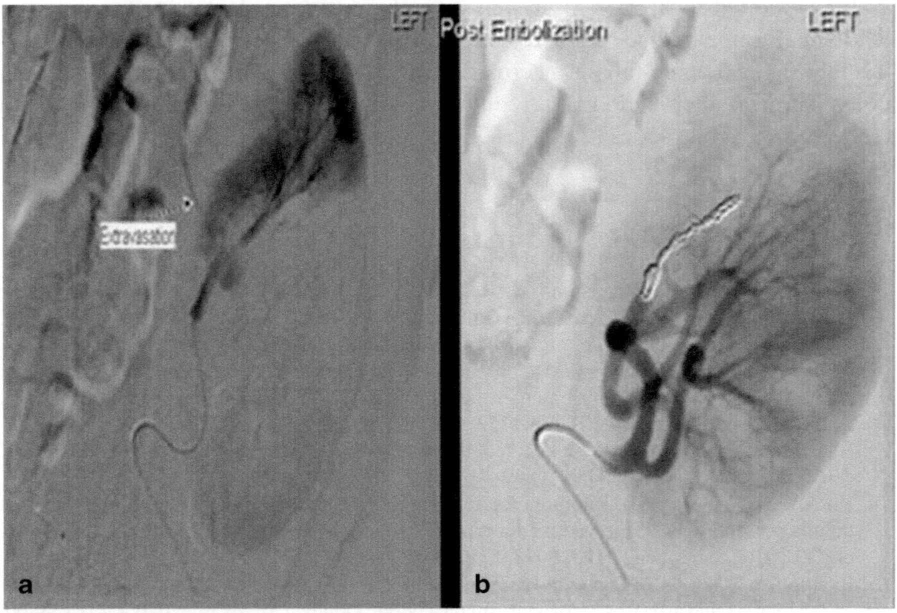

Fig. 10.5 The injured branch of the renal artery. (**a**) Pre-embolization. (**b**) Post-embolization. (From Rajagopal P et al. [20]. Creative Commons Attribution License)

Reports on kidney allograft loss are exceptional. In one of them, the cause of the trauma was the patient's cat jumping on his abdomen 1 week before his presentation to the hospital where he was found to have a large subcapsular hematoma on CT-scan (grade II) and developed acute page kidney few days later [18].

Another factor worth noting is the possible occurrence of an iatrogenic injury of a transplant kidney during cesarean delivery. This warning is justified by the increased number of childbearing women receiving a transplant kidney nowadays. Moreover, a systematic review and meta-analysis showed that the cesarean rate in post-renal transplant women was higher than in the general American population, with values of 56.9% and 31.9%, respectively [22]. This fact was observed to an even greater extent in a Norwegian national cohort study which found that post-kidney transplant pregnant women had a fivefold increased risk of undergoing cesarean section compared with the non-transplanted pregnant women [23].

However, despite the increased number of cesarean sections, iatrogenic injuries to the renal graft or ureter are seldom reported. One of the discussed cases mentioned a laceration of the renal graft during traction, which was treated with pressure and renorrhaphy using a 3-0 pledgeted prolene [24].

Before closing this chapter, it should be remembered that spontaneous renal allograft rupture is by far more frequently encountered than traumatic injury. Fortunately, it is still a rare phenomenon occurring in 0.3–3% of cases of renal transplantations [25].

It is reported to happen at around 2 weeks post-transplantation. Incriminated etiological factors include acute rejection as the main cause, followed by renal vein thrombosis, and acute tubular necrosis. It is a life-threatening condition requiring urgent surgical intervention and frequently ending up in graft nephrectomy, which reached 70% in one series [26].

References

1. Schmidlin FR, Iselin CE, Naimi A, Rohner S, Borst F, Farshad M, Niederer P, Graber P. The higher injury risk of abnormal kidneys in blunt renal trauma. Scand J Urol Nephrol. 1998;32(6):388–92. https://doi.org/10.1080/003655998750015151.
2. Becker AB, Baig MB, Becker AM. Conservative management of a grade V injury to an ectopic pelvic kidney following blunt trauma to the lower abdomen: a case report. J Med Case Rep. 2010;4:224. https://doi.org/10.1186/1752-1947-4-224.
3. Hani MA, Sallami S, Ben Achour J, Zoghlami A, Najah N. Trauma of an ectopic kidney. A case report. Tunis Med. 2004;82(1):69–71.
4. Ho SW, Yeh YT, Yeh CB. Rupture of ectopic pelvic dysplastic kidney after blunt abdominal trauma presenting as left lower quadrant pain. J Emerg Med. 2013;44(2):e173–5. https://doi.org/10.1016/j.jemermed.2012.02.072. Epub 2012 Aug 24.
5. Ibrahimi A, Zahdi O, Dergamoun H, Ziani I, El Sayegh H, Benslimane L, Lekehal B, Nouini Y. Traumatic renal artery pseudoaneurysm on a pelvic kidney. J Med Vasc. 2020;45(3):158–60. https://doi.org/10.1016/j.jdmv.2020.03.003. Epub 2020 Mar 27.
6. Jindal T, Kamal MR, Mukherjee S, Mandal SN, Karmakar D. Management of an iatrogenic injury in a crossed ectopic kidney without fusion. Korean J Urol. 2014;55(8):554–6. https://doi.org/10.4111/kju.2014.55.8.554. Epub 2014 Aug 8.
7. Asanad K, Remulla D, Nassiri N, Nabhani J. Grade IV renal laceration in a 13-year-old boy with cross-fused renal ectopia. Urology. 2020;145:243–6. https://doi.org/10.1016/j.urology.2020.06.011. Epub 2020 Jun 20.
8. Kim SW, Rudick DH, Cohen EL. Crossed fused renal ectopia presenting with blunt trauma. Urology. 1978;12(1):69–70. https://doi.org/10.1016/0090-4295(78)90372-2.
9. Gibson GR. Ruptured horseshoe (fused) kidney: a review and report of a case with traumatic renal hypertension. J Urol. 1964;92:374–6. https://doi.org/10.1016/s0022-5347(17)63971-5.
10. Cortese F, Fransvea P, Marcello R, Saputelli A, Lepre L, Gioffrè A, Sganga G. Challenging case of horseshoe kidney double fracture. Int J Surg Case Rep. 2017;41:158–61. https://doi.org/10.1016/j.ijscr.2017.08.070. Epub 2017 Oct 10.
11. Krutsri C, Singhatas P, Sumpritpradit P, Chaijareenont C, Viseshsindh W, Thampongsa T, Choikrua P. Traumatic blunt force renal injury in a diseased horseshoe kidney with successful embolization to treat active bleeding: a case report and literature review. Case Rep Urol. 2020;2020:8897208. https://doi.org/10.1155/2020/8897208.
12. Boninsegna E, Simonini E, Crosara S, Sozzi C, Colopi S. Horseshoe kidney blunt trauma with double laceration: endovascular management. Vasc Endovasc Surg. 2020;54(7):643–5. https://doi.org/10.1177/1538574420940091. Epub 2020 Jul 8.
13. Lai CC, Fan WC, Chao CM, Liu WL, Hou CC. Traumatic rupture of a renal angiomyolipoma. J Emerg Med. 2012;43(5):e339–40. https://doi.org/10.1016/j.jemermed.2011.05.059. Epub 2011 Aug 25
14. Hsu YP, Chen RJ, Fang JF, Lin BC. Traumatic rupture of renal angiomyolipoma managed with angioembolization followed by elective surgery: a report of two cases. J Trauma. 2005;59(3):737–41.
15. Tsai CK, Lin YT, Lin TC. Traumatic rupture of bilateral huge renal angiomyolipomas in tuberous sclerosis complex. J Trauma. 2010;69(2):477. https://doi.org/10.1097/TA.0b013e318180a428.

16. Coulshed SJ, Caterson RJ, Mahony JF. Traumatic infarct at the lower pole of a renal transplant secondary to seat belt compression. Nephrol Dial Transplant. 1995;10(8):1464–5.
17. McHugh PP, Clifford TM, Johnston TD, Banerjee AS, Gedaly R, Jeon H, Ranjan D. Seatbelt injury resulting in functional loss of a transplanted kidney. Prog Transplant. 2008;18(3):199–202. https://doi.org/10.1177/152692480801800309.
18. Takahashi K, Prashar R, Putchakayala KG, et al. Allograft loss from acute page kidney secondary to trauma after kidney transplantation. World J Transplant. 2017;7(1):88–93. https://doi.org/10.5500/wjt.v7.i1.88.
19. Papadakis G, Dost S, Kunduzi B, Olsburgh J, Brown C, Mamode N, Karydis N. High-grade blunt traumatic rupture of kidney transplant: is conservative management an option? Ann R Coll Surg Engl. 2022;104(4):e113–5. https://doi.org/10.1308/rcsann.2021.0167. Epub 2021 Nov 26.
20. Rajagopal P, Chughtai SA, Khan S, Ali A. Traumatic injury to renal allograft. Literature review and case series. Trauma renal transplant recipient. A case report. Int J Collab Res Internal Med Public Health. 2019;11(1). https://www.iomcworld.org/articles/traumatic-injury-to-renal-allograft-literature-review-and-case-series-trauma-in-renal-transplant-recipient-a-case-report-18959.html#ai.
21. Martínez-Mier G, García-Almazán E, Esselente-Zetina N, et al. Blunt trauma in kidney transplant with preservation of renal function. Cir Cir. 2006;74(3):205–8.
22. Deshpande NA, James NT, Kucirka LM, Boyarsky BJ, Garonzik-Wang JM, Montgomery RA, Segev DL. Pregnancy outcomes in kidney transplant recipients: a systematic review and meta-analysis. Am J Transplant. 2011;11(11):2388–404. https://doi.org/10.1111/j.1600-6143.2011.03656.x. Epub 2011 Jul 27.
23. Majak GB, Sandven I, Lorentzen B, Vangen S, Reisaeter AV, Henriksen T, Michelsen TM. Pregnancy outcomes following maternal kidney transplantation: a national cohort study. Acta Obstet Gynecol Scand. 2016;95(10):1153–61.
24. Gordon CE, Tatsis V. Shearing-force injury of a kidney transplant graft during cesarean section: a case report and review of the literature. BMC Nephrol. 2019;20:94. https://doi.org/10.1186/s12882-019-1281-6.
25. Shahrokh H, Rasouli H, Zargar MA, Karimi K, Zargar K. Spontaneous kidney allograft rupture. Transplant Proc. 2005;37(7):3079–80. https://doi.org/10.1016/j.transproceed.2005.07.054.
26. Szenohradszky P, Smehák G, Szederkényi E, Marofka F, Csajbók E, Morvay Z, Ormos J, Iványi B. Renal allograft rupture: a clinicopathologic study of 37 nephrectomy cases in a series of 628 consecutive renal transplants. Transplant Proc. 1999;31(5):2107–11. https://doi.org/10.1016/s0041-1345(99)00277-8.

Part II

Ureteral Trauma

The kidneys are essential for life, and ureters are essential for the kidneys. This is enough to understand that damage to these thin and waving tubules may turn your life into a nightmare.

Introduction to Ureteral Trauma

Many researchers have credited Mr. Alfred Poland for the first reported cases of ureteral trauma in 1869. However, some of the cases described by Mr. Poland were published earlier by other authors whom he clearly credited. He gave a detailed account of six cases of traumatic ureteral rupture from blunt and penetrating trauma with multiple associated injuries, and only two of them survived their injuries. For those who succumbed, the diagnosis was confirmed only through autopsy. One of the victims was the Archbishop of Paris who was wounded on 29th June 1848 by a musket ball and died after 18 h. [1] The autopsy revealed a division of the upper ureter with widespread urinary extravasation, as well as a division of the spine at the L3 level, and the ball was found in the psoas muscle [1].

Today, despite 150 years having elapsed, Mr. Poland's report is not outdated. **Ureteric trauma is still very rare**. However, due to the tremendous multiplication of surgical procedures for the last half-century (endourological, gyneco-obstetrical, and colorectal interventions), ureteral injury has become **mostly iatrogenic nowadays** and external trauma with penetrating agents is very rare as are blunt injuries such as deceleration in RTA or blows. When caused by external trauma, ureteric injuries are generally associated with other organs injury and are often missed. From whatever cause, they have no immediate specific manifestations, making their

[1] Further research on the biography of Bishops and Archbishops of Paris confirmed this fact, identifying the victim as Monsignor Denis-Auguste Affre, but there is a little discrepancy in the dates of his death [2].

diagnosis delayed in many instances, with significant early-, mid-term, or late complications, including pain, urinary leak and urinoma, abscess with fever and sepsis, peritonitis, uremia, ureteral stricture with loss of the ipsilateral kidney, and death.

Iatrogenic ureteral injury increases the length of the hospital stay for the patient. In the USA, this caused an estimated overcharge of the treatment bill by an additional $31,000 [3], and 45% of ureteric injuries during gynecological procedures are subjected to litigation against the institutions in Canada [4].

Timely recognition of a ureteral injury is therefore of paramount importance if one aims at avoiding the grim consequences in the patient's general health and a lawsuit in the courts. This is compulsory during surgical interventions where preoperative preventive measures should be taken, and a low threshold of clinical suspicion is mandatory. But it remains very challenging in external or non-iatrogenic trauma (penetrating or blunt) where the dramatic presentation and the frequent association with other intra-abdominal or bony trauma usually mask the ureteral damage during the early post-traumatic period.

References

1. Poland A. On rupture of the ureter. Guy's Hosp Rep. 1869;14(85):85–98. https://books.google.com.om/books?id=Ky1TAAAAcAAJ&printsec=frontcover&hl=ar&source=gbs_ge_summary_r&cad=0#v=onepage&q&f=false.
2. https://fr.wikipedia.org/wiki/Liste_des_%C3%A9v%C3%AAques_puis_archev%C3%AAques_de_Paris.
3. Halabi WJ, Jafari MD, Nguyen VQ, Carmichael JC, Mills S, Pigazzi A, Stamos MJ. Ureteral injuries in colorectal surgery: an analysis of trends, outcomes, and risk factors over a 10-year period in the United States. Dis Colon Rectum. 2014;57(2):179–86. https://doi.org/10.1097/DCR.0000000000000033.
4. Jacob GP, Vilos GA, Al Turki F, et al. Ureteric injury during gynaecological surgery—lessons from 20 cases in Canada. Facts Views Vis Obgyn. 2020;12(1):31–42. Published 2020 May 7.

11 Anatomy of the Ureter

11.1 General Aspects

The ureter is a retroperitoneal tubular structure that measures 25–30 cm, with a diameter of 1.5–6 mm, and connects the kidney to the bladder. It is a continuation of the renal pelvis, which is rightly called by some anatomists ureteral pelvis rather than renal pelvis with regard to the embryological origin of the collecting system arising from the ureteric bud.

The ureter is a contractile conduit whose wall is made up of three main layers [1]

- An inner mucosal layer lined by a transitional epithelium (urothelium) that is identical to the lining of the renal pelvicalyceal system, the bladder, and the proximal urethra.
- An intermediate muscular coat made of interweaving and interlacing smooth muscle fibers allowing peristaltic movements.
- An outer adventitial layer adherent to the posterior parietal peritoneum and containing a network of blood vessels and fatty tissue.

Urologists classically divide the ureter into three segments: **The lumbar or proximal or upper ureter** overlying the lumbar vertebrae above the sacro-iliac joint, **the mid-ureter** overlying the sacro-iliac joint, and **the pelvic or distal or lower ureter** below the sacro-iliac joint. However, it has been proposed to simplify the description into two segments of approximately equal length: **abdominal and pelvic segments** being arbitrarily demarcated by the pelvic brim. Finally, the international anatomical terminology of the ureter describes three parts: **the abdominal, the pelvic, and the intramural segments** [1, 2].

The ureter has three anatomical narrowings

- at the pelviureteric junction,

S. A. AL-Mamari, *Urogenital Trauma: A Practical Guide*, https://doi.org/10.1007/978-981-99-6171-9_11

- at the pelvic brim, where it is compressed by the bones and the iliac vessels, and,
- and at the uretero-vesical junction, which is the narrowest segment.

Functionally, these hollow structures have intrinsic peristaltic movements initiated by pacemakers located in the renal pelvis and transmitted up to the ureteric orifices from where the urine can be seen intermittently effluxing on cystoscopy. The ureteral peristalsis was described in 1869 by the German Physiologist and polymath Theodor Wilhelm Engelmann (1843–1909), who made the same conclusion for intrinsic heart beating and proposed to consider the whole ureter as a functional syncytium [3, 4].

11.2 Course

In the retroperitoneum, the ureter generally lies close to the tips of the transverse processes of the lumbar vertebrae. However, this position varies normally among individuals because of the mobility of the upper half of the ureter, being sometimes more medial or lateral [2].

Cadaveric studies have confirmed the relative mobility of the ureter bathing in the perirenal fat, but they also showed that it becomes firmly fixed to the anterior aspect of the psoas major muscle distally from the crossing point of the gonadal vessels [5]. Due to this cranial mobility, the ureter may exhibit various degrees of kinking observable on CT-urography. The kinking can be classified into grade 1 (mild), grade 2 (moderate), and grade 3 (severe) [5]. In the same individual, the mechanism of intermittent kinking of the cranial portion to the crossing level is caused by the adaptation of the ureter to the kidney ascent and descent during respiration while the caudal portion remains relatively fixed [5].

Regardless of the kinking, the normal ureter's course is not straightforward; after a descent in front of the psoas fascia, it leaves the psoas major muscle and turns medially, and crosses the pelvic brim by lying anterior to the bifurcation of the common iliac artery. Then its pelvic segment runs first in a posterolateral direction close to the lateral wall of the pelvic cavity, anteriorly to the internal iliac artery, then turns at the level of the ischial spine and travels anteromedially above the pelvic floor before entering the trigonal region on the posterior bladder wall [1].

11.3 Topography

(a) Posterior relations: These are similar on both sides and for both sexes. The abdominal ureter descends in front of the genitofemoral nerve (or its genital and femoral branches) on the anterior aspect of the psoas major muscle that separates it from the tips of the lumbar transverse processes. At the level of the pelvic brim, the common iliac artery lies behind the ureter.

(b) Anterior relations:
  - Right ureter: The abdominal segment is crossed by the lower end of the root of the small intestinal mesentery, the right gonadal vessels, the right colic vessels, and ileocolic vessels. The upper end is in proximity to the second part of the duodenum.
  - Left ureter: The upper end is crossed by the body of the pancreas. The abdominal segment is crossed by the left gonadal vessels, the left colic vessels, and the sigmoid vessels embedded in the mesocolon.

Within the pelvic cavity, the ureter travels postero-lateral to the bladder and its relations depend on the gender. In male subjects, it is crossed anteriorly by the vas deferens traveling from lateral to medial. In females, it is crossed superiorly by the uterine artery [1, 2] (Figs. 11.1 and 11.2). Near the bladder, the terminal ureter is covered by the **muscular layer of Waldeyer** and its 1.2–2.5-cm intramural segment runs obliquely through the bladder wall coalescing with bundles of the detrusor muscle to end with the ureteric orifice [2].

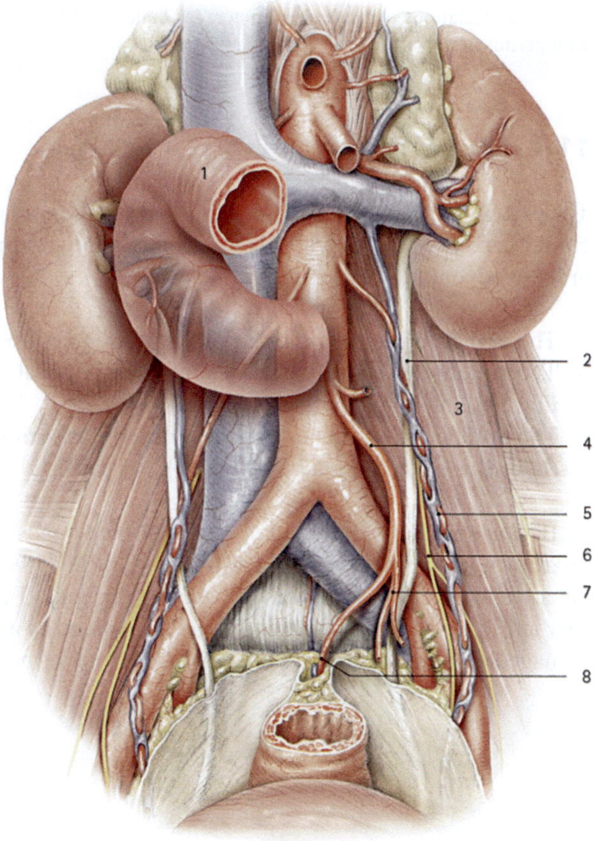

Fig. 11.1 The retroperitoneal space with the anatomical structures surrounding the left and the right ureter. 1, duodenum; 2, ureter; 3, psoas; 4, inferior mesenteric artery; 5, testicular/ovarian artery and vein; 6, genitofemoral nerve—femoral and genital branches; 7, sigmoid arteries; 8, superior rectal artery. (From Fröber R [2], with permission from John Wiley and Sons)

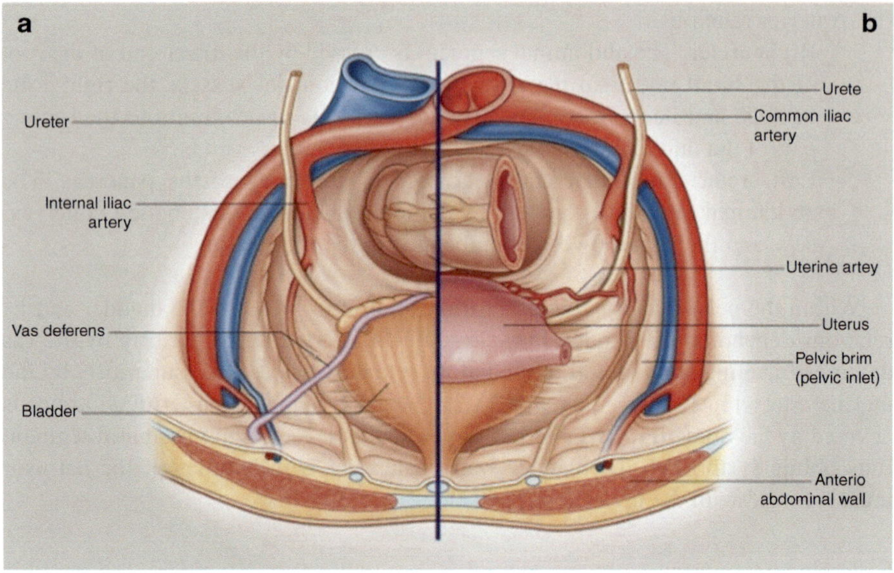

Fig. 11.2 Relations of intrapelvic ureter; (**a**) male, (**b**) female. (From Mahadevan, V. (2019) [1], with permission from Elsevier)

11.4 Blood Supply

The ureter has a segmental or staged blood supply with different sources, distributed cranio-caudally, forming a rich and delicate longitudinal anastomosis in the peri-ureteric adventitia [1, 2] (Figs. 11.3 and 11.4):

- The upper third: ureteric branch of the ipsilateral renal artery.
- The middle third: small branches from the gonadal artery, and from the common iliac and internal iliac arteries.
- The intrapelvic segment: branches from the superior and inferior vesical arteries (branches of the internal iliac artery).

Because of the rich collateral circulation and anastomosis, it is possible to cauterize or ligate a single arteriole as it travels through the so-called mesoureter before entering the ureteral wall without causing necrosis (Fig. 11.5). However, unnecessary and excessive mobilization should be avoided as more arterial sources might be damaged and cause ischemia, increasing the risk of postoperative ureteric stricture.

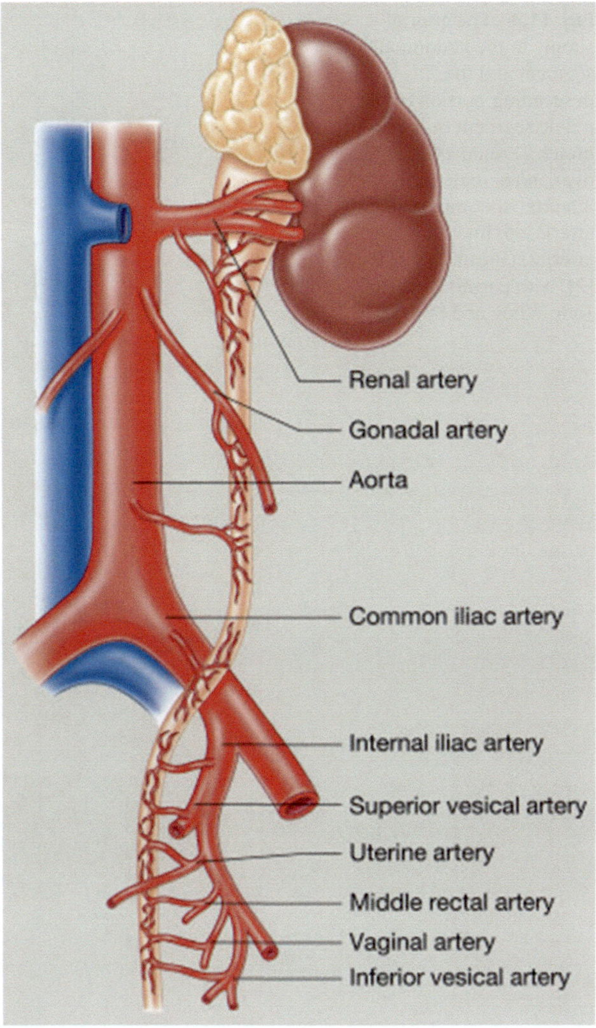

Fig. 11.3 Arterial supply of ureter. (From Mahadevan V [1], with permission from Elsevier)

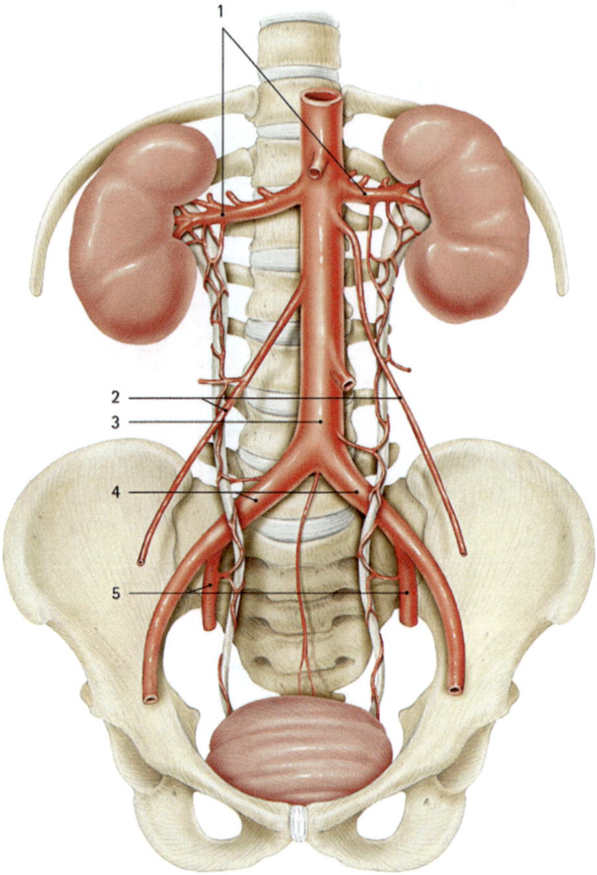

Fig. 11.4 The arterial supply to the abdominal segment and the descending portion of the pelvic segment of the ureter. 1, renal arteries; 2, ovarian/testicular arteries; 3, aorta; 4, common iliac arteries; 5, internal iliac arteries. (From Fröber R [2], with permission from John Wiley and Sons)

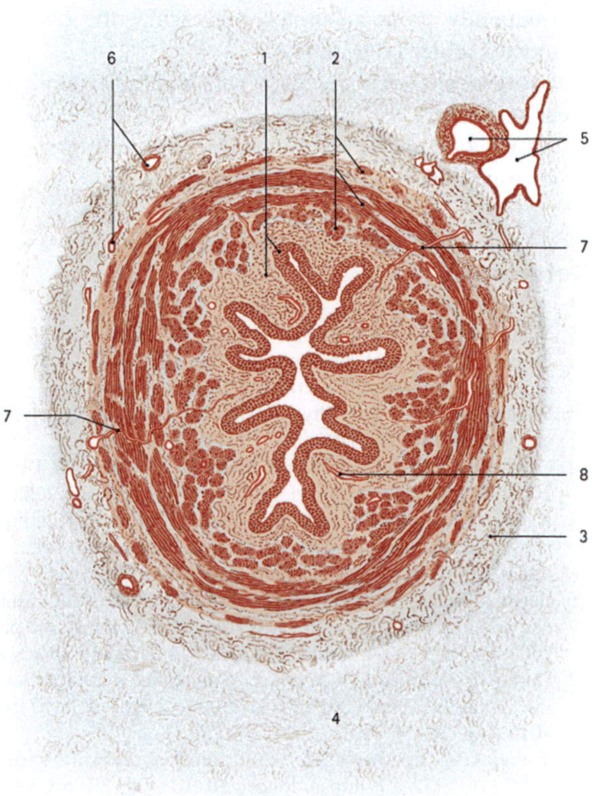

Fig. 11.5 The nutrient vascular structures in a schematic illustration of a microscopic transverse section of the ureter. 1, mucosa; 2, muscle coat; 3, adventitia; 4, mesoureter; 5, supplying artery and vein; 6, adventitial vascular plexus; 7, perforating arteries; 8, mucosal vascular plexus. (From Fröber R [2], with permission from John Wiley and Sons)

11.5 Congenital Abnormalities

The ureteral congenital abnormalities can be summarized as follows [6–8]

- **Uretero-pelvic junction obstruction**: This is the most common congenital ureteral abnormality with an incidence of 1 in 1000–1500 newborns.
- **Double ureter or ureteral duplication**: May be partial or complete.
- **Primary vesicoureteral reflux**: The most common cause of antenatal hydronephrosis (40%).
- **Primary megaureter**.
- **Ectopic ureter**: Complete ureteral duplication is found in 70% of ectopic ureters. In complete ureteral duplication with separate ureteral orifices in the bladder, the **Weigert-Meyer law**[1] states that the ureter connected to the upper pole moi-

[1]Carl Weigert (1845–1904) and Robert Meyer (1864–1947) were two German pathologists. Weigert described the caudal termination of the ureter from the upper moiety in 1877 [9] and Meyer described the medial termination of the same in 1907 [10] compared to the ureter draining the lower moiety.

ety opens into the bladder medial and inferior to the orifice of the ureter draining the lower renal moiety. Moreover, the ureter draining the upper pole moiety is frequently prone to ureterocele, while the one draining the lower moiety is mostly subjected to reflux.

– **Ureterocele**: About 75% of ureteral duplications are associated with ureterocele.
– **Retrocaval ureter** (or more correctly pre-ureteric vena cava).
– **Ureteral folds, valves, and strictures**.

References

1. Mahadevan V. Anatomy of the kidney and ureter. Surgery (Oxford). 2019;37(7):359–64.
2. Fröber R. Surgical anatomy of the ureter. BJU Int. 2007;100(4):949–65. https://doi.org/10.1111/j.1464-410X.2007.07207.x.
3. Engelmann TW. Zur Physiologie des Ureter. Pflüger Arch. 1869;2:243–93. https://doi.org/10.1007/BF01628404.
4. Osman F, Romics I, Nyírády P, Monos E, Nádasy GL. Ureteral motility. Acta Physiol Hung. 2009;96(4):407–26. https://doi.org/10.1556/APhysiol.96.2009.4.2. PMID: 19942548
5. Kamo M, Nozaki T, Yoshida K, Tateishi U, Akita K. Kinking of the upper ureter in CT urography: anatomic and clinical significance. Surg Radiol Anat. 2016;38(10):1115–21. https://doi.org/10.1007/s00276-016-1689-7. Epub 2016 May 9
6. Berrocal T, López-Pereira P, Arjonilla A, Gutiérrez J. Anomalies of the distal ureter, bladder, and urethra in children: embryologic, radiologic, and pathologic features. Radiographics. 2002;22(5):1139–64. https://doi.org/10.1148/radiographics.22.5.g02se101139.
7. Dorko F, Tokarčík J, Výborná E. Congenital malformations of the ureter: anatomical studies. Anat Sci Int. 2016;91(3):290–4. https://doi.org/10.1007/s12565-015-0296-8. Epub 2015 Aug 19
8. Young DW, Lebowitz RL. Congenital abnormalities of the ureter. Semin Roentgenol. 1986;21(3):172–87. https://doi.org/10.1016/0037-198X(86)90018-0.
9. Weigert C. Über einige Bildungsfehler der Ureteren. Archiv für pathologische Anatomie und Physiologie und für klinische Medizin. 1877;70:490–501.
10. Meyer R. Zur Anatomie und Entwicklungsgeschichte der Ureterverdoppelung. Archiv für pathologische Anatomie und Physiologie und für klinische Medizin. 1907;187:408–34.

12 Epidemiology of Ureteral Injuries

Non-iatrogenic ureteral injury is a very rare event occurring in only 3 per 10,000 trauma admissions [1].

To substantiate this rarity, it is enough to mention that a French review of over 43,000 Road Traffic Accident (RTA) cases showed 199 cases of urogenital trauma (UGT), but not a single ureteral trauma was recorded [2]. With a larger French study including 162,690 RTA victims, 963 UGT (0.59%) were detected, and a total of five ureteric injuries were recorded (0.003% of total RTA trauma, or 0.5% of UGT) [3]. Further enlargement was achieved through a 4-year analysis of the American NTDB identifying 582 ureteral injuries out of 22,706 UGT, representing 2.56% [1]. This study showed that, contrary to renal trauma, penetrating causes are more frequent than blunt ones and comprise 61.5% of ureteral injuries.

A single-institution experience showed an even more striking predominance of penetrating injuries in ureteral trauma reaching 96.5%, with a great proportion arising from gunshots (91%), while stab wounds occurred in only 5.5%. Blunt injuries, mainly due to motor vehicle accidents (MVA), were an extremely rare cause of ureteral injury (3.5%) in this study [4].

Like renal trauma, penetrating ureteral trauma has a higher incidence of associated injuries in intraabdominal organs. The overall associated injuries in ureteral trauma are present in 90.4% of cases [5]. Most encountered associations are injuries to the small bowel (46%), the large bowel (44%), and the vessels (38%). However, blunt trauma is associated with a higher incidence of bony pelvic injuries (20%) [1].

Another NTDB review showed that even blunt traumatic ureteral injuries expose to serious outcomes, as 66.7% of the patients were unstable and 34.7% had high-grade ureteral injuries. Confirming the rarity of ureteral injuries and especially those arising from blunt traumas, only 147 blunt traumatic ureteral injuries were recruited over a 10-year period [6].

There is a male predominance in ureteral injury reaching 84%. The proportion of males is even greater when specifying to study to penetrating injuries with 91% vs. 73% for blunt injuries. Most of the victims are young with a mean age of 31 years [1].

S. A. AL-Mamari, *Urogenital Trauma: A Practical Guide*,
https://doi.org/10.1007/978-981-99-6171-9_12

Ultimately, as already stated above, it is important to remember that iatrogenic complications (surgery and radiation therapy) are the most frequent causes of ureteral injuries accounting for 80%, while non-iatrogenic or external violence or accidents account for 20% only [7]. Among iatrogenic causes, Gynecologic procedures are incriminated in 64–82% of cases, followed by colorectal, vascular, and urological surgeries [8]. Of course, the innumerable minor ureteral injuries caused by endourological procedures are not taken into account here.

References

1. Siram SM, Gerald SZ, Greene WR, Hughes K, Oyetunji TA, Chrouser K, Cornwell EE 3rd, Chang DC. Ureteral trauma: patterns and mechanisms of injury of an uncommon condition. Am J Surg. 2010;199(4):566–70. https://doi.org/10.1016/j.amjsurg.2009.11.001.
2. Paparel P, N'diaye A, Laumon B, Caillot J-L, Perrin P, Ruffion A. The epidemiology of trauma of the genitourinary system after traffic accidents: analysis of a register of over 43,000 victims. BJU Int. 2006;97(2):338–41. https://doi.org/10.1111/j.1464-410x.2006.05900.x.
3. Terrier JE, Paparel P, Gadegbeku B, Ruffion A, Jenkins LC, N'Diaye A. Genitourinary injuries after traffic accidents: analysis of a registry of 162,690 victims. J Trauma Acute Care Surg. 2017;82(6):1087–93. https://doi.org/10.1097/TA.0000000000001448.
4. Best CD, Petrone P, Buscarini M, Demiray S, Kuncir E, Kimbrell B, Asensio JA. Traumatic ureteral injuries: a single institution experience validating the American Association for the Surgery of Trauma-Organ Injury Scale grading scale. J Urol. 2005;173(4):1202–5. https://doi.org/10.1097/01.ju.0000155526.37963.ef.
5. Pereira BM, Ogilvie MP, Gomez-Rodriguez JC, et al. A review of ureteral injuries after external trauma. Scand J Trauma Resusc Emerg Med. 2010;18:6. https://doi.org/10.1186/1757-7241-18-6.
6. Mendonca SJ, Jessica Pan SM, Li G, Brandes SB. Real-world practice patterns favor minimally invasive methods over ureteral reconstruction in the initial treatment of severe blunt ureteral trauma: A National Trauma Data Bank Analysis. J Urol. 2021;205(2):470–6. https://doi.org/10.1097/JU.0000000000001347.
7. Elliott SP, McAninch JW. Ureteral injuries: external and iatrogenic. Urol Clin N Am. 2006;33(1):55–66. https://doi.org/10.1016/j.ucl.2005.11.005.
8. Gild P, Kluth LA, Vetterlein MW, Engel O, Chun FKH, Fisch M. Adult iatrogenic ureteral injury and stricture-incidence and treatment strategies. Asian J Urol. 2018;5(2):101–6. https://doi.org/10.1016/j.ajur.2018.02.003.

13 Etiology and Mechanisms of Ureteral Trauma

The ureter is relatively well protected from external trauma by many factors: vermiform shape, small diameter, mobility, retroperitoneal location with an anterior bowel cushion, and a posterior psoas muscle shield. The other side of the coin is that the ureter travels in close proximity to uterine, iliac, inferior mesenteric, and sigmoid vessels, as well as the cervix, the colon, and the rectum exposing it to the risk for iatrogenic injuries during gynecological or colorectal surgeries [1].

For the sake of clarity, it is important to divide the etiology into two categories: iatrogenic and non-iatrogenic trauma.

13.1 Iatrogenic Injuries

This is the most common cause of ureteral injury and may occur during endourological procedures, open or laparoscopic gynecological, colorectal, and vascular surgeries, and to a lesser degree as a delayed complication of chemoradiation therapy.

The iatrogenic ureteric injury may occur either after direct physical trauma, i.e., abrasion, perforation, section, ligation, crush, or coagulation, or indirectly due to secondary ischemia provoked by large-caliber endourological instruments, extrinsic devascularization, or thermal injury during open or laparoscopic surgery [1]. The mechanism of injury comprises four types: laceration, ligation (stitches or clips), devascularization, and energy-induced (monopolar cautery bears more risks) [2] (Fig. 13.1a, b).

In general, iatrogenic agents most commonly injure the pelvic ureter while non-iatrogenic and especially penetrating trauma mostly damage the proximal ureter [3].

Indeed, iatrogenic injuries involve the distal, the middle, and the proximal third of the ureter in 91%, 7%, and 2%, respectively [4].

The iatrogenic causes may be further subdivided as follows:

S. A. AL-Mamari, *Urogenital Trauma: A Practical Guide*,
https://doi.org/10.1007/978-981-99-6171-9_13

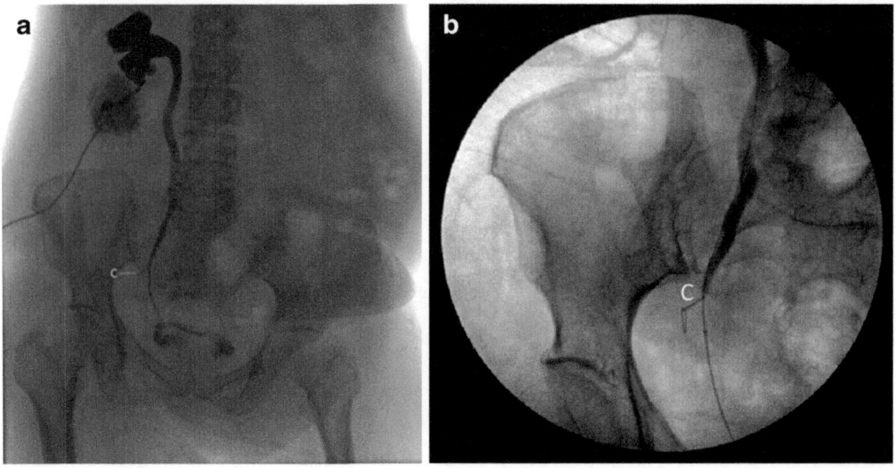

Fig. 13.1 (**a**, **b**) Antegrade nephrostogram in a 54-year woman with a history of radical abdominal hysterectomy and bilateral salpingo-oophorectomy for endometrial cancer followed by chemotherapy. She developed partial obstruction of right kidney caused by a metallic clip (C) inadvertently applied on the distal right ureter during the hysterectomy

13.1.1 Endourological Procedures

They were reported to be the most frequent cause of iatrogenic ureteral injuries accounting for 42% in a series of 156 cases, followed by gynecological surgeries with 34% [4]. However, most of the endourological complications are minor, diagnosed intraoperatively, and timely managed with a better prognosis. In addition, a large number of them have a low clinical significance and remain underreported, thus leaving gynecological causes to take the lion's part in iatrogenic causes according to recent studies [1].

A prospective study of 437 patients who underwent ureteroscopy for stones revealed the occurrence of ureteral wall injury of various grades in 30.4% [5]. Here again, it is important to notice that many of these injuries consisted of mucosal abrasions and perforations which are self-limited and well-managed with a good prognosis. The most catastrophic complication of endourology is ureteral avulsion, but this is a very rare event, being reported in less than 1% of procedures only [6].

During a ureteroscopy performed for calculi, the injury might be caused by the insertion of a guidewire, the push of the semi-rigid ureteroscope, the in-situ lithotripsy with whatever energy (Swiss Lithoclast, Holmium-Laser, etc..), the retrieval of a stone that scratches the ureteral wall during its descent, or the insertion of a ureteral access sheath.

A recent review has shown the following incidence of ureteroscopic complications: mucosal erosions and false passages (0.13–9.5%), perforations (0.3–7.4%), and avulsion (0.04–0.9%) [7]. Ureteral avulsion occurs mostly during an attempt to retrieve a stone that is too large to pass through the ureteral lumen, or during the

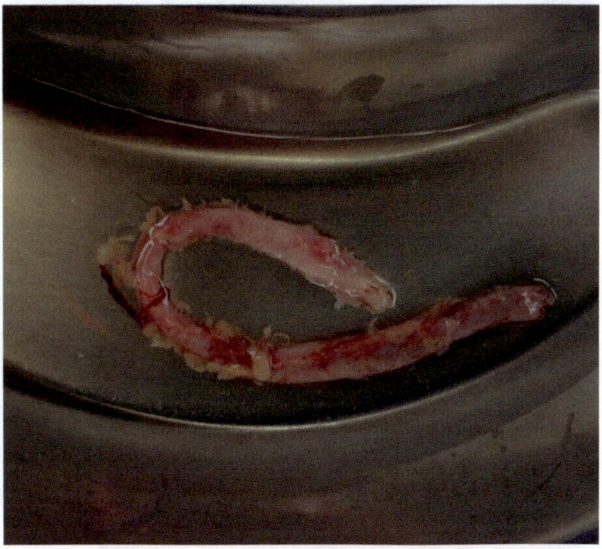

Fig. 13.2 Complete avulsion of the right ureter with preexisting strictures during a rigid ureteroscopy performed for an upper ureteric stone in a 75-year-old man. (Courtesy Kurian George, Retiree from the Urology Department, The Royal Hospital, Muscat, Oman)

insertion of a semi-rigid ureteroscope that is too large to be safely negotiated through the ureter. Sometimes even a small ureteroscope might avulse the ureter if forcibly pushed against a diseased fibrotic and strictured ureter (Fig. 13.2).

Ureteral wall injury by ureteral access sheath may consist of superficial lesions (39.9%), deeper lesions (17.6%), or circumferential perforation (4.7%) [7].

13.1.2 Gynecological Procedures (Cesarean Section, Hysterectomy)

Here the risk factors for ureteric injury are obesity, previous laparotomic pelvic surgery, pelvic adhesions, large pelvic tumors, and unexpected intra-operative bleeding [8] (Fig. 13.3a–c). Most ureteral injuries during gynecological procedures are diagnosed only after discharge from the hospital (70%) resulting in litigation in 45% of the cases [8].

A systematic review recruiting 140,444 gynecologic laparoscopic surgeries for benign indications showed 0.08% of ureteral injury, and these were more often unrecognized intraoperatively [9]. A more specific study showed incidences of 1.3 ureteric injuries per 1000 cases of total abdominal hysterectomy and 0.2 injuries per 1000 cases of vaginal hysterectomy, with or without bilateral salpingo-oophorectomy [10]. In this review, laparoscopic hysterectomy was associated with the highest incidence of ureteral injury reaching 7.8 per 1000 procedures.

There is also a correlation between the types of gynecological interventions and the location of ureteral injury [11] (Fig. 13.4).

In developing countries, obstetrical injuries are frequent causes of vesicovaginal fistulas. The alarm was recently sounded about the surge of uterovaginal fistulas

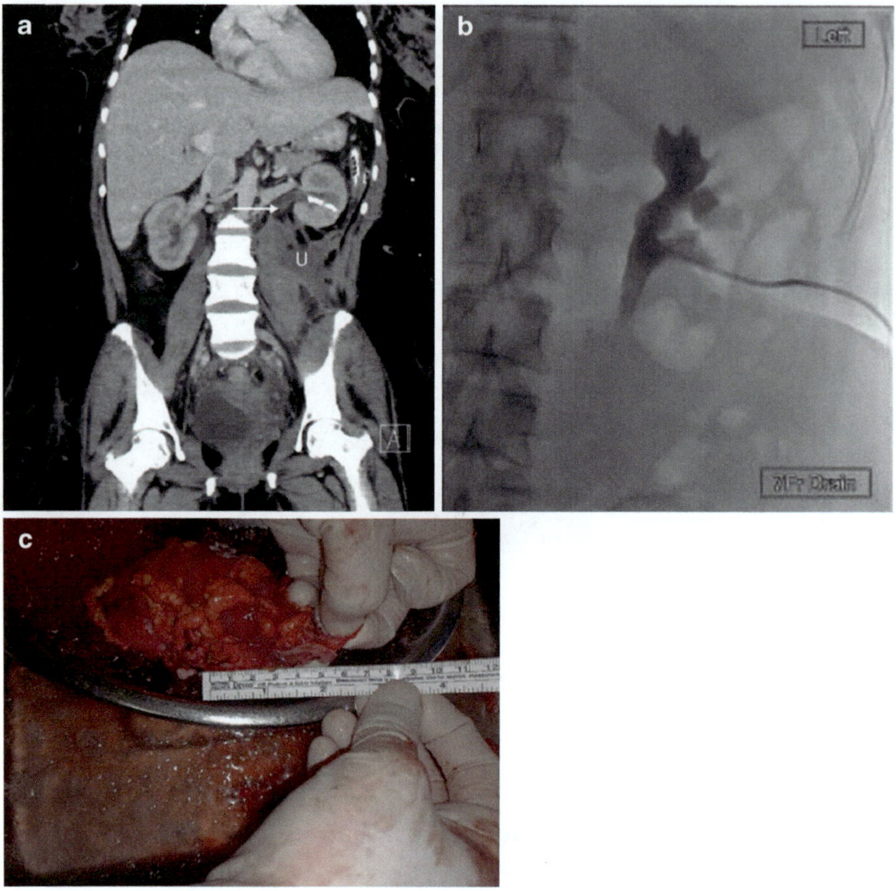

Fig. 13.3 Pan-ureteral injury with devitalization of the left ureter in a 36-year woman during cesarean section complicated with severe bleeding that prompted a hysterectomy and packing in a regional hospital. She later underwent repeated laparotomies for recurrent bleeding, as well as embolization and ligation of the left internal iliac artery. The ureteral injury was initially managed with ligation at the remaining viable stump and nephrostomy. (**a**) Coronal CT showing the nephrostomy tube in situ with dilated proximal ureter ending abruptly at the level of ligation (arrow) and a urinoma (U). (**b**) Antegrade nephrostogram demonstrating the left pelvicalyceal system and the short ureteral stump. (**c**) Four months after the injury, the left kidney was harvested after a tedious open approach through a flank incision. A short ureter (5.5 cm) is seen during the back-table preparation of the graft for autotransplantation in the right iliac fossa. (Courtesy Feroz Amir Zafar, Urology, the Royal Hospital, Muscat, Oman)

secondary to emergency cesarean sections for prolonged labors, abdominal hysterectomies, and vaginal hysterectomies [12].

Colpopexy also carries a potential risk to the ureter, as shown by a cadaveric study [13].

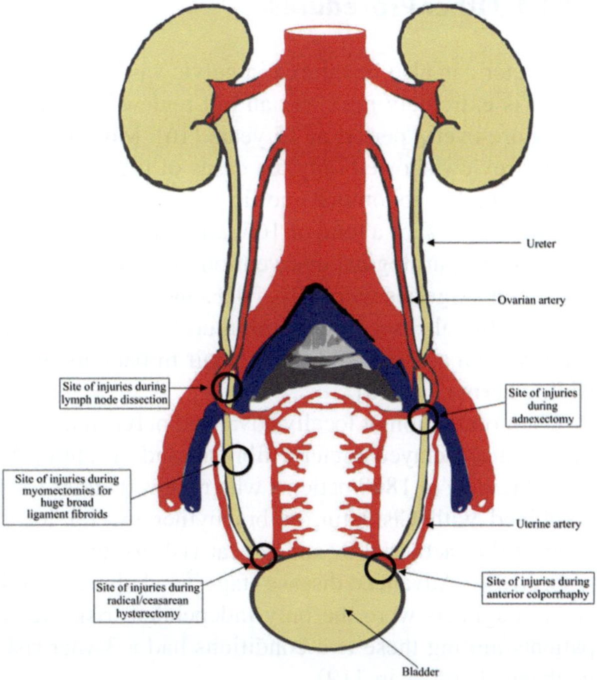

Fig. 13.4 The common sites of ureteral injuries. (From Ade-Ojo IP et al. [11]. International Journal of Women's Health 2021, 13, 895–902. Originally published by and used with permission from Dove Medical Press Ltd.)

13.1.3 Colorectal Procedures

A nationwide retrospective study in the United States conducted over a decade and recruiting 2,165,848 **colorectal surgical procedures** showed a total of 6027 ureteral injuries equivalent to **0.28%**. It was also noticed that this rate was higher in the second half of the decade than in the first decade, with respective rates of 0.31% vs. 0.25%, probably because of the trend to operate on more complex cases, such as sigmoidectomy for complicated diverticulitis with adhesions, or surgery on cancer after neoadjuvant chemoradiotherapy [14]. It is estimated that colorectal procedures (such as low anterior resection and abdominoperineal resection) account for 9% of iatrogenic ureteral injuries [15].

The risk factors associated with colorectal surgery are rectal cancer diagnosis, presence of intra-operative adhesions, metastatic cancer, malnutrition or weight loss, and teaching institutions [14]. On the contrary, some factors such as laparoscopic procedures, as opposed to the open counterpart, surgery on the transverse and right colons, as opposed to left colon and recto-sigmoid segments, didn't appear to be associated with ureteral injuries [14].

13.1.4 Other Procedures

The ureter can also be injured in pelvic vascular surgery. Nonetheless, this complication is extremely rare, and an old review documented only 23 cases in English Literature over a period of 25 years [16]. Moreover, a 20-year retrospective multicentric review showed only ten cases of ureteral injury in relation to vascular surgery, namely abdominal aortic aneurysm repair and aorto-femoral bypass, representing 6% of a total of 165 iatrogenic ureteric injuries in the same period [4]. In this series, urological interventions were the first causes, followed by Gynae and colorectal surgeries with 42%, 34%, and 26%.

Exceptional cases of ureteral injuries have also been reported in routine general surgery such as inguinal hernia repair in patients with a congenital abnormality or sliding hernia [17, 18].

Chemoradiation of locally advanced pelvic malignancies is also known to potentially cause delayed ureteric fibrosis and stricture. An EMBRACE collaborative group[1] review of 1860 patients who received either External beam radiation therapy combined with Cisplatin, or brachytherapy, for locally advanced cervix cancer, showed that actuarial 3- and 5-year risk for ureteral stricture was 1.7% and 2.1% respectively. Advanced disease stage T3–4 along with the presence of hydronephrosis at diagnosis were the only independent risk factors for ureteral stricture, and patients uniting these two conditions had a 3-year risk of 11.5%, which remained unchanged at 5 years [19].

13.2 Non-iatrogenic or External Trauma

As already mentioned above, penetrating injuries are more frequent than blunt trauma among non-iatrogenic causes.

A series of 20 patients with penetrating ureteric injuries showed that 18 of them were due to gunshot (90%) and only two were caused by stabbing (10%), and none was diagnosed before an emergency laparotomy that was performed for associated injuries [20].

Abdomen gunshot wound has been estimated to involve the ureter in 2–5% of the time, through two mechanisms: either by a direct transection of the ureter in the pathway of the projectile, or disruption of its blood supply in blast injury, resulting in necrosis [21]. This combined mechanism results in extensive damage to the ureter. By contrast, stab wounds account for only 5% of ureteral injuries in the United States and cause only short-segment damage to the ureter [21] (Table 13.1).

[1] EMBRACE: Image-guided intensity modulated **E**xternal beam radiochemotherapy and **MR**I-based adaptive **BRA**chytherapy in Locally advanced **CE**rvical cancer.

Table 13.1 Mechanism of ureteral trauma

Mechanism of ureteral injuries	*n* (total 582)	Percentage
Blunt trauma	**224**	**38**
Motor vehicle collision	110	19
Pedestrian	25	4
Motorcyclist	18	3
High fall	15	3
Low fall	8	1
Cyclist	3	<1
Other	45	8
Penetrating trauma	**358**	**62**
Gunshot wound	316	54
Stab	29	5
Other	13	2

From Siram SM [21], with permission from Elsevier

13.3 "Spontaneous Ureteral Rupture"

At first glance, this entity seems off-topic in this book. But the concept of spontaneous rupture remains a subject of controversy, raising some interest here. Despite having been described for nearly one century [22], there are still extremely rare cases of spontaneous ureteral rupture in the literature. No clear underlying causes have been found. Attempts to explain their mechanism include stone impaction, malignancy, old neglected trauma, extracorporeal shockwave lithotripsy, idiopathic retroperitoneal fibrosis, and other factors proceeding through obstruction and/or dilatation [23–25]. Some cases of spontaneous ureteral rupture of the ureter have been described after an uncomplicated vaginal delivery, and the authors hypothesized that the downward pressure exerted on the bladder during active labor creates traction on the ureter [26]. Nonetheless, despite all the attempted explanations, there are cases of spontaneous ureteral rupture which are not associated with none of the above factors (tumor, stone, history of trauma, obstruction, etc.), validating therefore the concept of "spontaneous rupture" [27].

References

1. Gild P, Kluth LA, Vetterlein MW, Engel O, Chun FKH, Fisch M. Adult iatrogenic ureteral injury and stricture-incidence and treatment strategies. Asian J Urol. 2018;5(2):101–6. https://doi.org/10.1016/j.ajur.2018.02.003.
2. Delacroix SE Jr, Winters JC. Urinary tract injures: recognition and management. Clin Colon Rectal Surg. 2010;23(2):104–12. https://doi.org/10.1055/s-0030-1254297.
3. Engelsgjerd JS, LaGrange CA. Ureteral injury 2021. In: StatPearls [Internet]. Treasure Island (FL): StatPearls Publishing; 2022.
4. Selzman AA, Spirnak JP. Iatrogenic ureteral injuries: a 20-year experience in treating 165 injuries. J Urol. 1996;155(3):878–81. https://doi.org/10.1016/s0022-5347(01)66332-8.

5. Karakan T, Kilinc M, Demirbas A, Hascicek A, Doluoglu O, Yucel M, Resorlu B. Evaluating of ureteral wall injuries with endoscopic grading system and analysis of the predisposing factors. J Endourol. 2016;30:375. https://doi.org/10.1089/end.2015.0706.
6. Burks FN, Santucci RA. Management of iatrogenic ureteral injury. Ther Adv Urol. 2014;6(3):115–24. https://doi.org/10.1177/1756287214526767.
7. De Coninck V, Keller EX, Somani B, Giusti G, Proietti S, Rodriguez-Socarras M, Rodríguez-Monsalve M, Doizi S, Ventimiglia E, Traxer O. Complications of ureteroscopy: a complete overview. World J Urol. 2020;38(9):2147–66. https://doi.org/10.1007/s00345-019-03012-1. Epub 2019 Nov 20
8. Jacob GP, Vilos GA, Al Turki F, et al. Ureteric injury during gynaecological surgery—lessons from 20 cases in Canada. Facts Views Vis Obgyn. 2020;12(1):31–42. Published 2020 May 7
9. Wong JMK, Bortoletto P, Tolentino J, Jung MJ, Milad MP. Urinary tract injury in gynecologic laparoscopy for benign indication: a systematic review. Obstet Gynecol. 2018;131(1):100–8. https://doi.org/10.1097/AOG.0000000000002414.
10. Gilmour D, Das S, Flowerdew G. Rates of urinary tract injury from gynecologic surgery and the role of intraoperative cystoscopy. Obstet Gynecol. 2006;92:1366–77.
11. Ade-Ojo IP, Tijani O. A review on the etiology, prevention, and management of ureteral injuries during obstetric and gynecologic surgeries. Int J Womens Health. 2021;13:895–902. https://doi.org/10.2147/IJWH.S330060. PMID: 34621135; PMCID: PMC8491787
12. Lawal O, Bello O, Morhason-Bello I, Abdus-Salam R, Ojengbede O. Our experience with iatrogenic ureteric injuries among women presenting to University College Hospital, Ibadan: a call to action on trigger factors. Obstet Gynecol Int. 2019;2019:6456141. https://doi.org/10.1155/2019/6456141. PMID: 30881457; PMCID: PMC6387707
13. Siff LN, Jallad K, Hickman LC, Walters MD. Surgical anatomy of the uterosacral ligament colpopexy. Urogynecology. 2018;24(5):380–2. https://doi.org/10.1097/SPV.0000000000000461.
14. Halabi WJ, Jafari MD, Nguyen VQ, Carmichael JC, Mills S, Pigazzi A, Stamos MJ. Ureteral injuries in colorectal surgery: an analysis of trends, outcomes, and risk factors over a 10-year period in the United States. Dis Colon Rectum. 2014;57(2):179–86. https://doi.org/10.1097/DCR.0000000000000033.
15. St Lezin M, Stoller M. Surgical ureteral injuries. Urology. 1991;38:497–506.
16. Dalsing MC, Bihrle R, Lalka SG, Cikrit DF, Sawchuk AP. Vascular surgery-associated ureteral injury: zebras do exist. Ann Vasc Surg. 1993;7(2):180–6. https://doi.org/10.1007/BF02001013. PMID: 8518136
17. Hwang CM, Miller FH, Dalton DP, Hartz WH. Accidental ureteral ligation during an inguinal hernia repair of patient with crossed fused renal ectopia. Clin Imaging. 2002;26(5):306–8. https://doi.org/10.1016/s0899-7071(02)00437-0.
18. Eziyi AK, Etonyeaku AC, Olajide AO, Adejumobi MO. Herniorrhaphy: an unusual cause of ureteral injury in Nigeria. Clin Case Rep. 2014;2(6):247–9. https://doi.org/10.1002/ccr3.98.
19. Fokdal L, Tanderup K, Pötter R, Sturdza A, Kirchheiner K, Chargari C, Jürgenliemk-Schulz IM, Segedin B, Tan LT, Hoskin P, Mahantshetty U, Bruheim K, Rai B, Kirisits C, Lindegaard JC, EMBRACE Collaborative Group. Risk factors for ureteral stricture after radiochemotherapy including image guided adaptive brachytherapy in cervical cancer: results from the EMBRACE studies. Int J Radiat Oncol Biol Phys. 2019;103(4):887–94. https://doi.org/10.1016/j.ijrobp.2018.11.006. Epub 2018 Nov 10
20. Fraga GP, Borges GM, Mantovani M, Ferreira U, Laurito TL, Netto NR Jr. Penetrating ureteral trauma. Int Braz J Urol. 2007;33(2):142–8., discussion 149–50. https://doi.org/10.1590/s1677-55382007000200003.
21. Siram SM, Gerald SZ, Greene WR, Hughes K, Oyetunji TA, Chrouser K, Cornwell EE 3rd, Chang DC. Ureteral trauma: patterns and mechanisms of injury of an uncommon condition. Am J Surg. 2010;199(4):566–70. https://doi.org/10.1016/j.amjsurg.2009.11.001.
22. Sidney S. Spontaneous ureteral rupture with peri-ureteral abscess formation. Am J Surg. 1939;45(1):139–41. ISSN 0002-9610. https://doi.org/10.1016/S0002-9610(39)90390-9.
23. Eken A, Akbas T, Arpaci T. Spontaneous rupture of the ureter. Singap Med J. 2015;56(2):e29–31. https://doi.org/10.11622/smedj.2015029.

24. Liu S, Lin J, Huang C, Tsai I. Spontaneous rupture of the ureter mimicking acute appendicitis: two case reports. JACME. 2011;1:61–3.
25. Ay D, Yencilek E, Celikmen MF, Akkas M, Ekci B. Spontaneous rupture of ureter: an unusual cause of acute abdominal pain. Am J Emerg Med. 2012;30(390):e1–2.
26. Ratkowski KL, Lin M, Bhalla S. Spontaneous ureteral injury. Appl Radiol. 2018;47:38–9.
27. Aggarwal G, Adhikary SD. Spontaneous ureteric rupture, a reality or a faux pas? BMC Urol. 2016;16:37. https://doi.org/10.1186/s12894-016-0158-2.

Presentation, Symptoms, Imaging, Grading, and Complications of Ureteral Injuries

14

14.1 Presentation and Symptoms

The urologist is often called to the operating theater by gynecologists or colorectal surgeons suspecting a ureteral injury. More rarely the call comes from an endocrinological surgeon performing adrenalectomy and para-aortic lymphadenectomy, or a vascular surgeon. The patient may also be referred to the urologist 1 or 2 days after a surgical procedure because of severe localized loin and flank pain and tenderness, with or without signs of peritoneal irritation, that have prompted an ultrasonographic study revealing ipsilateral hydronephrosis.

However, as a urologist, you are likely to end your career without being involved in the emergency department for suspected ureteral injury after blunt or penetrating trauma. Not surprisingly and very logically, priority is given there by the trauma team to other life-threatening injured organs, and the ureteric trauma will become obvious only when imaging investigations will show urinary leak or signs of obstruction and hydronephrosis.

Depending on the delay in the presentation, the patient may develop fever and sometimes abscess formation in infected urinoma. A female patient may also present with a vaginal urinary leak. Hematuria (microscopic and macroscopic) occurs in only 44–53% of the cases of ureteral injury [1, 2].

14.2 Imaging

Historically intravenous urography (IVU) was the imaging modality of choice to evaluate the ureters. Now like in kidney trauma, it has been superseded by **computerized-tomography urography (CTU)**. However, the choice of the best imaging modality practically depends on the scenarios [3–5]:

S. A. AL-Mamari, *Urogenital Trauma: A Practical Guide*,
https://doi.org/10.1007/978-981-99-6171-9_14

1. Intra-operative suspicion of ureteric injury: The patient is already in the Operating theater and is under general or spinal anesthesia, **retrograde urography is the best choice, and is indeed the most sensitive imaging means for the detection of ureteral trauma.**
2. Post-operative suspicion of ureteric injury suggested by specific complaints and complications (pain, tenderness, raised creatinine, fever, inflammatory markers, etc.): **Ultrasonography is the most rapid test to orient the diagnosis but has limited sensitivity and specificity**. If the suspicion of ureteral injury is strengthened by the ultrasonographic findings (ipsilateral hydronephrosis, free fluid in the retroperitoneal or intraperitoneal cavity), **a CTU will be the best imaging modality to ascertain the diagnosis, harboring high specificity and sensitivity.**
3. In a patient presenting with a history of trauma, either penetrating or blunt, the first imaging modality is **an abdominal and pelvic multi-detector CT (MDCT) images or a contrast-enhanced CT (CECT) scan of the abdomen** which will provide a view of the whole post-trauma damage. If the CECT-scan raised suspicion of ureteral injury but provides unclear images of the anatomy, delayed-phase images, namely a CTU should be requested [4, 5].
4. Sometimes the patient might have an obvious obstruction or leak in the ureter suggestive of ligation or transection, respectively, for which a percutaneous nephrostomy (PCN) has already been performed. When a further definition of the lesion is necessary, the ideal modality here is an **antegrade urography or pyelography performed through the PCN tube, technically known as antegrade nephrostogram (ANG).**

After an initial non-contrast phase, CTU comprises three phases following IV-contrast injection [5] (Fig. 14.1):

- Vascular (angiographic or corticomedullary) phase: at 25–40 s after IV-contrast injection.
- Nephrographic (parenchymal) phase: at 75–90 s after IV-contrast injection,
- Urographic (excretory) phase: at 3–5 min after IV-contrast injection.

MR urography has a limited value in the evaluation of a suspected injured ureter because it doesn't add much information compared to a CT scan, is not widely distributed, is not cost-effective, and is time-consuming and therefore not suitable in an emergency setting. However, being radiation-free, it can be useful for selected cases such as pregnant women and children, with a reservation for the latter category who would require general anesthesia for the completion of the investigation.

As mentioned above, ultrasonography is only useful in the primary assessment of the kidney for any hydronephrosis suggestive of ureteric obstruction, and for the visualization of a free fluid collection compatible with a urinoma. However, it has no value in the direct identification of a ureteric injury.

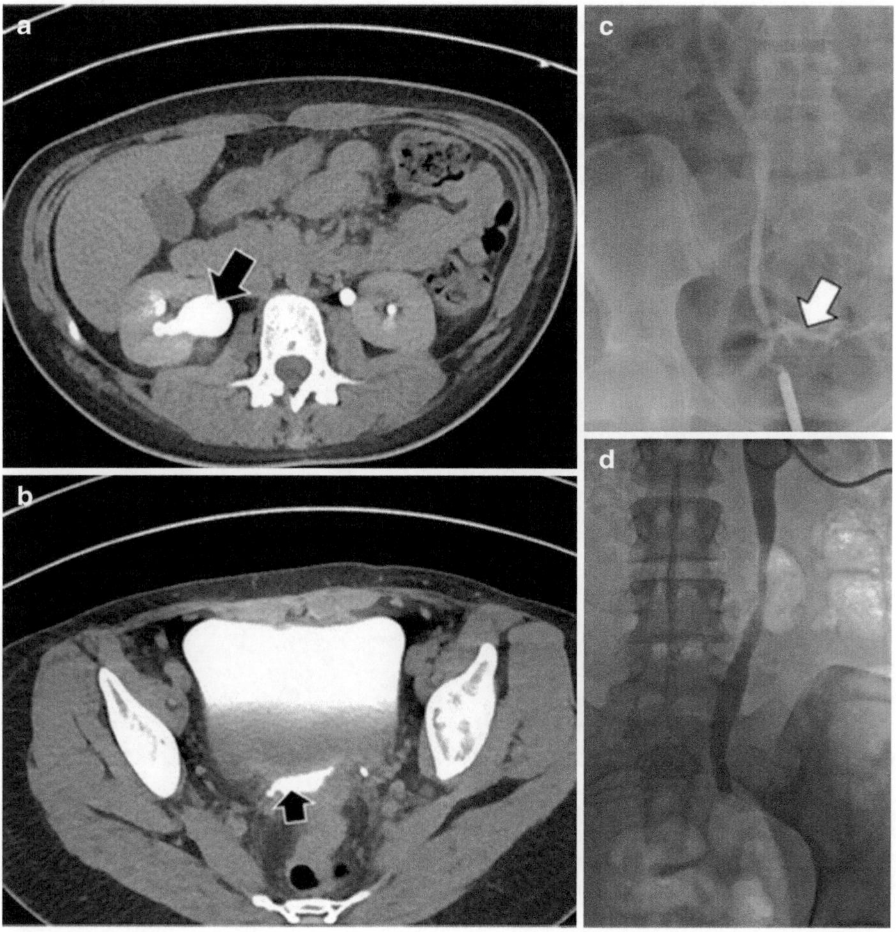

Fig. 14.1 A 50-year-old woman presents with pain and fever after transabdominal hysterectomy. Excretory-phase CTU image shows right hydronephrosis (arrow, **a**) and a leak of contrast from the right distal ureter (arrow, **b**). (**c**) Retrograde pyelography confirmed right ureteral transection with a leak of contrast (arrow) (grade 3 injury). (**d**) Antegrade pyelography after percutaneous drainage of right hydronephrosis was performed for the management of the ureteral injury. (From Alabousi A. et al. [5], with permission from Springer)

14.3 Grading

The ureteral injuries are commonly described as per their anatomic location, being at the ureteropelvic junction, abdominal, or pelvic, or according to the timing of their diagnosis, being immediate (at the time of, or shortly after, the injury), or delayed [6]. The American Association for the Surgery of Trauma (AAST) classification is very widely used for kidney injury but is seldom utilized for ureteral

Table 14.1 AAST ureter injury scale

Grade	Injury type	Description of injury	AIS 90
I	Hematoma	Contusion or hematoma without devascularization	2
II	Laceration	Less than 50% transection	2
III	Laceration	50% or greater transection	3
IV	Laceration	Complete transection with less than 2 cm of devascularization	3
V	Laceration	Avulsion with greater than 2 cm of devascularization	3

Advance one grade for bilateral lesions up to grade III
From Moore et al. [7], with permission from Elsevier

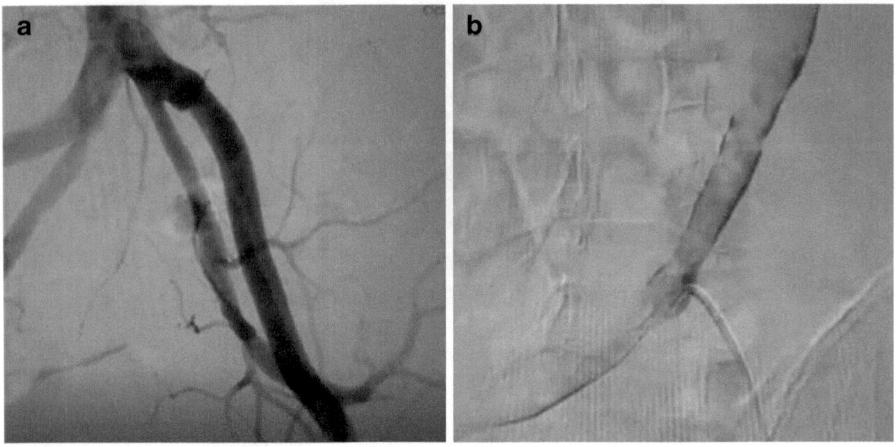

Fig. 14.2 (**a**) Left arteriogram showing contrast extravasating through the fistula tract in a 65-year-old male patient who underwent radical cystectomy with ureterocutaneostomy 15 months earlier. (**b**) The catheter entering the ureter through the fistula of the iliac artery. (From Jiang Z et al. [11]. Creative Commons Attribution 4.0 International License)

injuries and many Urologists are unfamiliar with it. It comprises the following grades [7] (Table 14.1):

Contrary to kidney trauma, the majority of reported ureteric injuries are intermediate and high grade (III and IV), but this might probably be due to underdiagnosis and underreporting of minor cases [8].

14.4 Complications of Ureteral Injury

Mild to moderate injuries caused by endourology might progress insidiously and give rise to delayed strictures with chronic hydronephrosis and progressive loss of kidney function. Serious ureteral injuries are associated with increased morbidity, hospital stay, and costs. Those subsequent to blunt or penetrating trauma are associated with higher mortality because of associated injuries to other organs. Regardless of other associated injuries, ureteral perforation alone causes anuria (if solitary kidney), uremia, urinoma, and ascites. In more severe cases, there might be abdominal compartment syndrome and death [9].

The presence of an indwelling DJ stent, major pelvic vascular or visceral surgeries may trigger an intense inflammatory response around the ureters ending in an arterio-ureteral fistula (AUF) [10, 11], a potentially life-threatening complication (Fig. 14.2). When considering all possible causes, hundreds of cases of AUF fistulae have been reported in the literature [12, 13]. A very recent comprehensive review included up to 445 patients with AUF and showed that the most common associated factors are chronic indwelling ureteral stents (80%) and a history of pelvic cancer (70%), the best diagnostic mean is angiography with 62% sensitivity, and the most predominant location is the common iliac artery ureteral crossing [14].

References

1. Medina D, Lavery R, Ross SE, Livingston DH. Ureteral trauma: preoperative studies neither predict injury nor prevent missed injuries. J Am Coll Surg. 1998;186(6):641–4. https://doi.org/10.1016/s1072-7515(98)00108-2.
2. Pereira BM, Ogilvie MP, Gomez-Rodriguez JC, Ryan ML, Peña D, Marttos AC, Pizano LR, McKenney MG. A review of ureteral injuries after external trauma. Scand J Trauma Resusc Emerg Med. 2010;18:6. https://doi.org/10.1186/1757-7241-18-6. PMID: 20128905; PMCID: PMC2830948
3. EAU Guidelines. Edn. presented at the EAU Annual Congress Amsterdam March 2022. ISBN 978-94-92671-16-5. https://d56bochluxqnz.cloudfront.net/documents/full-guideline/EAU-Guidelines-on-Urological-Trauma-2022_2022-03-24-104100_fwda.pdf.
4. Ramchandani P, Buckler PM. Imaging of genitourinary trauma. AJR Am J Roentgenol. 2009;192(6):1514–23. https://doi.org/10.2214/AJR.09.2470.
5. Alabousi A, Patlas MN, Menias CO, Dreizin D, Bhalla S, Hon M, O'Brien A, Katz DS. Multimodality imaging of the leaking ureter: why does detection of traumatic and iatrogenic ureteral injuries remain a challenge? Emerg Radiol. 2017;24(4):417–22. https://doi.org/10.1007/s10140-017-1507-5. Epub 2017 Apr 27
6. Engelsgjerd JS, LaGrange CA. Ureteral injury 2021. In: StatPearls [Internet]. Treasure Island (FL): StatPearls Publishing; 2022.
7. Moore EE, Shackford SR, Pachter HL, McAninch JW, Browner BD, Champion HR, Flint LM, Gennarelli TA, Malangoni MA, Ramenofsky ML, et al. Organ injury scaling: spleen, liver, and kidney. J Trauma. 1989;29(12):1664–6. https://doi.org/10.1016/S0039-6109(16)46589-8.
8. Best CD, Petrone P, Buscarini M, Demiray S, Kuncir E, Kimbrell B, Asensio JA. Traumatic ureteral injuries: a single institution experience validating the American Association for the Surgery of Trauma-Organ Injury Scale grading scale. J Urol. 2005;173(4):1202–5. https://doi.org/10.1097/01.ju.0000155526.37963.ef.
9. Katz R, Meretyk S, Gimmon Z. Abdominal compartment syndrome due to delayed identification of a ureteral perforation following abdomino-perineal resection for rectal carcinoma. Int J Urol. 1997;4(6):615–7. https://doi.org/10.1111/j.1442-2042.1997.tb00320.x.
10. Burks FN, Santucci RA. Management of iatrogenic ureteral injury. Ther Adv Urol. 2014;6(3):115–24. https://doi.org/10.1177/1756287214526767.
11. Jiang Z, Wang J, Cui J, et al. Arterioureteral fistula after radical cystectomy and ureterocutaneostomy: two case reports and a systematic literature review. BMC Urol. 2022;22:117. https://doi.org/10.1186/s12894-022-01071-y.
12. van den Bergh RC, Moll FL, de Vries JP, Lock TM. Arterioureteral fistulas: unusual suspects-systematic review of 139 cases. Urology. 2009;74(2):251–5. https://doi.org/10.1016/j.urology.2008.12.011. Epub 2009 Apr 10

13. Turo R, Hadome E, Somov P, Hamid B, Gulur DM, Pettersson BA, Awsare NS. Uretero-arterial fistula—not so rare? Curr Urol. 2018;12(1):54–6. https://doi.org/10.1159/000489419. Epub 2018 Jun 30. PMID: 30374282; PMCID: PMC6198778
14. Kamphorst K, Lock TMTW, van den Bergh RCN, Moll FL, de Vries JPM, Lo RTH, de Kort GAP, Bruijnen RCG, Dik P, Horenblas S, de Kort LMO. Arterio-ureteral fistula: systematic review of 445 patients. J Urol. 2022;207(1):35–43. https://doi.org/10.1097/JU.0000000000002241.

Management of Ureteral Injuries: Prevention, Conservative, and Minimally Invasive Management

15

The management of ureteral injuries depends on the causes, either iatrogenic, blunt, or penetrating trauma.

15.1 Prevention and Early Detection

This applies to iatrogenic ureteric injuries.

Obviously, in order to avoid ureteric damage during any open or laparoscopic surgery, the first critical point is to identify and clearly visualize the ureters and many techniques and tricks help achieve this goal:

1. *Pre-operative urteral catheter placement*: There is a controversy on whether the ureteric catheter prevents ureteric injury or just helps diagnose it once it has happened, or is not effective in none [1].

   A systematic review of the role of prophylactic ureteral catheters recruiting a total of 102,370 patients with ureteric stents/catheters versus 767,233 controls, without randomization, **paradoxically showed a higher rate of ureteric injuries in stented patients than in the controls**, which may retrospectively be attributed to a selection bias where the stented patients were selected based on a higher risk of ureteral injuries and more complex surgeries [2].

   A nationwide survey conducted among Swiss surgeons showed that 93.5% of them considered that ureteral stenting was useful in complex procedures, 56.9% of them admitted the use of stents at least once in the past year, and 54.5% of the participants considered only noninvasive techniques for identifying ureters in their regular daily practice [3].

   Anyway, to date, there is insufficient data to conclude about the effectiveness of the stents to decrease ureteric injury or increase intraoperative detection of ureteral injuries.

S. A. AL-Mamari, *Urogenital Trauma: A Practical Guide*,
https://doi.org/10.1007/978-981-99-6171-9_15

However, the European Association Of Urology (EAU) recommends the pre-operative prophylactic use of stents in high-risk cases (major procedures, large pelvic tumors, or history of previous surgery with distorted anatomy) [4].

Technology to enhance ureteric detection: Early clinical experience of lighted ureteral catheters was published in the mid-90s; however, they are still not widely distributed [5, 6].

A novel technology was recently introduced using stents coated with biocompatible fluorescent material (NICE: near-infrared coating of equipment) with conclusive results in pigs and human cadavers [7] (Figs. 15.1 and 15.2).

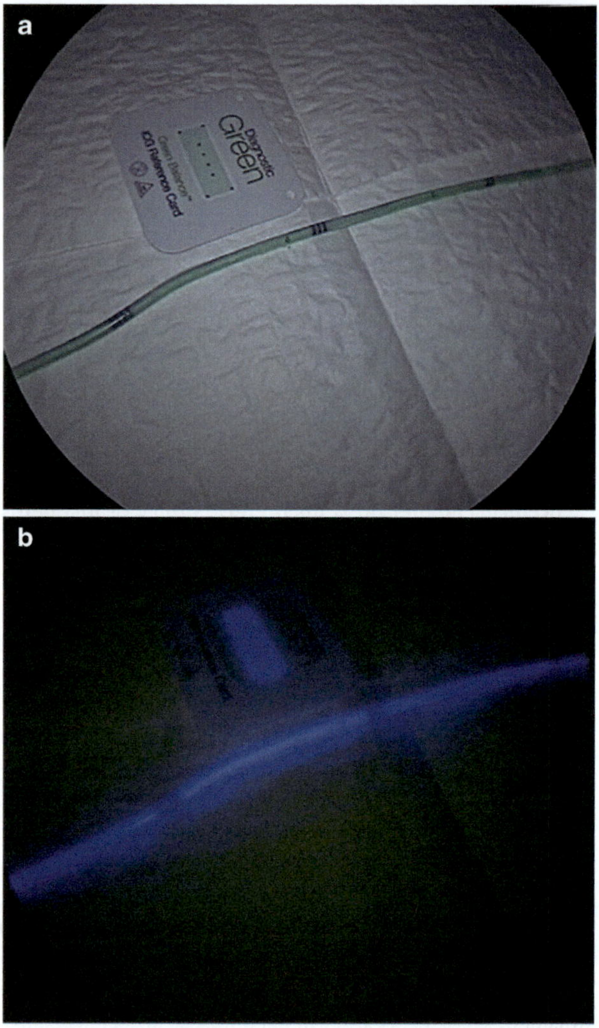

Fig. 15.1 (**a**, **b**) NICE-coated catheter demonstration under white light (**a**) and near-infrared light (**b**). (From Barberio et al. [7] Commons Creative License)

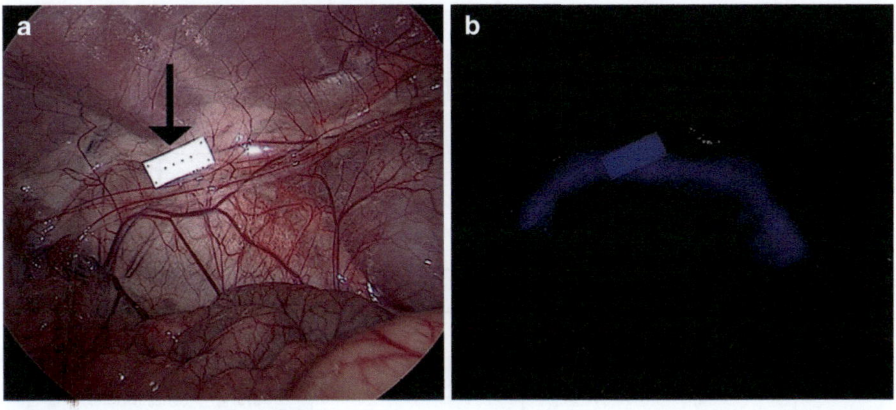

Fig. 15.2 Demonstration of a NICE-coated catheter under white light (**a**) and near-infrared mode (**b**). The arrow highlights the fluorescence reference card. Contrary to humans, the ureter is easily visible under white light in pigs due to the thin overlying tissues. (From Barberio et al. [7] Commons Creative License)

2. *No-stent tricks and technique*: Where no ureteric tube is used, the ureter may be identified through its characteristic vermiculations (peristalsis). If sluggish or at prolonged intervals, these reptations can be stimulated by gentle manual pressure, the so-called "**Kelly's sign**". There is also a promising rat model that showed perfect visualization of the ureters and their vasculatures after intravenous administration of sodium fluorescein and activation with a 530-nm light transmitter, with no stent use [8].
3. Finally, once a ureteric injury is suspected, **on-table IVP or an retrograde pyelography (RGP) or retrograde injection of methylene blue** are easy and effective diagnostic methods [9].

Regarding ureteral injuries in endourological procedures, the following recommendations should be considered [10]

- Use of small-sized instruments, i.e., to adapt the instruments to the patient's anatomy and not vice-versa.
- When the ureter is deemed narrow, leave a ureteral stent and retry the intervention after a few weeks, to allow time for passive ureteral dilatation.
- Use baskets with utmost care under direct vision.
- Fragment the ureteral stones from the center, far from the mucosa.

Abboudi et al. have suggested a practical algorithm to manage an intra-operatively suspected ureteric injury [11] (Fig. 15.3).

Notwithstanding the above recommendations of clearly visualizing the ureter to prevent injury and proceeding to its immediate repair or stenting if diagnosed intra-operatively, the situation may sometimes dictate priority to the patient survival in

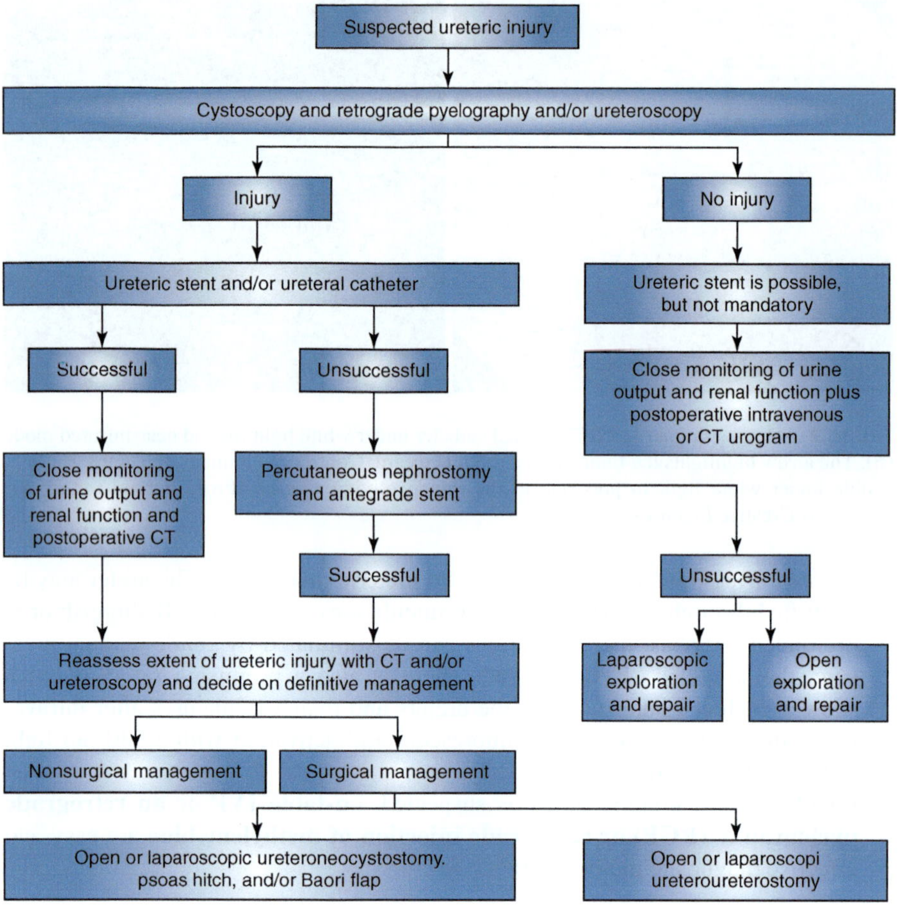

Fig. 15.3 A suggested schematic for the clinical management of an intraoperatively suspected ureteric injury. (From Abboudi H et al. [11], with permission from Springer Nature)

cases with severe bleeding and therefore a so-called **"damage-control strategy"** should be preferred, consisting of ligation of the damaged ureter and urinary diversion with a temporary nephrostomy, and a repair to be considered later [12].

15.2 Minimally Invasive Techniques in Ureteral Injury

1. **Percutaneous nephrostomy, antegrade or retrograde DJ stenting with or without balloon dilatation**: A review of post-open hysterectomy ureteral injury showed a successful first attempt stenting of 52.4% within a median time of 25 days. However, out of those who had successful stenting, only 27.3% had a resolution of the ureteral injury requiring no further intervention, and others required open delayed reconstruction [13] (Fig. 15.4a–d).

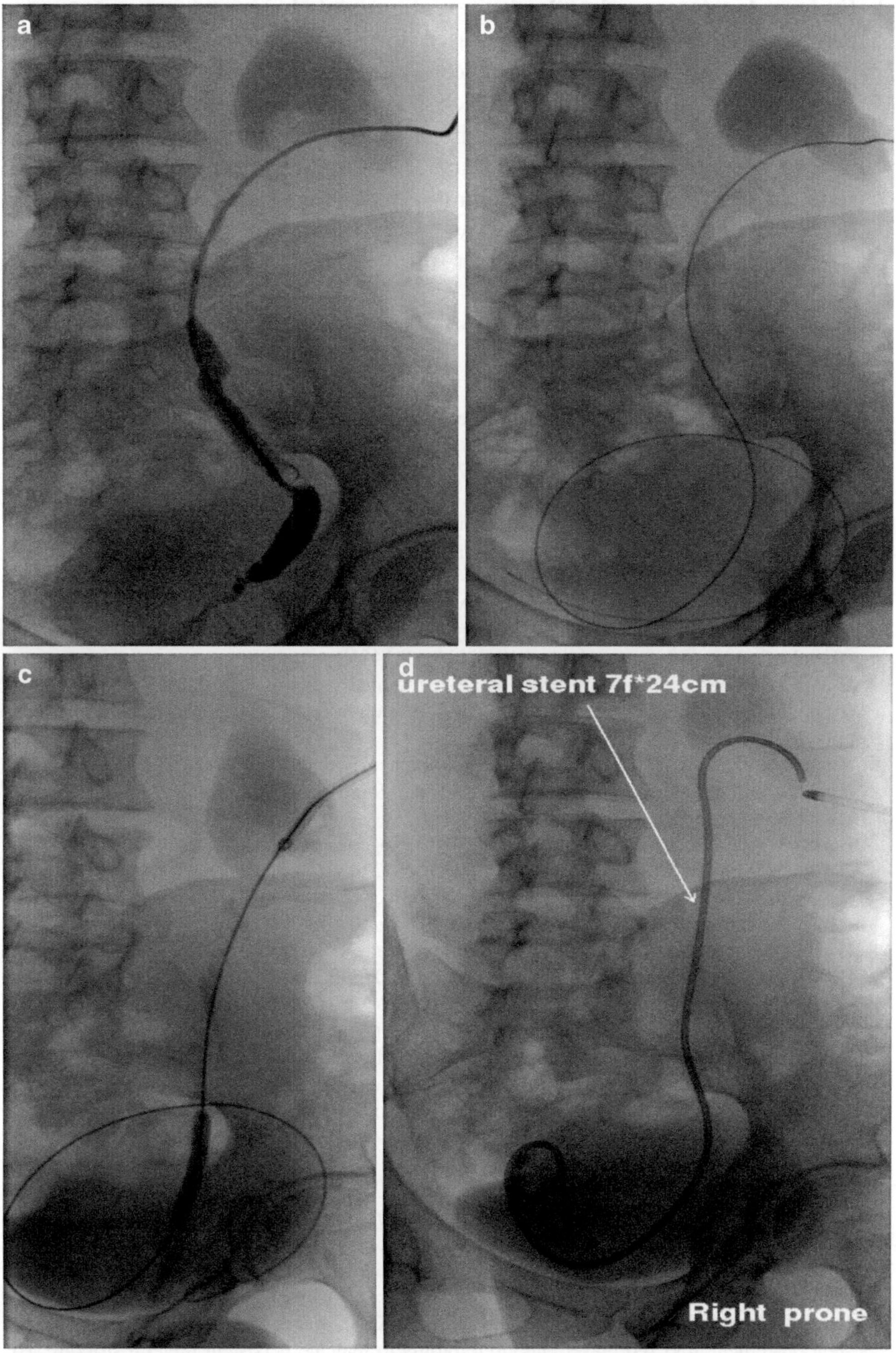

Fig. 15.4 (**a**–**d**) 38-year-old man with a history of right iatrogenic lower ureteric injury sustained during an endourological procedure. (**a**) Antegrade nephrostogram showing severely strictured distal right ureter (prone position). (**b**) Successful negotiation of a guidewire through the stricture. (**c**) Balloon dilatation of the stricture. (**d**) Successful antegrade insertion of the DJ stent. (Courtesy Mahmood Al Hajri, Interventional Radiologist, The Royal Hospital, Muscat, Sultanate of Oman)

2. **Endoureterotomy and endoscopic realignment:** Laser endoureterotomy and balloon dilatation are frequently used for short strictures with incomplete obstruction, but the risk of recurrence is very high. Scanty articles report successful results of this technique which is contraindicated in active infection, in strictures longer than 2 cm, and failure of endoureterotomy [14].

   Endoscopic realignment of the ureter has seldom been reported. A small series of eight patients with totally transected ureters showed successful results in six of them (75%) at a mean follow-up of 21.5 months. Larger series and longer follow-ups are required to validate this approach [15].

References

1. Chou MT, Wang CJ, Lien RC. Prophylactic ureteral catheterization in gynecologic surgery: a 12-year randomized trial in a community hospital. Int Urogynecol J Pelvic Floor Dysfunct. 2009;20(6):689–93. https://doi.org/10.1007/s00192-008-0788-3.
2. Croghan SM, Zaborowski A, Mohan HM, Mulvin D, McGuire BB, Murphy M, Galvin DJ, Lennon G, Quinlan D, Winter DC. The sentinel stent? A systematic review of the role of prophylactic ureteric stenting prior to colorectal resections. Int J Color Dis. 2019;34(7):1161–78. https://doi.org/10.1007/s00384-019-03314-1.
3. Douissard J, Meyer J, Ris F, Liot E, Morel P, Buchs NC. Iatrogenic ureteral injuries and their prevention in colorectal surgery: results from a nationwide survey. Color Dis. 2019;21(5):595–602. https://doi.org/10.1111/codi.14552.
4. EAU Guidelines. Edn. presented at the EAU Annual Congress Amsterdam. 2022. https://d56bochluxqnz.cloudfront.net/documents/full-guideline/EAU-Guidelines-on-Urological-Trauma-2022_2022-03-24-104100_fwda.pdf.
5. Senagore AJ, Luchtefeld M. An initial experience with lighted ureteral catheters during laparoscopic colectomy. J Laparoendosc Surg. 1994;4(6):399–403. https://doi.org/10.1089/lps.1994.4.399.
6. Burks FN, Santucci RA. Management of iatrogenic ureteral injury. Ther Adv Urol. 2014;6(3):115–24. https://doi.org/10.1177/1756287214526767.
7. Barberio M, Al-Taher M, Felli E, et al. Intraoperative ureter identification with a novel fluorescent catheter. Sci Rep. 2021;11:4501. https://doi.org/10.1038/s41598-021-84121-z.
8. Dip FD, Nahmod M, Anzorena FS, Moreira A, Sarotto L, Ampudia C, Kalaskar SN, Ferraina P, Rosenthal RJ, Wexner SD. Novel technique for identification of ureters using sodium fluorescein. Surg Endosc. 2014;28(9):2730–3. https://doi.org/10.1007/s00464-014-3519-5.
9. Delacroix SE Jr, Winters JC. Urinary tract injures: recognition and management. Clin Colon Rectal Surg. 2010;23(2):104–12. https://doi.org/10.1055/s-0030-1254297.
10. De Coninck V, Keller EX, Somani B, Giusti G, Proietti S, Rodriguez-Socarras M, Rodríguez-Monsalve M, Doizi S, Ventimiglia E, Traxer O. Complications of ureteroscopy: a complete overview. World J Urol. 2020;38(9):2147–66. https://doi.org/10.1007/s00345-019-03012-1.
11. Abboudi H, Ahmed K, Royle J, Khan MS, Dasgupta P, N'Dow J. Ureteric injury: a challenging condition to diagnose and manage. Nat Rev Urol. 2013;10:108–15.
12. Coccolini F, Moore EE, Kluger Y, et al. Kidney and uro-trauma: WSES-AAST guidelines. World J Emerg Surg. 2019;14:54. https://doi.org/10.1186/s13017-019-0274-x.
13. Morrow J, Curry D, Dooher M, Woolsey S. Minimally invasive management of delayed recognition iatrogenic ureteric injury. Ulster Med J. 2017;86(3):181–4.
14. Isogai M, Hamamoto S, Hasebe K, Iida K, Taguchi K, Ando R, Okada A, Yasui T. Dual ureteral stent placement after redo laser endoureterotomy to manage persistent ureteral stricture. IJU Case Rep. 2020;3(3):93–5. https://doi.org/10.1002/iju5.12152.
15. Liu C, Zhang X, Xue D, Liu Y, Wang P. Endoscopic realignment in the management of complete transected ureter. Int Urol Nephrol. 2014;46:335–40.

16 Reconstructive Techniques for Ureteral Injuries: Using Urinary Tract Tissues

Generally, patients presenting with penetrating wounds have associated injuries prompting urgent exploration without pre-diagnosis of any ureteral injury.

For blunt trauma, experience-based experts' opinion recommends managing severe blunt traumatic ureteral injuries **first** with minimally invasive methods such as PCN insertion and antegrade DJ stenting. Early ureteral reconstructive surgery is advised only when the patient must undergo laparotomy for associated injuries [1], and the use of ureteral stents is universally recommended after all surgical repairs [2–4] because it reduces leaks and prevents strictures.

As a general rule of thumb, injuries to the distal ureter (**caudal to the iliac vessels**) are better treated by reimplantation of the ureter into the bladder, the so-called **uretero-neocystostomy** because of the risk of impaired blood supply to the distal end, and injuries above this level are better addressed with an **end-to-end anastomosis** [2, 4].

If the ureteric injury is iatrogenic, its management further depends on whether it is diagnosed intraoperatively or not. When the injury is diagnosed intraoperatively, the management can be summarized as follows, depending on the anatomic location and the mechanism [5]:

- **Laceration or transection**: the two ends should be spatulated, then anastomosed without tension using 4/0 absorbable sutures in a watertight technique, and a **DJ stent should be left for 4–6 weeks**. This end-to-end ureteric anastomosis is technically called **ureteroureterostomy**.
- **Ligation**: The tying material should be removed, and a **DJ stent left for 4–6 weeks**. However, the ligated segment may suffer irreversible focal damage due to ischemia and develop a **secondary stricture** that should be ruled out with a follow-up imaging study (CT-urography), and treated to prevent ipsilateral renal atrophy.

S. A. AL-Mamari, *Urogenital Trauma: A Practical Guide*,
https://doi.org/10.1007/978-981-99-6171-9_16

Radiation therapy should not be forgotten among iatrogenic causes of ureteral injury. Either external beam radiation therapy (EBRT) or brachytherapy (for cervix cancer, for example) can cause ureteral ischemia, fibrosis, and stricture in a slow process that can only be diagnosed months or years after the treatment [6]. Hence, when one bears in mind this possible complication, imaging of the kidneys should be obtained for early detection of kidney and upper tract changes.

There are controversies about the timing for surgical correction of a ureteral injury discovered post-operatively. The debate is about operating immediately or placing a nephrostomy tube and waiting 6 weeks–3 months or even more until edema and inflammation subside. Some authors plead for the first attitude and others for the second [7, 8]. The debate is still on the table, and for most iatrogenic injuries, it has been suggested that the delay depends on the type and location of the ureteral injury and the general condition of the patients, the extent of the damage, and the pathologies for which the first surgery was performed (benign condition, malignancy, post-radiation, inflammatory disease). Some patients might need to be explored for immediate repair, while others might need to be kept on kidney drainage (nephrostomy), and the definitive management of the ureteral injury be deferred until optimal conditions prevail [8, 9].
Further techniques depend on the location and the extent of tissue loss.

16.1 Antegrade DJ Stenting

This is a very common procedure that should always be attempted for a short segment ureteric stricture and may be all that is needed for the treatment of the injury.

16.2 Endoureterotomy and Endoscopic Realignment

As mentioned in the previous chapter, this is seldom reported in the literature [10].

16.3 Ureteroneocystostomy

This is the technique of choice for damage to a small segment of the distal ureter, ideally 2–3 cm. It consists of a dissection of the ureter up to the injury site, then a section of the healthy ureter just proximal to the fibrotic segment which is ligated and left in situ. The healthy ureter is then spatulated and reimplanted into a different site of the bladder without tension, using a 4/0 absorbable suture material (Monocryl, Vicryl). The anastomosis should be performed in an anti-reflux way (see the techniques below) and stented for 3–6 weeks. This procedure has been successfully performed for decades using an open approach [11]. After a transient period of laparoscopic surgery which is a very challenging approach for the ureteroneocystostomy, there are now increasing reports of robotic-assisted procedures with excellent results after over a 20-month follow-up [12].

Many techniques of ureteroneocystostomy have been described in the 50s and 60s, and the main indication was then to treat patients with vesicoureteral reflux [13–18]. These techniques were further developed in the subsequent decades with the generalization of renal transplantations [19, 20], and they are generally eponymously referred to their inventors' or the first authors' names who published them. They all aim at creating a non-refluxing mechanism and can be roughly divided into two groups:

(a) *Intra-vesical technique*: Here the most famous are the Hutch technique (1952) [13] (Fig. 16.1), the Nipple or valve technique (1956) [14], the Ledbetter-Politano technique (1958) [15] (Fig. 16.2a–g), and the Taguchi technique (1971) [19] (Fig. 16.3a–d).
(b) *Extravesical technique*: The **Lich-Gregoir technique** (published by Lich et al. in 1961 [17] and by Gregoir et al. and 1964 [18]). The eponym "**de Campos Freire**" also applies to this technique since the publication of a successful Brazilian series of renal transplantation in 1974 [20] (Fig. 16.4a–i).

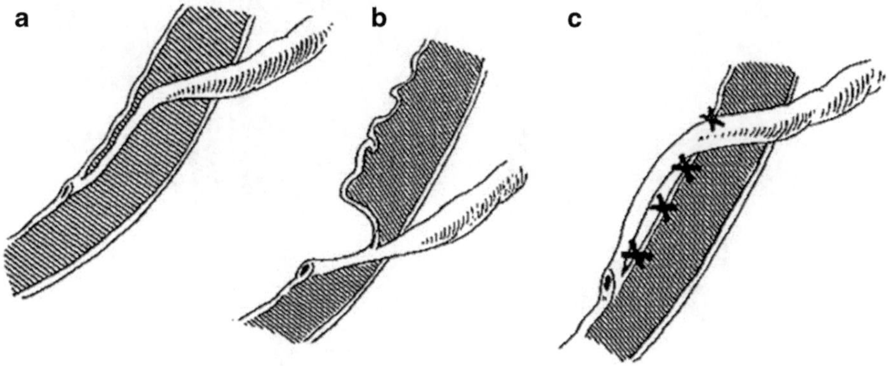

Fig. 16.1 (**a**) Course of normal ureter passing through a normal bladder. (**b**) Saccule above the ureteral orifice. Note how the course of the intramural ureter is altered. The saccule must have resulted from weakness of the detrusor muscle which normally lies under the intramural ureter. (**c**) Postoperative position of the ureter. The attachment at trigone has been preserved. A long intravesical ureter has been created. The defect in the bladder under the ureter has been firmly sutured. X marks indicate the position of the sutures. (From Hutch JA [13], with permission from Wolters Kluwer Health)

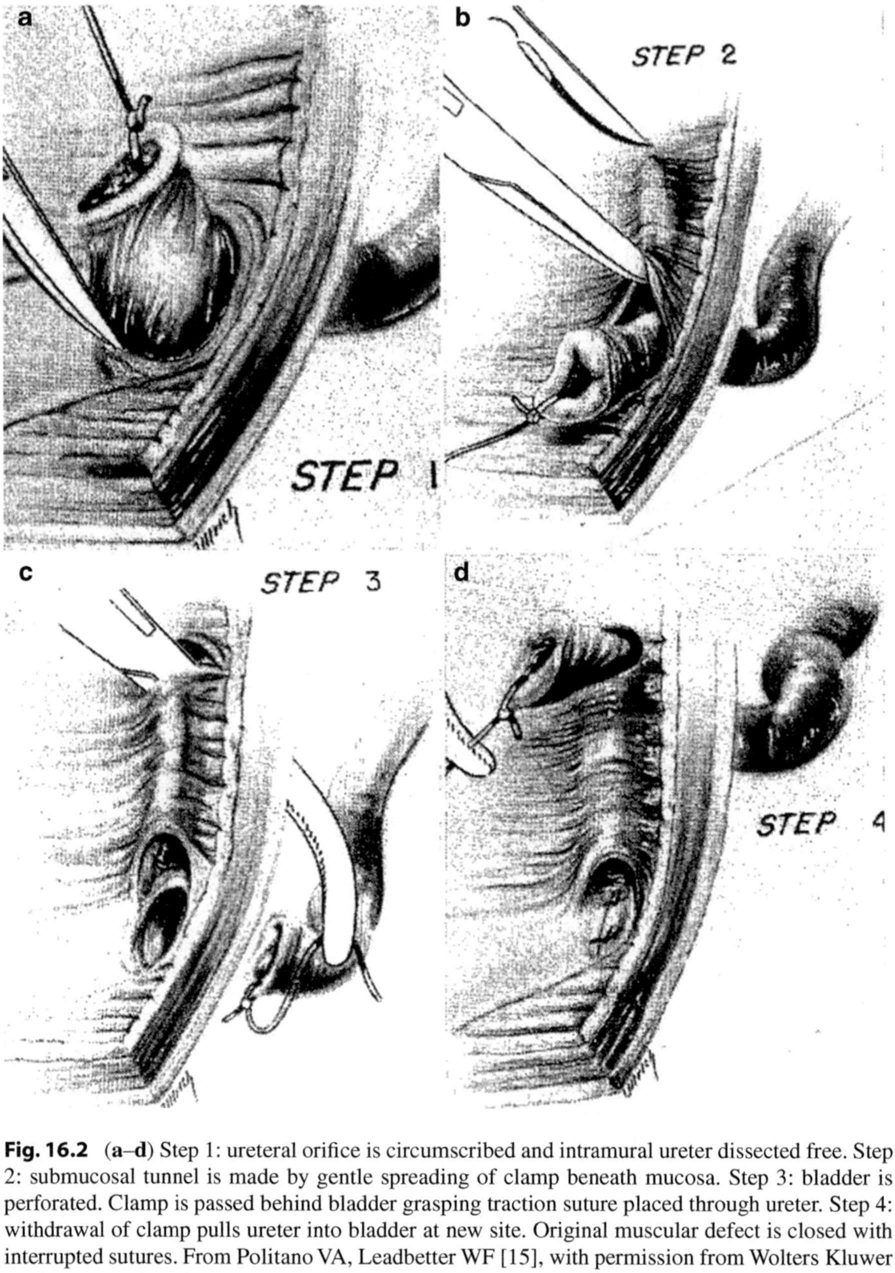

Fig. 16.2 (**a–d**) Step 1: ureteral orifice is circumscribed and intramural ureter dissected free. Step 2: submucosal tunnel is made by gentle spreading of clamp beneath mucosa. Step 3: bladder is perforated. Clamp is passed behind bladder grasping traction suture placed through ureter. Step 4: withdrawal of clamp pulls ureter into bladder at new site. Original muscular defect is closed with interrupted sutures. From Politano VA, Leadbetter WF [15], with permission from Wolters Kluwer Health. (**e–g**) Step 5: distal end of ureter is pulled through submucosal tunnel. Step 6: ureter has been pulled through tunnel and is ready for mucosa-to-mucosa anastomosis. Step 7: anastomosis completed by using several interrupted fine chromic sutures. (From Politano VA, Leadbetter WF [15], with permission from Wolters Kluwer Health)

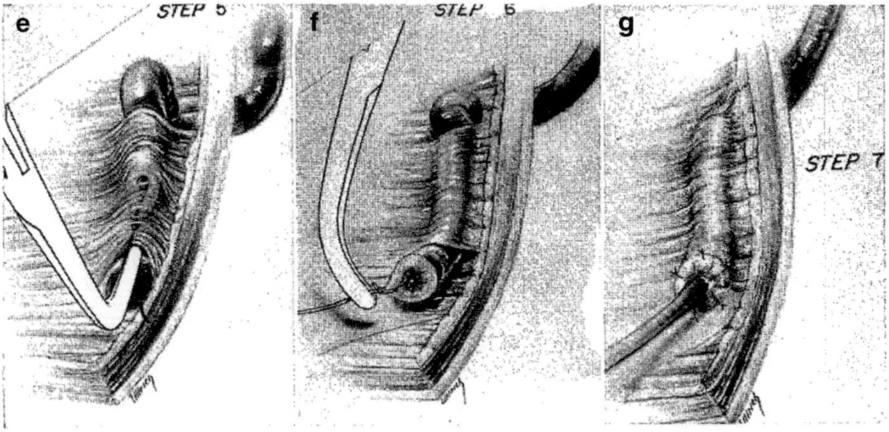

Fig. 16.2 (continued)

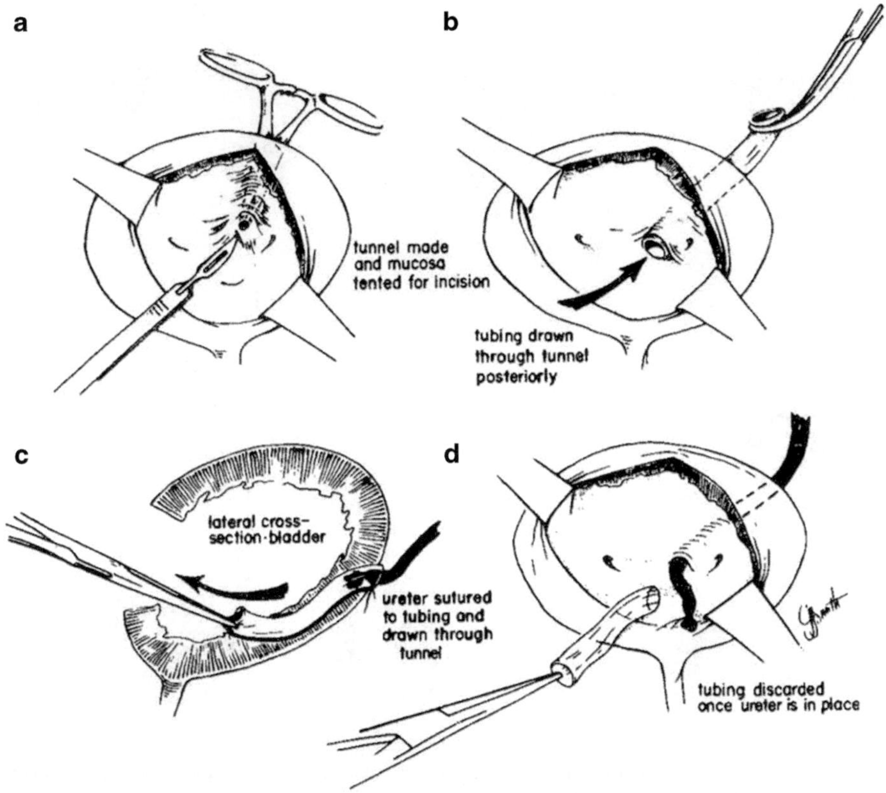

Fig. 16.3 (**a**–**d**) Technique for ureteral implantation. (From Taguchi Y et al. [19], with permission from Wolters Kluwer Health)

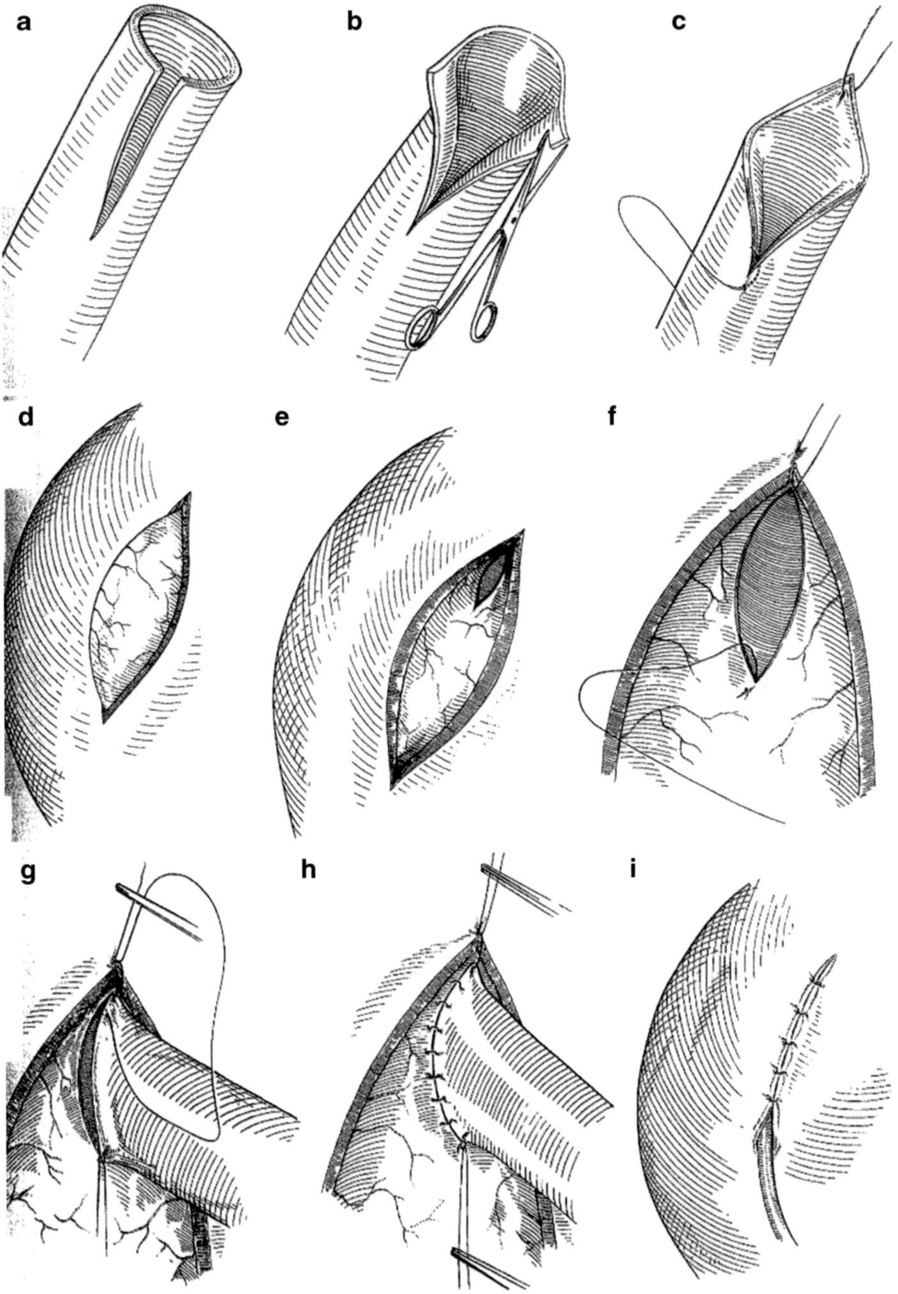

Fig. 16.4 (**a–c**) Spatulation of distal end of ureter and placement of sutures at each end of spatulated opening. (**d–f**) Preparation of muscular tunnel in the bladder. (**g–i**) Ureterovesical anastomosis and closure of muscular tunnel. (From Campos Freire Júnior et al. [20], with permission from Elsevier)

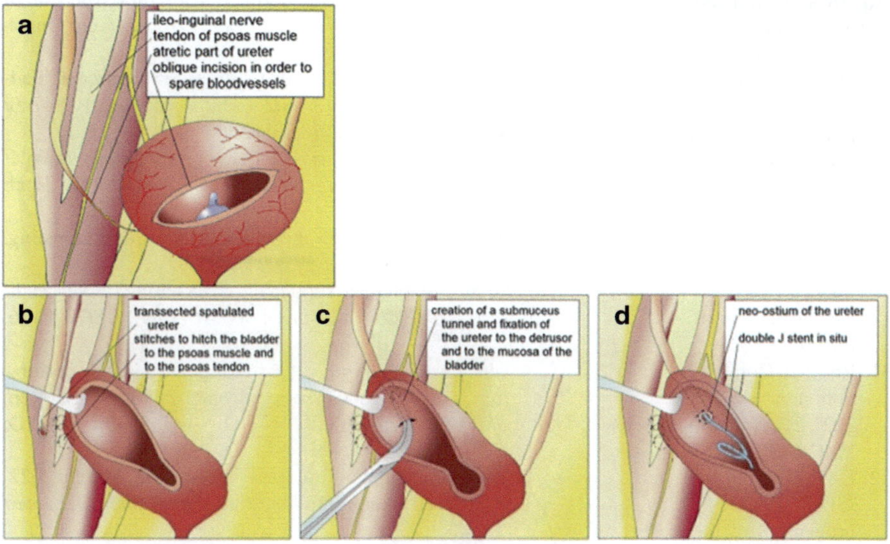

Fig. 16.5 (**a**) Mobilization of bladder dome, transection of urachus. Psoas muscles exposed. Ilioinguinal nerve identified. Oblique incision in order to spare blood vessels. (**b**) Atretic and obstructing part of ureter removed, fixation of the bladder to psoas muscles and to the tendon of the psoas muscle. (**c**) Creation of a submucosal tunnel, fixation of the ureter into the bladder wall. (**d**) Leaving a double J stent in situ. (From Groen VH et al. [25], Creative Commons License)

16.4 Psoas Hitch Associated with the Ureteroneocystostomy

This technique is reported to exist in the urology armamentarium for more than one century, having been described for the first time by Witzel in 1896 [21]. However, the name “Psoas hitch” was coined by Turner Warwick and Peter Worth in 1969 [22]. It helps to approximate the bladder to the ureter and to support the anastomosis. It is indicated when the anastomosis appears under tension and can be utilized to palliate up to a 10-cm defect of the distal ureter [23]. To be successful, this technique must ensure a tension-free anastomosis, an antireflux ureteral implantation through a long submucosal tunnel, and a straight non-kinking course of the implanted ureter at the entry point into the bladder [24]. In expert hands, the success rate of a psoas-hitch ureteroneocystostomy has been estimated to be 92–96.7% [24, 25] (Fig. 16.5a–d).

16.5 Uretero-Ureterostomy

This procedure applies to any level of the ureter provided the damaged segment is short to allow tension-free anastomosis of both ends. It also proceeds through a spatulation of both ends, the use of 4/0 absorbable suture materials, and stenting [26] (Fig. 16.6). It has traditionally been performed through an open approach. Nowadays many centers are publishing successful results using laparoscopic and robotic approaches. It is a

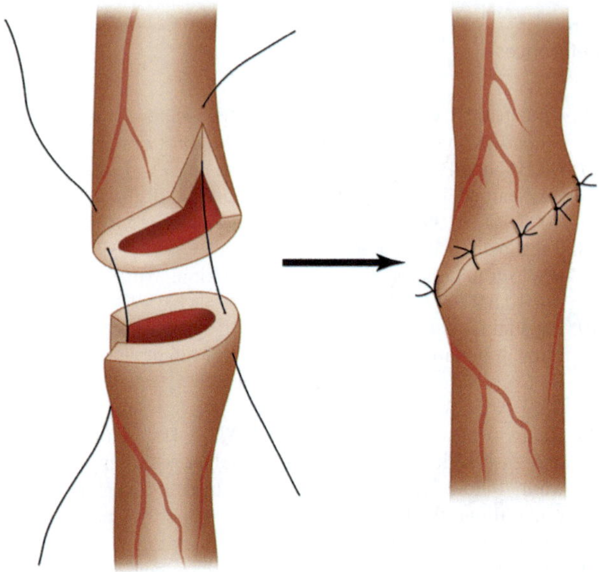

Fig. 16.6 Spatulated, end-to-end anastomosis of the ureter using interrupted absorbable, synthetic suture. (From Shah NL and Fred Muhletaler M [26], with permission from Springer Nature)

valuable approach for various indications (malignancy, trauma) provided the defect doesn't exceed 5 cm and was recently shown to have a high success rate (95%) in terms of kidney protection after a median follow-up time of 62 months [27].

16.6 Ureterocalycostomy

This technique can be understood as the proximal counterpart of a ureteroneocytostomy. However, it is a far rarer and more complex procedure. **Its traditional indication is a congenital pelvi-ureteric obstruction with an intra-renal pelvis**. Yet, it can also be helpful in injured PUJ and proximal ureter where there is no possibility of an end-to-end anastomosis (uretero-ureterostomy) with the distal healthy ureter. The latter is then anastomosed to the lower calyx using a 4/0 absorbable suture. A 73–90% success rate was published in various series [28, 29].

16.7 Boari Flap

This eponym has been given after **Achille Boari**, an Italian Urological surgeon in Ferrara (North Italy) who dedicated his career to surgery. He first described the technique of bladder flap on a dog to palliate a large loss of the lower ureter in 1894 [30, 31]. It took nearly 40 years more until this canine experience was revived by **Spies et al.** in 1933 at the Yale Institute [32]. The first human experience is attributed to **Nelse Ockerblad** who performed this technique on a 44-year-old woman in 1936 in Kansas City (Missouri). Hereafter is the encouraging message left by N. Ockerblad to posterity while publishing his case in 1947 after the successful completion of his surgery and an uneventful 10-year follow-up [33]:

I believe I was the first to make use of this ingenious flap method of performing a ureteral implantation into the bladder in a human being. It is a method which is practical and can be used whenever the ureter is too short to be implanted by any of the better-known procedures. It does not seem to matter how the bladder flaps are made, nor just where the base of the flap is located, nor yet the direction the flap may take. The flap should not be too narrow as it will shrink. There seems to be ample blood supply.

While paying tribute to Dr. N. Ockerblad for this great and exceptional surgical and artistic achievement and saluting his optimism, his positive attitude, and his inspiring message, we should at the same time temper his exaltation because the size and position of the base to achieve a good length and the direction of the flap are important aspects in the final success of the reconstruction (see further discussion below).

The flap is indicated for defects of around 5–10 cm and is traditionally utilized for distal or mid-ureteric damage [34] (Figs. 16.7, 16.8a–c). However, cases have been published of extended Boari flaps reaching the upper ureter and even replacing a panureteric stricture up to the renal pelvis [35–37] (Figs. 16.9, 16.10, and 16.11).

The advantage of the bladder flap is to avoid bowel-related complications. **A minimum of 4 cm of the flap base breadth is required to maintain a good blood supply of the flap and the ratio length/base should not exceed 3**. If a greater length of the flap is desired, a useful artifice consists of fashioning an oblique or "S" shaped flap [36]. Also, a good bladder capacity is a prerequisite for Boari flap as the subtraction of

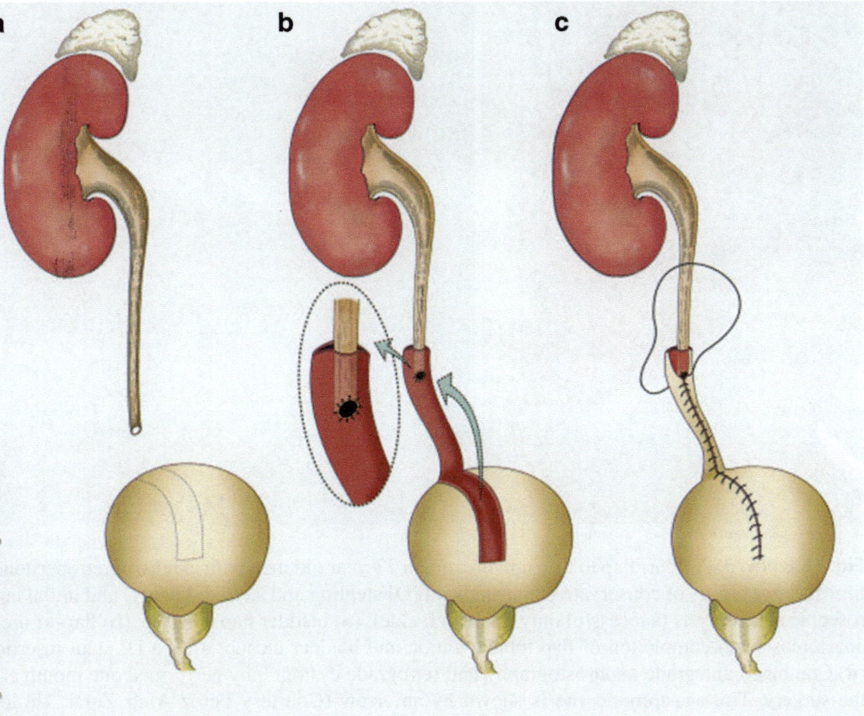

Fig. 16.7 Boari flap. (From Pereira BM et al. [34]. Creative Commons Attribution License)

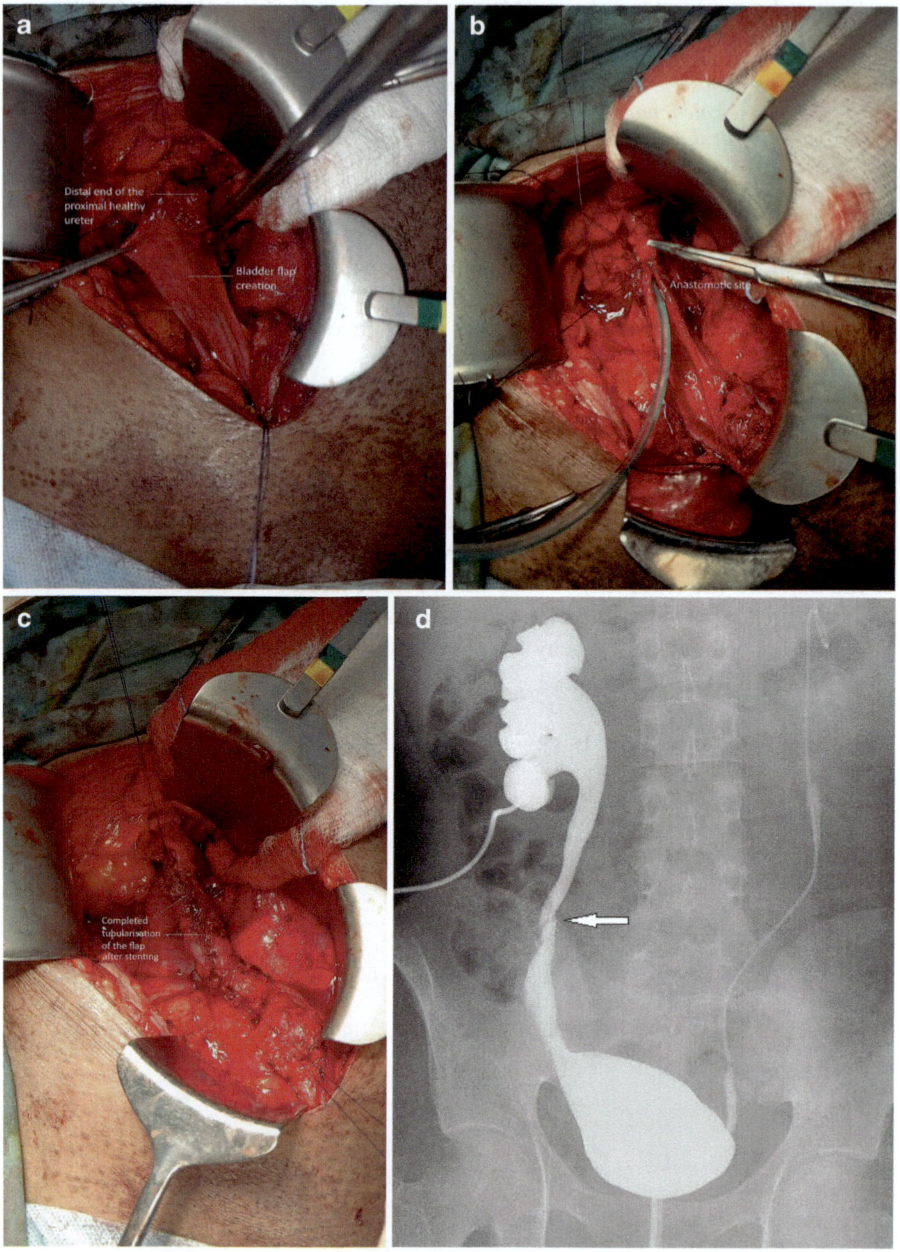

Fig. 16.8 (**a**–**d**) A Boari flap to the right ureter in a 22-year old man with extensive retroperitoneal fibrosis after failure of conservative management (DJ stenting and steroid therapy) and initial laparoscopic adhesiolysis (successful only on the left side). (**a**) bladder flap creation, (**b**) flap-to-ureter anastomosis, (**c**) completion of flap tubularization and bladder closure after a DJ stent insertion. (**d**) Combined antegrade nephrostography and retrograde cystography performed one month after the surgery. The anastomotic site is shown by an arrow (Courtesy Feroz Amir Zafar, Urology Department, The Royal Hospital, Muscat, Oman)

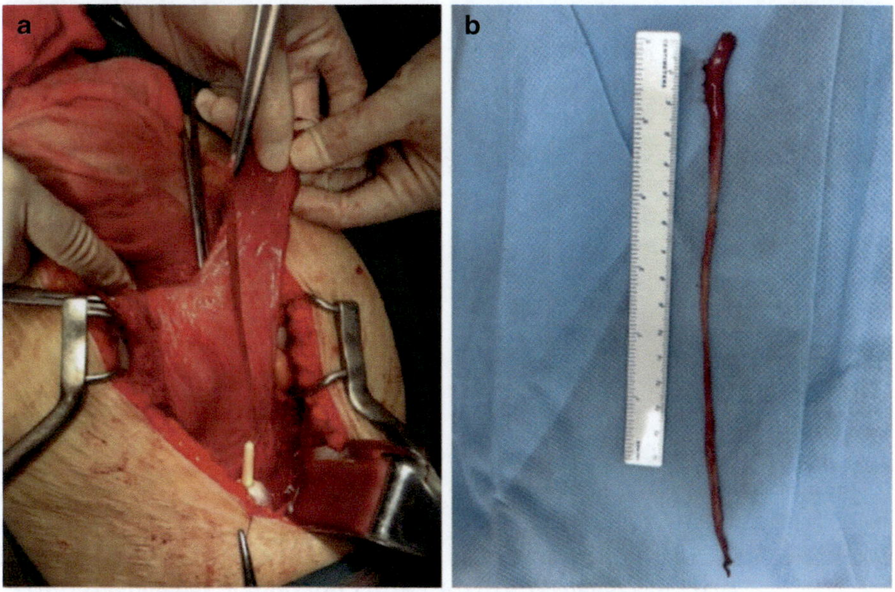

DOI: 10.12998/wjcc.v10.i34.12610 **Copyright** ©The Author(s) 2022.

Fig. 16.9 A completely avulsed ureter. (**a**) A long isolated devitalized ureter was noticed within the bladder intraoperatively. (**b**) The full-length avulsed ureter. (From Zhong MZ et al. [37], with permission from the Authors)

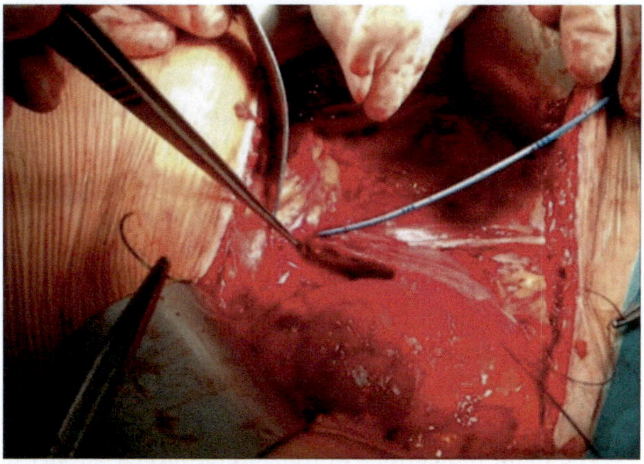

Fig. 16.10 Intraoperative view of an extended Boari flap procedure. (From Grzegółkowski P et al. [35], with permission from the Polish Urological Association)

the flap will inevitably reduce the initial capacity. And when one wants to create a very long flap (e.g., 20–22 cm), the bladder capacity should not be inferior to 300 mL [36].

When performing a Boari flap, renal mobilization with downward nephropexy can be useful to help increase the chance of tension-free anastomosis in proximal ureteric injuries [38]. Failure of a Boari flap is generally attributed to the compromised blood supply and will manifest as necrosis, stricture, or dehiscence at the anastomotic site.

There are increasing reports on successful performances of Boari flaps using laparoscopic or robotic-assisted approaches [39].

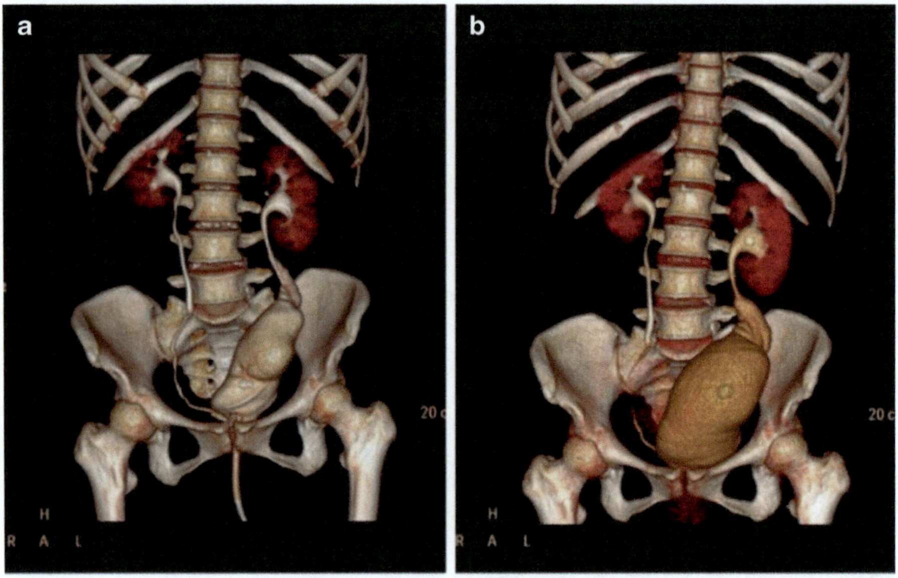

DOI: 10.12998/wjcc.v10.i34.12610 **Copyright** ©The Author(s) 2022.

Fig. 16.11 Postoperative computed tomography urography. (**a**, **b**) Computed tomography urography three-dimensional reconstruction at 14 days (**a**) and 2 months postoperatively (**b**). Note that bladder volume is visibly larger at 2 months postoperatively. (From Zhong MZ et al. [37], with permission from the Authors)

16.8 Transuretero-Ureterostomy

The first clinical experience of this technique has been described by Charles C. Higgins in 1935 in a 25-year-old man [40] and the first series was published by Hodges et al. in 1963 reporting on a total of 32 patients [41].

It consists of the transposition of one ureter whose distal part is damaged to the contralateral counterpart in an end-to-side manner. It is performed transperitoneally after an oblique opening of the mesentery of the small bowel through an avascular line to access the retroperitoneum. A study has shown that the rate of transposition is almost balanced between both directions (right to left in 47.6% and left to right in 52.4%) and showed sustained improvement of the renal function and 96.4% patency of the anastomosis after a mean follow-up of nearly 6 years [42].

The main indications of transureteroureterostomy are: long lower ureteric stricture, proximal ureteric stricture, ectopic ureter, iatrogenic or traumatic lower ureteric injuries, malignant lesions of the pelvis (prostate, bladder, gynecological, colorectal, liposarcoma, etc.) invading the lower ureter, [42, 43].

Rare indications include: ectopic ureter, ureteric duplication, small capacity bladder (following excision of large diverticulae, posterior urethral valves, gross vesicoureteric reflux) requiring ureteric reimplantation (anticipating an inadequate space to tunnel both ureters in the bladder wall), dilated ureters with non-compliant bladder (here the distal part of the donor ureter can be used to augment the bladder and function as a catheterizable conduit, and its proximal part will be anastomosed to the recipient counterpart) [43].

The contraindications of transureteroureterostomy include a history of extensive pelvic irradiation, the presence of reflux or distal partial obstruction of the recipient's ureter, retroperitoneal fibrosis with the risk of reduced vascular supply to the anastomotic site, unsolved calculus disease on either side and marked size disparity between the two ureters, especially when the recipient one is smaller than the donor [44].

Sandoz et al. have preconized the following golden principles for a successful transureteroureterostomy: site of the anastomosis at 2–4 cm above the pelvic brim (here the ureters are closer to each other and the recipient ureter has a straight course at this point), a minimum of 1.5 cm for the recipient ureterostomy parallel to the line of the ureter, preservation of the periureteric fat on the recipient side to prevent adhesions, postoperative retroperitoneal drainage, preservation of a good blood supply to the donor ureter which should join the recipient counterpart tangentially rather than perpendicularly, and insertion of a ureteral stent [44, 45] (Figs. 16.12, 16.13, 16.14, and 16.15a, b).

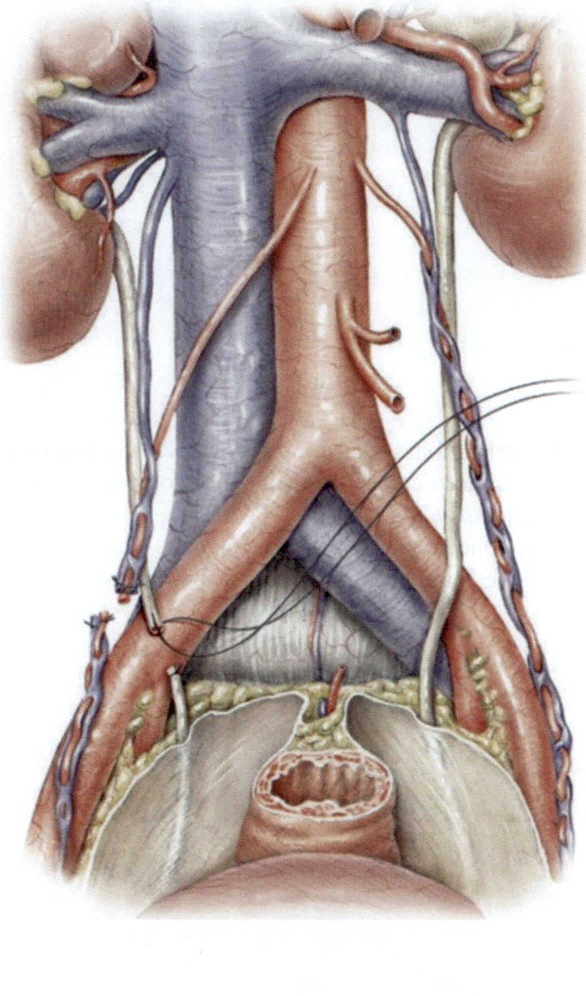

Fig. 16.12 The donor ureter is ligated distally and divided proximal to the ligature. The ureter is spatulated on its medial surface to create a 2-cm opening and tagged with a stay suture that will be used for gentle traction. The donor ureter is dissected proximally. **The gonadal vessels are divided between ligatures so they will swing medially with the donor ureter**. The donor ureter is swung over the great vessels towards the recipient ureter. (From Barry JM [45], with permission from John Wiley and Sons)

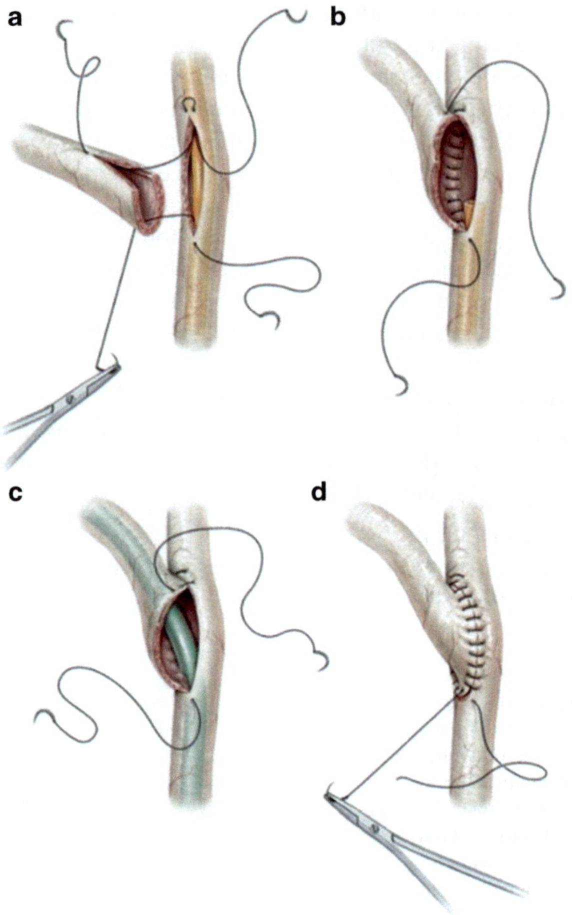

Fig. 16.13 (a–d) 5/0 monofilament stay sutures are placed side-by-side in the recipient ureter at the proposed longitudinal ureterotomy. The recipient ureter is incised with a no. 15 blade and the incision is extended with Pott scissors to match the opening in the donor ureter; 5/0 absorbable monofilament sutures are placed at either end of the recipient ureterotomy and into the heel and toe of the donor ureter. The anastomosis is started posteriorly and completed by a running 5/0 absorbable suture over a DJ stent. (From Barry JM [45], with permission from John Wiley and Sons)

Complications: Anastomotic leak, sepsis, fibrosis, reflux to the recipient side kidney, uretero-cutaneous fistula, anastomotic stricture, and hydronephrosis on the unaffected side [44, 46].

The concern of placing the opposite contralateral healthy ureter at risk must always be borne in mind and one must consider performing this technique when

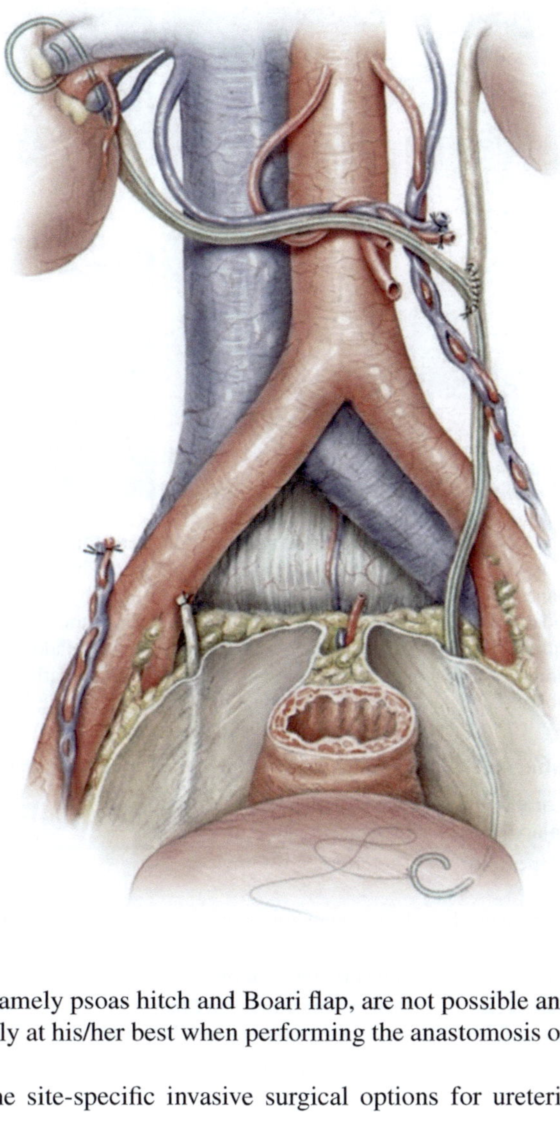

Fig. 16.14 General view after the anastomosis. (From Barry JM [45], with permission from John Wiley and Sons)

other less risky approaches, namely psoas hitch and Boari flap, are not possible and the surgeon must be technically at his/her best when performing the anastomosis on the non-diseased ureter.

Table 16.1 summarizes the site-specific invasive surgical options for ureteric injury/stricture [47].

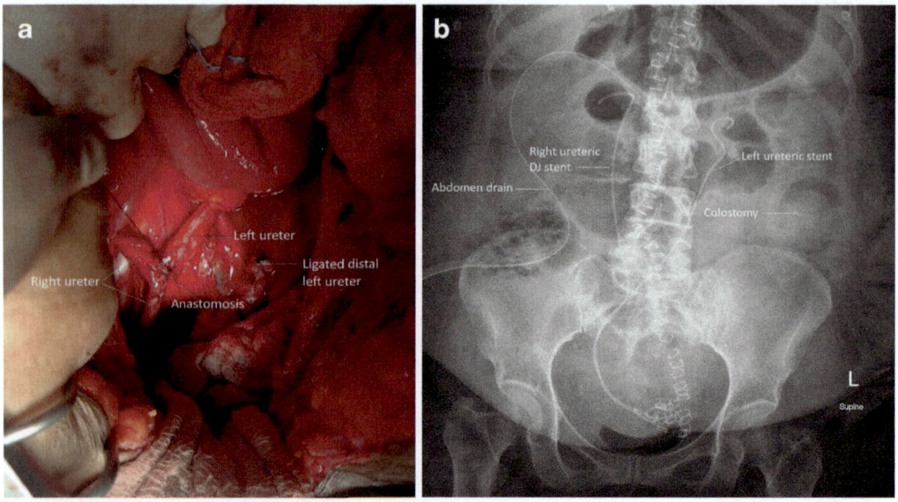

Fig. 16.15 (**a**–**b**) Left-to-right transureteroureterostomy in a 50-year-old woman with metastatic rectal carcinoma after extensive palliative and cytoreductive surgery (left hemicolectomy and permanent colostomy). The carcinoma was invading and obstructing a long segment of the left mid and distal ureter. The healthy proximal left ureter was too short for a uretero-vesical reimplantation and a Boari flap was not considered an option as the bladder capacity was small with concern of tumour infiltration of the posterior wall. (**a**) An intraoperative view after completion of the anastomosis. (**b**) A post-operative abdomen radiography showing DJ stents inserted into both ureters

Table 16.1 Site-specific management options for ureteral injuries

Location of injury	First-line repair options	Second-line repair options
Upper third	Ureteroureterostomy	Transureteroureterostomy; ureterocalycostomy
Middle third	Ureteroureterostomy	Transureteroureterostomy; Boari flap
Lower third	Direct reimplantation	Psoas hitch
Complete ureteral loss	Ileal interposition (see Chap. 17); autotransplantation (see Chap. 18)	Nephrectomy

From Abboudi H et al. [47], with permission from Springer Nature

References

1. Mendonca SJ, Jessica Pan SM, Li G, Brandes SB. Real-world practice patterns favor minimally invasive methods over ureteral reconstruction in the initial treatment of severe blunt ureteral trauma: a National Trauma Data Bank Analysis. J Urol. 2021;205(2):470–6. https://doi.org/10.1097/JU.0000000000001347. Epub 2020 Sep 8
2. Coccolini F, Moore EE, Kluger Y, et al. Kidney and uro-trauma: WSES-AAST guidelines. World J Emerg Surg. 2019;14:54. https://doi.org/10.1186/s13017-019-0274-x.
3. EAU Guidelines. Edn. presented at the EAU Annual Congress Amsterdam March 2022. ISBN 978-94-92671-16-5. https://d56bochluxqnz.cloudfront.net/documents/full-guideline/EAU-Guidelines-on-Urological-Trauma-2022_2022-03-24-104100_fwda.pdf.

4. Morey AF, Brandes S, Dugi DD 3rd, et al. Urotrauma: AUA guideline. J Urol. 2014;192:327. (amended 2020)
5. Delacroix SE Jr, Winters JC. Urinary tract injures: recognition and management. Clin Colon Rectal Surg. 2010;23(2):104–12. https://doi.org/10.1055/s-0030-1254297.
6. Fokdal L, Tanderup K, Pötter R, Sturdza A, Kirchheiner K, Chargari C, Jürgenliemk-Schulz IM, Segedin B, Tan LT, Hoskin P, Mahantshetty U, Bruheim K, Rai B, Kirisits C, Lindegaard JC, EMBRACE Collaborative Group. Risk factors for ureteral stricture after radiochemotherapy including image guided adaptive brachytherapy in cervical cancer: results from the EMBRACE studies. Int J Radiat Oncol Biol Phys. 2019;103(4):887–94. https://doi.org/10.1016/j.ijrobp.2018.11.006. Epub 2018 Nov 10
7. Onwudiegwu U, Makinde O, Badejo O, Okonofua F, Ogunniyi S. Ureteric injuries associated with gynecologic surgery. Int J Gynecol Obstet. 1991;34:235–8. https://doi.org/10.1016/0020-7292(91)90355-9.
8. Wijaya T, Lo TS, Jaili S, Wu P-Y. The diagnosis and management on ureteric injury after laparoscopy. Gynecol Minim Invasive Ther. 2015;4:29. https://doi.org/10.1016/j.gmit.2015.02.003.
9. Lee RA, Symmonds RE. Ureterovaginal fistula. Am J Obstet Gynecol. 1971;109(7):1032–5. https://doi.org/10.1016/0002-9378(71)90286-9.
10. Liu C, Zhang X, Xue D, Liu Y, Wang P. Endoscopic realignment in the management of complete transected ureter. Int Urol Nephrol. 2014;46:335–40.
11. Paick JS, Hong SK, Park MS, Kim SW. Management of postoperatively detected iatrogenic lower ureteral injury: should ureteroureterostomy really be abandoned? Urology. 2006;67(2):237–41. https://doi.org/10.1016/j.urology.2005.08.041. Epub 2006 Jan 25
12. Dirie NI, Wang S. Robot-assisted laparoscopic ureteroneocystostomy in adults: a single surgeon experience and literature review. Asian J Urol. 2020;7(1):37–44. https://doi.org/10.1016/j.ajur.2019.10.005.
13. Hutch JA. Vesico-ureteral reflux in the paraplegic: cause and correction. J Urol. 1952;68(2):457–69. https://doi.org/10.1016/s0022-5347(17)68223-5.
14. Flynn P, Goodwin WE, Grey DN. Experimental methods of ureteroneocystostomy: experiences with the ureteral intussusception to produce a nipple or valve. Trans West Sect Am Urol Assoc. 1956;23:129–38. discussion, 139
15. Politano VA, Leadbetter WF. An operative technique for the correction of vesicoureteral reflux. J Urol. 1958;79(6):932–41. https://doi.org/10.1016/s0022-5347(17)66369-9.
16. Paquin AJ Jr. Ureterovesical anastomosis: the description and evaluation of a technique. J Urol. 1959;82:573–83. https://doi.org/10.1016/s0022-5347(17)65934-2.
17. Lich R Jr, Howerton LW, Davis LA. Recurrent urosepsis in children. J Urol. 1961;86:554. https://doi.org/10.1016/S0022-5347(17)65219-4.
18. Gregoir W, Vanregemorter G. Le Reflux vesico-ureteral congenital [congenital vesico-ureteral reflux]. Urol Int. 1964;18:122–36. https://doi.org/10.1159/000279233.
19. Taguchi Y, Klauber GT, MacKinnon KJ. Implantation of transplant ureters: a technique. J Urol. 1971;105(2):194–5. https://doi.org/10.1016/s0022-5347(17)61491-5.
20. de Campos FG Jr, de Góes GM, de Campos Freire JG. Extravesical ureteral implantation in kidney transplantation. Urology. 1974;3(3):304–8. https://doi.org/10.1016/s0090-4295(74)80108-1.
21. Witzel O. Extraperitoneale ureterocystostomie mit schragkanalbildung. Zentralbl Gynakol. 1896;20:296–303.
22. Warwick RT, Worth PH. The psoas bladder-hitch procedure for the replacement of the lower third of the ureter. Br J Urol. 1969;41(6):701–9. https://doi.org/10.1111/j.1464-410x.1969.tb09981.x.
23. Manassero F, Mogorovich A, Fiorini G, Di Paola G, De Maria M, Selli C. Ureteral reimplantation with psoas bladder hitch in adults: a contemporary series with long-term followup. Sci World J. 2012;2012:379316. https://doi.org/10.1100/2012/379316. Epub 2012 Jul 31. PMID: 22919311; PMCID: PMC3417182
24. Riedmiller H, Becht E, Hertle L, Jacobi G, Hohenfellner R. Psoas-hitch ureteroneocystostomy: experience with 181 cases. Eur Urol. 1984;10:145–50. https://doi.org/10.1159/000463777.

25. Groen VH, Lock MTWT, de Angst IB, et al. Psoas hitch procedure in 166 adult patients: the largest cohort study before the laparoscopic era. BJUI Compass. 2021;2:331–7. https://doi.org/10.1111/bco2.85.
26. Shah NL, Fred Muhletaler M. Kidney and ureter. In: Skandalakis LJ, editor. Surgical anatomy and technique. Cham: Springer; 2021. https://doi.org/10.1007/978-3-030-51313-9_25.
27. Pisters PW, Ranasinghe W, Wei W, et al. Long-term renal functional outcomes following ureteroureterostomy performed during multi-organ resection for non-urothelial cancers. BJUI Compass. 2021;2:348–54. https://doi.org/10.1111/bco2.88.
28. Mesrobian HG, Kelalis PP. Ureterocalicostomy: indications and results in 21 patients. J Urol. 1989;142(5):1285–7. https://doi.org/10.1016/s0022-5347(17)39058-4.
29. Osman T, Eltahawy I, Fawaz K, Shoeib M, Elshawaf H, El Halaby R. Ureterocalicostomy for treatment of complex cases of ureteropelvic junction obstruction in adults. Urology. 2011;78(1):202–7. https://doi.org/10.1016/j.urology.2011.01.044. Epub 2011 Mar 25
30. Boari A. Contribute sperementalc alla plastica delle uretere. Atti Accad Med Ferrara. 1894;14:444.
31. Graziano ME, Thompson P. The story of the Boari flap. J Urol. 2008;179:309–9.
32. Spies JW, Yermooten VD, Wilson CS. Ureterovesical anastomosis: an experimental study. Proc Soc Exp Biol Med. 1933;30(4):426–7. https://doi.org/10.3181/00379727-30-6510.
33. Ockerblad NF. Reimplantation of the ureter into the bladder by a flap method. J Urol. 1947;57(5):845–7. https://doi.org/10.1016/s0022-5347(17)69714-3.
34. Pereira BM, Ogilvie MP, Gomez-Rodriguez JC, Ryan ML, Peña D, Marttos AC, Pizano LR, McKenney MG. A review of ureteral injuries after external trauma. Scand J Trauma Resusc Emerg Med. 2010;18:6. https://doi.org/10.1186/1757-7241-18-6. PMID: 20128905; PMCID: PMC2830948
35. Grzegółkowski P, Lemiński A, Słojewski M. Extended Boari-flap technique as a reconstruction method of total ureteric avulsion. Cent Eur J Urol. 2017;70:188–91.
36. Rajaian S, Murugavaithianathan P, Krishnamurthy K, Murugasen L. Extended Boari-flap reconstruction in isolated tuberculous pan-ureteral stricture. Urol Ann. 2020;12(1):87–9. https://doi.org/10.4103/UA.UA_165_18.
37. Zhong MZ, Huang WN, Huang GX, Zhang EP, Gan L. Long-term results of extended Boari flap technique for management of complete ureteral avulsion: a case report. World J Clin Cases. 2022;10(34):12610–6. https://doi.org/10.12998/wjcc.v10.i34.12610. PMID: 36579100; PMCID: PMC9791534
38. Mauck RJ, Hudak SJ, Terlecki RP, Morey AF. Central role of Boari bladder flap and downward nephropexy in upper ureteral reconstruction. J Urol. 2011;186(4):1345–9. https://doi.org/10.1016/j.juro.2011.05.086.
39. White C, Stifelman M. Ureteral reimplantation, psoas hitch, and Boari flap. J Endourol. 2020;34(S1):S25–30. https://doi.org/10.1089/end.2018.0750.
40. Higgins C. Transureteroureteral anastomosis: report of a clinical case. J Urol. 1935;34:349.
41. Hodges CV, Moore RJ, Lehman TH, Behnam AM. Clinical experiences with transureteroureterostomy. J Urol. 1963;90:552–62. https://doi.org/10.1016/s0022-5347(17)64453-7.
42. Iwaszko MR, Krambeck AE, Chow GK, Gettman MT. Transureteroureterostomy revisited: long-term surgical outcomes. J Urol. 2010;183(3):1055–9. https://doi.org/10.1016/j.juro.2009.11.031. Epub 2010 Jan 21
43. Manjunath DA, Radhakrishna V, Vepakomma D. Transureteroureterostomy in children: a retrospective study. Am J Clin Exp Urol. 2021;9(2):163–9. Published 2021 Apr 15
44. Sandoz IL, Paull DP, MacFarlane CA. Complications with transureteroureterostomy. J Urol. 1977;117(1):39–42. https://doi.org/10.1016/s0022-5347(17)58329-9.
45. Barry JM. Surgical atlas transureteroureterostomy. BJU Int. 2005;96(1):195–201. https://doi.org/10.1111/j.1464-410X.2005.05552.x.
46. Ehrlich RM, Skinner DG. Complications of transureteroureterostomy. J Urol. 1975;113(4):467–73. https://doi.org/10.1016/s0022-5347(17)59502-6.
47. Abboudi H, Ahmed K, Royle J, et al. Ureteric injury: a challenging condition to diagnose and manage. Nat Rev Urol. 2013;10:108–15. https://doi.org/10.1038/nrurol.2012.254.

Reconstructive Techniques for Ureteral Injuries: Using Extra-Urinary Autologous Tissues

17

Here the humans' genius has crossed a milestone compared to all the previously described techniques. Now it is not about reconstructing the urinary tract with other urinary tissues, but it is about utilizing non-urinary autologous materials to achieve this goal. Many candidate grafts have been tried for this purpose including fallopian tubes in females, blood vessels, fashioned peritoneal tubes, etc. but all failed.

The French Surgeon Chaput published an experience of uretero-colic anastomosis to treat a uretero-vaginal fistula in 1893 [1]. This was redescribed by Christian Fenger in a booklet detailing all the knowledge gained at that time about ureteric surgery. Fenger is also credited as the first to propose by writing a technique to reconstruct the ureter using a small bowel loop without interrupting its mesentery [2, 3]. d'Urso and de Fabii are reported to have performed the first ileal substitution of the ureter in dogs in 1900 [3].

The first human experience of an ileal ureter was published in 1906 by Shoemaker who replaced the ureter of an 18-year-old woman with an ileal loop interposition [4]. However, it took half a century for the technique to be popularized by Charles Wells and Willard Goodwin et al. in 1956 and 1959, respectively [5, 6]. Since then, many series and case reports on this technique have been published, but the world's largest series is probably that of A Kocot et al. who published 157 cases performed in a single institution (Wurzburg, Germany) in 2017 with a mean follow-up of 54.1 months [7].

1. Ileal ureter

   As shown by the above historical data, only the ileum stood the test of time to finally be regarded as the most suitable tissue for ureteric replacement today. The so-called **ileal ureter reconstruction** is used for a long-segment ureteral injury/stricture for which other reconstructions (namely Boari flap, psoas hitch) are not feasible. Its principle is isolating a segment of ileum from the intestinal tract while maintaining its mesentery, i.e., blood supply, and

S. A. AL-Mamari, *Urogenital Trauma: A Practical Guide*,
https://doi.org/10.1007/978-981-99-6171-9_17

suturing it to the upper ureter or renal pelvis proximally and to the bladder distally or rarely to the distal ureteric segment if viable [8].

(a) **Indications**: Recurrent calculi, ureteral stricture, fistula, congenital obstruction of the ureter, extensive ureteral injury, retroperitoneal fibrosis, tuberculosis, ureteral carcinoma in a solitary kidney [3, 7, 9–11].

(b) **Contraindications**: inflammatory bowel disease, post-radiation, incontinence, bladder neck obstruction, neurogenic bladder, metastatic cancer, renal failure, and hepatic dysfunction [3, 7, 9, 10].

(c) **Technical aspects of the ileal ureter reconstruction**: The lumen of the selected ileal segment must first be reduced before reconstruction using staplers (GIA) or 4/0 resorbable sutures. Practically, it can be tailored over a 12-Fr Foley's. The peristalsis direction must be maintained and the proximal end of the fashioned tube is anastomosed to the proximal ureter or the renal pelvis, using a 4/0 resorbable suture, in an end-to-end manner and the distal end will be anastomosed either to the bladder using one of the techniques described in the ureteroneocystoplasty (Lich-Gregoir extravesical nonrefluxing, for example) or to the spatulated cephalic end of the lower ureter segment if healthy, using the uretero-ureterostomy technique.

If there is bilateral ureteric damage, both sides can be reimplanted into a common isoperistaltic ileal segment end-to-endwise using the Wallace technique uniting the two ureteric ends, or separately end-to-sidewise after closing the proximal end of the ileal segment, and the distal end of the ileum segment will be anastomosed to the dome of the bladder in an anti-reflux manner (e.g. Lich-Gregoir technique) (Figs. 17.1, 17.2, and 17.3). The reconstructions are stented for 3–6 weeks, a drain is left in situ for a few days, and a urethral catheter is kept indwelling for 10–14 days [7, 8, 10, 12].

The combination of an ileal ureter and a Boari flap allows the use of a shorter ileal segment [8] (Fig. 17.4).

(d) **Complications of an ileal ureter**: Paralytic ileus, recurrent UTI with pyelonephritis, renal deterioration, ileovesical stricture, mucus obstruction, fistula, stone formation, pancreatitis, metabolic acidosis, diarrhea, and transient hepatic encephalopathy [3, 7, 9, 10, 12]. The rate of anastomotic stricture and fistula (ileal uretero-enteric or enterovaginal fistula) is estimated to be 3.3% and 6.6%, respectively, after a mean follow-up of 36 months [12]. Metabolic acidosis is an expected complication but a recent series of 23 patients showed that metabolic acidosis occurred only in the unique patient who underwent bilateral ileal ureter replacement and not in the 22 others [8].

(e) **Results**. The results of an ileal ureter in maintaining or improving the renal function depends on the published series, varying from 75–76% for some [11, 12] to 83–95% of patients for others after various mean follow-ups of 36–65 months [7–9]. Kocot et al. observed a significant improvement in upper urinary tract dilatation in 86% of their 157 patients [7]. In a series of 14 patients, the most common site of ureteric injury was the lower and mid-ureteric segments

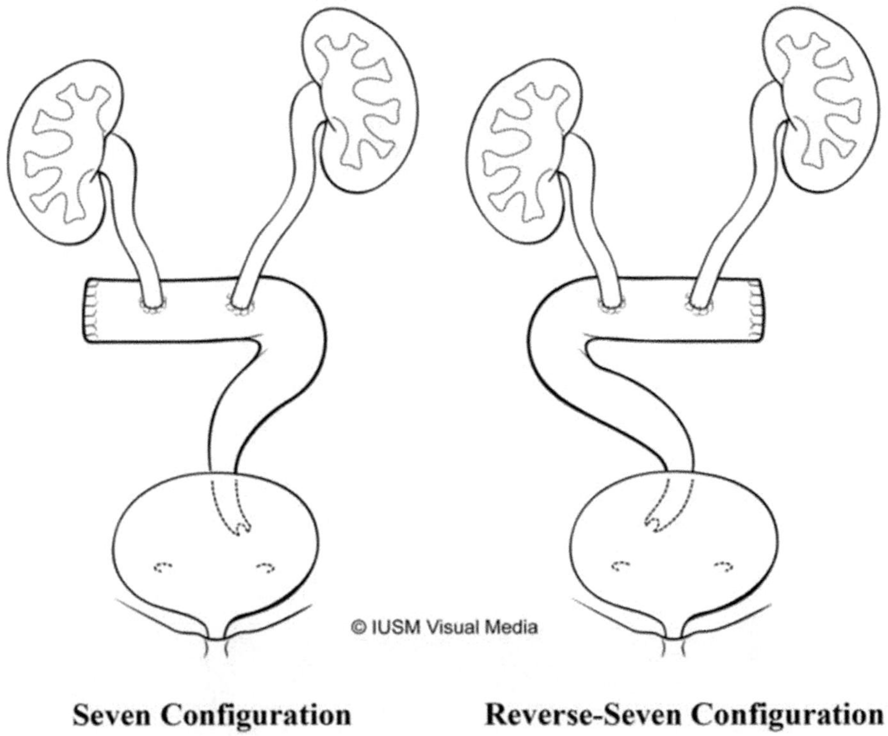

Fig. 17.1 Seven and reverse seven configurations of bilateral ureteral reimplantation into a common ileal segment. (From Armatys SA et al. [12], with permission from Wolters Kluwer Health)

and the mean length of the mobilized ileum was 11.2 cm [11]. The average nadir serum creatinine levels were 1.57 mg/dL and 1.37 mg/dL pre-operatively and at 12 months postoperatively, respectively [10].

2. Buccal mucosa grafting.

   This technique is very popular for urethral stricture, but only scanty publications exist for ureteric replacement. The use of buccal mucosa for the ureter was first described by Naude in Cape Town, South Africa, in 1999, and can be performed as an onlay or a tubularized graft wrapped with omentum [13]. There have been a few small series published since then [14, 15]. There is even a small reported series of 4 patients who underwent robotic-assisted ureteral buccal reconstructions with buccal mucosa with 100% success after a median follow-up of 15.5 months [16].
3. *Replacement by the gonadal vein*: An initial cadaveric model with partial ureteric replacement using a gonadal vein was published in 2019 with promising results. The obvious advantage is the course of the gonadal vein parallel to the

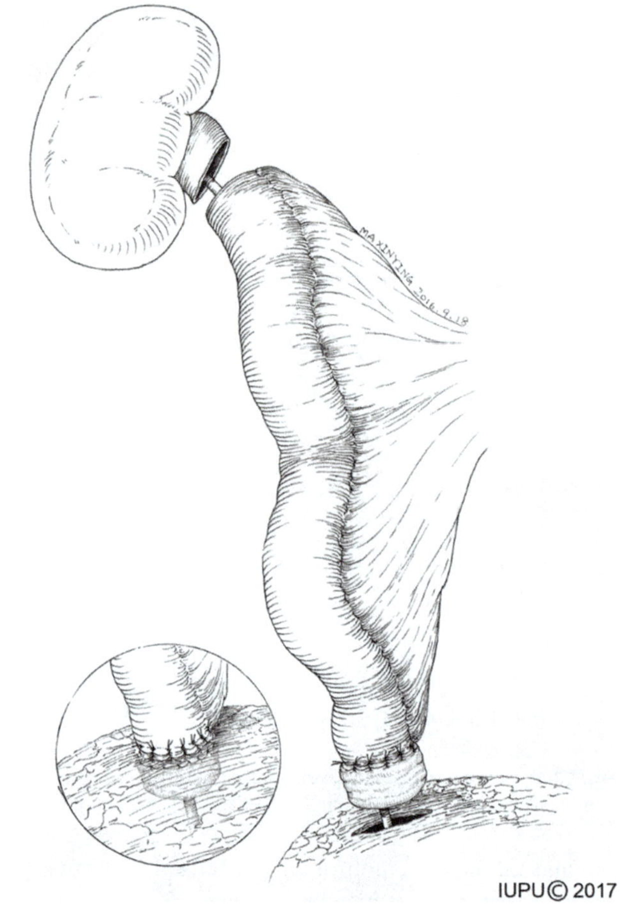

Fig. 17.2 The anti-reflux nipple valve for ileal ureter substitution. (From Zhong W et al. [8]. Creative Commons Attribution 4.0 International License)

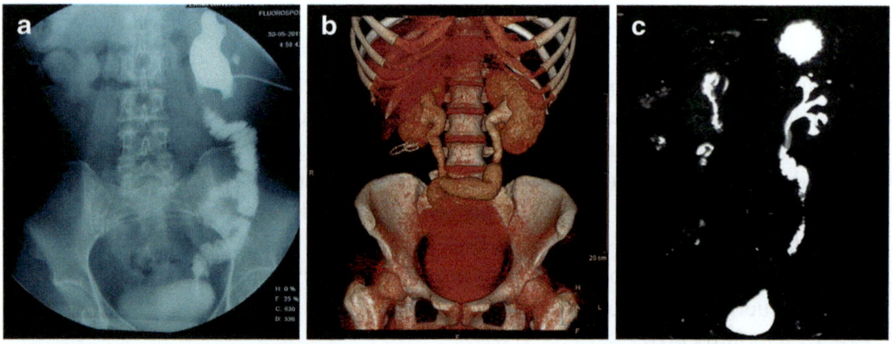

Fig. 17.3 Different types of ureteral replacement. (**a**) Unilateral ileal ureter replacement, (**b**) bilateral ileal ureter replacement, (**c**) combined ileal–ureter substitution and Boari flap–psoas hitch. (From Zhong W et al. [8]. Creative Commons Attribution 4.0 International License)

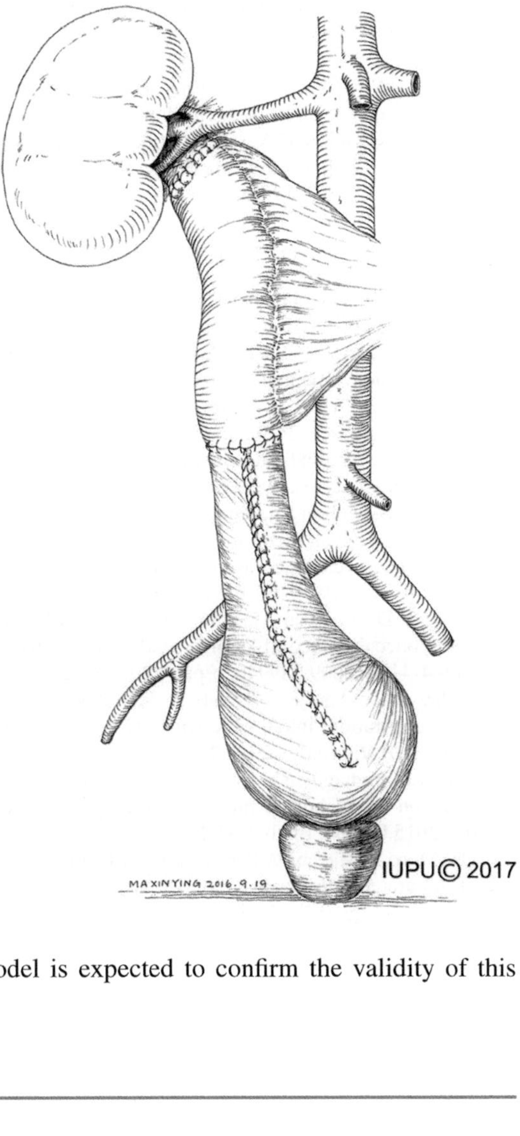

Fig. 17.4 The combination of ileal ureter replacement and Boari flap–psoas hitch technique. (From Zhong W et al. [8]. Creative Commons Attribution 4.0 International License)

ureter. An animal (porcine) model is expected to confirm the validity of this autologous graft [17].

References

1. Chaput. Bulletins et Mémoires de la Société de Chirurgie de Paris, Tome XIX, 1893;309.
2. Fenger CI. Surgery of the ureter. Ann Surg. 1894;20(3):257–96. https://doi.org/10.1097/00000658-189407000-00042.
3. Mattos RM, Smith JJ 3rd. Ileal ureter. Urol Clin N Am. 1997;24(4):813–25. https://doi.org/10.1016/s0094-0143(05)70422-5.
4. Shoemaker J. Discussie op voordracht van JM van Damn over interaabdominale plastiken. Ned Tijdschr Geneesk. 1911:836. PubMed | Google Scholar; Yang WH

5. Wells CA. The use of the intestine in urology, omitting ureterocolic anastomosis. Br J Urol. 1956;28(4):335–50.; discussion, 406–16. https://doi.org/10.1111/j.1464-410x.1956.tb04783.x.
6. Goodwin WE, Winter CC, Turner RD. Replacement of the ureter by small intestine: clinical application and results of the ileal ureter. J Urol. 1959;81:406–18.
7. Kocot A, Kalogirou C, Vergho D, Riedmiller H. Long-term results of ileal ureteric replacement: a 25-year single-centre experience. BJU Int. 2017;120(2):273–9. https://doi.org/10.1111/bju.13825. Epub 2017 Mar 21
8. Zhong W, Hong P, Ding G, et al. Technical considerations and outcomes for ileal ureter replacement: a retrospective study in China. BMC Surg. 2019;19:9. https://doi.org/10.1186/s12893-019-0472-1.
9. Verduyckt FJ, Heesakkers JP, Debruyne FM. Long-term results of ileum interposition for ureteral obstruction. Eur Urol. 2002;42(2):181–7. https://doi.org/10.1016/s0302-2838(02)00266-x.
10. Pamecha Y, Shelke U, Patil B, Patwardhan S, Kini S. Use of ileum for complex ureteric reconstruction: assessment of long-term outcome, complications, and impact on renal function. Urol Ann. 2018;10(4):369–74. https://doi.org/10.4103/UA.UA_5_18.
11. Boxer RJ, Fritzsche P, Skinner DG, Kaufman JJ, Belt E, Smith RB, Goodwin WE. Replacement of the ureter by small intestine: clinical application and results of the ileal ureter in 89 patients. J Urol. 1979;121(6):728–31. https://doi.org/10.1016/s0022-5347(17)56972-4.
12. Armatys S, Mellon M, Beck S, Koch M, Foster R, Bihrle R. Use of ileum as ureteral replacement in urological reconstruction. J Urol. 2009;181:177–81.
13. Naude JH. Buccal mucosal grafts in the treatment of ureteric lesions. BJU Int. 1999;83(7):751–4. https://doi.org/10.1046/j.1464-410x.1999.00019.x.
14. Kroepfl D, Loewen H, Klevecka V, Musch M. Treatment of long ureteric strictures with buccal mucosal grafts. BJU Int. 2010;105(10):1452–5. https://doi.org/10.1111/j.1464-410X.2009.08994.x. Epub 2009 Oct 28
15. Badawy AA, Abolyosr A, Saleem MD, Abuzeid AM. Buccal mucosa graft for ureteral stricture substitution: initial experience. Urology. 2010;76(4):971–5.; discussion 975. https://doi.org/10.1016/j.urology.2010.03.095.
16. Zhao LC, Yamaguchi Y, Bryk DJ, Adelstein SA, Stifelman MD. Robot-assisted ureteral reconstruction using buccal mucosa. Urology. 2015;86(3):634–8. https://doi.org/10.1016/j.urology.2015.06.006. Epub 2015 Jun 26
17. Dal Moro F, Macchi V, Porzionato A, Mandato FG, De Caro R. RUG technique: replacement of the ureter with gonadal vein. A cadaveric study. Minerva Urol Nefrol. 2019;71(1):85–91. https://doi.org/10.23736/S0393-2249.18.03261-7. Epub 2018 Nov 7. PMID: 30421594

Renal Autotransplantation, Evolving Techniques, and Tissue Engineering

18

18.1 Renal Autotransplantation

The first renal autotransplantation was performed by Hardy in 1963 on a 64-year man whose right ureter was severed during aortic aneurysm surgery. The patient had first a nephrostomy performed, and the ipsilateral kidney could not be sacrificed since the left kidney was hydronephrotic [1].

(a) *Indications*: **These are not limited to ureteric damages**. A large series of 108 patients showed that most of the patients (62%) underwent this procedure to allow extracorporeal (back table) repair of complex renal artery lesions. **Ureteric indications were present in 25% of patients only**, while malignancy (extracorporeal partial nephrectomy for bilateral renal cell carcinoma (RCC) or RCC in solitary kidneys) was the third group of indications with 13% of patients [2]. The ureteric indications can be summarized by damages or conditions not amenable to the previously described techniques in solitary anatomic or functioning kidneys: trauma, iatrogenic injuries, atonic ureter, and urinary undiversion [2, 3].
(b) *Technical aspects*: Renal autotransplantation is performed according to the same principles of donor nephrectomy and living donor allograft kidney transplantation. An open approach can be chosen through the traditional lombotomy, or through a transperitoneal route. A transperitoneal laparoscopic technique can also be utilized [4]. The kidney is harvested with a good length of vessels and is immediately perfused and cooled in a back table, where further vascular preparation is completed. The ureter is evaluated and the decision for the subsequent technique is made depending on the available ureteral length. A Gibson incision is then made to create the kidney bed and skeletonize the recipient's vessels. The vascular anastomosis is made to the external iliac vessels using 6/0 Prolene and the continuity of the urinary tract is generally restored by ureteroneocystostomy, ureteroureterostomy, or pyeloureterostomy, if there is a persistent viable ureter proximally or distally [2, 3, 5]. However, when there is no

S. A. AL-Mamari, *Urogenital Trauma: A Practical Guide*,
https://doi.org/10.1007/978-981-99-6171-9_18

viable ureter at all (panureteral stricture of complete avulsion), the continuity can be re-established through a pyelovesicostomy preferably through a Boari flap [6, 7] (Figs. 18.1, 18.2 and 18.3).

(c) *Complications*: With the exception of rejection, all classical complications of renal transplantation can be excepted here: delayed graft function, vascular thrombosis, urinary tract infection and sepsis, fever of unknown origin, surgical site infection and abscess, urinoma, lymphocele, segmental infarction, pneumonia, artery stenosis, incisional hernia, pseudoaneurysm, anastomotic stricture, graft infection, and chronic wound pain [4].

(d) *Results*: Excellent long-term outcome is observed with 87–92% having good renal function after 1.5–14 years [2, 3].

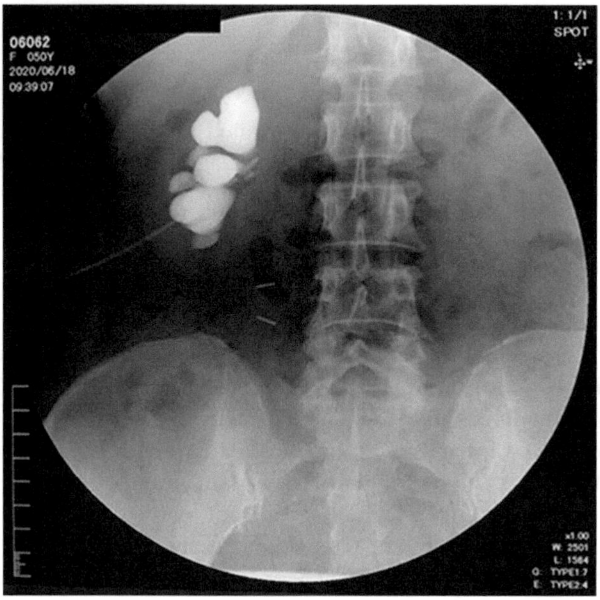

Fig. 18.1 A 50-year-old woman with a history of ureteral avulsion during ureteroscopy for removal of proximal right ureteral stone. Consequently, she underwent a laparoscopic right ureteral re-implantation and stone removal. An antegrade nephrostogram performed 3 months later demonstrated hydronephrosis with retained contrast in the collecting system of the right kidney. There is no contrast visualized within the right ureter. Two clips can be identified along the anatomical path of the right ureter. (From Pham NH et al. [7], Research and Reports in Urology 2021, 13, 733–737. Originally published by and used with permission from Dove Medical Press Ltd.)

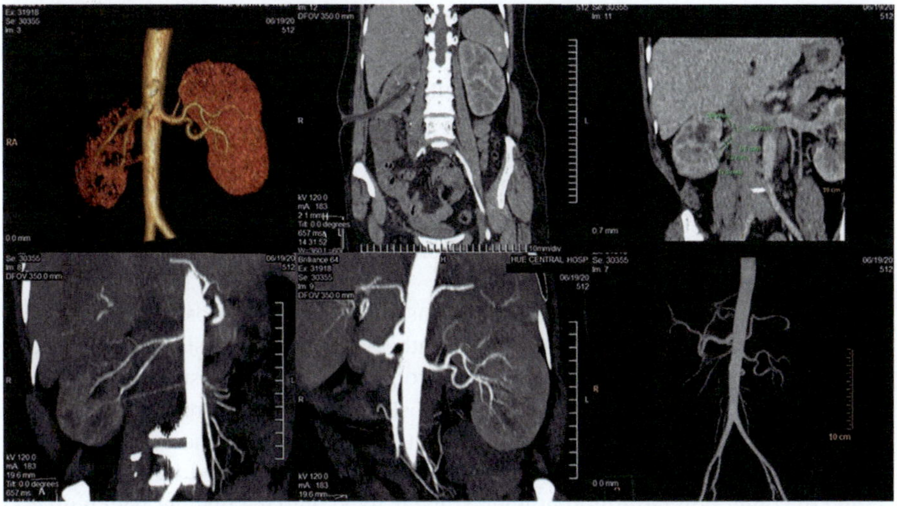

Fig. 18.2 Abdomen and pelvis CT scan with intravenous contrast demonstrates two main renal arteries. There is contralateral renal hypertrophy with preserved renal parenchyma on the ipsilateral side. (From Pham NH et al. [7], Research and Reports in Urology 2021, 13, 733–737. Originally published by and used with permission from Dove Medical Press Ltd.)

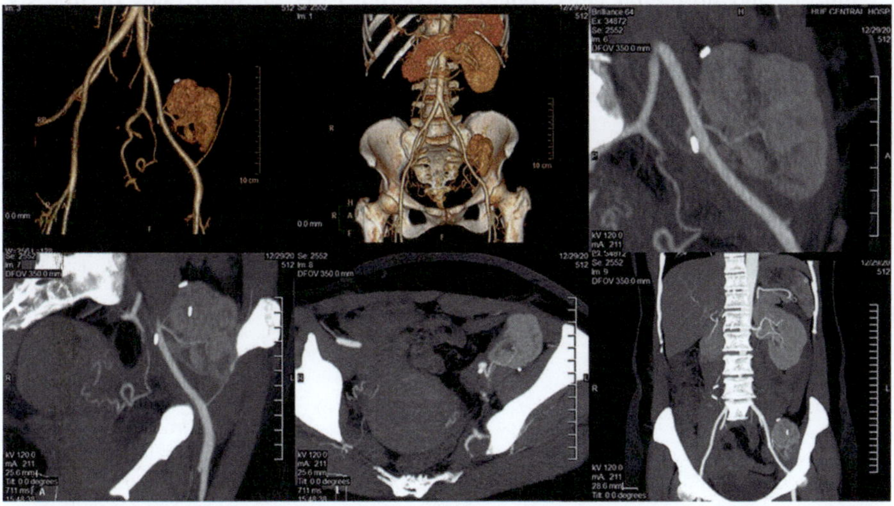

Fig. 18.3 Abdomen and pelvis CT scan 6 months after surgery (the kidney seems to be smaller because the slices are not via the main axis of the kidney). (From Pham NH et al. [7], Research and Reports in Urology 2021, 13, 733–737. Originally published by and used with permission from Dove Medical Press Ltd.)

18.2 Evolving Techniques and Tissue Engineering

1. *Artificial ureters*: The concept of subcutaneous nephron-vesical bypass (SNVB) was introduced more than two decades ago with promising results. The initial results using a silicone-PTFE prosthesis in this minimally invasive procedure showed encouraging results as a better alternative to permanent nephrostomy drainage, rendering the patient bagless [8]. Newer prostheses are made of an outer sheath of polyester over an inner silicone tube (Detour™, *Mentor-Porgès*) with equally satisfactory results [9, 10].

   The procedure starts with percutaneous insertion of the prosthesis under general anesthesia through an Amplatz sheath. A large-bore plastic hollow tube is used to create a subcutaneous tunnel from the loin to the suprapubic region (Fig. 18.4a–c). After the passage of the prosthesis, the large bore tube is removed. A Pfannenstiel incision is then performed to connect the prosthesis to the bladder through a small cystotomy: the inner silicone tube is inserted into the bladder, and the outer polytetrafluoroethylene tube is fixed onto the bladder wall with 4–0 Vicryl sutures.
2. *Tissue engineering for ureteral substitutes*: The progress of tissue engineering for ureteral substitutes has faced many challenges related to the nature of the ideal scaffold. Initially, acellular scaffolds such as small intestinal submucosa (SIS), collagen, or Gore-Tex, were tried in animal models to regenerate smooth muscle and urothelial cells, but the experience led to high rates of fibrosis. Further trials incorporated cell seeding of acellular scaffolds, including various candidates: primary smooth muscle or urothelial cells, mesenchymal or adipose-derived stem cells. There is still a long way to success, but ongoing research raises some hope [11].

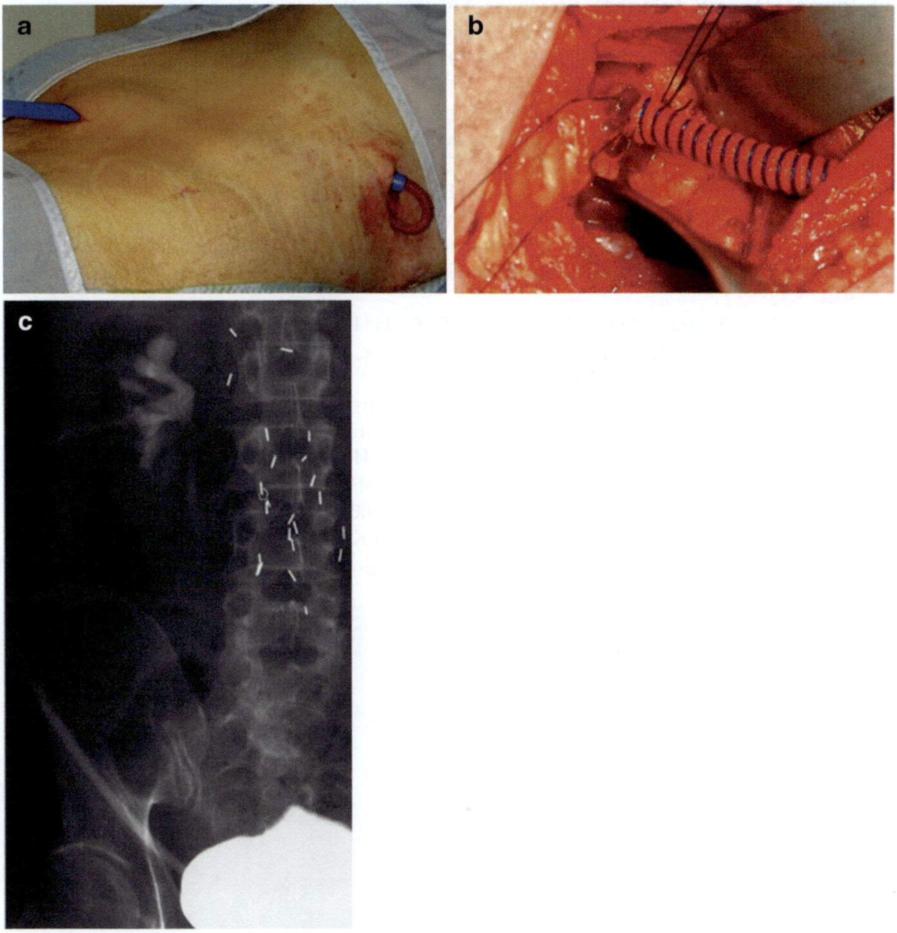

Fig. 18.4 (**a**) A large-bore plastic hollow tube is used to create a subcutaneous tunnel from the loin to the suprapubic region. (**b**) The bladder is accessed through a Pfannenstiel rectus splitting incision, and a small open cystotomy is performed following retrograde bladder distension. The inner silicone tube, with a few small perforations, is inserted into the bladder, and the outer polytetrafluoroethylene tube is secured onto the bladder wall with 4–0 Vicryl sutures. (**c**) Cystogram confirming the patency of the stent with free reflux of contrast from the bladder into the collecting system with no leaks. (From Lloyd SN et al. [10], with permission from Elsevier)

References

1. Hardy JD. High ureteral injuries. Management by autotransplantation of the kidney. JAMA. 1963;184:97–101. https://doi.org/10.1001/jama.1963.03700150051008.
2. Novick AC, Jackson CL, Straffon RA. The role of renal autotransplantation in complex urological reconstruction. J Urol. 1990;143(3):452–7. https://doi.org/10.1016/s0022-5347(17)39988-3.
3. Bodie B, Novick AC, Rose M, Straffon RA. Long-term results with renal autotransplantation for ureteral replacement. J Urol. 1986;136(6):1187–9. https://doi.org/10.1016/s0022-5347(17)45278-5.

4. Ruiz M, Hevia V, Fabuel JJ, Fernández AA, Gómez V, Burgos FJ. Kidney autotransplantation: long-term outcomes and complications. Experience in a tertiary hospital and literature review. Int Urol Nephrol. 2017;49(11):1929–35. https://doi.org/10.1007/s11255-017-1680-1. Epub 2017 Aug 21
5. Voelzke B. Overview of traumatic and iatrogenic ureteral injury. https://ykhoa.org/d/topic.htm?path=overview-of-traumatic-and-iatrogenic-ureteral-injury.
6. Tonyali S, Haberal HB, Bilen CY, Aki FT. Feasibility of Boari bladder flap procedure in patients with heterotrophic renal transplant. Exp Clin Transplant. 2019;17(5):599–603. https://doi.org/10.6002/ect.2018.0395. Epub 2019 May 2
7. Pham NH, Visser WR, Phan-Huu QV, Hampton LJ. Renal autotransplantation for the treatment of complete ureteral loss: a case report. Res Rep Urol. 2021;13:733–7. https://doi.org/10.2147/RRU.S328832.
8. Jabbour ME, Desgrandchamps F, Angelescu E, Teillac P, Le Duc A. Percutaneous implantation of subcutaneous prosthetic ureters: long-term outcome. J Endourol. 2001;15(6):611–4. https://doi.org/10.1089/089277901750426391.
9. Andonian S, Zorn KC, Paraskevas S, Anidjar M. Artificial ureters in renal transplantation. Urology. 2005;66(5):1109. https://doi.org/10.1016/j.urology.2005.05.012.
10. Lloyd SN, Tirukonda P, Biyani CS, Wah TM, Irving HC. The detour extra-anatomic stent—a permanent solution for benign and malignant ureteric obstruction? Eur Urol. 2007;52(1):193–8. https://doi.org/10.1016/j.eururo.2006.11.008. Epub 2006 Nov 13
11. Gild P, Kluth LA, Vetterlein MW, Engel O, Chun FKH, Fisch M. Adult iatrogenic ureteral injury and stricture-incidence and treatment strategies. Asian J Urol. 2018;5(2):101–6. https://doi.org/10.1016/j.ajur.2018.02.003.

Part III
Urinary Bladder Injury

The bladder is not just a reservoir. It is also a guardian devoted to the protection of the kidneys. With time it has become even smarter, preserving your dignity, and relieving your desires. Furthermore, out of altruism, it spends less time crying from its own injury but might mourn all its life a spinal cord or other neurological trauma.

Introduction to Urinary Bladder Trauma

Features of a well-functioning bladder are known, namely a good storage capacity under low pressure and complete emptying upon voluntary commands without reflux. However, there seems to be an unknown critical advantage granted to mankind by the bladder: we probably owe our survival to the urinary bladder! Indeed, a recent simulation model has shown that the increased storage capacity of the urinary bladder has a linear correlation with the species' separation from prey to predator and overall survival since primitive species do not have such capacity, leaving continuous urine scents and increasing the trail detection rate by their predators [1].

The bladder is relatively protected by the pelvic wall. Therefore, its injury is rare. And when this occurs in blunt trauma (such as in MVA), it is generally associated with a pelvic shield fracture. The bladder may also be injured by penetrating agents during an assault but is more frequently subjected to injury during surgeries, especially colorectal and gyneco-obstetrical procedures [2].

When suspected, bladder injuries are easy to confirm and also generally easy to repair, and their healing is excellent. However, in some instances, they can be missed due to diverted attention toward more appalling associated injuries that represent an immediate risk to the patient's life. The delay in the diagnosis and repair of a bladder injury is detrimental to the patient's health and frequently gives rise to life-threatening complications. This delay, already blameworthy in the context of external trauma becomes a tragedy if the injury has occurred during a surgical act.

From there, the surgeons come down from their pedestals and the lawyers take the stage.

Finally, it should be borne in mind that iatrogenic injuries also prolong patients' hospital stays and increase medical costs which can reach exorbitant amounts. It is worth remembering that the total economic impact of medical errors, in general, has been estimated to reach 1 trillion per year in the USA and one should better be inspired not to play any role in it [3]. **Praemonitus praemunitus (forewarned is forearmed).**

References

1. McCarthy M, McCarthy L. The evolution of the urinary bladder as a storage organ: scent trails and selective pressure of the first land animals in a computational simulation. SN Appl Sci. 2019;1:1727. https://doi.org/10.1007/s42452-019-1692-9.
2. Cohen AJ, Packiam VT, Nottingham CU, Pariser JJ, Faris SF, Bales GT. Iatrogenic bladder injury: national analysis of 30-day outcomes. Urology. 2016;97:250–6. https://doi.org/10.1016/j.urology.2016.05.002. Epub 2016 May 12.
3. Andel C, Davidow S, Hollander M, Moreno D. The economics of health care quality and medical errors. J Health Care Finance. 2012;39:39–50.

Anatomy of the Urinary Bladder 19

19.1 Embryology

The bladder mostly derives from the **mesoderm**. The partition of the cloaca by the urorectal septum takes place **between the 4th and 7th weeks**. Producing the **primitive urogenital sinus** ventrally and the anorectal canal dorsally. The primitive urogenital sinus undergoes further division into a **cranial vesical part** that is continuous with the **allantois**, a **middle pelvic part**, and a **caudal phallic part**. The bladder mainly arises from the vesical part and the **trigone** develops from the caudal ends of the mesonephric ducts which connect to the posterior bladder wall. The middle pelvic part of the primitive urogenital sinus will give rise to **the bladder neck, the male prostatic urethra, and the entire female urethra**. The **urachus** develops from the allantois' anterior portion [1–4] (Fig. 19.1).

S. A. AL-Mamari, *Urogenital Trauma: A Practical Guide*,
https://doi.org/10.1007/978-981-99-6171-9_19

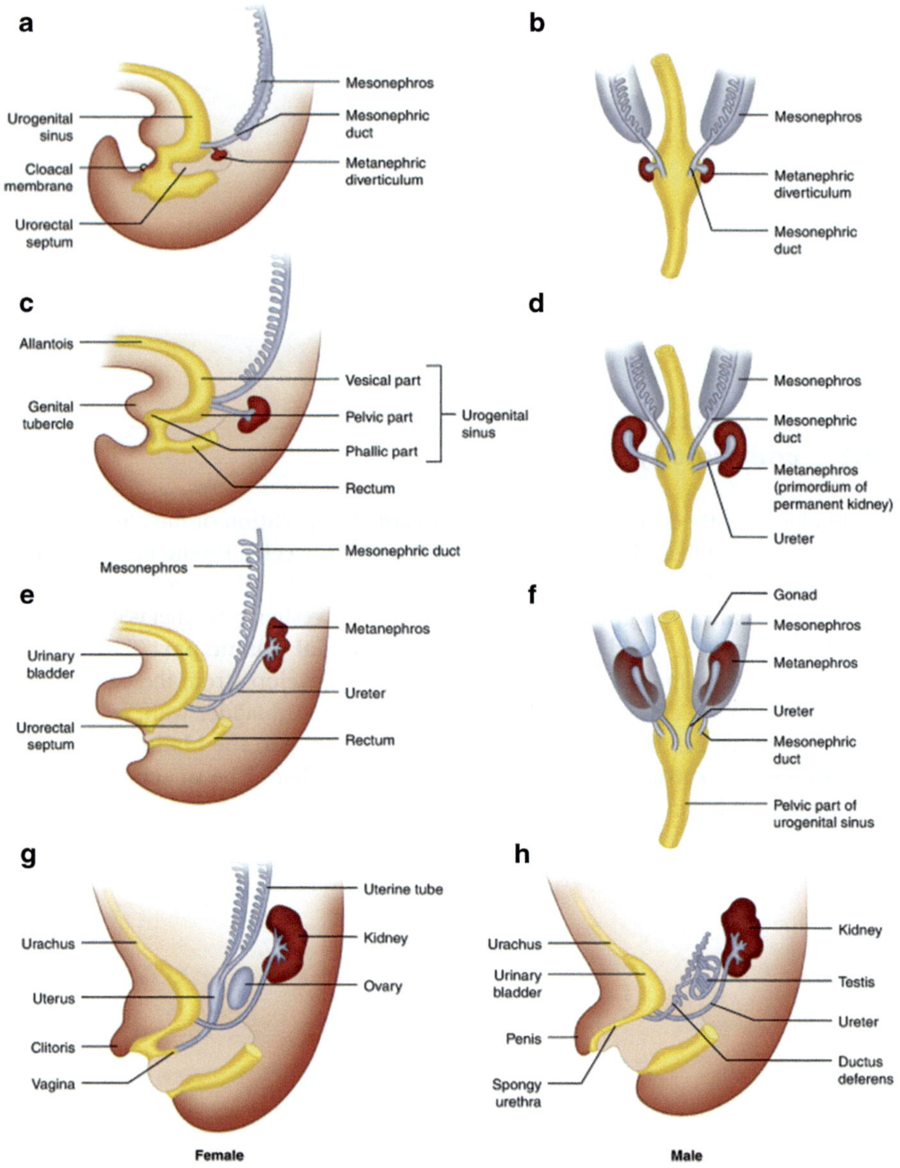

Fig. 19.1 Diagram depicting the sequential division of the cloaca into the urogenital sinus and the rectum, as well as the development of the urinary bladder and urethra. The association between the developing kidneys and gonads, as well as their relationships to the cloaca, urogenital sinus, and bladder are shown. Panels (**a**, **c**, **e**, **g**, **h**) are lateral views. Panels (**b**, **d**, **f**) are dorsal views. (From Kassab GH et al. [4], with permission from Springer)

19.2 General Aspects

The urinary bladder is an extraperitoneal hollow viscus, having a tetrahedral shape while empty, and becoming globular on repletion. In adults, it occupies the true or lesser pelvis when empty, and with filling, it develops toward the greater pelvis and may even reach the lower abdominal cavity. However, in neonates and infants, it lies in the lower abdomen even when empty because the pelvic cavity is relatively small and shallow at these ages. It is estimated that the pelvis acquires sufficient volume and depth to accommodate the bladder only by the age of 7–8 years and that this viscus becomes a true intrapelvic organ on emptiness only at puberty [5].

The bladder can be divided into two components on each side of a horizontal line passing at the level of the ureteral orifices: a **body** lying above this line and a **base formed by the trigone and bladder neck.** The body contains fascicles of myofibrils in random directions. The base forms the bladder outlet in addition to the urethra and the striated urethral sphincter or rhabdosphincter.

The wall of the bladder base is formed by the following layers from inside-outside: a superficial mucosal coat, a submucosa, a muscle coat that is continuous with the detrusor of the bladder body, the serosa in some areas or the adventitia in others, and the perivesical fat. The mucosa is made of **transitional epithelium** and a **basement membrane**. The submucosal coat is an areolar connective tissue also referred to as the **lamina propria**. The muscular coat is also referred to as **muscularis propria** and is made of **three layers**: an inner longitudinal, a middle circular, and an outer longitudinal. **The serosa is just a visceral reflection of the peritoneum. Therefore, it covers only the bladder dome** (superior surface and the upper lateral surfaces). The **adventitia** is a connective tissue encountered on the remaining walls not covered by the peritoneal serosa. The **perivesical fat** surrounds either the serosa or the adventitia.

Contrary to men, an anatomic smooth-muscle sphincter at the bladder neck is not obvious in women. Anyway, in either gender, the function of the bladder neck in the maintenance of continence is not clearly determined because this faculty is preserved after the destruction or opening of the bladder neck [6].

19.3 Topography

The bladder is in relation to the following organs and structures [5, 7, 8] (Figs. 19.2, 19.3 and 19.4):

- Superiorly: the pelvic peritoneum, covering the dome of the bladder and being densely attached to its surface, and coils of the small intestine and the sigmoid loop.
- Postero-superiorly: the anteverted body of the uterus in females.
- Anteriorly: the pubis, the **median umbilical ligament** (the obliterated remnant of the urachus). Between the pubis and the bladder is the **Retzius space** which extends laterally and contains loose perivesical fat and connective tissue. This

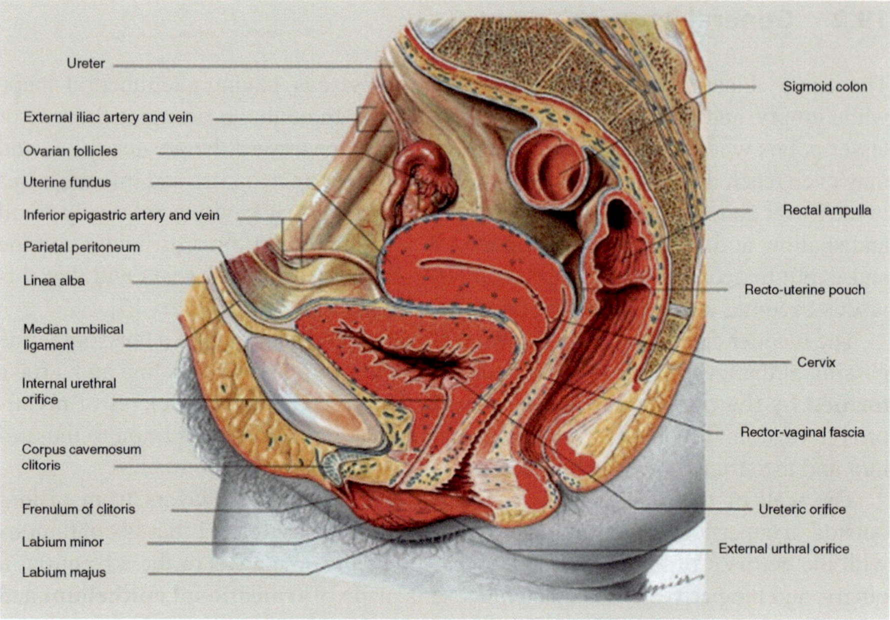

Fig. 19.2 Sagittal view of female pelvic cavity showing relations of urinary bladder and relationship of the peritoneum to the bladder. (From Mahadevan V [5], with permission from Elsevier)

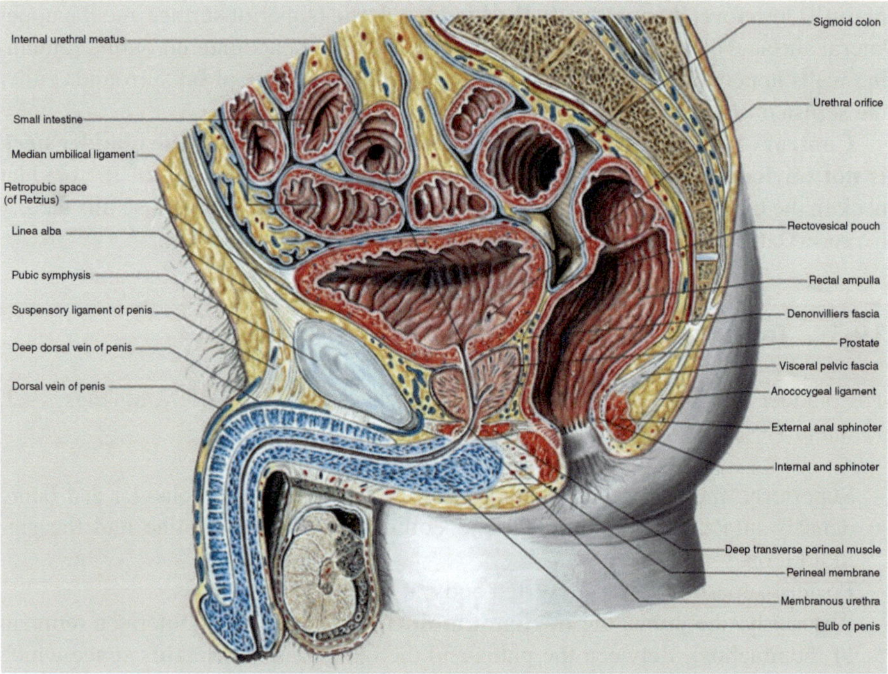

Fig. 19.3 Sagittal view of male pelvic cavity showing relations of urinary bladder and the various segments of the urethra. (From Mahadevan V [5], with permission from Elsevier)

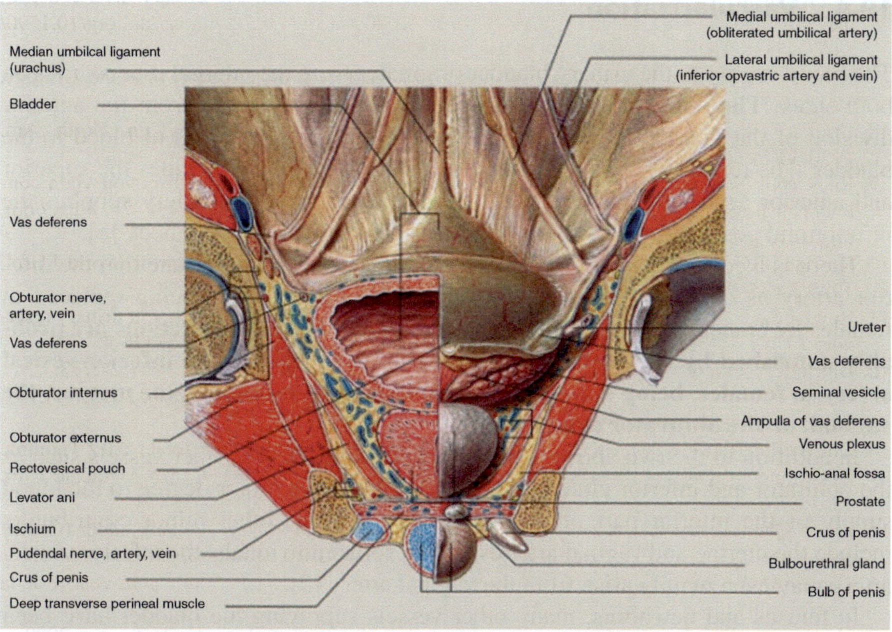

Fig. 19.4 Coronal view of male pelvic cavity (viewed from behind) showing lateral and inferior relations of urinary bladder, and relationship of peritoneum to the bladder. (From Mahadevan V [5], with permission from Elsevier)

space is particularly important as it is one of the potential sites for urine or blood collection in bladder trauma.

– Posteriorly: the rectum, the vasa deferentia, and the seminal vesicles in males; the vagina and the cervix in females. It receives the ureters at its lateral angles.
– Infero-laterally: the levator ani and obturator internus muscles.
– Inferiorly: the prostate in males, and the pelvic fascia in females.

During cystoscopy, a transversal mucosal fold called the **interureteric bar or Mercier's bar** runs between the two ureteric orifices which are located posteriorly and separated by 3 cm on emptiness or 5 cm on repletion [5].

As suggested by its name, the trigone is a triangular area situated between the ureteric and the urethral orifices. **Contrary to the mucosa of the bladder body, the trigone has a smooth surface and is the least mobile part of the bladder, being firmly fixed to the upper surface of the prostate in males and to the anterior vaginal wall in females**. In chronic bladder outlet obstruction, characteristic trabeculations, sacculations, and even pseudodiverticula appear on the bladder body due to muscle hypertrophy and mucosa herniation [5, 7].

19.4 Vascularization

The blood supply to the urinary bladder originates from the internal iliac arteries on both sides. **The superior and inferior vesical arteries** derive from the anterior division of the internal iliac artery and are the principal suppliers of blood to the bladder. The territory supplied by the superior vesical artery includes the superior and anterior aspects of the bladder, while the inferior vesical artery supplies the inferior and posterior aspects of the bladder, including the bladder neck [5].

There is a controversy among anatomists since some authors state that the inferior artery as described above is specific to the male gender, being replaced in females by branches of the vaginal or uterine artery. **The contradictions are probably nourished by the multiple variations of the origin of the inferior vesical artery in females, being either the internal iliac, the umbilical, the uterine, the vaginal, or the obturator artery** [9].

In addition to the two abovementioned main contributors, other vessels such as the obturator and inferior gluteal arteries contribute to a minor degree to the blood supply of the inferior part of the bladder. In females, other minor contributors include the uterine and vaginal arteries, and in some individuals, the inferior vesical artery may even mainly arise from the vaginal artery [5].

In fetuses and newborns, many other vessels supplying the bladder have been described in addition to the superior and inferior vesical arteries: urachal artery, middle vesical artery, vesico-deferential (males), and uterine (females) arteries [10].

The venous drainage of the urinary bladder starts with a rich, delicate valveless plexus, circumferentially situated around the lower part of the bladder which is called the **perivesical venous plexus**. In males, this plexus is continuous with the extracapsular peri-prostatic venous plexus lying at the anterior and lateral aspects of the prostate. In females, it is continuous with the plexus around the intra-pelvic vagina and at the base of the broad ligament of the uterus. The perivesical venous plexus coalesces and gives rise to larger veins that accompany the vesical arteries and drain into the internal iliac veins bilaterally [5].

19.5 Innervation of the Bladder

The urinary bladder is supplied by three types of **efferent nerve fibers** [2, 11, 12] (Fig. 19.5):

(a) Parasympathetic: Arising from the sacral roots S2–S4, these fibers are contained in the pelvic splanchnic nerves. They stimulate urination through detrusor muscle contraction.
(b) Sympathetic: Exiting from T12–L2, they are conveyed by the superior and inferior hypogastric nerve. They are responsible for the relaxation of the detrusor muscle.

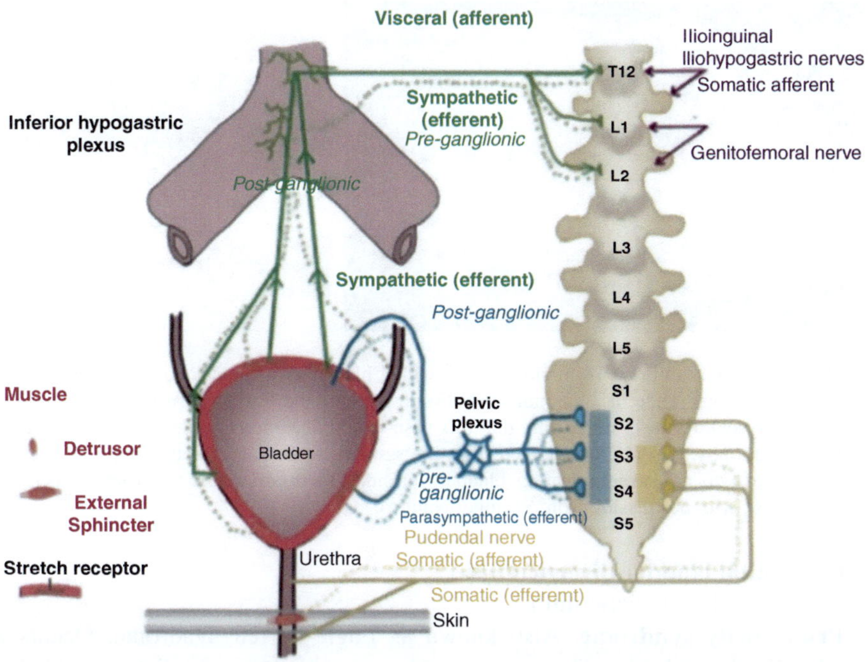

Fig. 19.5 Illustration of three separate contributions to bladder innervation, thoracolumbar, sacral visceral, and sacral somatic, each of which contains both afferent and efferent fibers. (From Dellon AL and Herati AS [12], with permission from Georg Thieme Verlag KG)

(c) Somatic: Originating from the Onuf's nucleus[1] at S2–S4, they travel through pudendal nerves up to the external urethral sphincter, and control the voluntary micturition.

There are also **sensory or afferent nerve fibers** that convey messages related to stretch and pain (bladder distension) from mechanoreceptors in the bladder wall to the central nervous system (up to the brain cortex). These fibers travel through the hypogastric and pelvic splanchnic nerves.

19.6 Congenital Malformations [4, 13, 14]

- **Bladder exstrophy**: 0.002% births. Constantly associated with epispadias.
- **Megacystis**: neurodysplastic disease, due to abnormal or deficient innervation, leading to a bladder dilatation over 7 cm in diameter in the fetus and the newborn. Incidence: 0.06–0.30% in the first trimester with male-to-female ratio of 8:1.

[1]The Onuf's nucleus is named after the American Neurologist Bronislaw Onuf Onufrowicz (1863–1928), who first discovered it in New York in 1899.

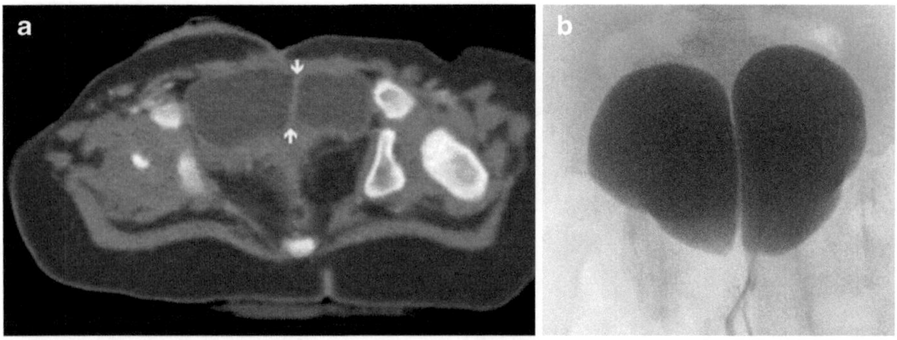

Fig. 19.6 (**a**) CT scan in an 18-month-old girl with a history of a cloacal exstrophy variant with an imperforate anus. There is a sagittal separation traversing the bladder (arrows). Note the wide pubic symphyseal diastasis suggesting that this case would accurately be described as a covered duplicate exstrophy. (**b**) VCUG obtained from the same patient after catheterizing both urethras demonstrating two noncommunicating bladders in side-to-side orientation. (From Wise L and Wyers M [16], with permission from Springer Nature)

- **Congenital bladder diverticulitis**.
- **Vesicourachal diverticulum.**
- **Prune belly syndrome**: Also known as Eagle-Barrett syndrome. Occurs in 0.004% of live births. This syndrome describes a massively distended bladder with incomplete emptying, associated with thin overlying abdominal wall muscles. Nearly always occurring in males, in association with undescended testes.
- **Urofacial syndrome**: Also called Ochoa syndrome as it was first described by Bernardo Ochoa, a Colombian Physician [15]. This extremely rare abnormality consists of detrusor contractions against an incompletely opened bladder outflow with a characteristic grimace when smiling or laughing, that rather resembles crying.
- **Duplicated bladder**: Complete bladder duplication is extremely rare with approximately 70 cases reported in the literature. Its frequency is roughly equal in both genders. It may be associated with other malformations such as cloacal exstrophy with an imperforate anus as well as duplication of other pelvic viscera (vagina, uterus, and urethra) [16] (Fig. 19.6a, b).
- **Bladder agenesis**: Fewer than 70 cases reported in the literature.
- **Megacystis-microcolon-intestinal hypoperistalsis syndrome.**

References

1. Ntoulia A, Papadopoulou F, Benz-Bohm G. Urinary tract embryology, anatomy, and anatomical variants. In: Riccabona M, editor. Pediatric urogenital radiology. Cham: Springer; 2018. https://doi.org/10.1007/978-3-319-39202-8_7.
2. Shermadou ES, Rahman S, Leslie SW. Anatomy, abdomen and pelvis, bladder. In: StatPearls [Internet]. Treasure Island (FL): StatPearls Publishing; 2022.

3. Liaw A, et al. Development of the human bladder and ureterovesical junction. Differentiation. 2018;103:66–73.
4. Kassab GH, et al. Urinary tract. In: Paltiel HJ, Lee EY, editors. Pediatric ultrasound. Cham: Springer; 2021. https://doi.org/10.1007/978-3-030-56802-3_17.
5. Mahadevan V. Anatomy of the lower urinary tract. Surgery (Oxford). 2016;34(7):318–25. https://doi.org/10.1016/j.mpsur.2016.04.001.
6. de Groat WC, Yoshimura N. Anatomy and physiology of the lower urinary tract. Handb Clin Neurol. 2015;130:61–108. https://doi.org/10.1016/B978-0-444-63247-0.00005-5.
7. Ellis H. Anatomy of the urinary bladder, prostate, and male urethra. Surgery (Oxford). 2005;23(3):97–8. https://doi.org/10.1383/surg.23.3.97.63118.
8. Hickling DR, Sun TT, Wu XR. Anatomy and physiology of the urinary tract: relation to host defense and microbial infection. Microbiol Spectr. 2015;3(4):2012. https://doi.org/10.1128/microbiolspec.UTI-0016-2012. PMID: 26350322; PMCID: PMC4566164
9. de Treigny OM, Roumiguie M, Deudon R, de Bonnecaze G, Carfagna L, Chaynes P, Rimailho J, Chantalat E. Anatomical study of the inferior vesical artery: is it specific to the male sex? Surg Radiol Anat. 2017;39(9):961–5. https://doi.org/10.1007/s00276-017-1828-9. Epub 2017 Feb 22
10. Shehata R. The arterial supply of the urinary bladder. Acta Anat (Basel). 1976;96(1):128–34. https://doi.org/10.1159/000144666.
11. Yoshimura N, Chancellor MB. Neurophysiology of lower urinary tract function and dysfunction. Rev Urol. 2003;5(Suppl 8):S3–S10. PMID: 16985987; PMCID: PMC1502389
12. Dellon AL, Herati AS. Review of bladder pain and referred T12–L2 input as one etiology for interstitial cystitis. J Reconstr Microsurg Open. 2019;4:e58–63.
13. Woolf AS, Lopes FM, Ranjzad P, Roberts NA. Congenital disorders of the human urinary tract: recent insights from genetic and molecular studies. Front Pediatr. 2019;7:136. https://doi.org/10.3389/fped.2019.00136. PMID: 31032239; PMCID: PMC6470263
14. Sandulescu SM, Vicol RM, Serban A, Carp AV, Cristian V. Congenital anomalies of urinary tract and anomalies of fetal genitalia. In: Congenital anomalies—from the embryo to the neonate. IntechOpen; 2018. https://doi.org/10.5772/intechopen.73641.
15. Ochoa B, Gorlin RJ. Urofacial (ochoa) syndrome. Am J Med Genet. 1987;27(3):661–7. https://doi.org/10.1002/ajmg.1320270320.
16. Wise L, Wyers M. Duplicated bladder. Pediatr Radiol. 2010;40(Suppl 1):11. https://doi.org/10.1007/s00247-010-1810-8.

20 Epidemiology, Etiology, and Mechanism of Urinary Bladder Injury

Due to its relative anatomical protection in the bony pelvis, the bladder is less frequently injured in blunt or penetrating trauma than the kidneys.

A 10-year study recruiting 15,169 adult patients who sustained blunt abdominal trauma showed an occurrence of bladder ruptures in 54 patients of them (**0.35%**) [1]. A 5-year review of the US National Trauma Data Bank (NTDB) revealed 8565 cases of bladder trauma with **85% being caused by blunt trauma**. **In 46% of the cases, there was an associated pelvic fracture, particularly one of the pubic rami**, and in 15% there were at least two other intra-abdominal injuries [2]. Males are predominant with 63–75%, and the average age is 38.9% [1, 2].

Conversely, another NTDB review of 31,380 patients with pelvic fracture showed that 1444 (4.6%) had a genitourinary injury, and sole injuries of the bladder were more common (3.39%) than urethral (0.94%) or combined bladder-urethra injuries (0.19%) [3].

Nearly similar results were reported in a level I trauma center showing 4.2% of lower urinary tract injuries out of 5518 cases of blunt trauma associated with a pelvic injury [4].

Extraperitoneal bladder ruptures are more common among patients with pelvic fractures than those without pelvic fractures, with 39.1% and 14.7%, respectively, and the presence of pelvic fractures in patients with lower urinary tract injury is associated with increased overall injuries severity and portends increased rates of inpatient complications and longer hospital stays [4, 5].

Motor vehicle accidents or collisions (VMAs or MVCs) are the most common cause of bladder blunt trauma accounting for 50.5%, followed by pedestrian-cars accidents and falls from height with 29.1% and 14.5%, respectively [6–8].

MVC is also the most frequent mechanism causing pelvic injuries, associated or not with genitourinary injury (GUI), and injured pedestrians and motorcyclists have a statistically higher percentage of pelvic fractures with associated GUI [3]. Falls are other causes of pelvic fractures; however, they are seldom associated with GUI

S. A. AL-Mamari, *Urogenital Trauma: A Practical Guide*,
https://doi.org/10.1007/978-981-99-6171-9_20

(5.12%) [3]. Fullness of the bladder makes it susceptible to rupture even from mild trauma such as a fall after tripping on stairs. Alcohol consumption is a particularly important risk factor here as it rapidly fills up the bladder, reduces the concentration of the individual, and slower his/her reflex to cushion the fall with his/her hands.

More infrequently do bladder injuries result from a penetrating injury during assaults (fire guns, stabbing) accounting for 14–49% depending on the published series [6]. Herein gunshot wounds represent the great majority (88%) of causes. Conversely, bladder injury has been reported to be present in 3.6% of abdominal gunshot injuries and is also associated with 13% of penetrating injuries of the rectum and 20% of penetrating injuries to the buttock [9]. Contrary to blunt bladder injuries which are mostly associated with pelvic fracture, penetrating bladder injuries are mostly associated with small bowel and rectum injuries [10].

A non-negligible etiological group is made of iatrogenic bladder injuries occurring in 1.8–13.8 per 1000 surgeries [6]. Out of over a million and half of the surgical interventions recorded in the US National Surgical Quality Improvement Program database, there were 1685 (0.11%) cases of bladder injuries [11].

It has been proposed to divide iatrogenic bladder injuries into those arising from cystoscopic procedures and those occurring during open or laparoscopic surgery carried out in the vicinity of the bladder [12]. The first group includes procedures such as cystolitholapaxy, transurethral resection of bladder tumor (TURBT), and transurethral resection of the prostate (TURP), and the second one comprises gynecological, colorectal, general, and urological surgeries.

Bladder injuries are reported to occur in 0.36% of gynecological interventions, 0.35% of open colorectal surgeries, and 0.08% of general surgery [11].

Risk factors of iatrogenic bladder or ureteral injury in gynecological surgeries include prior abdominal surgery or laparotomy, history of cesarean section, endometriosis, adhesions of any origin, broad ligament fibroids, high blood loss during surgery provoking panic and blind mass ligation, and low-volume surgeons, in addition to complete placenta praevia and accrete, which are specific risk factors in cesarean section [13, 14].

In a single institution, it was found that out of 127 patients with nonendoscopic iatrogenic bladder injuries, they were more women than men (87% vs. 13%), the mean age was 51 years, the most associated risk factors were prior surgery, presence of inflammation, and increased tumor burden [15]. **This study also showed that gyneco-obstetrical surgery caused the highest percentage of injuries (65%)**, followed by general surgery and non-endoscopic urologic procedures with 22%, and 13%, respectively. **Among gyneco-obstetrical procedures, hysterectomy is the most incriminated cause followed by cesarean section. The incidence of bladder injury during cesarean section has been evaluated to be 0.08–0.94%, and the risk increases with repeat surgeries** [16–18]. This apparently low incidence should be taken with caution when one knows that over 30% of deliveries in the United States occur through a cesarean section [19] and that the current estimated birth number in this country is over 3.6 million per year [20].

In cesarean sections, the inadvertent bladder cutting or laceration may occur either during entry into the peritoneal cavity (bladder not emptied, or presence of adhesions), during the bladder flap creation, or during uterine incision or fetal extraction. The bladder may also be included in the suture of the uterine incision, arising in the development of a secondary vesicovaginal or vesicouterine fistula [13] (Fig. 20.1a, b).

Bladder injury during a cesarean section can be considered non-negligent or defendable in scenarios of postoperative adhesions, abnormal anatomy, or in a fully dilated cervix with the fetal head lying deep in the pelvis. However, injuries occurring without anatomic abnormalities are considered technical mishaps, and non-recognition and repair of any injury intra-operatively might be litigated as negligence [18]. An exception to this rule is where there is a placenta praevia or accreta with massive life-threatening bleeding, where the immediate purpose is to control the hemorrhage by packing and/or ballooning with the plan to take back the patient after 1–2 days for reevaluation and completion of the treatment [21].

Many tricks have been proposed to prevent bladder injury during cesarean section, including bladder catheterization, Pfannenstiel incision as opposed to a midline sub-umbilical one, prevention of adhesions by careful handling and closure of the tissues and correct hemostasis, double layers suturing of the uterus, sharp incision of the adhesions as opposed to blunt dissection using gauzes, etc. However, the creation of a bladder flap, the type of uterine incision, the exteriorization of the uterus after fetus delivery, and the closure of the peritoneum are controversial in preventing adhesions. Indeed, most bladder injuries occur during the creation of the bladder flap [16]. It is traditionally recommended to catheterize and empty the bladder to avoid injury. However, a paradoxical approach was recently proposed by a

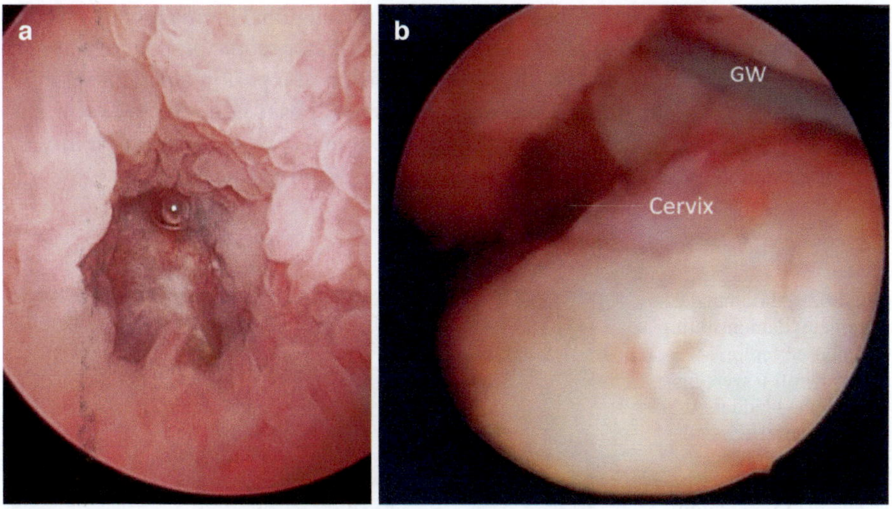

Fig. 20.1 (**a**) Cystoscopy showing a 2-cm large vesico-vaginal fistula at the posterior vesical wall in a 39-year old lady 2 months after a cesarean section. (**b**) Vaginoscopy showing a guide wire exiting through the fistula into the upper third of the vagina just below the uterine cervix (same patient discussed in the Fig. 22.1a, b. (Courtesy Feroz Amir Zafar, Urology, the Royal Hospital, Muscat, Oman)

randomized controlled trial that demonstrated the effectiveness of cystoinflation with 300 mL normal saline to well expose the bladder for safe adhesiolysis in repeated cesarean sections [22].

The risk factors associated with bladder injury during trans-urethral cystoscopic procedures, namely TURBT and TURP, have not been specifically studied. However, based on the experience, one can assume that these include large tumor size, high stage of the tumor requiring deeper resection, location of the tumor at bladder dome where the wall is the thinnest and most vulnerable, or at the lateral walls where there is a high likelihood of an **obturator reflex**, and the limited surgeon experience. Spinal anesthesia doesn't prevent obturator reflexes. Therefore, if general anesthesia is not used, and the tumor site is in the lateral bladder wall, a nerve block should be considered. A prospective study has evaluated a technique of **obturator nerve block** using 2% Lidocaine injected through the thigh inter-adductor approach in the Lithotomy position showing an efficacy of 94% out of 542 cases [23]. Another prospective study showed that the use of the **combination of spinal anesthesia with obturator nerve block** was an effective safety measure to reduce obturator reflex and prevent bladder perforation during resection of lateral wall tumor, either for monopolar or bipolar TURBT [24]. Furthermore, a comparison between bipolar and monopolar TURBT without the use of a nerve block did not show any superiority of the former in the prevention of obturator block and bladder injury [25]. Interestingly, microscopic and immunohistochemical studies of the bladder tissue from patients who developed bladder perforation during TURBT permitted to rule out an intrinsic deficiency in the bladder wall structure, leaving the main responsibility to the surgical technique [26].

Rare causes of iatrogenic bladder injuries include inguinal hernia repair, vascular surgery (femoral–femoral bypass graft) (Fig. 20.2), laparoscopic procedures (appendicectomy, nephrectomy, etc.) with too-low insertion of a port in a patient with full bladder (Fig. 20.3), sling operation for incontinence, positioning the reservoir during artificial sphincter or penile prosthesis, transvaginal oocytes retrieval for in-vitro fertilization, and even a simple catheter insertion [27–31].

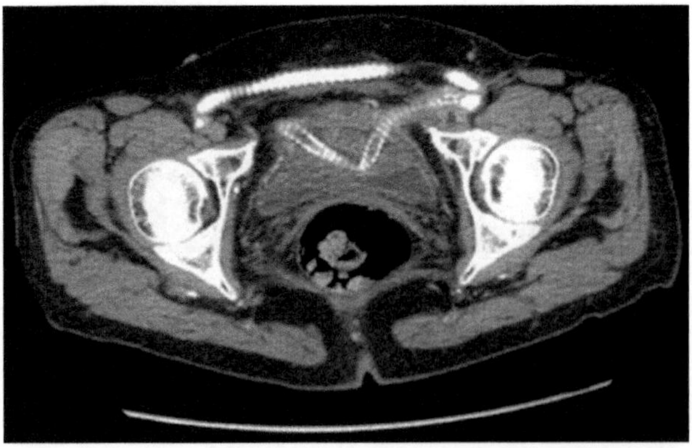

Fig. 20.2 Abdominal CT angiogram demonstrating a thrombosed femoral-femoral graft traversing through the bladder. A patent femoral-femoral graft is seen in the subcutaneous tissue. (From Nakamura LY et al. [28], with permission from Elsevier)

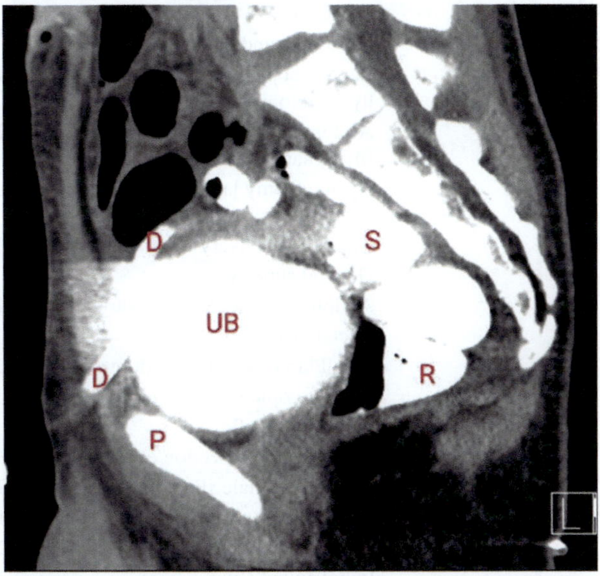

Fig. 20.3 Sagittal plane of a CT-urography in a 13-year-old boy who underwent an emergency laparoscopic surgery for a perforated appendix 24 h earlier. A 5-mm port was inserted too low near the pubis (P) with no urinary catheterization. It transpierced the bladder at the antero-superior aspect, and this event was unnoticed during all the procedure. A drain was introduced through the same port at the end of the operation. The alert was sounded the next day when excessive fluid was noted in the drain bag with high creatinine concentration, prompting this CT-urography showing the drain (D) crossing the urinary bladder (UB). The contrast seen in the sigmoid colon (S) and the rectum (R) was from the initial CT scan study with IV and oral contrast performed to diagnose the perforated appendix at presentation. (Courtesy Mohamed Abdul Salam Al-Qadri, General Surgery, The Royal Hospital, Muscat, Oman)

Table 20.1 gives an overview of the incidence of bladder trauma in various surgical procedures [32].

Finally, before closing this chapter, let's mention some exceptional cases of spontaneous intraperitoneal bladder rupture that have been reported in the literature, secondary to prostatic adenoma with urinary retention and bladder distention, and also in near term pregnancies, during childbirth, or after a normal delivery. This is considered an extremely rare event with an incidence of 1:126,000 deliveries but has a high mortality rate of 50% due to delayed management [33–36]. Underlying pathologies such as cystitis, diverticulum, and tumors are suggested to explain the bladder fragility and the pressure exerted by a gravid uterus or an acutely distended bladder are the triggering factors.

Table 20.1 Incidence of iatrogenic bladder trauma during various procedures

Procedure	Percentage (%)
Obstetrics and gynecology	
Laparoscopic/robotic radical hysterectomy (malignant)	4.19–4.59
Abdominal radical hysterectomy (malignant)	2.37
Hysterectomy laparoscopic/abdominal/vaginal (benign)	0.1–2.5
Caesarean delivery	0.08–0.94
General surgery	
Abdominal cytoreductive surgery	4.5
Rectal procedures	0.27–0.41
Small/large bowel procedures	0.12–0.14
Laparoscopic inguinal hernia repair	0.04–0.14
Urology specific	
Transurethral resection of the bladder	3.5–58
Retropubic male sling	8.0–19
Mid-urethral sling (retropubic route)	4.91–5.5
Transvaginal mesh surgery	2.84
Pubovaginal sling	2.8
Laparoscopic sacrocolpopexy	1.9
Mid-urethral sling (transobturator route)	1.61
Burch colposuspension	1.0–1.2
Native tissue colporrhaphy	0.53

From the EAU guidelines [32], with permission from the EAU

References

1. Matlock KA, Tyroch AH, Kronfol ZN, McLean SF, Pirela-Cruz MA. Blunt traumatic bladder rupture: a 10-year perspective. Am Surg. 2013;79(6):589–93. https://doi.org/10.1177/000313481307900619.
2. Deibert CM, Spencer BA. The association between operative repair of bladder injury and improved survival: results from the National Trauma Data Bank. J Urol. 2011;186(1):151–5. https://doi.org/10.1016/j.juro.2011.03.002. Epub 2011 May 14
3. Bjurlin MA, Fantus RJ, Mellett MM, Goble SM. Genitourinary injuries in pelvic fracture morbidity and mortality using the National Trauma Data Bank. J Trauma. 2009;67(5):1033–9. https://doi.org/10.1097/TA.0b013e3181bb8d6c.
4. Johnsen NV, Dmochowski RR, Young JB, Guillamondegui OD. Epidemiology of blunt lower urinary tract trauma with and without pelvic fracture. Urology. 2017;102:234–9. https://doi.org/10.1016/j.urology.2016.11.015. Epub 2016 Dec 30
5. Kang L, Geube A. Bladder trauma. In: StatPearls [Internet]. Treasure Island (FL): StatPearls Publishing; 2022. https://www.ncbi.nlm.nih.gov/books/NBK557875/.
6. McGeady JB, Breyer BN. Current epidemiology of genitourinary trauma. Urol Clin N Am. 2013;40(3):323–34. https://doi.org/10.1016/j.ucl.2013.04.001. Epub 2013 Jun 12. PMID: 23905930; PMCID: PMC4016766

7. Ford D, Palma J, Robinson J. Traumatic bladder rupture in a paratrooper. Mil Med. 2009;174(6):662–5. https://doi.org/10.7205/milmed-d-02-5108.
8. Ami S, Ina D, Yair G. Ruptured urinary bladder after a 'simple' fall. Am J Med. 2018;132:e11. https://doi.org/10.1016/j.amjmed.2018.08.010.
9. Gomez RG, Ceballos L, Coburn M, Corriere JN Jr, Dixon CM, Lobel B, McAninch J. Consensus statement on bladder injuries. BJU Int. 2004;94(1):27–32. https://doi.org/10.1111/j.1464-410X.2004.04896.x. PMID: 15217426
10. Pereira BM, de Campos CC, Calderan TR, Reis LO, Fraga GP. Bladder injuries after external trauma: 20 years experience report in a population-based cross-sectional view. World J Urol. 2013;31(4):913–7. https://doi.org/10.1007/s00345-012-0871-8. Epub 2012 Apr 28
11. Cohen AJ, Packiam VT, Nottingham CU, Pariser JJ, Faris SF, Bales GT. Iatrogenic bladder injury: national analysis of 30-day outcomes. Urology. 2016;97:250–6. https://doi.org/10.1016/j.urology.2016.05.002. Epub 2016 May 12
12. Esparaz AM, Pearl JA, Herts BR, LeBlanc J, Kapoor B. Iatrogenic urinary tract injuries: etiology, diagnosis, and management. Semin Intervent Radiol. 2015;32(2):195–208. https://doi.org/10.1055/s-0035-1549378. PMID: 26038626; PMCID: PMC4447880
13. Radu VD, Pristavu AI, Vinturache A, Onofrei P, Socolov DG, Carauleanu A, Boiculese L, Scripcariu SI, Costache RC. Risk factors for urological complications associated with caesarean section—a case-control study. Medicina (Kaunas). 2022;58(1):123. https://doi.org/10.3390/medicina58010123. PMID: 35056431; PMCID: PMC8779572
14. Adelman MR, Bardsley TR, Sharp HT. Urinary tract injuries in laparoscopic hysterectomy: a systematic review. J Minim Invasive Gynecol. 2014;21:558. https://doi.org/10.1016/j.jmig.2014.01.006.
15. Cordon BH, Fracchia JA, Armenakas NA. Iatrogenic nonendoscopic bladder injuries over 24 years: 127 cases at a single institution. Urology. 2014;84(1):222–6. https://doi.org/10.1016/j.urology.2014.03.028. Epub 2014 May 22
16. Tarney CM. Bladder injury during cesarean delivery. Curr Womens Health Rev. 2013;9(2):70–6. https://doi.org/10.2174/157340480902140102151729. PMID: 24876830; PMCID: PMC4033551
17. Salman L, Aharony S, Shmueli A, Wiznitzer A, Chen R, Gabbay-Benziv R. Urinary bladder injury during cesarean delivery: maternal outcome from a contemporary large case series. Eur J Obstet Gynecol Reprod Biol. 2017;213:26–30. https://doi.org/10.1016/j.ejogrb.2017.04.007. Epub 2017 Apr 5
18. Manidip P, Soma B. Cesarean bladder injury—obstetrician's nightmare. J Fam Med Prim Care. 2020;9(9):4526–9. https://doi.org/10.4103/jfmpc.jfmpc_586_20. PMID: 33209757; PMCID: PMC7652199
19. Martin JA, Hamilton BE, Ventura SJ, Osterman MJ, Kirmeyer S, Mathews TJ, Wilson EC. Births: final data for 2009. Natl Vital Stat Rep. 2011;60(1):1–70.
20. https://www.prb.org/articles/u-s-births-increased-in-2021-but-dont-call-it-a-comeback/
21. Caliskan E, Tan O, Kurtaran V, Dilbaz B, Haberal A. Placenta previa percreta with urinary bladder and ureter invasion. Arch Gynecol Obstet. 2003;268(4):343–4. https://doi.org/10.1007/s00404-002-0402-8. Epub 2002 Oct 15
22. Saaqib S, Iqbal A, Naheed M, Saeed T, Khalid M. A randomized controlled trial of cystoinflation to prevent bladder injury in the adhesive disease of multiple caesarean sections. Sci Rep. 2020;10(1):15297. https://doi.org/10.1038/s41598-020-71132-5. PMID: 32943657; PMCID: PMC7499421
23. Pladzyk K, Jureczko L, Lazowski T. Over 500 obturator nerve blocks in the lithotomy position during transurethral resection of bladder tumor. Cent Eur J Urol. 2012;65(2):67–70. https://doi.org/10.5173/ceju.2012.02.art2. Epub 2012 Jun 12. PMID: 24578931; PMCID: PMC3921785
24. Bolat D, Yarimoglu S, Aydin ME. Monopolar versus bipolar transurethral resection of lateral wall-located bladder cancer under obturator nerve block: a single center prospective randomized study. Int Braz J Urol. 2021;47(3):584–93. https://doi.org/10.1590/S1677-5538.IBJU.2020.0568. PMID: 33621007; PMCID: PMC7993959.

25. Ozer K, Horsanali MO, Gorgel SN, Ozbek E. Bladder injury secondary to obturator reflex is more common with plasmakinetic transurethral resection than monopolar transurethral resection of bladder cancer. Cent Eur J Urol. 2015;68(3):284–8. https://doi.org/10.5173/ceju.2015.565. Epub 2015 Sep 26. PMID: 26568867; PMCID: PMC4643702
26. Poletajew S, Ilczuk T, Krajewski W, et al. Bladder perforation during transurethral resection of bladder tumour is not a result of a deficient structure of the bladder wall. World J Surg Oncol. 2020;18:216. https://doi.org/10.1186/s12957-020-01992-8.
27. Ee TX, Toh WL, Chan JKY. Rare surgical complication of in vitro fertilisation treatment: bladder injury during oocyte retrieval. J Med Cases. 2021;12(3):102–6. https://doi.org/10.14740/jmc3632. Epub 2021 Jan 19. PMID: 34434438; PMCID: PMC8383583
28. Nakamura LY, Ferrigni RG, Stone WM, Fowl RJ. Urinary bladder injuries during vascular surgery. J Vasc Surg. 2010;52(2):453–5. https://doi.org/10.1016/j.jvs.2010.02.261. Epub 2010 Jun 11
29. Minaglia S, Ozel B, Klutke C, Ballard C, Klutke J. Bladder injury during transobturator sling. Urology. 2004;64(2):376–7. https://doi.org/10.1016/j.urology.2004.04.030.
30. Poola S, Mohan A. A Foley fallacy: a case of bladder rupture after "Routine" Foley catheter placement. Case Rep Urol. 2018;2018:7978126. https://doi.org/10.1155/2018/7978126. PMID: 30643662; PMCID: PMC6311248
31. Roy SP, Combes AD, Perera DS. A very rare case report of an iatrogenic bladder perforation in a young female with concurrent Fitz–Hugh–Curtis syndrome. J Surg Case Rep. 2021;2021(5):rjab218. https://doi.org/10.1093/jscr/rjab218. PMID: 34055300; PMCID: PMC8153801
32. EAU Guidelines. Edn. presented at the EAU Annual Congress Amsterdam March 2022. ISBN 978-94-92671-16-5. https://uroweb.org/guidelines/urological-trauma/chapter/urogenital-trauma-guidelines.
33. Ibrahimi A, Dergamoun H, Ziani I, Makhoukhi ZEBE, Sayegh HE, Benslimane L, Nouini Y. Successful conservative management of a spontaneous intraperitoneal urinary bladder rupture secondary to benign prostatic hyperplasia: a case report. Pan Afr Med J. 2021;38:268. https://doi.org/10.11604/pamj.2021.38.268.26684. PMID: 34122695; PMCID: PMC8179998
34. Peters PC. Intraperitoneal rupture of the bladder. Urol Clin N Am. 1989;16(2):279–82.
35. Qiao P, Tian D, Bao Q. Delayed diagnosis of spontaneous bladder rupture: a rare case report. BMC Womens Health. 2018;18:124. https://doi.org/10.1186/s12905-018-0616-y.
36. Diana V, Bhargavi K. Spontaneous isolated bladder rupture following normal delivery. Int J Reprod Contracept Obstet Gynecol. 2018;7:1638–40.

Anatomopathology of Urinary Bladder Injury

21

Four anatomopathological entities of the bladder injury are described [1–5]:

- Bladder contusions
- Extraperitoneal rupture
- Intraperitoneal rupture
- Mixed or combined bladder ruptures

1. In *bladder contusions*, the damage is either limited to the mucosa, including or not the muscular coat, but without breaching the serosa/adventitia for injuries arising intravesically (during endourological procedures such as TURBT), or inversely lacerating the serosa/adventitia while the muscular and mucosa layers are spared for extra-vesical trauma (penetrating agents, surgical operations). In either case, there is no complete rupture of the bladder wall, and consequently, no urinary leak occurs. This entity almost always remains undiagnosed, and its incidence is therefore unknown, though it is probably the most common anatomopathological form [2].
2. *Extraperitoneal bladder ruptures* are reported to mostly occur in association with **pelvic fractures**, due to penetration by bone spicules, or to shear forces and distortion of the bladder wall as a contrecoup mechanism following ligamentous injury, and their proportion is estimated to be **55–78%** according to multiple series. As logically expected, extraperitoneal rupture concerns any part of the bladder below the peritoneal reflection, be it on the anterior, lateral, or posterior walls. Furthermore, extraperitoneal bladder injuries are divided into two types: simple and complex. In the former, the contrast extravasation is limited to the pelvic extraperitoneal space. In the complex type, there are large extraperitoneal bladder ruptures associated with a rupture of the superior fascia of the urogenital diaphragm, allowing the urine leak to spread through Dartos, Colles, and Scarpa's fasciae which are continuous with the urogenital diaphragm (Fig. 21.1).

S. A. AL-Mamari, *Urogenital Trauma: A Practical Guide*,
https://doi.org/10.1007/978-981-99-6171-9_21

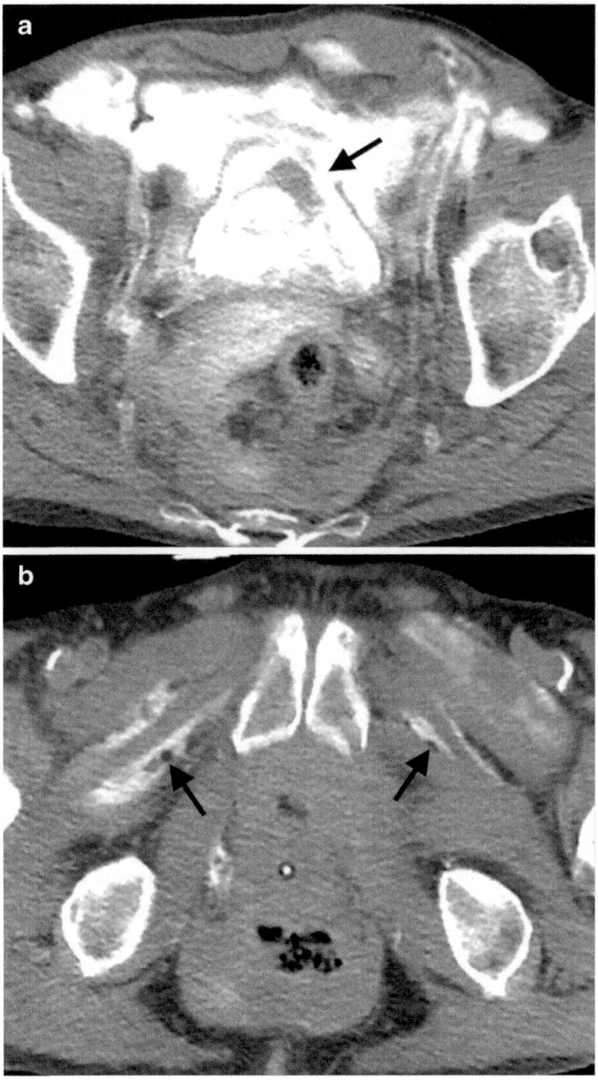

Fig. 21.1 Complex extraperitoneal bladder rupture. (**a**) Axial CT cystographic image shows a defect in the anterior bladder wall (arrow) with contrast extravasation in the extraperitoneal space beyond the pelvis. (**b**) Axial CT cystographic image at more inferior level shows contrast extravasation into soft tissue in bilateral thighs (arrow). (From Wongwaisayawan S [8], with permission from Springer Nature)

Therefore, the urine will extravasate into the scrotum through the inguinal canal, the perineum, the penis, and the thighs via the obturator foramen, or into the anterior abdominal wall, or even retroperitoneally as high as the perinephric region [2, 6–8].

3. *Intraperitoneal ruptures* occur mainly with high-energy blows directly hitting an overdistended bladder and their proportion is around **17–39%**. Here the injury is located above the peritoneal reflection, mainly on the bladder dome which is the weakest point of the bladder wall [8] (Fig. 21.2).

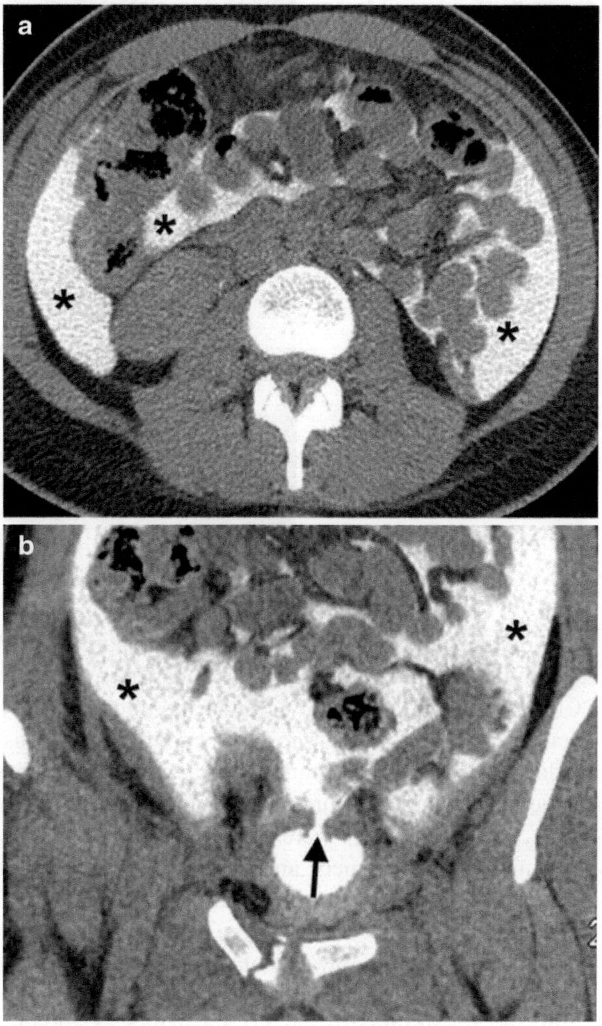

Fig. 21.2 Intraperitoneal bladder rupture. (**a**) Axial CT cystographic image shows large amount of contrast material in bilateral paracolic gutters and between the mesenteric folds (*). (**b**) Coronal CT cystographic image shows a defect at the bladder dome (arrow) with contrast extravasation in bilateral paracolic gutters (*). (From Wongwaisayawan S [8], with permission from Springer Nature)

4. *Combined intra- and extraperitoneal ruptures* of the bladder are possible and their occurrence is estimated to be 5–8% of all bladder ruptures.

In intraperitoneal bladder ruptures the urine leaks into the abdominal cavity and is absorbed by the peritoneal membrane, leading to an increase in blood urea nitrogen and creatinine, as well as electrolytes and metabolic imbalances (hyperchloremic metabolic acidosis, hypernatremia, hyperkalemia) [2, 5, 7]. In either intra- or extra-peritoneal bladder rupture, there is decreased urine output.

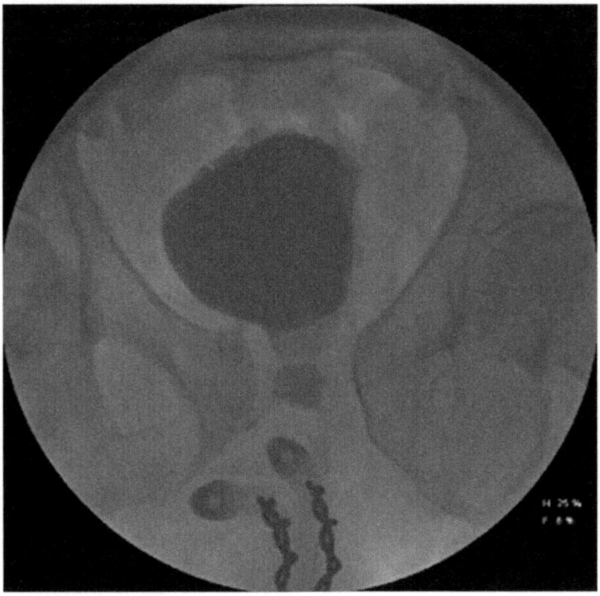

Fig. 21.3 Cystogram of a patient with a bladder neck and prostatic injury and a relatively small cavity. The patient also has a malleable penile implant. (From Mundy and Andrich [9], with permission from John Wiley and Sons)

A distinct and extremely rare anatomopathological entity consists of bladder neck injury. To date, the largest series has been published by Mundy and Andrich in 2010 comprising a total of 15 men recruited over a 15-year period [9]. They all occurred after pelvic fractures. Only 5 of the 15 cases had lesions confined to the bladder neck and the prostatic urethra, while others were more complex, extending to the subprostatic urethra often with posterior urethral rupture (Figs. 21.3 and 21.4). Two of the cases were particularly severe with simultaneous complete transection of the bladder neck and of the membranous urethra leaving a freely floating prostate (Fig. 21.5). After this series, a few smaller series and isolated case reports have been published here and there [3, 10].

It is important to know that bladder neck injury is more common in children due to the relatively unprotected anatomy of the bladder. And the rare cases reported in adults are longitudinal (vertical) consisting of a bladder and prostatic injury. Few cases of transversal (horizontal) bladder neck transection have been reported in children but are extremely rare in adults [11, 12] (Fig. 21.6a–c).

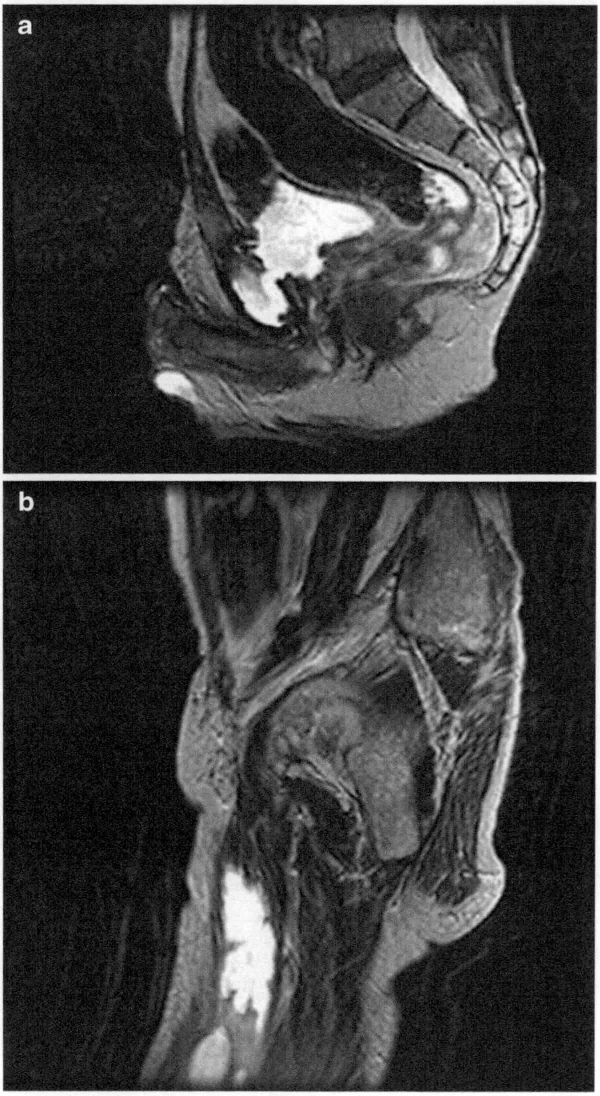

Fig. 21.4 (**a**, **b**) MRI of a patient with a bladder neck and prostatic injury and cavitation spreading down into the thigh. (From Mundy and Andrich [9], with permission from John Wiley and Sons)

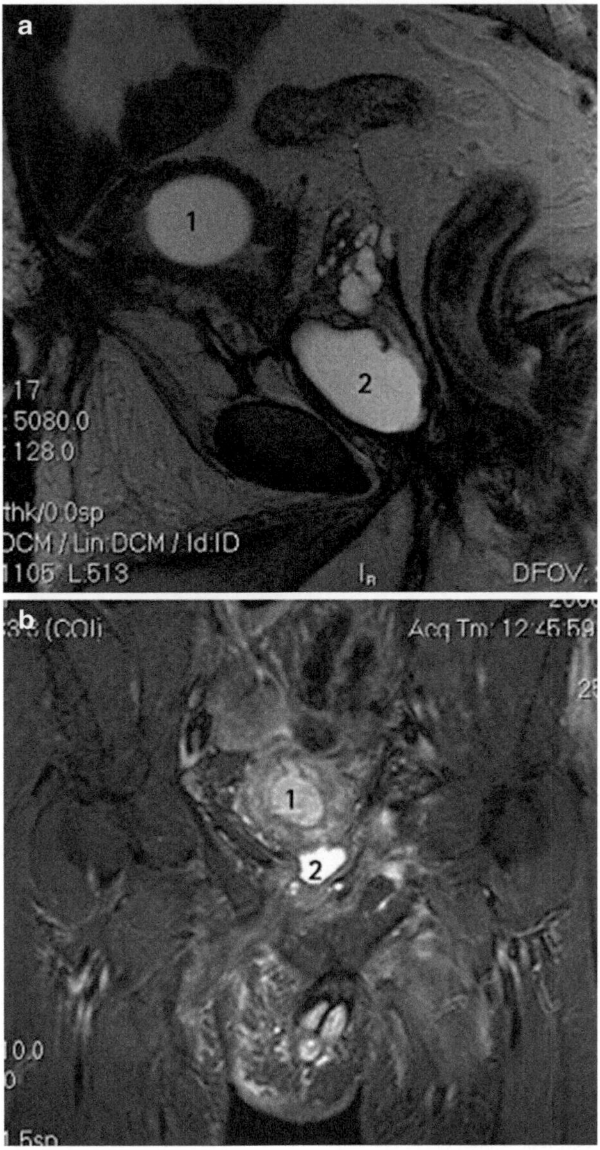

Fig. 21.5 Representative MRI of the two patients with a transected bladder neck above and a transected membranous urethra below a sequestered prostate. In each case 1 = bladder and 2 = prostatic urethra. (**a**) sagittal view in patient 1; (**b**) coronal view in patient 2. (From Mundy and Andrich [9], with permission from John Wiley and Sons)

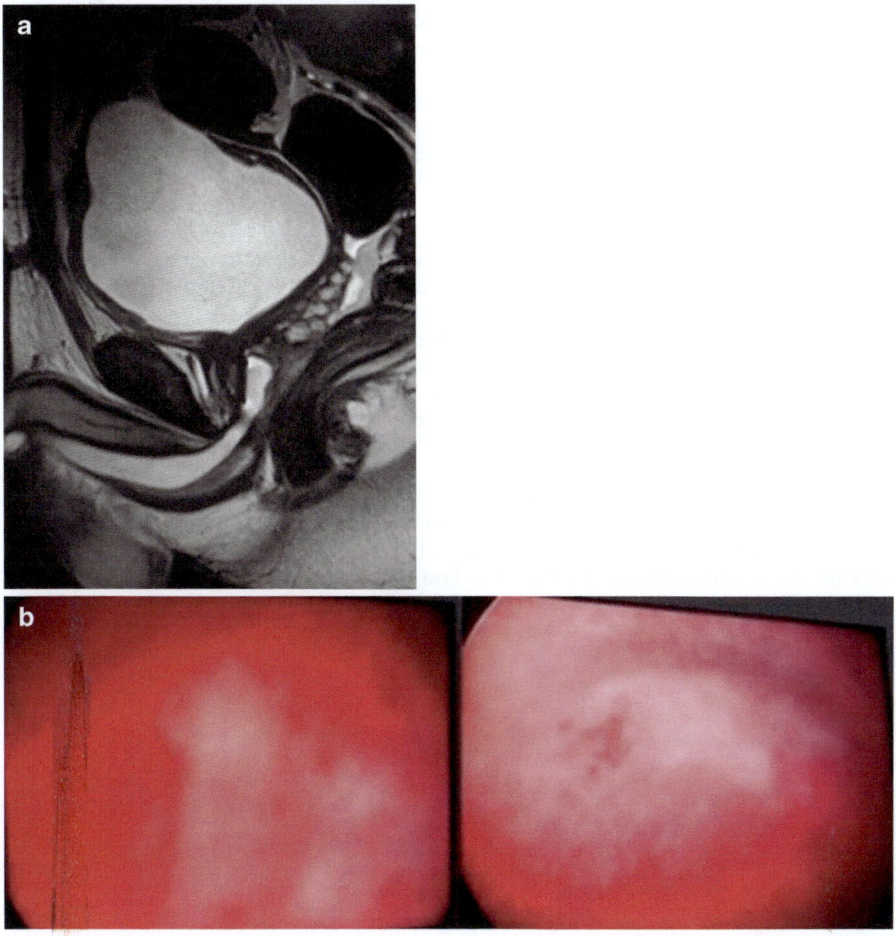

Fig. 21.6 (**a**) MRI pelvis showing complete transection noted at junction of bladder neck and proximal prostatic urethra. From Gite VA et al. [12], with permission from Elsevier. (**b**, **c**) SPC scopy and urethroscopy image. (From Gite VA et al. [12], with permission from Elsevier)

References

1. McGeady JB, Breyer BN. Current epidemiology of genitourinary trauma. Urol Clin N Am. 2013;40(3):323–34. https://doi.org/10.1016/j.ucl.2013.04.001. Epub 2013 Jun 12. PMID: 23905930; PMCID: PMC4016766
2. Gomez RG, Ceballos L, Coburn M, Corriere JN Jr, Dixon CM, Lobel B, McAninch J. Consensus statement on bladder injuries. BJU Int. 2004;94(1):27–32. https://doi.org/10.1111/j.1464-410X.2004.04896.x. PMID: 15217426
3. Kong JP, Bultitude MF, Royce P, Gruen RL, Cato A, Corcoran NM. Lower urinary tract injuries following blunt trauma: a review of contemporary management. Rev Urol. 2011;13(3):119–30. PMID: 22114545; PMCID: PMC3222924

4. Matlock KA, Tyroch AH, Kronfol ZN, McLean SF, Pirela-Cruz MA. Blunt traumatic bladder rupture: a 10-year perspective. Am Surg. 2013;79(6):589–93. https://doi.org/10.1177/000313481307900619.
5. Kang L, Geube A. Bladder trauma. In: StatPearls [Internet]. Treasure Island (FL): StatPearls Publishing; 2022.
6. Ramchandani P, Buckler PM. Imaging of genitourinary trauma. AJR Am J Roentgenol. 2009;192(6):1514–23. https://doi.org/10.2214/AJR.09.2470.
7. Brandes S, Borrelli J Jr. Pelvic fracture and associated urologic injuries. World J Surg. 2001;25(12):1578–87.
8. Wongwaisayawan S, Krishna S, Sheikh A, Kaewlai R, Schieda N. Imaging spectrum of traumatic urinary bladder and urethral injuries. Abdom Radiol (NY). 2021;46(2):681–91. https://doi.org/10.1007/s00261-020-02679-0. Epub 2020 Jul 28
9. Mundy AR, Andrich DE. Pelvic fracture-related injuries of the bladder neck and prostate: their nature, cause and management. BJU Int. 2010;105(9):1302–8. https://doi.org/10.1111/j.1464-410X.2009.08970.x. Epub 2009 Oct 28
10. Lv R, Jin C, Shu H, et al. Bladder neck reconstruction in girls' pelvic fracture bladder neck avulsion and urethral rupture. BMC Urol. 2020;20:179. https://doi.org/10.1186/s12894-020-00741-z.
11. Sawant AS, Kapadnis LA, Kumar V, Pawar P, Tamhankar AS. Paediatric post-traumatic bladder neck distraction injury: case series. J Clin Diagn Res. 2017;11(2):PR03–4. https://doi.org/10.7860/JCDR/2017/20782.9244. Epub 2017 Feb 1
12. Gite VA, Singal A, Nikose JV, Jain HM. Post traumatic isolated bladder neck transection: unreported and undescribed injury. Urol Case Rep. 2017;17:67–9. https://doi.org/10.1016/j.eucr.2017.12.001.

Presentation, Diagnostic Investigations, and Grading of Urinary Bladder Injury

22

22.1 Presentation

In a patient who sustained a pelvic or abdominal, blunt or penetrating injury, the presence of a bladder injury is often suggested by the following classical triad of symptoms [1]:

- **gross hematuria,**
- **suprapubic or abdominal pain or tenderness, and,**
- **difficulty or inability to void.**

Hematuria is the most common symptom being present in 100% of cases of bladder injury. However, in less than 5% of cases, it might only be microscopic [2].

The physical examination of the patient has to be carefully performed in penetrating injuries, especially after a gunshot, where the entrance and exit wounds should be identified in the lower abdomen, the perineum, or the buttocks.

For the iatrogenic causes, intraoperative bladder injuries are generally easily recognized and repaired without delay. About 80% of injuries are recognized during surgery as the result of direct visualization of the injury site, either during extravesical surgery (open or laparoscopic) or cystoscopies. Additionally, during non-cystoscopic abdominal or pelvic procedures, suspicion of a bladder injury may be raised by the presence of urine in the operative field, or air in the urinary bag, or more directly by visualization of the Foley catheter [3].

When one doesn't directly observe a bladder perforation during cystoscopic procedures (chiefly transurethral resection of bladder tumour (TURBT), but also transurethral resection of the prostate (TURP)), this can be suspected through a newly appearing abdominal distension, or difficulty in maintaining bladder distension with the irrigation fluid, or mismatch between the instillated and the drained fluid with the latter appearing significantly low.

S. A. AL-Mamari, *Urogenital Trauma: A Practical Guide*,
https://doi.org/10.1007/978-981-99-6171-9_22

22.2 Investigations

22.2.1 Conventional Cystography

Immediate retrograde cystography is absolutely indicated and is the mainstay of diagnosis in blunt trauma patients who are hemodynamically stable and present with the classic combination of pelvic fracture and gross hematuria [4–7].

However, this procedure should be performed only after the exclusion of an associated urethral injury which can be suspected when one observes blood at the external urethral meatus. Moreover, retrograde cystography can be spared for patients with isolated hematuria or pelvic fracture alone [4, 5, 8]. This reduces possible hazards to the patient and saves time and money.

Cystography might be postponed in a scenario of pelvic fracture with massive bleeding requiring angiographic embolization because the extravasated contrast material in the pelvis is likely to impair the accuracy of the angiography [6].

Microscopic hematuria is a poor indicator of bladder rupture and even its association with a pelvic fracture constitutes only a relative indication for retrograde cystogram, as is the presence of gross hematuria without pelvic fracture. A retrospective study including 721 cases of blunt pelvic fracture has demonstrated that hematuria values <30 RBC/HPF are poorly correlated with the presence of bladder injury. This study also refined pelvic fracture characteristics that predict a high likelihood of bladder injury, namely diastasis of the pubic symphysis >1 cm, and fracture of the obturator ring with displacement >1 cm. No patient with an isolated acetabular fracture was shown to have a bladder injury [9]. Conversely, out of 31 patients with gross hematuria after blunt pelvic trauma, only those who had a concomitant pelvic fracture (26%) were found to have a bladder injury in a randomized prospective study [10].

The accuracy of cystography has been estimated to be 85–100% according to published series. For optimal results, the bladder should be filled with at least 300–400 mL of diluted contrast medium. False-negative results are due to inadequate distention of the bladder and absence of post-drainage films because small anterior or posterior extravasations might be covered by the full bladder in an anteroposterior picture and would not become obvious until the bladder is emptied [11–13] (Fig. 22.1a, b).

One of the explanations for false-negative cystograms has been suggested to be small-caliber bullet wounds where the omentum or blood clots might plug the breach [11]. Other causes of false negative are pelvic hematoma not leaving space for the contrast to freely extravasate, contraction of the detrusor muscle provisionally sealing a small perforation, presence of a Foley catheter balloon blocking a small tear, gravity, impossibility to turn the patient in a prone position in pelvic trauma (missing a small breach in the anterior vesical wall) [14].

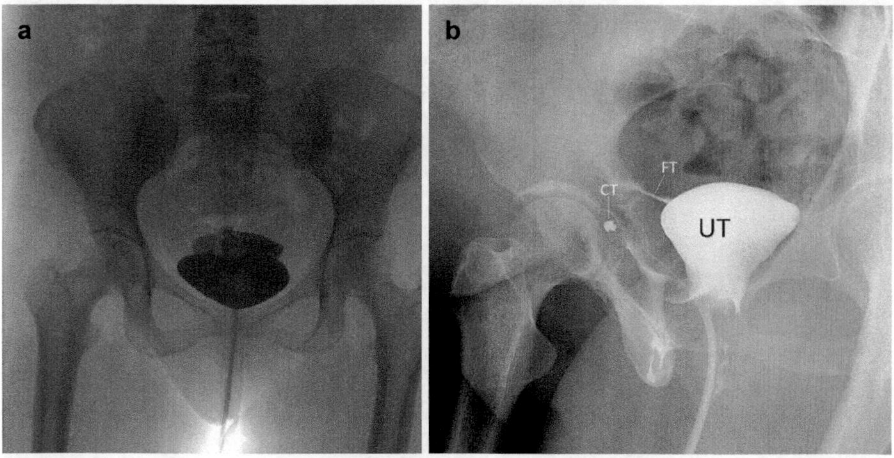

Fig. 22.1 (**a**, **b**) Post-cesarean section in a 39-year old woman with persistent upper vesico-vaginal fistula (same patient discussed in the Figure 20.1a, b). (**a**) Double-contour image on an antero-posterior conventional cystography. (**b**) Lateral view after emptying the bladder showing contrast filling the uterus (UT) and one of the fallopian tube (FT). The vesical catheter tip (CT) is seen anteriorly to the uterus and some contrast is seen flowing freely through the vagina. (Courtesy Ashraf Abdelsalam Al Ozeni, Urology, The Royal Hospital, Muscat, Oman)

22.2.2 CT-Cystography

CT-cystography is another valuable means to diagnose a bladder perforation and is better performed after intra-vesical contrast instillation. This has been proved to have an accuracy comparable to that of a conventional cystography in diagnosing bladder injuries [15] (Fig. 22.2a–d).

Out of 234 patients, a level I trauma center found a nearly 100%-overall sensitivity and specificity of CT cystography in diagnosing bladder rupture, and the addition of sagittal and coronal images from the multiplanar reformation is particularly useful in identifying the site of the lesion [16].

Expert panels recommend either technique (standard cystography or CT-cystography) for bladder injury diagnosis when the patient presents with gross hematuria or pelvic fracture associated with microscopic hematuria, taking into account the advantages and drawbacks of each (time, cost) [5]. CT-cystography has the advantage to avoid confusion with overlying bone fragments caused by pelvic fractures, spine boards, or clothing artifacts.

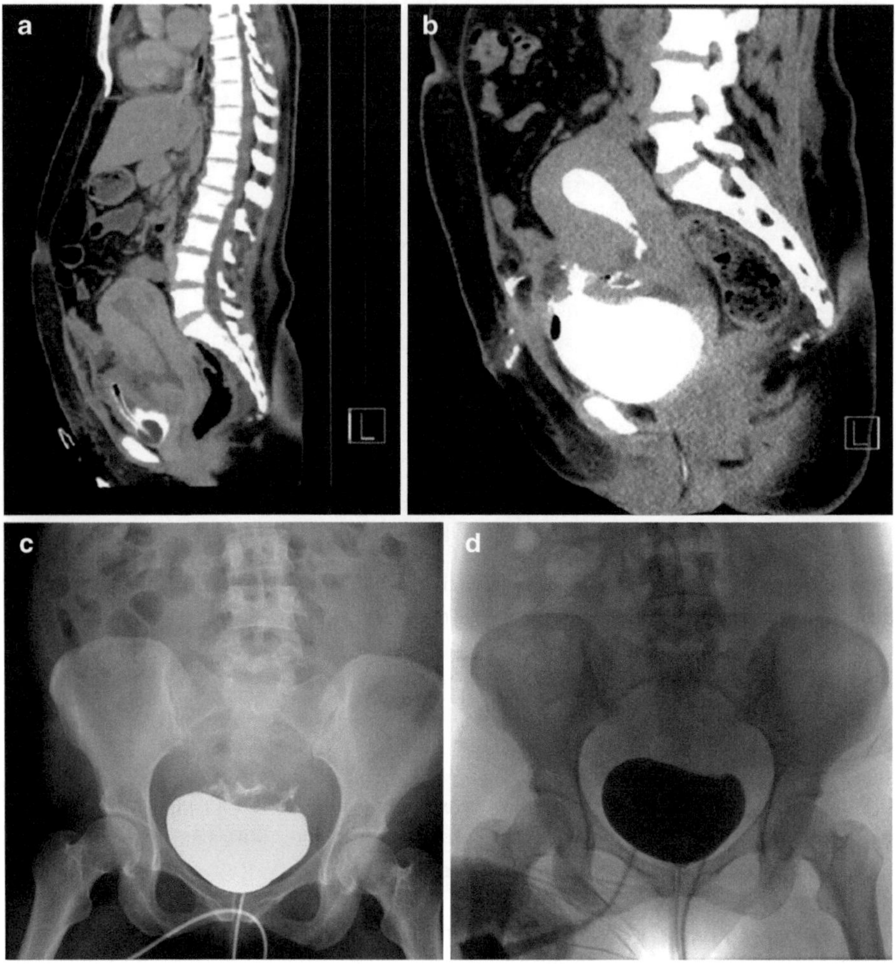

Fig. 22.2 (**a**, **b**) CT cystography showing vesicouterine fistula 2 weeks after a cesarean section in placenta accreta during which the bladder was severely damaged and immediately repaired. The fistula was treated conservatively with an indwelling catheter. (**c**) Cystogram at 2 weeks shows persistent leakage. (**d**) Follow-up conventional cystography at 6 weeks showing complete healing

22.2.3 CT-Urography

A CT-urography after intra-vesical contrast instillation, combined with IV and oral contrast for a whole abdomen examination is a time-saving procedure when one wants to evaluate associated abdominal viscera injuries and obviate the need for a separate conventional retrograde-cystography. However, a CT-cystography with only IV contrast and passive physiological bladder filling with catheter clamping is not recommended due to a high rate of false-negative results. Needless to say, the use of traditional Intravenous pyelography (IVP) is obsolete, especially for this indication [6, 11, 17–20].

22.2.4 Intraoperative Means

In the setting of iatrogenic bladder injury during laparoscopic or open abdominal or pelvic surgery, the diagnosis can be readily made by the direct observation of the breach and the intra-vesical catheter. In unclear cases where the suspicion is raised by a sudden increase of intraperitoneal fluid (urine), decreased urine output in the urinary bag, or unexplained hematuria, an intravenous injection of indigo carmine can be used or, more rapidly a retrograde intravesical instillation of diluted methylene blue [6].

22.2.5 Other Techniques

(a) "**Sentinel clot sign**": This concept has been introduced to help in diagnosing abdominal viscera trauma through CT observation of a focal high-density clotted blood adjacent to an organ, and showed high sensitivity and specificity in predicting an injury of that organ [21]. In this study, the sentinel clot was the only clue of injury in 9% of splenic trauma cases and 32% of bowel or mesenteric injuries. A subsequent study has demonstrated the value of this concept in refining the radiological diagnosis of intraperitoneal bladder rupture following blunt trauma. Herein a sentinel clot abutting the bladder dome showed a high correlation with an injury at this level [22].
(b) **Pneumo-CT-Cystography:** CT scan of a gas-distended bladder followed by a 3-D virtual reconstruction has permitted to mimic a cystoscopy with high accuracy in patients with small bladder tumors. This technique was therefore referred to as **CT-cystoscopy** [23, 24]. A recent application of this technique using 150–300 mL of intra-vesical air insufflation rather than contrast material combined with an Intravenous contrast-enhanced CT has been proposed for bladder rupture detection, as a so-called **pneumo-CT-cystography** [14]. Further studies with larger cohorts are required to confirm the accuracy of this technique.

22.2.6 Grading of Bladder Injury

In routine clinical practice, the American Association for the Surgery of Trauma (AAST) grading system is not used for bladder injury as frequently as for kidney trauma [25] (Table 22.1). However, it is of paramount importance for every Urologist to have a sound knowledge of the main characteristic of each grade of bladder trauma, as this impacts survival and can lead to fatal outcomes if incorrectly or not timely managed.

A radiologic classification system has also been proposed to help analyze the different patterns of extravasation, including the atypical ones, but is seldom used [26] (Table 22.2). This grading is interesting with regard to the description of radiological features of the injury, but has to be interpreted with caution as the

Table 22.1 AAST for bladder injury

Grade	Injury	Description	AIS-90
I	Hematoma Laceration	Intramural hematoma Partial thickness	2 3
II	Laceration	Extraperitoneal bladder wall laceration <2 cm	4
III	Laceration	Extraperitoneal ≥2 cm or intraperitoneal <2 cm bladder wall laceration	4
IV	Laceration	Intraperitoneal bladder wall laceration ≥2 cm	4
V	Laceration	Intraperitoneal or extraperitoneal laceration extending into bladder neck or ureteral orifice (trigone)	4

From Moore EE [25], with permission from Elsevier

Table 22.2 Patterns of extravasation in bladder injuries

Type	Injury	Radiographic appearances (cystography)
1	Bladder contusion	Normal
2	Intraperitoneal (IP) rupture	Ill-defined contrast extravasation surrounding loops of bowel and in the paracolic gutters and pouch of Douglas
3	Interstitial bladder injury (rare)	Contrast dissects into bladder wall, causing irregularity or defect; no contrast extravasation
4	Extraperitoneal (EP) rupture	
	Simple	Contrast is limited to the perivesical space with linear streaks or a sunburst pattern
	Complex	The pelvic floor is breeched and contrast may track up the peritoneal space and appear as an IP rupture; extravasation may extend to scrotum, penis, and anterior abdominal wall
5	Combined IP and EP	Combination of type 2 and 4

Adapted from Sandler CM et al. [26]

presentation is not strictly in accordance with the severity and the prognosis of the lesion. This is illustrated by the fact that an intraperitoneal rupture is described as type 2 while a simple extraperitoneal rupture is labeled as type 4.

References

1. Guttmann I, Kerr HA. Blunt bladder injury. Clin Sports Med. 2013;32:239–46.
2. Brandes S, Borrelli J Jr. Pelvic fracture and associated urologic injuries. World J Surg. 2001;25(12):1578–87.
3. Esparaz AM, Pearl JA, Herts BR, LeBlanc J, Kapoor B. Iatrogenic urinary tract injuries: etiology, diagnosis, and management. Semin Intervent Radiol. 2015;32(2):195–208. https://doi.org/10.1055/s-0035-1549378.
4. Morey AF, Brandes S, Dugi DD 3rd, Armstrong JH, Breyer BN, Broghammer JA, Erickson BA, Holzbeierlein J, Hudak SJ, Pruitt JH, Reston JT, Santucci RA, Smith TG 3rd, Wessells H, American Urological Assocation. Urotrauma: AUA guideline. J Urol. 2014;192(2):327–35. https://doi.org/10.1016/j.juro.2014.05.004. Epub 2014 May 20. PMID: 24857651; PMCID: PMC4104146

5. Yeung LL, McDonald AA, Como JJ, Robinson B, Knight J, Person MA, Lee JK, Dahm P. Management of blunt force bladder injuries: a practice management guideline from the Eastern Association for the Surgery of Trauma [Erratum in: J Trauma Acute Care Surg 2019 Aug;87(2):511]. J Trauma Acute Care Surg. 2019;86(2):326–36. https://doi.org/10.1097/TA.0000000000002132.
6. Coccolini F, Moore EE, Kluger Y, et al. Kidney and uro-trauma: WSES-AAST guidelines. World J Emerg Surg. 2019;14:54. https://doi.org/10.1186/s13017-019-0274-x.
7. https://uroweb.org/guidelines/urological-trauma/chapter/urogenital-trauma-guidelines.
8. Morey AF, Iverson AJ, Swan A, Harmon WJ, Spore SS, Bhayani S, Brandes SB. Bladder rupture after blunt trauma: guidelines for diagnostic imaging. J Trauma. 2001;51(4):683–6. https://doi.org/10.1097/00005373-200110000-00010.
9. Avey G, Blackmore CC, Wessells H, Wright JL, Talner LB. Radiographic and clinical predictors of bladder rupture in blunt trauma patients with pelvic fracture. Acad Radiol. 2006;13(5):573–9. https://doi.org/10.1016/j.acra.2005.10.012.
10. Fuhrman GM, Simmons GT, Davidson BS, Buerk CA. The single indication for cystography in blunt trauma. Am Surg. 1993;59(6):335–7.
11. Corriere JN, Sandler CM. Bladder rupture from external trauma: diagnosis and management. World J Urol. 1999;17:84–9.
12. Carroll PR, McAninch JW. Major bladder trauma: the accuracy of cystography. J Urol. 1983;130(5):887–8. https://doi.org/10.1016/s0022-5347(17)51551-7.
13. Cass AS. False negative retrograde cystography with bladder rupture without pelvic fracture. J Urol. 1984;124:168–9.
14. Trinci M, Cirimele V, Cozzi D, Galluzzo M, Miele V. Diagnostic accuracy of pneumo-CT-cystography in the detection of bladder rupture in patients with blunt pelvic trauma. Radiol Med. 2020;125(10):907–17. https://doi.org/10.1007/s11547-020-01190-2. Epub 2020 Apr 9
15. Peng MY, Parisky YR, Cornwell EE 3rd, Radin R, Bragin S. CT cystography versus conventional cystography in evaluation of bladder injury. AJR Am J Roentgenol. 1999;173(5):1269–72. https://doi.org/10.2214/ajr.173.5.10541103.
16. Chan DP, Abujudeh HH, Cushing GL Jr, Novelline RA. CT cystography with multiplanar reformation for suspected bladder rupture: experience in 234 cases. AJR Am J Roentgenol. 2006;187(5):1296–302. https://doi.org/10.2214/AJR.05.0971.
17. Gomez RG, Ceballos L, Coburn M. Consensus statement on bladder injuries. BJU Int. 2004;94(1):27–32.
18. Vaccaro JP, Brody JM. CT cystography in the evaluation of major bladder trauma. Radiographics. 2000;20(5):1373–81. https://doi.org/10.1148/radiographics.20.5.g00se111373.
19. Ramchandani P, Buckler PM. Imaging of genitourinary trauma. AJR Am J Roentgenol. 2009;192(6):1514–23. https://doi.org/10.2214/AJR.09.2470.
20. Rehm CG, Mure AJ, O'Malley KF, Ross SE. Blunt traumatic bladder rupture: the role of retrograde cystogram. Ann Emerg Med. 1991;20(8):845–7. https://doi.org/10.1016/s0196-0644(05)81424-6.
21. Orwig D, Federle MP. Localized clotted blood as evidence of visceral trauma on CT: the sentinel clot sign. AJR Am J Roentgenol. 1989;153:747–9.
22. Shin SS, Jeong YY, Chung TW, Yoon W, Kang HK, Kang TW, Shin HY. The sentinel clot sign: a useful CT finding for the evaluation of intraperitoneal bladder rupture following blunt trauma. Korean J Radiol. 2007;8(6):492–7. https://doi.org/10.3348/kjr.2007.8.6.492.
23. Vining DJ, Zagoria RJ, Liu K, Stelts D. CT cystoscopy: an innovation in bladder imaging. AJR Am J Roentgenol. 1996;166(2):409–10. https://doi.org/10.2214/ajr.166.2.8553956.
24. Gualdi GF, Casciani E, Rojas M, Polettini E. Cistoscopia virtuale delle neoplasie della vescica. Esperienza preliminare [Virtual cystoscopy of bladder neoplasms. Preliminary experience]. Radiol Med. 1999;97(6):506–9. Italian
25. Moore EE, Shackford SR, Pachter HL, McAninch JW, Browner BD, Champion HR, Flint LM, Gennarelli TA, Malangoni MA, Ramenofsky ML, et al. Organ injury scaling: spleen, liver, and kidney. J Trauma. 1989;29(12):1664–6. https://doi.org/10.1016/S0039-6109(16)46589-8.
26. Sandler CM, Hall JT, Rodriguez MB, Corriere JN Jr. Bladder injury in blunt pelvic trauma. Radiology. 1986;158:633–8.

Treatment of Urinary Bladder Injury: Conservative Approach, Direct Repairs, and Reconstructive Techniques Using Urinary Tract Tissues

23

Bladder rupture is a potentially fatal event if not timely diagnosed and repaired. Except for some cases of complex bladder base and bladder neck injuries, the repair of this hollow viscus is generally technically easy and less challenging than that of a kidney, ureter, or urethra.

The management of bladder injury differs from other urinary system trauma in the following aspects:

- Renal trauma management is mainly conservative and intervention is only indicated upon patient hemodynamic instability. When intervention is required, it first consists of a minimally invasive procedure (angioembolization) and when an open exploration is required, it often results in nephrectomy, and rarely partial nephrectomy.
- Ureteric injury can be temporarily managed by urinary diversion with a percutaneous nephrostomy until further treatment. Sometimes an antegrade DJ stenting can be inserted without the need for invasive surgery. When surgical repair is necessary, it might require complex reconstructive techniques as discussed in the previous chapter.
- We will see in the next section of this book that urethral rupture is provisionally managed with a suprapubic catheter until an elective repair is performed, which potentially involves complex techniques.

Contrary to the above injuries, and with the exception of a simple extraperitoneal injury, bladder ruptures have no alternative than urgent surgical repair. Fortunately, bladder repair is generally a simple procedure and seldom requires complicated reconstructive techniques. Usually, the intervention is carried out through an open procedure and the detection of the bladder site injury is generally easy [1] (Fig. 23.1). The laparoscopic approach is also an option for selected intraperitoneal cases in expert hands, with the advantage of lower morbidity and a shorter hospital stay [2, 3] (Fig. 23.2).

S. A. AL-Mamari, *Urogenital Trauma: A Practical Guide*,
https://doi.org/10.1007/978-981-99-6171-9_23

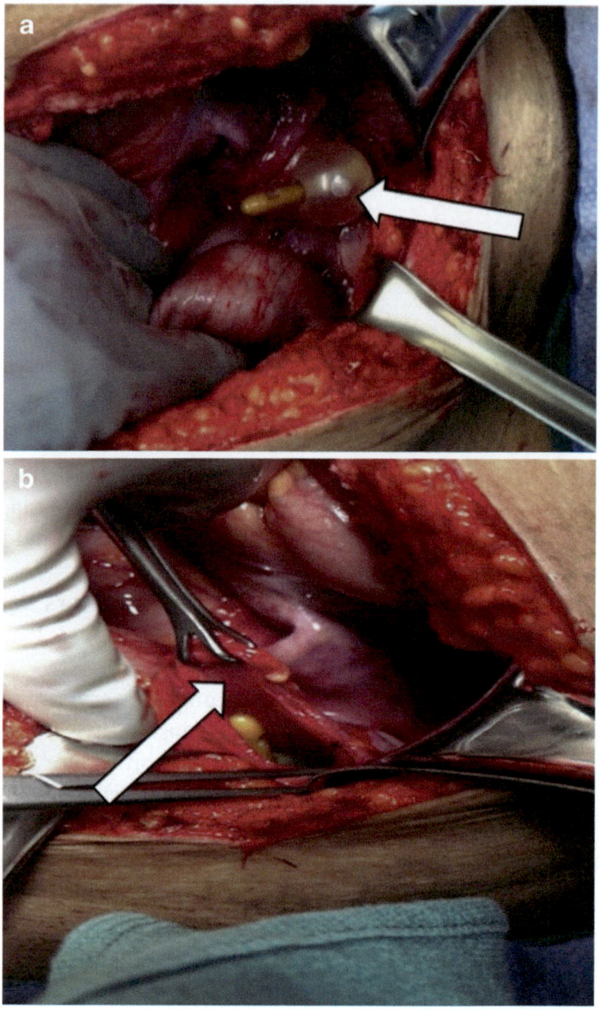

Fig. 23.1 (**a**) Intraoperative view of low midline laparotomy showing ruptured bladder dome with bladder catheter and inflated balloon. (**b**) Ruptured bladder wall held with Babcock forceps. (From Elkbuli A et al. [1]. Open-access article under the CC BY license)

The principles of management of a bladder trauma are based on the anatomopathology of the lesion, being either extraperitoneal or intraperitoneal, or mixed.

Bladder hematoma or rupture with an **extraperitoneal urinary leak** should be first addressed with conservative management consisting of indwelling drainage and prophylactic antibiotics. In large peri-vesical hematoma with distortion of the bladder, the catheter should be maintained until significant hematoma resorption and near normalization of the bladder anatomy is achieved. Additionally, since the patient will frequently have an associated pelvic fracture, the catheter should be kept until he/she ambulates [4, 5]. More than 85% of bladder injuries kept on indwelling catheter heal by the 10th day, and nearly all heal within 3 weeks [4, 6].

A rupture with **intraperitoneal or mixed urinary leak** calls for urgent intervention which should be performed through a midline laparotomy incision, followed by

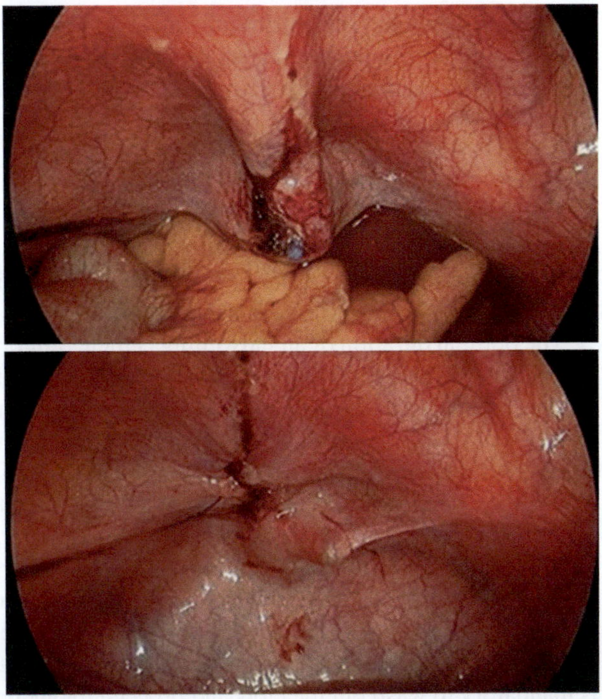

Fig. 23.2 Intraoperative photo showing the tip of Foley catheter protruding through the bladder wall and subsequent repair. (From Roy SP et al. [3], with permission from Oxford University Press)

suction of the effused urine, watertight repair of the bladder breach using absorbable sutures in two layers (mucosa-muscular layers and serosa), and intraperitoneal drain. The two-layer closure remains very popular among surgeons despite there being no evidence of its superiority over a watertight single-layer technique [7]. Some rare cases of small uncomplicated intra-peritoneal bladder perforations that occur during endoscopic procedures (TURBT) can be managed conservatively under closed observation and antibiotic prophylaxis [7].

In the exclusion of bladder rupture with obvious massive intraperitoneal urine extravasation, and in the absence of randomized studies, experts have reached a consensus on when to proceed to surgical repair in extra-peritoneal rupture, either through minimally invasive or open surgery [4–8]:

- Inadequate bladder drainage, either due to catheter block by a clot or persistent extravasation.
- Concomitant pelvic hollow viscus injury (vagina, rectum).
- Severe bladder neck injury or avulsion.
- Patients undergoing internal fixation for a pelvic fracture should have a bladder repair to avoid urinary extravasation and contamination/infection of orthopedic implants.
- Finally, any patient undergoing laparotomy for extra-urological injuries should have his/her bladder evaluated if suspicions are present (hematuria, mechanism of trauma, low urine output, suprapubic pain/tenderness), and repaired.

– Other indications: all penetrating injuries, ureteric orifice involvement in the bladder injury, bony fragments compressing or incrusted in the bladder, and failed conservative management, such as persistent urine extravasation, continuous bleeding, or occurrence of an abscess.

Technically, domal and anterior lacerations can be directly repaired, but posterior wall, trigonal, and bladder neck wounds should be approached transvesically through an anterior midline book-opening vertical incision of the bladder, thus avoiding disturbance of the pelvic hematoma and a perilous peri-vesical dissection with risk of life-threatening hemorrhage.

The optimal duration of an indwelling catheter after bladder repair is not codified by current guidelines. However, a 7–14-day duration is commonly preached and observed. Placement of a suprapubic catheter should only be indicated by the presence of complex bladder neck injury or associated urethral trauma where urethral catheterization is contra-indicated. It should not be a routine practice since it doesn't add to the effective drainage of a urethral catheter in the majority of cases while increasing unnecessarily the morbidity and hospital duration [5, 8].

In the extremely rare cases of bladder injury due to iatrogenic injury where the bladder is pierced by a sharp and thin instrument, such as during oocyte retrieval, or SLING surgery for incontinence, there might be severe bleeding out of proportion to the needle passage. In these cases, intravesical insertion of a three-way catheter is mandatory to wash out the clots and proceed to bladder irrigation. If this management fails, the patient should be taken for cystoscopy under general anesthesia, the clot should be removed with an Ellik evacuator, and the bleeding sites (entrance and exit) be examined and eventually fulgurated.

In cases of bladder neck transection, an immediate suprapubic catheter should be inserted but there is controversy about the optimal timing of the definitive operation. On the one hand, an immediate repair might be justified because these injuries do not have a spontaneous tendency to heal. On the other hand, delaying the intervention for a few months (generally three) to avoid disturbance of the blood clot and massive bleeding is also a defendable strategy. The repair is performed after a sub-umbilical incision (midline, or inverted "Y" incision, or Pfannenstiel) [9]. The patient can also undergo a combined vaginal and transpubic approach while in a lithotomy position [10]. The retropubic area is approached after releasing fibrosis, and a segment of the pubic bone may need to be cut for better exposure of the atretic bladder neck and the proximal urethra [10]. The bladder is opened horizontally at the level of the bladder neck. A metallic sound is inserted retrogradely to identify the prostatic urethra end which is then longitudinally opened with a knife. The peri-urethral fibrous tissue is excised and the proximal ureteral end is spatulated. Now an end-to-side anastomosis is performed over an indwelling silicone catheter. If the defect is too long, a T-shaped incision is made at the anterior bladder wall to create two well-vascularized flaps (around 1.3–3 cm long and 1–2 cm wide). These flaps are positioned downwards to augment the ventral part of the bladder neck and proximal urethra. A safety suprapubic catheter (SPC) is replaced and a drain is left in the Retzius space before closing the abdominal wall [9, 10] (Figs. 23.3 and 23.4).

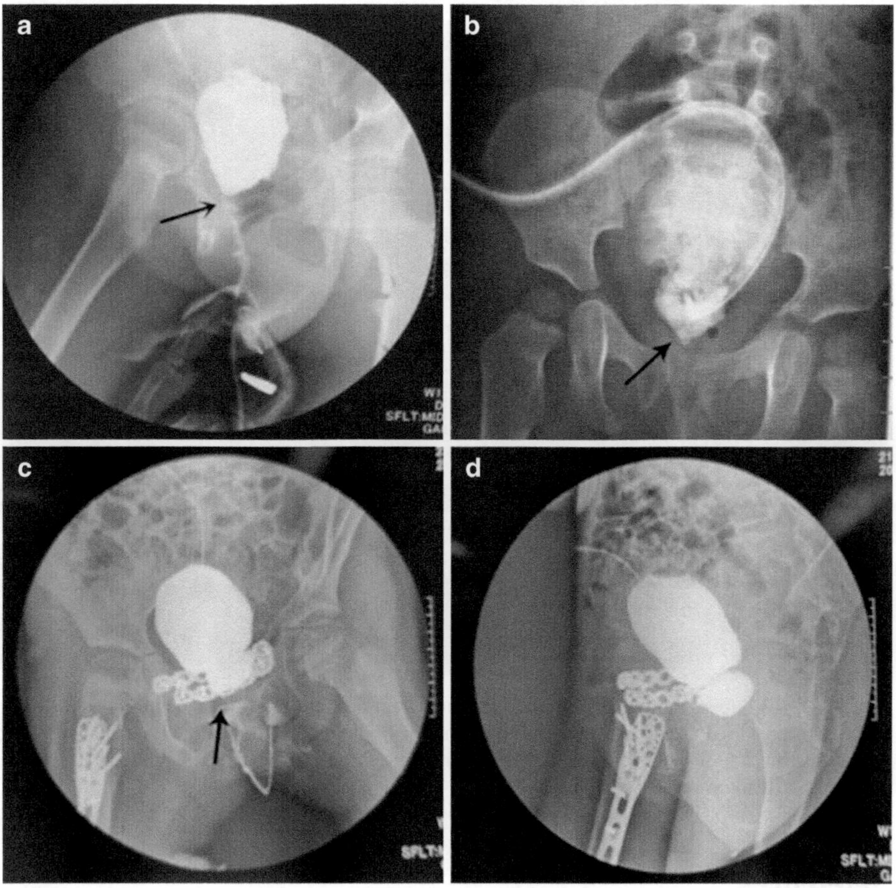

Fig. 23.3 (**a**–**c**) Preoperative voiding cystourethrography showed complete atresia of the bladder neck in a young girl with a history of pelvic fracture bladder neck avulsion and urethral rupture; (**d**) preoperative voiding cystourethrography showed vesicovaginal fistula. (From Rong Lv et al. [10]. Creative Commons Attribution 4.0 International License)

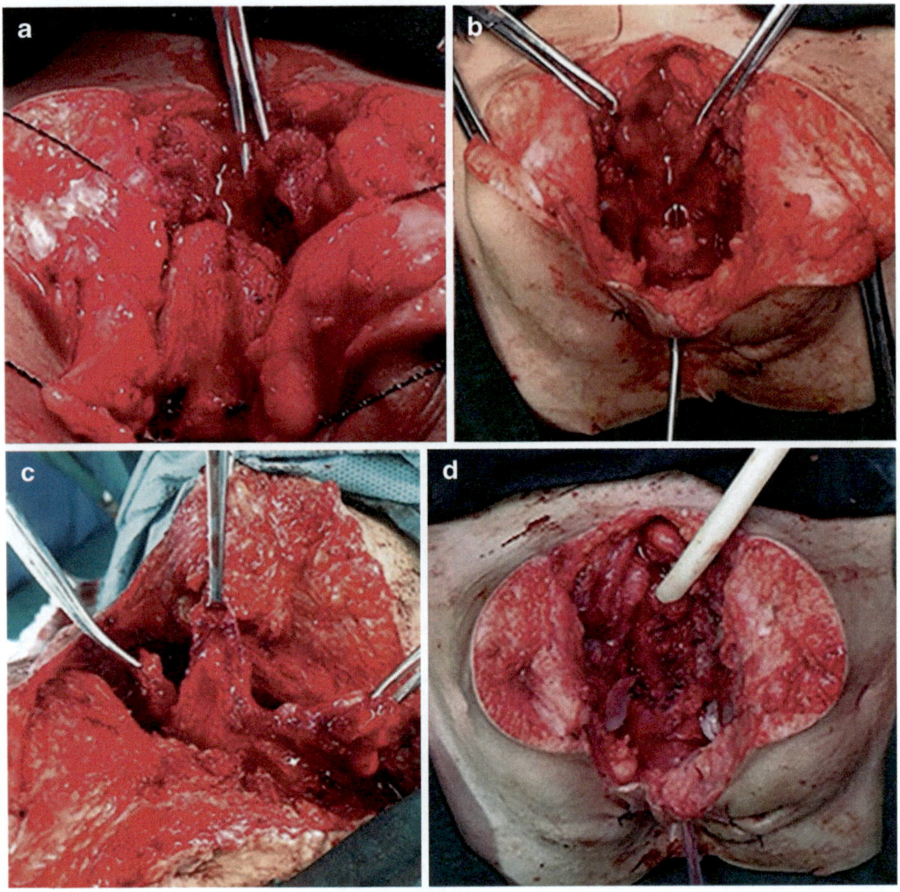

Fig. 23.4 (**a**) Pubectomy with Gigli saw; (**b**) the defect between the atretic bladder neck and the obstructed proximal urethra is 1 cm; (**c**) acquiring the bladder flap from the anterior bladder wall; (**d**) reconstruction of the bladder neck and proximal urethra. (From Rong Lv et al. [10]. Creative Commons Attribution 4.0 International License)

References

1. Elkbuli A, Ehrhardt JD, Hai S, McKenney M, Boneva D. Management of blunt intraperitoneal bladder rupture: case report and literature review. Int J Surg Case Rep. 2019;55:160–3. https://doi.org/10.1016/j.ijscr.2019.01.038. Epub 2019 Feb 1. PMID: 30739872; PMCID: PMC6369329
2. Culhane J, Syed JR, Siddiqui S. Minimally invasive management versus open surgery in the treatment of penetrating bladder injuries: a retrospective cohort study. BMC Urol. 2021;21:138. https://doi.org/10.1186/s12894-021-00900-w.
3. Roy SP, Combes AD, Perera DS. A very rare case report of an iatrogenic bladder perforation in a young female with concurrent Fitz–Hugh–Curtis syndrome. J Surg Case Rep.

2021;2021(5):rjab218. https://doi.org/10.1093/jscr/rjab218. PMID: 34055300; PMCID: PMC8153801

4. Gomez RG, Ceballos L, Coburn M. Consensus statement on bladder injuries. BJU Int. 2004;94(1):27–32.
5. Morey AF, Brandes S, Dugi DD 3rd, Armstrong JH, Breyer BN, Broghammer JA, Erickson BA, Holzbeierlein J, Hudak SJ, Pruitt JH, Reston JT, Santucci RA, Smith TG 3rd, Wessells H, American Urological Assocation. Urotrauma: AUA guideline. J Urol. 2014;192(2):327–35. https://doi.org/10.1016/j.juro.2014.05.004. Epub 2014 May 20. PMID: 24857651; PMCID: PMC4104146
6. Kong JP, Bultitude MF, Royce P, Gruen RL, Cato A, Corcoran NM. Lower urinary tract injuries following blunt trauma: a review of contemporary management. Rev Urol. 2011;13(3):119–30. PMID: 22114545; PMCID: PMC3222924
7. EAU Guidelines. Edn. presented at the EAU Annual Congress Amsterdam March 2022. ISBN 978-94-92671-16-5. https://uroweb.org/guidelines/urological-trauma/chapter/urogenital-trauma-guidelines.
8. Mahat Y, Leong JY, Chung PH. A contemporary review of adult bladder trauma. J Inj Violence Res. 2019;11(2):101–6. https://doi.org/10.5249/jivr.v11i2.1069. Epub 2019 Apr 13. PMID: 30979861; PMCID: PMC6646823
9. Gite VA, Singal A, Nikose JV, Jain HM. Post traumatic isolated bladder neck transection: unreported and undescribed injury. Urol Case Rep. 2017;17:67–9. https://doi.org/10.1016/j.eucr.2017.12.001. PMID: 29379741; PMCID: PMC5782400
10. Lv R, Jin C, Shu H, et al. Bladder neck reconstruction in girls' pelvic fracture bladder neck avulsion and urethral rupture. BMC Urol. 2020;20:179. https://doi.org/10.1186/s12894-020-00741-z.

24 Treatment of Bladder Injury: Reconstructive Surgery Using Extraurinary Autologous Tissues

Unlike the ureter and the urethra, one particularity of the bladder function is its full dependence on sympathetic, parasympathetic, and somatic nerve supplies integrity. The bladder often suffers from spine, sacral plexus, or pelvic nerves injuries, and its dysfunction represents a direct threat to the kidneys. There are multiple reconstructive techniques that the human genius has invented to alleviate neurogenic cystopathy or to palliate a congenital abnormality or a cystectomy performed for various reasons such as muscle-invasive bladder cancer. With the exception of a cutaneous urostomy, they all use bowel segments (mostly the terminal ileum) with their intact mesenteries to refashion the bladder, augment its capacity, or just drain out the urine through the abdominal wall. **Although this topic deviates somehow from the subject treated in this book, as the underlying problem is mainly a congenital, neurological, or oncological pathology, a succinct overview of the techniques alluded to above would not be superfluous. Indeed, the following case report would solely justify this additional effort: inadvertent cystectomy has occurred during a cesarean section complicated with severe hematuria necessitating urgent hysterectomy** [1]. The entire body of the bladder and lower ureters were removed along with the uterus leaving only the bladder neck and part of the trigone. The management included immediate cutaneous ureterostomy and elective bladder augmentation with a catheterizable continent stoma using the appendix.

1. ***Techniques proper for neurogenic bladder and congenital abnormalities***: In these techniques, the bladder is preserved, and stratagems are carried out to increase its capacity and ensure drainage.
   (a) **Augmentation enterocystoplasty** simply called **bladder augmentation**: This technique utilizes a detubularized patch of the terminal ileum to cover a sagittally bivalved bladder. It is indicated in small bladder capacity with poor compliance, in refractory overactive bladder, in infective and inflammatory disorders (TB, Schistosomiasis), after radiation therapy, etc. In childhood, it is performed for congenital abnormalities such as bladder

S. A. AL-Mamari, *Urogenital Trauma: A Practical Guide*,
https://doi.org/10.1007/978-981-99-6171-9_24

exstrophy or epispadias. It is also preferred over an ileal conduit in the setting of renal transplantation when the recipient has bladder dysfunction [2, 3].

(b) **Mitrofanoff appendicovesicostomy**: This technique was introduced in 1976 and published in 1980 by the French pediatric urologist Paul Mitrofanoff as a continent catheterizable diversion anastomosing the appendix tip to the bladder and its base to the skin in children with neurogenic bladder. The cystostomy thus created was combined with a closure of the bladder neck at the same time. Bladder augmentation is often performed along with a Mitrofanoff appendicovesicostomy [4–6] (Fig. 24.1a–d).

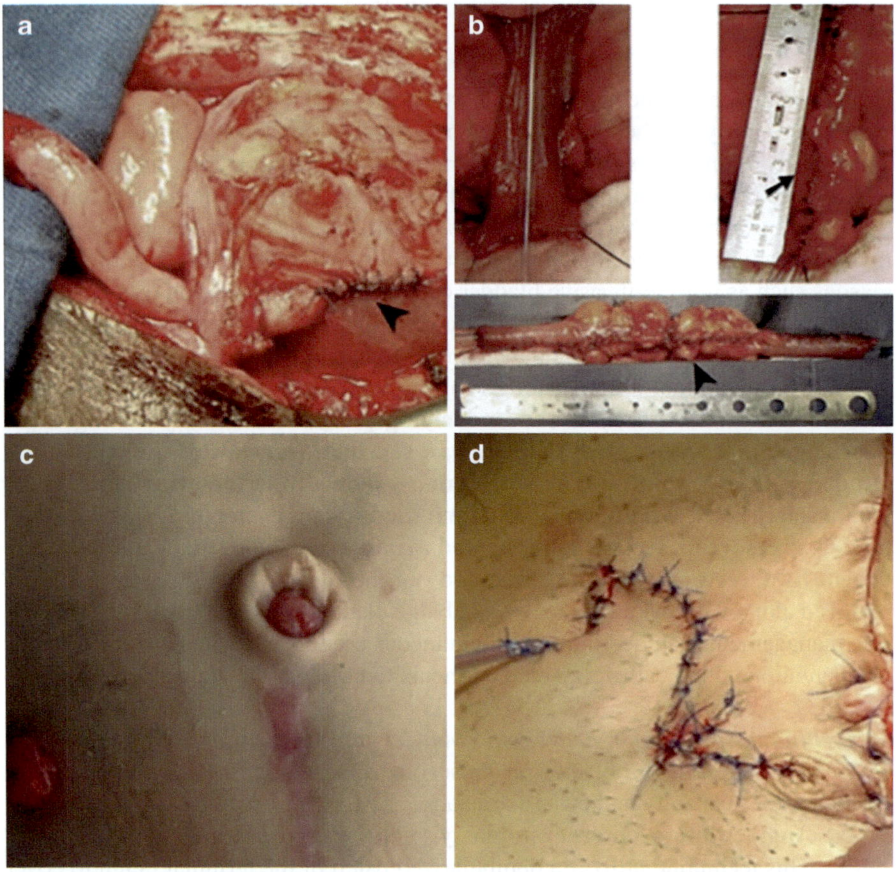

Fig. 24.1 (**a**) Appendicovesicostomy with the Mitrofanoff principle showing an anti-reflux extravesical reimplantation technique (arrow head) as the anti-incontinence mechanism. (**b**) Continent urinary diversion with the Mitrofanoff principle using an ileal segment for a transverse ileal tube (Yang-Monti) (arrow) and a double tube (Monti technique) (arrow head). (**c**) Umbilical stoma in a patient who underwent an Appendicovesicostomy and Malone antegrade continence enema (MACE) procedure. (**d**) V-Quadrilateral-Z (VQZ) plasty stoma in a patient with a complex urethral stricture. (From Chavarriaga J et al. [6]. Creative Commons Attribution License)

Many techniques arose utilizing the Mitrofanoff principle with other gastro-intestinal segments than the appendix [5, 6]:

- **Yang-Monti tube**: Uses a detubularized 2–3 cm ileal segment, and transversally retubularized over a 14–18 Fr catheter. One end of the tube is tunneled submucosally and anastomosed to the bladder while the other end is attached to the skin as a stoma.
- Other tissue sources include coecum associated with the appendix, stomach, ureter, etc.

2. ***Techniques after cystectomy***. Here the bladder has been removed and the challenge consists of its replacement whenever possible, or just of urine drainage.
   (a) **Cutaneous urostomy**: This is an exception in this chapter as it doesn't utilize extra-urinary tissue. When the bladder has been removed and there is no suitable bowel segment to create a diversion or the patient is not fit for a major reconstruction, the ureters can be brought directly through the abdominal wall to the skin. This is considered a better alternative to permanent percutaneous nephrostomy [7].
   (b) **Ileal conduit urinary diversion**: This incontinent diversion is very popular and is used for all patients undergoing a radical cystectomy who are unfit for bladder replacement (neo-bladder). The most popular is the **Bricker technique** where the spatulated ureters are reimplanted separately in an end-to-side technique to the proximal end of a 12–20 cm ileal conduit whose distal end is anastomosed to the abdominal skin through the rectus muscle sheath [8]. The two ureters may also be anastomosed conjointly in an end-to-end fashion on the proximal end of the ileal conduit, according to Wallace technique. Jejunal and colonic conduits can also be used, but are associated with more metabolic disturbances.

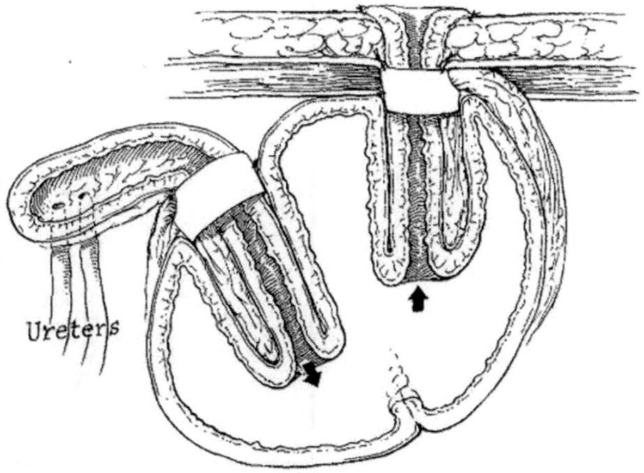

Fig. 24.2 The Kock pouch: completed ileal reservoir in situ. (From Kock NG et al. [9], with permission from Wolters Kluwer Health)

(c) **Continent cutaneous diversion:**

- **Kock pouch:** It is made of a reservoir fashioned from a 60–70 cm ileal segment, having an afferent limb connected to the ureters and an efferent limb connected to the skin through a catheterizable stoma [9] (Fig. 24.2).

- **Indiana pouch:** Developed at Indiana University (Michigan, USA), it consists of a reservoir fashioned from a detubularized coecum and a segment of the ascending colon. The ureters are tunneled and implanted along the cecal tenia to ensure an antireflux mechanism while the plicated terminal ileum and the ileocecal valve provide incontinence to the catheterizable stoma [10–12] (Fig. 24.3).

(d) **Orthotopic bladder substitution:** This is also known as neo-bladder, and is made from a detubularized long ileal segment (50–60 cm) which is roughly refashioned as a sphere and anastomosed proximally to the ureters and distally to the urethra. Its continence relies on the natural external urethral sphincter. Many techniques have been proposed for the creation of a neo-bladder and are referred to by eponyms: Camey-Leduc (U- and Z-shaped), Hautmann (W-shaped), Kock, Studer, Abol-Enein and Ghoneim, the Vescica Ileale

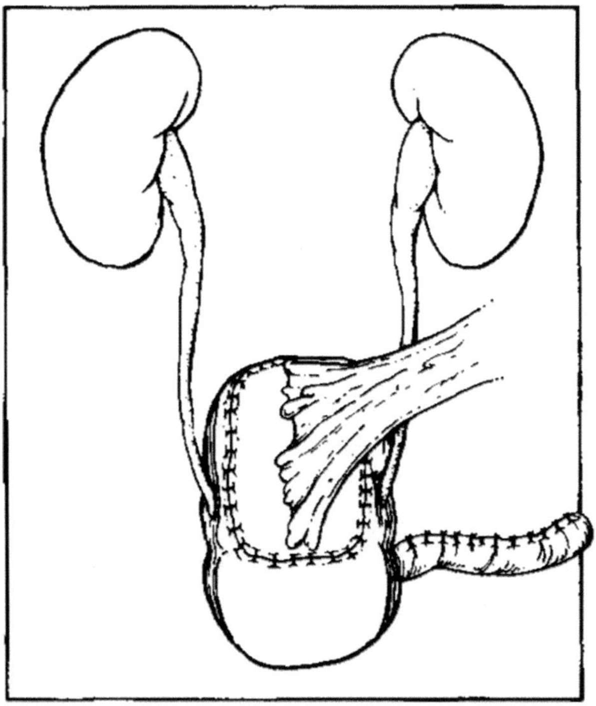

Fig. 24.3 The Indiana pouch. Diagrams illustrate the technique for anastomosis of the ureters to the cecum along the tenia. (From Rowland RG [10], with permission from Springer Nature)

Padovana (circular shape), etc. Mainz and Le Bag pouches are characteristically fashioned from ileocolonic segments while the Reddy pouch is made of the sigmoid colon [13–17].

(e) **Ureterosigmoidostomy:** Published for the first time in 1857 by Mr. Simon, this technique was first performed in a child with bladder exstrophy [18]. The ureters are anastomosed end-to-side to the sigmoid colon in an anti-reflux manner (Coffey, Petit-Leadbetter, Mainz) with the obvious advantages of obviating the need for a stoma, hence providing better cosmetic results. The continence is ensured by the anal sphincter. Besides other complications such as chronic diarrhea, the increased incidence of colorectal cancer associated with this technique has caused it to be disregarded for many decades before regaining some interest due to the ease of its performance through newly developed minimally invasive approaches [19, 20].

24.1 Future Perspectives

The unlimited human genius was not satisfied with surgical reconstruction alone but did imagine ways to recreate a new bladder or produce tissues that would mimic a natural reservoir. Hence the concept of tissue engineering and regenerative medicine. The used scaffolds are biomaterials that are roughly divided into three categories [21–25]:

- natural matrices, including collagen,
- acellular tissue matrices, such as bladder submucosa,
- synthetic matrices, such as poly(lactic-*co*-glycolic acid) (PLGA), Teflon, silicon.

There is still a long way to the successful production of a bladder or any other biological organ (pancreas, kidney, etc.) with desired characteristics and properties. Nonetheless, human determination and abnegation will not stop until success, and the advent of nanotechnology will surely stimulate further research and open doors to unsuspected achievements.

References

1. Alahmadi M, Ghazi AA. Case reported for iatrogenic cystectomy during cesarean delivery. Urol Case Rep. 2020;31:101180. https://doi.org/10.1016/j.eucr.2020.101180.
2. Biers SM, Venn SN, Greenwell TJ. The past, present and future of augmentation cystoplasty. BJU Int. 2012;109(9):1280–93. https://doi.org/10.1111/j.1464-410X.2011.10650.x. Epub 2011 Nov 25
3. Veeratterapillay R, Thorpe AC, Harding C. Augmentation cystoplasty: contemporary indications, techniques and complications. Indian J Urol. 2013;29(4):322–7. https://doi.org/10.4103/0970-1591.120114.
4. Mitrofanoff P. Trans-appendicular continent cystostomy in the management of the neurogenic bladder. Chir Pediatr. 1980;21:297–305.

5. Veeratterapillay R, Morton H, Thorpe AC, Harding C. Reconstructing the lower urinary tract: the Mitrofanoff principle. Indian J Urol. 2013;29(4):316–21. https://doi.org/10.4103/0970-1591.120113.
6. Chavarriaga J, Fernández N, Campo MAO, Bolivar J, Patiño G, Perez J. Self-perception, quality of life and ease of catheterization in patients with continent urinary diversion with the mitrofanoff principle. Int Braz J Urol. 2020;46(5):743–51. https://doi.org/10.1590/S1677-5538.IBJU.2019.0388.
7. Kearney GP, Docimo SG, Doyle CJ, Mahoney EM. Cutaneous ureterostomy in adults. Urology. 1992;40(1):1–6. https://doi.org/10.1016/0090-4295(92)90426-w.
8. Bricker EM. Bladder substitution after pelvic evisceration. Surg Clin North Am. 1950;30(5):1511–21. https://doi.org/10.1016/s0039-6109(16)33147-4.
9. Kock NG, Nilson AE, Nilsson LO, Norlén LJ, Philipson BM. Urinary diversion via a continent ileal reservoir: clinical results in 12 patients. J Urol. 1982;128(3):469–75. https://doi.org/10.1016/s0022-5347(17)53001-3.
10. Rowland RG, Mitchell ME, Bihrle R. The cecoileal continent urinary reservoir. World J Urol. 1985;3:185–90. https://doi.org/10.1007/BF00326991.
11. Rowland RG, Mitchell ME, Bihrle R, Kahnoski RJ, Piser JE. Indiana continent urinary reservoir. J Urol. 1987;137(6):1136–9. https://doi.org/10.1016/s0022-5347(17)44428-4.
12. Bihrle R. The Indiana pouch continent urinary reservoir. Urol Clin N Am. 1997;24:773.
13. Chang DT, Lawrentschuk N. Orthotopic neobladder reconstruction. Urol Ann. 2015;7(1):1–7. https://doi.org/10.4103/0974-7796.148553.
14. Couvelaire R. Le réservoir iléal de substitution après la cystectomie totale chez l'homme [substitute ileal reservoir following total cystectomy in the male]. J Urol Medicale Chir. 1951;57(6):408–17.
15. Lilien OM, Camey M. 25-year experience with replacement of the human bladder (Camey procedure). J Urol. 1984;132(5):886–91. https://doi.org/10.1016/s0022-5347(17)49934-4.
16. Camey M, Le Duc A. L'enterocystoplastie avec cystoprostatectomie totale pour cancer de la vessie. Ann Urol. 1979;13:114.
17. Hautmann RE. Ileale Ersatzblasen [Ileal bladder substitute]. Urologe A. 2008 . German;47(1):33–4. https://doi.org/10.1007/s00120-007-1606-0.
18. Simon C. Ektopia vesicae: operation for diverting the orifices of the ureters into the rectum: temporary success; subsequent death; autopsy. Lancet. 1857;2:568–70. https://doi.org/10.1016/S0140-6736(02)63646-3.
19. Przydacz M, Corcos J. Revisiting ureterosigmoidostomy, a useful technique of urinary diversion in functional urology. Urology. 2018;115:14–20. https://doi.org/10.1016/j.urology.2018.01.003. Epub 2018 Jan 31
20. Hansen MH, Hayn M, Murray P. The use of bowel in urologic reconstructive surgery. Surg Clin N Am. 2016;96(3):567–82. https://doi.org/10.1016/j.suc.2016.02.011.
21. Atala A, Bauer SB, Soker S, Yoo JJ, Retik AB. Tissue-engineered autologous bladders for patients needing cystoplasty. Lancet. 2006;367:1241–6. https://doi.org/10.1016/S0140-6736(06)68438-9.
22. Atala A. Tissue engineering of human bladder. Br Med Bull. 2011;97:81–104. https://doi.org/10.1093/bmb/ldr003.
23. Aboushwareb T, Atala A. Stem cells in urology. Nat Clin Pract Urol. 2008;5:621–31. https://doi.org/10.1038/ncpuro1228.
24. Soler R, Fullhase C, Atala A. Regenerative medicine strategies for treatment of neurogenic bladder. Therapy. 2009;6(2):177–84. https://doi.org/10.2217/14750708.6.2.177.
25. Subramaniam R. Regenerative medicine in bladder reconstructive surgery. Eur Urol Suppl. 2016;16:23. https://doi.org/10.1016/j.eursup.2016.10.005.

25 Prognosis, Complications, and Follow-Up of Bladder Injury

A well-repaired bladder rupture has an excellent prognosis since this organ has a good blood supply which allows rapid and complete healing.

However untreated or poorly treated cases carry a grim prognosis because of the complications arising from the bladder injury itself or from the associated organs trauma. A population-based review recruiting 111 patients with AAST bladder injury grade ≥ II who underwent laparotomy showed a complication rate of 38% and a mortality rate of 11% either due to associated injuries or complications of mismanaged bladder injury, and patients with systemic, non-urinary complications were more prone to a fatal outcome (26.2% of 42 patients) than the non-complicated cases (1.4% of 69 patients) [1]. The authors found that ISS >25, systolic pressure <90 mmHg, a revised trauma score (RTS) <7.84, and the presence of a pelvic fracture were the most important predictors for complications in bladder trauma [1]. The same mortality rate (11%) was found in a 10-year population study at a level I center [2].

An National Trauma Data Bank (NTDB) review showed that surgical bladder repair reduces in-patient mortality by 59%, and factors associated with increased mortality were African-American and native American races, presence of pelvic injuries, penetrating trauma, and multiple abdominal injuries [3].

Suboptimal bladder wall repair with continuous peri-vesical urine extravasation may give rise to abdominal wound dehiscence. Missed urinary extravasation gives rise to urinary ascites, ileus, abdominal distension, dyspnea, sepsis, localized pelvic abscess, or generalized peritonitis.

Complications surely arise from delayed diagnosis and treatment or from suboptimal repair, but also depend on the anatomopathology of the injury [4–7]:

- For intraperitoneal urine leak: electrolytes imbalance, urea reabsorption, and uremia.

S. A. AL-Mamari, *Urogenital Trauma: A Practical Guide*, https://doi.org/10.1007/978-981-99-6171-9_25

- If there is a simple and isolated bladder rupture, the complications consist of persistent hemorrhage (haematuria or increased perivesical or intravesical hematoma), the occurrence of urinary infection, decreased bladder capacity, and rarely a secondary bladder pseudodiverticulum at the breach due to mucosa healing without muscular layer repair.
- In a massive rupture, over-debridement during repair may decrease bladder capacity and cause urinary urgency.
- Delay in the bladder neck, vagina, and rectum repair causes urinary incontinence or stricture, vesicovaginal or vesica-rectal fistula, and stricture.
- Bladder neuropathy due to major injury to the sacrum, sacral roots, or pelvic nerves. If it is only neuropraxia, temporary intermittent self-catheterization may be an effective solution. If the sacral plexus damage is permanent, it will result in a hypotonic neurogenic bladder, with most likely an associated erectile dysfunction.

For extraperitoneal bladder injuries, a large prospective multicentric study conducted in the United States, including 157 patients showed that 43% of them underwent an operative repair in the initial management and revealed the following complications classified by whether the patients were operated on (OP) or not (NOP): Overall complications (23% NOP vs. 19% OP), pelvic infection/Urinoma (1% NOP vs. 6% OP), persistent urinary extravasation (18% NOP vs. 13% OP), urinary tract to skin fistula (1% NOP vs. 4% OP), non-union of the pelvic fracture (1% NOP vs. 1% OP), hardware infection/removal (4% NOP vs. 7% OP), et pelvic osteomyelitis (0% NOP vs. 3% OP) [8]. This study also showed that bladder neck injury and combined urethral trauma are the only statistically significant predictors of complications. While this study supports the concept of conservative management in extraperitoneal bladder injury, the non-statistical difference in the complications profile between the two groups must be interpreted with caution due to selection bias in the management decision, and one can logically assume that patients in the operated group had more complex injuries [8].

A follow-up retrograde cystography performed at 10–14 days to ascertain bladder healing before catheter removal has been advocated by many authors and expert boards [9]. **However, the Eastern Association for the Surgery of Trauma limited the indications for this study only to patients with a moderate or high risk of a urinary leak, namely those who had a repaired complex intra-peritoneal or extra-peritoneal bladder injury or those who presented with a simple extra-peritoneal leak treated conservatively.** The panel recommended against follow-up cystography in low-risk patients, defined as those who benefited from an operative repair of simple intraperitoneal or extraperitoneal bladder ruptures, estimating that 999 out of 1000 cystographies in these patients would be unnecessary [10].

References

1. Pereira BM, de Campos CC, Calderan TR, Reis LO, Fraga GP. Bladder injuries after external trauma: 20 years experience report in a population-based cross-sectional view. World J Urol. 2013;31(4):913–7. https://doi.org/10.1007/s00345-012-0871-8. Epub 2012 Apr 28
2. Matlock KA, Tyroch AH, Kronfol ZN, McLean SF, Pirela-Cruz MA. Blunt traumatic bladder rupture: a 10-year perspective. Am Surg. 2013;79(6):589–93. https://doi.org/10.1177/000313481307900619.
3. Deibert CM, Spencer BA. The association between operative repair of bladder injury and improved survival: results from the National Trauma Data Bank [Erratum in: J Urol. 2012 May;187(5):1938]. J Urol. 2011;186(1):151–5. https://doi.org/10.1016/j.juro.2011.03.002. Epub 2011 May 14
4. Gomez RG, Ceballos L, Coburn M. Consensus statement on bladder injuries. BJU Int. 2004;94(1):27–32.
5. Simon LV, Sajjad H, Lopez RA, Burns B. Bladder rupture. In: StatPearls [Internet]. Treasure Island (FL): StatPearls Publishing; 2022.
6. Kong JP, Bultitude MF, Royce P, Gruen RL, Cato A, Corcoran NM. Lower urinary tract injuries following blunt trauma: a review of contemporary management. Rev Urol. 2011;13(3):119–30.
7. Kang L, Geube A. Bladder trauma. In: StatPearls [Internet]. Treasure Island (FL): StatPearls Publishing; 2022.
8. Anderson RE, Keihani S, Moses RA, et al. Current management of extraperitoneal bladder injuries: results from the Multi-Institutional Genito-Urinary Trauma Study (MiGUTS). J Urol. 2020;204(3):538–44. https://doi.org/10.1097/JU.0000000000001075. Epub 2020 Apr 7. PMID: 32259467; PMCID: PMC8717861
9. Morey AF, Brandes S, Dugi DD 3rd, Armstrong JH, Breyer BN, Broghammer JA, Erickson BA, Holzbeierlein J, Hudak SJ, Pruitt JH, Reston JT, Santucci RA, Smith TG 3rd, Wessells H, American Urological Assocation. Urotrauma: AUA guideline. J Urol. 2014;192(2):327–35. https://doi.org/10.1016/j.juro.2014.05.004. Epub 2014 May 20. PMID: 24857651; PMCID: PMC4104146
10. Yeung LL, McDonald AA, Como JJ, Robinson B, Knight J, Person MA, Lee JK, Dahm P. Management of blunt force bladder injuries: a practice management guideline from the Eastern Association for the Surgery of Trauma [Erratum in: J Trauma Acute Care Surg 2019 Aug;87(2):511]. J Trauma Acute Care Surg. 2019;86(2):326–36. https://doi.org/10.1097/TA.0000000000002132.

Part IV
Urethral Injuries

An injured and obstructed urethra can be compared to a tunnel collapsing just before the prisoners escape after the unlimited risks and tremendous efforts to dig it. Yet the distress of the patient unable to void would still be greater given the agonizing physical pain and direct repercussions to his health.

Introduction to Urethral Injury

Urethral injuries account for only 4% of genitourinary trauma [1, 2]. Nonetheless, they are probably the most abundantly studied topic of all urinary tract traumatology because of multiple controversies in their management, and the growing interest of surgeons and researchers in their challenging surgical approach [3]. Indeed, arguments start from the embryology of the urethra up to the classification and management of its injuries.

The importance of the urethra can be summarized as being the sole final outlet of the whole urinary transportation system which starts from the collecting renal tubules, and, for males, the exit channel for semen during ejaculation.

The urethra is anatomically divided into two parts, the posterior and the anterior, and this classification has a great bearing on the causes, mechanisms, and management of its injury. Its posterior part is very difficult to access through open procedures, being confined in an exiguous space between the pubic symphysis and rami, the vagina and uterine cervix in females, and the rectum in males. Unlike the bladder, and to a lesser degree the ureter, the urethra has very few reserve tissues to overcome losses.

The posterior urethra is protected by the pubic bones. However, in **pelvic fracture or dislocation** which is mostly caused by **road traffic accidents (RTA)**, this protective shield instantly turns into a severing sword or a shredding lever. Replacing the old term **"pelvic fracture urethral distraction defects" (PFUDD)** introduced by Turner-Warwick [4], the concept of "**pelvic fracture urethral injury" (PFUI)** is frequently used nowadays to refer to this anatomopathological entity as current evidence shows that these injuries are not usually complete nor they are necessarily distracted [5].

The anterior urethra is protected by the corpus spongiosum of the penis, and its pendulous part is generally spared from violent blunt trauma such as those arising from RTA and falling astride. It is however exposed to stab injuries, gunshots, animal or human bites, and iatrogenic injuries. The bulbar part of the anterior urethra is the segment most prone to straddle injuries and also pays a bitter price to iatrogenic trauma.

Historically, urethral injury was almost always fatal because of the inability to pass urine, the hematoma, and the secondary urine extravasation and infection. With the progress of modern medicine, urethral injuries not only are no longer fatal per se but also rarely jeopardize renal function since a rapid suprapubic catheterization is an easy, effective, and safe way to protect the upper urinary tract. Nonetheless, injury to the urethra exposes the patient to prolonged morbidity related to the mechanism (pelvic fracture) and other possible associated injuries (rectum, vagina, penis) and yields a high rate of functional complications (urinary incontinence, impotence).

The diagnosis of urethral injury is mainly reached through retrograde urethrography which can be combined with an antegrade urethrography in patients with complete disruption of the urethra provisionally treated with an SPC.

The repair of posterior urethral injuries requires a complex technique where there is almost no room for a pedicled graft or a free flap and efforts have to be made to approximate the urethral ends even when the gaps are long, by mobilizing the bulbar urethra. However, repair of anterior urethral injuries with long gaps is frequently performed using various interposition of inlay or onlay grafts.

The average total cost of the management of a urethral injury and stricture widely varies from publications and depends on the management strategies. It was estimated to be as low as $3000 for a simple anterior stricture requiring a mere urethrotomy/urethral dilatation, to as high as around $170,000 for a complex posterior urethral injury repair [6–10]. It is important to remember that this cost does not include the loss of productivity and quality of life.

References

1. McGeady JB, Breyer BN. Current epidemiology of genitourinary trauma. Urol Clin North Am. 2013;40(3):323–34. https://doi.org/10.1016/j.ucl.2013.04.001. Epub 2013 Jun 12.
2. Alwaal A, Zaid UB, Blaschko SD, Harris CR, Gaither TW, McAninch JW, Breyer BN. The incidence, causes, mechanism, risk factors, classification, and diagnosis of pelvic fracture urethral injury. Arab J Urol. 2015;13(1):2–6. https://doi.org/10.1016/j.aju.2014.08.006. Epub 2014 Sep 16.

3. Barbagli G, Sansalone S, Djinovic R, Romano G, Lazzeri M. Current controversies in reconstructive surgery of the anterior urethra: a clinical overview. Int Braz J Urol. 2012;38(3):307–16; discussion 316. https://doi.org/10.1590/s1677-55382012000300003.
4. Turner-Warwick RT. Principles of urethral reconstruction. In: Wesbter G, Kirby R, King L, editors. Reconstructive urology. Oxford: Blackwell Scientific Publications; 1993. p. 609–42.
5. Gómez RG, Mundy T, Dubey D, El-Kassaby AW, Firdaoessaleh, Kodama R, Santucci R. SIU/ICUD consultation on urethral strictures: pelvic fracture urethral injuries. Urology. 2014;83(3 Suppl):S48–58. https://doi.org/10.1016/j.urology.2013.09.023. Epub 2013 Nov 8.
6. Tausch TJ, Lotan Y, Zhao L, Morey AF. Decision analysis model comparing cost of management strategies for pelvic fracture urethral injuries. Urol Pract. 2016. https://doi.org/10.1016/j.urpr.2016.07.004.
7. Johnsen NV, Penson DF, Reynolds WS, Milam DF, Dmochowski RR, Kaufman MR. Cost-effective management of pelvic fracture urethral injuries. World J Urol. 2017;35(10):1617–23. https://doi.org/10.1007/s00345-017-2022-8. Epub 2017 Feb 22.
8. Rourke KF, Jordan GH. Primary urethral reconstruction: the cost minimized approach to the bulbous urethral stricture. J Urol. 2005;173(4):1206–10. https://doi.org/10.1097/01.ju.0000154971.05286.81.
9. Osterberg EC, Murphy G, Harris CR, Breyer BN. Cost-effective strategies for the management and treatment of urethral stricture disease. Urol Clin North Am. 2017;44(1):11–7. https://doi.org/10.1016/j.ucl.2016.08.002.
10. Greenwell TJ, Castle C, Andrich DE, MacDonald JT, Nicol DL, Mundy AR. Repeat urethrotomy and dilation for the treatment of urethral stricture are neither clinically effective nor cost-effective. J Urol. 2004;172(1):275–7. https://doi.org/10.1097/01.ju.0000132156.76403.8f.

26 Anatomy of the Urethra

26.1 Embryology of the Urethra

The cloacal membrane appears between the fourth and the fifth week and separates the cloaca from the amniotic cavity. Furthermore, the urorectal septum divides the cloaca into the urogenital sinus and the hindgut, the former being the precursor of the bladder and posterior urethra [1].

The development of the spongy urethra proceeds through three stages: a solid epithelial plate, a deep urethral groove, and a fused urethra [2]. Herein a grooved **urethral plate** was observed to develop from proximal to distal at 6 weeks and to be completely fused by 8 weeks. The glanular urethra development starts also at 6 weeks and is a longer process evolving in four stages: a solid epithelial plate (sixth week), a blind central canal (13th week), a deep glanular groove (14th week), and the floor from the preputial lamella (14th week) [2].

The distinction between the male and female genital systems is triggered once the gonad assumes characteristics of the testis or ovary in the eighth week of gestation. However, the external genital organs acquire specific sexual characteristics only from the 11th or 12th week [3].

The penile urethra was proposed to arise from the fusion of the urogenital swellings with primary luminization, whereas the glandular urethra was created by secondary luminization of the epithelial cord formed by the fusion of the arms of the genital tubercle, i.e., the glans [4].

An interesting theory, **"the double zipper hypothesis"**, states that the human male urethra develops through two mechanisms: **an initial "opening zipper"** that produces distal canalization of the solid urethral plate resulting in the urethral groove, which proceeds through a high rate of epithelial proliferation, and a subsequent **"closing zipper"** that consists of a fusion of the two epithelial surfaces of the urethral groove, resulting in the distal extension of the penile urethra [5].

Critical events have been described for the normal development of the urethra and genitals: (a) development of the external genitalia, (b) cloacal membrane fate,

S. A. AL-Mamari, *Urogenital Trauma: A Practical Guide*, https://doi.org/10.1007/978-981-99-6171-9_26

and (c) distal urethra formation [6]. Hypospadias occurs when there is a faulty ventral opening of the urethra as a result of either a defect in the external genitalia or in the distal urethra formation.

Does the urethral plate arise from the ectoderm, the mesoderm, or the endoderm?

There are ongoing controversies not only about the origin of the urethral plate but also concerning its role in the development of the urethra. However, most embryologists believe that the epithelial urethral plate is **formed by the proliferation of the endoderm** of the anterior cloacal wall, and **grows anteriorly in the mesoderm** of the genital tubercle while **remaining in contact with the ectoderm** covering the caudal median surface of the tubercle at the cloacal groove [7].

Even if you manage to comprehend the aforementioned sentence, you still won't be off the hook, as the role of the urethral plate is also up for debate. Some consider it to be the precursor of the sole glandular urethra while most of the penile urethra would develop from the urogenital sinus, and others state that it is the precursor of the whole penile urethra [7]. However, **a consensus exists on the fact that the urethral plate disintegrates creating the urethral groove which is then transformed into the urethra by fusion of the urethral folds which are present on the sides of the groove**. Yet again, this theory is challenged by some studies which deny the existence of a groove and folds, calling for revisiting the concept of hypospadias itself since this is considered to result from the failure of the fusion of the folds [8]. Hynes and Fraher found that the urethral plate is a mere temporary apposition of the walls of the phallic cloaca in the distal shaft and proximal glans and that the formation of the entire urethra results from a proximo-distal movement of waves of subepithelial migration and fusion of paramedian folds of mesoderm. They described **four pairs of folds** being involved in its formation, namely **urethral, frenular, preputial, and lacunar** which act in a similar manner to form their corresponding portions [9].

26.2 Gross Anatomy of the Male Urethra

Contrary to its female counterpart, the male urethra has a double function: it plays a key function in micturition as the terminal anatomical channel for urine elimination, but also has an essential role in the male reproductive system by conveying the semen emitted during ejaculation. It is a relatively long tubular structure whose length is about 22 cm in the adult male with no significant correlation with the patient's height, weight, body mass index, or age [10].

There are many subdivisions of the male urethra based on embryologic, topographic, anatomic, and clinical criteria. One of the proposals is to divide the urethra according to the surrounding organs or structures. Hence three portions can be described, namely the **prostatic, membranous, and spongy urethra**, in relation to the prostate gland, the urogenital diaphragm, and the corpus spongiosum, respectively [11].

However, most frequently, the male urethra is divided into two parts: The **posterior** urethra (prostatic and membranous urethra) and the **anterior** or spongy urethra (bulbar, penile urethra or pendulous urethra, fossa navicularis, and glandular urethra). The **urethral meatus** is the exiting orifice of the urethra at the tip of the penis. A pre-prostatic urethra is also described as a very short segment, 0.5–1.5 cm long, embedded within the wall of the urinary bladder before entering the prostate. It is lined by the same transitional epithelium or urothelium covering the bladder lumen. It is surrounded by the internal urethral sphincter made of thickened involuntary circular smooth muscle.

Hereafter is a brief description of the different urethral parts [12–15]:

1. **Prostatic urethra**: Found within the prostate, measures 3–4 cm. **It is the widest portion of the male urethra and contains many structures or appendices**: the urethral crest, seminal colliculus, prostatic utricle, verumontanum, and the orifices of the prostatic ducts. The entrance of the prostatic utricle lies between the two orifices of the ejaculatory ducts. The verumontanum is an important anatomic landmark serving as the distal limit during prostatic resection to preserve the voluntary striated sphincter which lies just distal to it. It is a prominent structure visible at the posterior distal prostatic urethra which can also be seen as a filling defect in urethrography. The prostatic urethra is lined by a continuation of the **urothelium** from the bladder and the upper urinary tract. The urothelium of the prostatic urethra is in direct contact with the glandular and stromal tissue of the periurethral zone of the prostate.
2. **Membranous urethra**: It is short, measuring 1–2.5 cm in length. It begins immediately below the prostate and ends just above the penile bulb. It passes through the deep perineal pouch, and the perineal membrane and **is surrounded by the external urethral sphincter, which is longer anteriorly and whose fibers do not meet posteriorly**. Posteriorly the membranous urethra is in close contact with the bulbourethral or Cowper's glands. It is lined by a **pseudostratified columnar epithelium**. **It is closely and intimately attached anteriorly to the pubis by the suspensory ligaments**.
3. **Anterior or Spongy urethra**: This is the longest segment of the urethra, traveling within the corpus spongiosum of the penis. It has an average length of 15 cm and comprises two widenings at the bulb of the penis and in the glans penis where it forms the **fossa navicularis**. Bulbourethral and urethral glands empty in this portion and can be visualized in urethrography as small dots. It is lined by a **pseudostratified columnar epithelium** up to the terminal portion which is lined by a **stratified squamous epithelium**. **Five layers** can be seen in a cross-section of the anterior urethra: **urethral epithelium, lamina propria, corpus spongiosum, tunica albuginea, and Buck's fascia**. The **bulbar urethra** measures 3–4 cm, is located within the bulbospongiosus muscle and extends from the urogenital diaphragm to the penoscrotal junction. The **penile urethra** measures about 15 cm, is entirely surrounded by the corpus spongiosum, and dilates as the **fossa navicularis** within the glans penis before ending by the **external meatus** (Fig. 26.1).

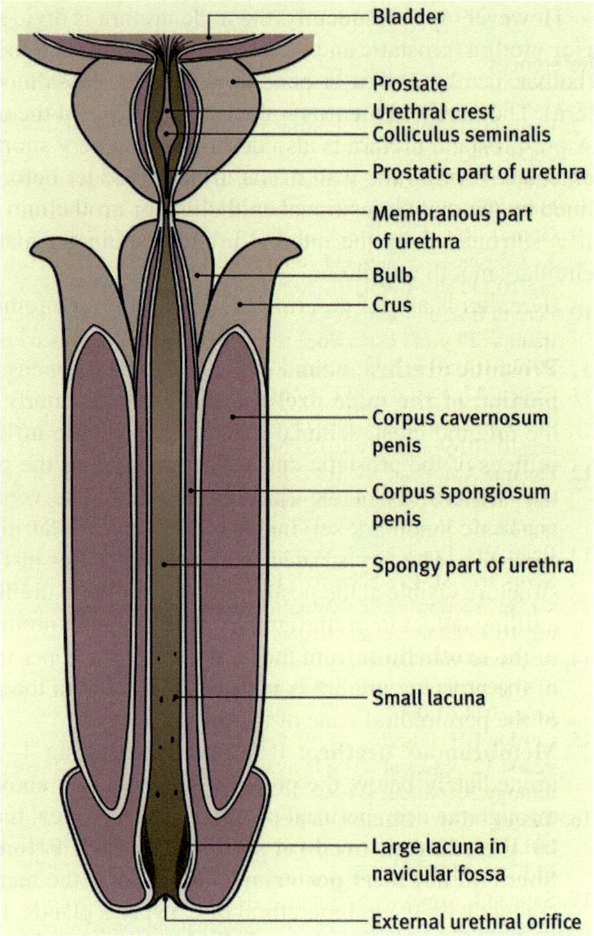

Fig. 26.1 The whole length of the lumen of the male urethra exposed by an incision extending into it from its dorsal aspect. (From Ellis H [15], with permission from Elsevier)

Females have only the posterior urethra, the anterior one being replaced by the labia minora resulting from the persistent separation of the urethral folds on the ventral surfaces of the genital tubercle [16].

Unlike other epithelia (e.g., gastrointestinal epithelium), **the urethral wall lacks a supporting muscularis mucosa**. Therefore, anteriorly it lies directly on the vascular erectile corpus spongiosum contained within the tight Buck's fascia. This direct contact exposes the corpus spongiosum to urine inundation once the urethral epithelium is breached. Thus, whenever the patient tries to void, the extravasation will increase inside the corpus spongiosum and the pressure might rupture Buck's fascia, allowing further urine extravasation and hematoma to reach the Colles' fascia, with a characteristic perineal butterfly bruising [17, 18].

26.3 Urethral Blood Supply

The urethra passes through several compartments in the perineum, therefore receiving blood supply from different sources: **the inferior vesical artery, bulbourethral artery, and the internal pudendal artery**. Moreover, the anterior urethra and its surrounding corpus spongiosum receive blood from both antegrade and retrograde streams mainly from the **bulbar and dorsal arteries** which arise from the **common penile artery**. The common penile artery is a continuation of the **internal pudendal artery** which divides into **bulbar, urethral, and dorsal arteries**: the bulbar arteries are responsible for the antegrade flow to the urethra and corpus spongiosum, and the dorsal arteries provide the retrograde blood supply starting from the glans [12, 13].

The venous drainage is organized distally from a plexus within the spongy glans that develops into periurethral veins running within the corpus spongiosum and communicating with the deep dorsal vein via multiple circumflex veins. Proximally these veins unite at **Santorini's plexus** proximal to the pubic bone and adjacent to the prostate [13].

26.4 Congenital Urethral Abnormalities

Congenital urethral abnormalities are rare but their anatomopathological forms are multiple [1, 19]:

1. *Hypospadias*: This pathology is characterized by abnormal development of the urethral fold and the ventral prepuce resulting in the urethral opening developing on the ventral aspect proximal to the penile tip. Hypospadias is classified as anterior (70%) (glandular and subcoronal), middle (distal and proximal penile and midshaft), and posterior (penoscrotal, scrotal, and perineal) [20]. The incidence of hypospadias varies from 1/200 to 1/300 boys. The embryological mechanism of hypospadias is not well understood, and many theories exist stating that it results from the failure of formation of the various primary urethral folds or from their non-fusion with their counterparts, or from a defect in the cloacal membrane. Moreover, the chordee associated with hypospadias is believed to arise from a failure of the increase in volume in the phallic length and the persistence of the urethral plate [9].
2. *Posterior urethral valves* (PUV): Occur in 1/5000–8000 newborn boys, and can have grim consequences such as bilateral renal obstruction, bladder dysfunction, vesicoureteral reflux, bilateral upper tract dilatation (hydroureteronephrosis) and renal damage [19] (Fig. 26.2). Hugh Hampton Young et al. proposed a classification of the PUV into three types in 1919 [21]:

   Type I valves (the most common): they develop from the verumontanum and extend distally attaching the lateral urethral walls as two leaflets (type Ia) or as a unicuspid leaflet (type Ib).

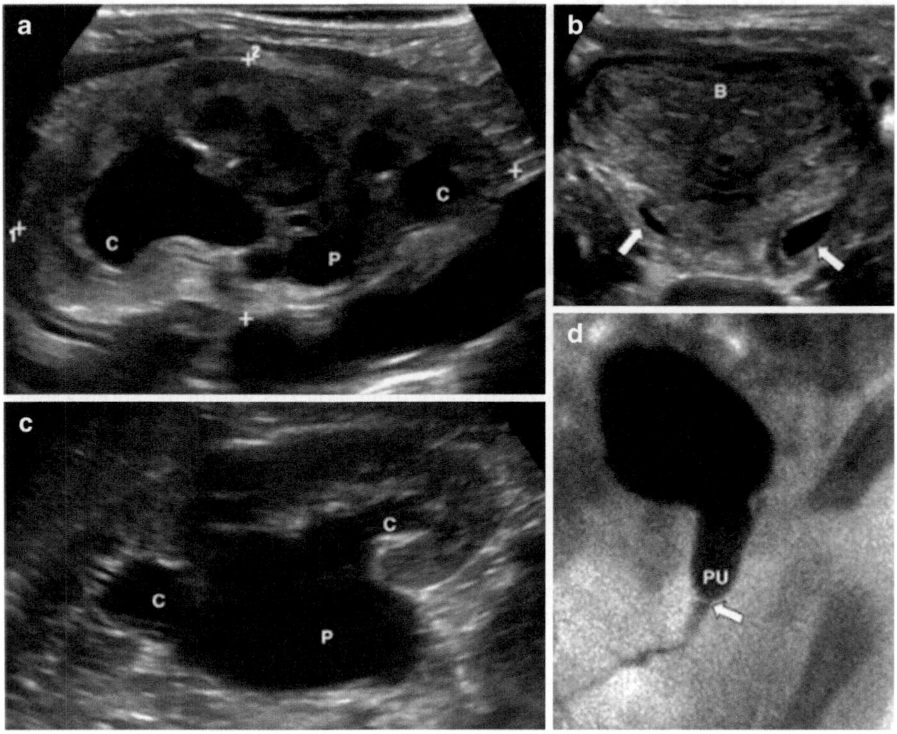

Fig. 26.2 Posterior urethral valves (PUV) in a 3-day-old male. Longitudinal grayscale ultrasound images of the right (**a**) and left (**b**) kidneys demonstrate dilation of the pelvicalyceal systems and right proximal ureter (U). *P* Renal pelvis, *C* calyx. (**c**) Transverse grayscale ultrasound image of the bladder (B) depicts severe wall thickening with dilation of the distal ureters (arrows). (**d**) VCUG image demonstrates marked dilation of the posterior urethra (PU). Arrow indicates the site of the valves. (From Kassab GH et al. [19], with permission from Springer Nature)

Type II valves: they extend from the bladder neck to the verumontanum. This type is no longer considered a valve, being regarded as a normal variant.

Type III valves: Appear as a diaphragm fixed on the whole circumference of the urethra, leaving a central hole. These are referred to as type IIIa, or type IIIb, if they are distal or proximal to the verumontanum, respectively. Cobb considered the type III valve merely as congenital urethral strictures, and they are sometimes referred to as Cobb's collar [22].

3. *Anterior urethral valves*: These rare anomalies have variable locations, distributed almost equally between the bulbar urethra (40%), the penoscrotal junction (30%), and the penile urethra (30%) [19].
4. *Prune-Belly Syndrome* (PBS): Also referred to by the eponym Eagle-Barret syndrome after the authors who first described it in 1950 [23]. Its incidence is estimated to be 3.8 per 100,000 live male births in the United States, and female occurrence is extremely rare, representing less than 5% of all PBS cases [24]. It is characterized by a triad comprising **deficient abdominal wall muscles,**

urinary tract anomalies, and cryptorchidism. Other associated abnormalities may also be present, including cardiac, intestinal, and musculoskeletal. There may be prostatic aplasia or hypoplasia causing dilatation of the prostatic urethra, and sometimes other anomalies such as megalourethra or urethral atresia of the penile urethra, or associated posterior urethral valves may be present. Patients with PBS and urethral obstruction do not survive [1].

5. *Epispadias*: In this malformation, the urethra opens on the upper surface or dorsum of the penis. Epispadias is rarely an isolated phenomenon, being frequently associated with bladder exstrophy in a so-called bladder exstrophy-epispadias complex (BEEC), with an estimated incidence of 2.4/100,000 and male-to-female ratio ranging from 1.5:1 to 6.0:1 [25].
6. *Other abnormalities*: Congenital urethral polyps, Mullerian ducts remnants, Cowper's syringocele, anterior urethral valves, urethral diverticula, megalourethra, urethral duplication, congenital urethroperineal fistula, etc. [1].

References

1. Levin TL, Han B, Little BP. Congenital anomalies of the male urethra. Pediatr Radiol. 2007;37:851–62. https://doi.org/10.1007/s00247-007-0495-0.
2. Hadidi AT, Roessler J, Coerdt W. Development of the human male urethra: a histochemical study on human embryos. J Pediatr Surg. 2014;49(7):1146–52. https://doi.org/10.1016/j.jpedsurg.2014.01.009. Epub 2014 Jan 31. PMID: 24952805.
3. Marshall FF. Embryology of the lower genitourinary tract. Urol Clin North Am. 1978;5(1):3–15. PMID: 347662.
4. van der Werff JF, Nievelstein RA, Brands E, Luijsterburg AJ, Vermeij-Keers C. Normal development of the male anterior urethra. Teratology. 2000;61(3):172–83. https://doi.org/10.1002/(SICI)1096-9926(200003)61:3<172::AID-TERA4>3.0.CO;2-B. PMID: 10661906.
5. Li Y, Sinclair A, Cao M, Shen J, Choudhry S, Botta S, Cunha G, Baskin L. Canalization of the urethral plate precedes fusion of the urethral folds during male penile urethral development: the double zipper hypothesis. J Urol. 2015;193(4):1353–9. https://doi.org/10.1016/j.juro.2014.09.108. Epub 2014 Oct 5. PMID: 25286011; PMCID: PMC4456085.
6. Kluth D, Fiegel HC, Geyer C, Metzger R. Embryology of the distal urethra and external genitals. Semin Pediatr Surg. 2011;20(3):176–87. https://doi.org/10.1053/j.sempedsurg.2011.03.003. PMID: 21708338.
7. Hynes PJ, Fraher JP. The development of the male genitourinary system: II. The origin and formation of the urethral plate. Br J Plast Surg. 2004;57(2):112–21. https://doi.org/10.1016/j.bjps.2003.08.018. PMID: 15037165.
8. Kluth D, Lambrecht W, Reich P. Pathogenesis of hypospadias—more questions than answers. J Pediatr Surg. 1988;23(12):1095–101. https://doi.org/10.1016/s0022-3468(88)80322-1. PMID: 3236174.
9. Hynes PJ, Fraher JP. The development of the male genitourinary system: III. The formation of the spongiose and glandar urethra. Br J Plast Surg. 2004;57:203–14.
10. Kohler TS, Yadven M, Manvar A, Liu N, Monga M. The length of the male urethra. Int Braz J Urol. 2008;34(4):451–4; discussion 455–6. PMID: 18778496. https://doi.org/10.1590/s1677-55382008000400007.
11. Orlandini SZ, Orlandini GE. Ultrastructure of human male urethra. Arch Androl. 1989;23(1):51–9. https://doi.org/10.3109/01485018908986789. PMID: 2675786.

12. Stoddard N, Leslie SW. Histology, male urethra. In: StatPearls [Internet]. Treasure island: StatPearls Publishing; 2022. PMID: 31194395.
13. Furr J, Gelman J. Functional anatomy of the male urethra for the reconstructive surgeon. In: Martins FE, Kulkarni SB, Köhler TS, editors. Textbook of male Genitourethral reconstruction. Cham: Springer; 2020. https://doi.org/10.1007/978-3-030-21447-0_2.
14. Humphrey PA. Male urethra and external genitalia anatomy. In: Brandes S, Morey A, editors. Advanced male urethral and genital reconstructive surgery. Current clinical urology. New York: Humana Press; 2014. https://doi.org/10.1007/978-1-4614-7708-2_2.
15. Ellis H. Anatomy of the urinary bladder, prostate, and male urethra. Gen Surg. 2005;23(3):97–8. https://doi.org/10.1383/surg.23.3.97.63118.
16. Martínez-Piñeiro L. Urethral trauma. In: Hohenfellner M, Santucci RA, editors. Emergencies in urology. Berlin: Springer; 2007. https://doi.org/10.1007/978-3-540-48605-3_23.
17. Mundy AR, Andrich DE. Urethral trauma. Part I: introduction, history, anatomy, pathology, assessment and emergency management. BJU Int. 2011;108(3):310–27. https://doi.org/10.1111/j.1464-410X.2011.10339.x. PMID: 21771241.
18. Chapple C, Barbagli G, Jordan G, Mundy AR, Rodrigues-Netto N, Pansadoro V, McAninch JW. Consensus statement on urethral trauma. BJU Int. 2004;93(9):1195–202. https://doi.org/10.1111/j.1464-410x.2004.04805.x. PMID: 15180604.
19. Kassab GH, et al. Urinary tract. In: Paltiel HJ, Lee EY, editors. Pediatric ultrasound. Cham: Springer; 2021. https://doi.org/10.1007/978-3-030-56802-3_17.
20. Bouty A, Ayers KL, Pask A, Heloury Y, Sinclair AH. The genetic and environmental factors underlying hypospadias. Sex Dev. 2015;9(5):239–59. https://doi.org/10.1159/000441988. Epub 2015 Nov 28. PMID: 26613581; PMCID: PMC5012964.
21. Young HH, Frontz WA, Baldwin JC. Congenital obstruction of the posterior urethra. J Urol. 3: 289–365, 1919. J Urol. 2002;167(1):265–7; discussion 268.
22. Cobb BG, Wolf JA Jr, Ansell JS. Congenital stricture of the proximal urethral bulb. J Urol. 1968;99(5):629–31. https://doi.org/10.1016/s0022-5347(17)62761-7. PMID: 5648559.
23. Eagle JF Jr, Barrett GS. Congenital deficiency of abdominal musculature with associated genitourinary abnormalities: a syndrome. Report of 9 cases. Pediatrics. 1950;6(5):721–36. PMID: 14797335.
24. Arlen AM, Nawaf C, Kirsch AJ. Prune belly syndrome: current perspectives. Pediatr Health Med Ther. 2019;10:75–81. https://doi.org/10.2147/PHMT.S188014.
25. Ludwig M, Ching B, Reutter H, Boyadjiev SA. Bladder exstrophy-epispadias complex. Birth Defects Res A Clin Mol Teratol. 2009;85(6):509–22. https://doi.org/10.1002/bdra.20557. PMID: 19161161.

Epidemiology of Urethral Injury

27

Urethral injuries are rare and account for 4% of genitourinary trauma according to many published series [1, 2]. Because of its length and reduced mobility, the male urethra is five times more likely to sustain an injury than the female urethra. The incidence of urethral injuries caused by urinary catheterization is estimated to be 3.2 per 1000 hospital patients [3].

Urethral stricture is a common disease encountered in adult men of all ages with an estimated prevalence of 229–627 per 100,000 males, and trauma has been reported to be the underlying cause in 9.6–36.1% of cases, others being infection, lichen sclerosus, iatrogenic (post-prostate cancer treatment, cystoscopic procedures, catheterization), post-circumcision meatal stenosis, and idiopathic [4]. The prevalence of urethral stricture disease of all etiologies seems to be higher in industrialized countries reaching 0.9% and in the United States alone, approximately 1.2 million patients sought medical care for this pathology between 2007 and 2012, i.e., in a 5-year period [5]. However, underreporting from developing countries might be a plausible explanation for this discrepancy.

Analysis of the Trauma Audit and Research Network (TARN) database (i.e., the national trauma registry for England and Wales) showed that the incidence of urethral injuries in major trauma is extremely low with only 165 patients identified over a 6-year period, equaling 1 per two million population per year, with over 90% being males. The most common circumstances were road traffic accidents, the overall mortality was 12%, and associated pelvic fractures were found in 82% and portended a two-fold increase in mortality [6]. Another TARN review recruiting over 12,000 motorcyclists admitted for trauma between January 2012 and December 2016 identified 6% with genitourinary injuries (GUI), the majority of whom sustained renal trauma, and only 0.2% had urethral injuries, including the front-riders and the pillion passengers [7].

An American level I trauma center registry covering a 15-year period recorded 5518 pelvic fracture cases, including 233 (4.2%) with lower urinary tract injury, of whom 71 patients (1.3%) had a urethral injury, almost all (70) being males. The

S. A. AL-Mamari, *Urogenital Trauma: A Practical Guide*,
https://doi.org/10.1007/978-981-99-6171-9_27

most common pelvic fracture type associated with urethral injury was pubic arch fractures (87%) and isolated acetabular fractures did not cause urethral injury [8].

A prospective study of 203 consecutive cases of male pelvic fractures showed 19% with urethral injury, 2.5% with bladder injury, and 6% with combined urethral and bladder injuries [9].

Although extremely rare, female urethral injuries associated with a pelvic fracture are not unheard of in the literature and a systematic review recorded 55 articles treating a total of 158 cases [10].

References

1. McGeady JB, Breyer BN. Current epidemiology of genitourinary trauma. Urol Clin North Am. 2013;40(3):323–34. https://doi.org/10.1016/j.ucl.2013.04.001. Epub 2013 Jun 12. PMID: 23905930; PMCID: PMC4016766.
2. Alwaal A, Zaid UB, Blaschko SD, Harris CR, Gaither TW, McAninch JW, Breyer BN. The incidence, causes, mechanism, risk factors, classification, and diagnosis of pelvic fracture urethral injury. Arab J Urol. 2015;13(1):2–6. https://doi.org/10.1016/j.aju.2014.08.006. Epub 2014 Sep 16. PMID: 26019970; PMCID: PMC4435767.
3. Kashefi C, Messer K, Barden R, Sexton C, Parsons JK. Incidence and prevention of iatrogenic urethral injuries. J Urol. 2008;179:2254–8.
4. Alwaal A, Blaschko SD, McAninch JW, Breyer BN. Epidemiology of urethral strictures. Transl Androl Urol. 2014;3(2):209–13. https://doi.org/10.3978/j.issn.2223-4683.2014.04.07. PMID: 26813256; PMCID: PMC4708169.
5. Osterberg EC, Murphy G, Harris CR, Breyer BN. Cost-effective strategies for the management and treatment of urethral stricture disease. Urol Clin North Am. 2017;44(1):11–7. https://doi.org/10.1016/j.ucl.2016.08.002. PMID: 27908365.
6. Battaloglu E, Figuero M, Moran C, et al. Urethral injury in major trauma. Injury. 2019;50(5):1053–7. ISSN 0020-1383.
7. Moss BF, Moss CE, Dervin P, Lawrence T, Jones S, Thomas S. High riding prostate: epidemiology of genitourinary injury in motorcyclists from a UK register of over 12,000 victims. Curr Urol. 2020;14(2):105–12. https://doi.org/10.1159/000499251. Epub 2020 Jun 23. PMID: 32774236; PMCID: PMC7390984.
8. Johnsen NV, Dmochowski RR, Young JB, Guillamondegui OD. Epidemiology of blunt lower urinary tract trauma with and without pelvic fracture. Urology. 2017;102:234–9. https://doi.org/10.1016/j.urology.2016.11.015. Epub 2016 Dec 30. PMID: 28043650.
9. Koraitim MM, Marzouk ME, Atta MA. Risk factors and mechanism of urethral injury in pelvic fractures. Br J Urol. 1996;77(6):876–80.
10. Patel DN, Fok CS, Webster GD, Anger JT. Female urethral injuries associated with pelvic fracture: a systematic review of the literature. BJU Int. 2017;120(6):766–73. https://doi.org/10.1111/bju.13989. Epub 2017 Sep 7. PMID: 28805298.

28 Etiology, Mechanisms, and Anatomopathology of Urethral Injury

An **old consensus** from WHO experts recommended the term **"stricture"** be used for the anterior urethra in cases with intrinsic corpus spongiosum fibrosis (spongiofibrosis) while the urethra remains in continuity. Conversely, they recommended the terms **"stenosis"** for the posterior urethra, and especially the term **"sphincter stenosis"** for simple continuity strictures of the membranous urethra (such as those from TURP or secondary to inflammations) or for those occurring after radical prostatectomy and urethra-vesical anastomosis, in order to emphasize that the distal urethral sphincter mechanism has not been destroyed although its function might be generally impaired to a variable extent. When there are more serious injuries of the posterior urethra (such as those arising from a pelvic fracture), the term **"PFUDD" (pelvic fracture urethral distraction defects)** was preferred [1].

However, this nomenclature is not yet strictly adhered to by all authors and will not be rigorously followed in this chapter. Moreover, as already mentioned in the introduction to this section, a more recent expert consensus has proposed to replace the term **"pelvic fracture urethral distraction defects (PFUDD)"** with **"pelvic fracture urethral injury (PFUI)"** as these injuries are not usually complete nor are they necessarily distracted [2].

The most frequent causes of urethral injury are iatrogenic: catheterization, urethrocystoscopic procedures, and procedures for female or male incontinence or for male sexual impotence. Other causes include falls, road traffic accidents, and penetrating agents (gunshot injuries, stabbing). Urethral trauma arising from falling astride particularly involves the bulbar urethra due to compression against the symphysis pubis while the RTA associated with pubic ramus fracture exposes to membranous urethra injury.

A 10-year study of nearly 1500 male patients with urethral stricture showed that the **iatrogenic causes were the most common etiology accounting for 38.6%**, including catheterization (16%), hypospadias repair (12%), and transurethral surgery (9%), etc. The second group of causes was idiopathic (35.8%), followed by lichen sclerosus (13.4%). **External trauma accounted for 11% of all causes** [3].

S. A. AL-Mamari, *Urogenital Trauma: A Practical Guide*,
https://doi.org/10.1007/978-981-99-6171-9_28

However, the proportion of trauma causes varies with the published series **between 9.6 and 36.1%** [4], and the association of urethral injuries with pelvic fractures varies **between 5 and 25%** [5].

Significant regional differences exist in the etiology and anatomical sites of urethral strictures between the western world and India. Thus, more penile strictures, fewer posterior urethral stenoses, and more iatrogenic causes, attributable to failed hypospadias repair, were found in the former, while more patients with lichen sclerosus and external trauma were recruited in India, where motor vehicle accidents (MVA) accounted for nearly 36% of urethral strictures compared with only 15% in the United States and Italy. In both groups the prevalence of infectious etiology was very low, accounting for only 1% of all causes [6].

While it is logical to hypothesize that the most common cause of anterior urethral injury is iatrogenic, mainly arising from traumatic Foley catheter insertion, it should be borne in mind however that this incidence cannot be reliably determined as these injuries are generally mild and underreported. A prospective study has shown an incidence of **3.2 urethral injuries per 1000 patients who underwent urethral catheterization**, and 100% of the patients complained of penile and/or perineal pain while 86% developed also penile bleeding. This incidence was significantly reduced, reaching 0.7 per 1000 patients, after the implantation of a nursing education program including basic urological anatomy, urethral catheter insertion techniques, and catheter safety [7].

A direct contusion is the most common cause of anterior urethral injury of clinical significance. This is mostly seen in **straddle-type injury**, and more rarely during **penile fracture**. The latter association varies geographically, ranging from 0–3% in Asia and the Middle East to 20–38% in the United States and Europe [8]. Straddle injury is the predominant mechanism of external urethral trauma, followed by pelvic fractures during RTA [8].

Penetrating injuries affect mostly the anterior urethra (bulbar and pendulous) and are mostly secondary to **civilian gunshot injuries**. Nevertheless, they are extremely rare, occurring only in 2.9% of a series of 309 patients with genitourinary tract gunshot injuries [9].

Children suffering from falls sustain more severe pelvic fractures and related urethral injuries than adults, and the insult results in a higher incidence of stricture formation, which is more likely to be proximal with a higher incidence of urinary incontinence [5].

A trauma registry study conducted at the Los Angeles County and University of Southern California trauma center during an 8-year period recruited 16,630 major blunt trauma, of whom 1545 (9.3%) sustained pelvic fractures, with a majority of males (60.6%). Bladder and urethra injuries were seen in 5.8% of cases. The circumstances of trauma were in decreasing order: motorcycle (15.5%), pedestrians (13.8%), falls from heights of >15 feet (12.9%), and automobile occupants (10.2%). Pedestrian and motorcycle accidents were also associated with more severe pelvic fractures compared to automobile occupants [10].

Motor vehicle collisions (MVCs) are the most common cause of pelvic fracture (68–84%) and the likelihood of subsequent urethral injuries here is four times higher than in falling from a height (6–25%) [5]. Pedestrians are also more likely to sustain pelvic fracture urethral injuries (PFUI) than motor vehicle occupants [10]. Less common causes of PFUI are slipping and falling astride, animal (horse) or machinery hit, and other industrial and mining accidents [5].

Non-iatrogenic posterior injuries in industrialized societies are approximately four times more frequent than anterior urethral injuries [8].

28.1 Anatomopathology of Posterior Urethral Injury

Posterior urethral injuries consist of a simple stretching of the membranous part in 25.5%, a partial rupture in 25.5–35%, and a complete rupture in 49–65% [11, 12]. In pelvic fracture, the number of broken rami parallels the risk of urethral injury [12].

Turner-Warwick categorized four end results of the PFUI [13]:

- No stricture, no sphincter damage
- No stricture, but distal sphincter damage
- Short supramembranous stricture, and little surrounding fibrosis and sphincter damage
- Complex posterior urethral strictures

The criteria of complexity were:

- stricture greater than 2 cm and surrounded by dense fibrosis after the organization of a pelvic floor hematoma,
- stricture of any length associated with extravasation diverticula, false passages or fistulas, and
- extensive sphincter damage (injury involves the bladder neck and the distal intrinsic urethral mechanisms).

In contrast, two factors were not counted in the complexity of the stricture: the completeness of the stricture with complete obliteration, and the presence of a pelvic fracture.

Contrary to the classical teaching, a cadaveric study has revealed that **most urethral disruptions in pelvic fractures occur distal to the external urinary sphincter**, and is provoked by a caudal and rostral displacement of the anterior pelvic ring and urogenital diaphragm complex, tearing the urogenital diaphragm off the urethra [14]. The same study also showed that these injuries measure an average of 3–4 cm, and are more significant dorsal than ventral. A prospective study of 20 cases of PFUI showed that, contrary to the general belief, **the injury consists of an avulsion of the membranous urethra from the bulbar urethra rather than a shearing through the membranous urethra, and therefore the external sphincter was not necessarily damaged**, as there was evidence of urethral sphincter function, either urodynamically (55%), endoscopically (65%), or functionally (85%) [15].

An NTDB review recruiting 31,380 patients with pelvic fractures showed that 1444 had associated genito-urinary injuries (4.6%) and bladder injury alone was more frequent (3.39%) than urethral injury (0.94%) or combined bladder and urethral injury (0.19%). Males were the most involved gender in the occurrence of pelvic fractures as well as in their association with GU injuries. This study also showed the following anatomopathological types of pelvic fractures among the patients who had a urethral injury: Pubis (49%), disruption of the pelvic circle (26%), acetabulum (23%), innominate/pelvic rim (11.3%), ilium (8.4%), Ischium (3.9%), and unspecified (10.1%) [16].

The anatomopathology of the posterior urethra has a linear correlation with the magnitude of trauma in pelvic fracture, progressing from simple stretching to partial or complete disruption at the bulbomembranous junction. Injuries to the prostatic urethra and bladder neck occur mostly in the pediatric population because the prostate is underdeveloped and poorly supported in this age category, while the female urethra usually suffers a partial tear of the anterior wall and rarely a complete disruption [17, 18]. Indeed, posttraumatic posterior urethral strictures in children were observed to be almost always distal to the verumontanum causing displacement in 44% of cases, and showed a high association with Malgaigne's fracture (35% of cases) and straddle fracture with or without diastasis of the sacroiliac joint (26%) [19].

Most PFUIs occur at the bulbomembranous junction, as a result of the rupture of ligamentous attachments during pelvic-ring disruption. Less frequently the urethra might also be directly injured by a bony fragment, an occurrence more likely to occur in women [18].

Total disruption of the supramembranous urethra is frequently associated with the disruption of the periprostatic venous plexus, resulting in a large hematoma that often displaces the prostate gland cephalad and posteriorly. Diastasis of the symphysis pubis with pubic arch separation may cause disruption of the membranous urethra with severance of the puboprostatic ligament as well as the urogenital diaphragm, and when a combined disruption of the urethra occurs at the level of the supramembranous urethra and the vesical neck, this will result in a **"free-floating"** prostate gland [20].

PFUIs generally lacerate the external sphincter mechanism at the level of the membranous urethra and jeopardize urinary incontinence which merely depends from now onwards on a competent bladder neck sphincter. **This fact is of paramount importance when one wants to perform urethroplasty as the re-establishment of the urethral channel might unmask incontinence**. This is one of the reasons behind a pre-operative urethrocystoscopy and cystography aiming at inspecting the bladder neck and predicting incontinence [21].

28.2 Mechanism of the Posterior Urethral Injury

A pelvic fracture may instantly produce a shearing force that avulses the apex of the prostate from the membranous urethra which is a rather fixed segment attached to the urogenital diaphragm [22]. Pokorny et al. have proposed four mechanisms for the PFUI [23]:

- The first and most common mechanism: diametric fracture with upward displacement of the hemipelvis and symphysis with secondary traction on the hypogastric wing attached to the base of the bladder and prostate. This fracture is generally caused by a force applied over the ipsilateral femur. The upwardly displaced symphysis ruptures the puboprostatic ligament and stretches the prostatomembranous urethra with or without rupture. However, the bulbous urethra is spared by this injury being fixed to the corpus spongiosum and central tendon.
- Second mechanism: This occurs in bilateral fracture of the superior and inferior pubic rami, causing a posteroinferior displacement of the intervening bony segment owing to a force acting over the pubis, with sudden retrocession of the urogenital diaphragm acting as guillotine against the membranous urethra.
- Third mechanism: This evolves through diastasis of the symphysis, rupture of the puboprostatic ligament, and tearing of the urogenital diaphragm from the contralateral bone. The diastasis pulls the membranous urethra in two opposite directions.
- Fourth mechanism: There is a direct injury of the posterior urethra by a bony spicule ejected during fractures of the pubis.

Pelvic ring disruptions are most commonly classified according to their instability, as they may be stable, rotationally unstable but vertically stable, or both

Table 28.1 Correlation of pelvic ring fracture classification and male or female LUTI

	Tile type			
Group (*n*)	A	B1	B2	C
Men (81)				
No LUTI (57)	3	21	6	27
LUTI (24)	0	7	4	13
Isolated bladder injury	0	2	2	2
PUI	0	5	2	7
CUD	0	0	0	4
Bladder + urethral injury	0	0	0	5
Bladder neck injury	0	0	0	3
Women (27)				
No LUTI (24)	0	3	6	15
LUTI (3)	0	0	1	2
Isolated bladder injury	0	0	1	2

LUTI lower urinary tract injury, *PUI* partial urethral injury, *CUD* complete urethral disruption
Reproduced from Andrich DE et al. [26]. Reproduced with permission from John Wiley and Sons

rotationally and vertically unstable [24]. Thus, rotationally unstable fractures are the most common cause of urethral injury while stable pelvic injuries are generally harmless to the urethra [24].

In 1988, Marvin Tile proposed a classification of pelvic disruptions aiming at guiding Orthopedicians in their decision for external fixation of pelvic ring fractures [25]. In 2007, Andrich et al. found the following association of lower urinary tract injuries with Tile's pelvic fracture grades [26] (Table 28.1).

28.3 Mechanism and Anatomopathology of Anterior urethral Injury

Contrary to the posterior urethra which is mostly associated with pelvic fractures sustained during an MVA, anterior urethral injury results from direct external blunt or penetrating trauma, and the **bulbous or bulbar urethra** is the most affected segment, being involved in 85%, as it is fixed beneath the pubic bone, while the pendulous urethra is freely mobile [22]. Straddle injuries mostly occur during work (builders), bicycle riding, and other sports (gymnastics such as pommel horse). An infrequent cause of urethral injury is a penile fracture (PF), and this association varies greatly with geographic entities, being lower in Asia and the Middle East (0–3%) than in the United States and Europe (20–38%) [8]. PF occurs when the phallus accidentally and forcibly strikes the female pubic ramus. Typically, there is a tear of the tunica albuginea covering the corpora cavernosa and the urethra is endangered when the tear extends into the corpus spongiosum [22].

Straddle-type injuries are blunt trauma caused by falling astride onto a hard surface as a home accident or during work, walking, or sports; they may arise also from a motor vehicle or bicycle accident or kicks to the perineum as an assault or during sports (football). During the impact, the bulbous urethra is crushed against the inferior pubic rami, resulting in its contusion or laceration.

Rarely anterior urethra injury can result from penetrating agents: firearms, stabbing, biting, or animal attacks such as cow horn injury (goring) [27].

Self-inflicted urethral injuries do also occur (stabbing, laceration, or insertion of foreign bodies) and will be developed at the end of this book in a special section.

Iatrogenic urethral injuries form an important group of causes [22]:

1. Prolonged or traumatic urethral instrumentation (Foley catheter insertion or retrieval without emptying the balloon): this disrupts the mucosa with urethral stricture as a late consequence mediated by inflammation and spongiofibrosis. It is mostly located at the bulbar urethra.
2. Repeated dilations and urethrotomies for stricture disease: this establishes a chronic inflammatory process and scarring.
3. Extracorporeal circulation during cardiac revascularization surgery: suspected causes are perioperative urethral catheterization and urethral ischemia.
4. bladder-drained pancreas transplantation and pancreas-kidney transplantation: there is urethral mucosa irritation by pancreatic enzymes.

5. Transurethral resection of the prostate (TURP): Urethral stricture occurs in 3.1–10% of patients, possibly as the consequence of abrasions by oversized resectoscopes, electrical transmission through the sheath with urethral burn, or post-operative urinary tract infections.
6. Transurethral microwave therapy (TUMT)
7. Radical prostatectomy: anastomotic urethra-vesical stricture (occurs in 7–17%)
8. Insertion of the needle during TOT or TVT.

The WHO consensus summarizes the causes of urethral injury as [1]:

1. Posterior urethra injuries:
   - Penetrating injuries: Gunshot wounds, stab wounds
   - PFUIs: road traffic accidents, falls from heights, industrial accidents
   - Iatrogenic injuries: endoscopic surgery (TURP), and radical prostatectomy
2. Anterior urethral injuries:
   - Blunt trauma: fall astride, kicks in the perineum, go-kart injuries, skateboarding
   - Penetrating trauma: gunshot/stab wounds
   - Sexual excess: penile fractures
   - Urethral foreign bodies
   - Constriction bands (seen in paraplegics, etc.)
   - Iatrogenic injuries: urethral catheters, penile surgery, endoscopic instrumentation

References

1. Chapple C, Barbagli G, Jordan G, Mundy AR, Rodrigues-Netto N, Pansadoro V, McAninch JW. Consensus statement on urethral trauma. BJU Int. 2004;93(9):1195–202. https://doi.org/10.1111/j.1464-410x.2004.04805.x. PMID: 15180604.
2. Gómez RG, Mundy T, Dubey D, El-Kassaby AW, Firdaoessaleh KR, Santucci R. SIU/ICUD consultation on Urethral strictures: pelvic fracture urethral injuries. Urology. 2014;83(3 Suppl):S48–58. https://doi.org/10.1016/j.urology.2013.09.023. Epub 2013 Nov 8. PMID: 24210734.
3. Palminteri E, Berdondini E, Verze P, De Nunzio C, Vitarelli A, Carmignani L. Contemporary urethral stricture characteristics in the developed world. Urology. 2013;81(1):191–6. https://doi.org/10.1016/j.urology.2012.08.062. Epub 2012 Nov 13. PMID: 23153951.
4. Alwaal A, Blaschko SD, McAninch JW, Breyer BN. Epidemiology of urethral strictures. Transl Androl Urol. 2014;3(2):209–13. https://doi.org/10.3978/j.issn.2223-4683.2014.04.07. PMID: 26813256; PMCID: PMC4708169.
5. Alwaal A, Zaid UB, Blaschko SD, Harris CR, Gaither TW, McAninch JW, Breyer BN. The incidence, causes, mechanism, risk factors, classification, and diagnosis of pelvic fracture urethral injury. Arab J Urol. 2015;13(1):2–6. https://doi.org/10.1016/j.aju.2014.08.006. Epub 2014 Sep 16. PMID: 26019970; PMCID: PMC4435767.
6. Stein DM, Thum DJ, Barbagli G, Kulkarni S, Sansalone S, Pardeshi A, Gonzalez CM. A geographic analysis of male urethral stricture aetiology and location. BJU Int. 2013;112(6):830–4. https://doi.org/10.1111/j.1464-410X.2012.11600.x. Epub 2012 Dec 18. PMID: 23253867.

7. Kashefi C, Messer K, Barden R, Sexton C, Parsons JK. Incidence and prevention of iatrogenic urethral injuries. J Urol. 2008;179(6):2254–7. https://doi.org/10.1016/j.juro.2008.01.108; discussion 2257–8. Epub 2008 Apr 18. PMID: 18423712.
8. McGeady JB, Breyer BN. Current epidemiology of genitourinary trauma. Urol Clin North Am. 2013;40(3):323–34. https://doi.org/10.1016/j.ucl.2013.04.001. Epub 2013 Jun 12. PMID: 23905930; PMCID: PMC4016766.
9. Najibi S, Tannast M, Latini JM. Civilian gunshot wounds to the genitourinary tract: incidence, anatomic distribution, associated injuries, and outcomes. Urology. 2010;76(4):977–81; discussion 981. PMID: 20605196. https://doi.org/10.1016/j.urology.2010.01.092.
10. Demetriades D, Karaiskakis M, Toutouzas K, Alo K, Velmahos G, Chan L. Pelvic fractures: epidemiology and predictors of associated abdominal injuries and outcomes. J Am Coll Surg. 2002;195(1):1–10. https://doi.org/10.1016/s1072-7515(02)01197-3. PMID: 12113532.
11. Webster GD, Mathes GL, Selli C. Prostatomembranous urethral injuries: a review of the literature and a rational approach to their management. J Urol. 1983;130(5):898–902. https://doi.org/10.1016/s0022-5347(17)51561-x. PMID: 6355512.
12. Koraitim MM, Marzouk ME, Atta MA. Risk factors and mechanism of urethral injury in pelvic fractures. Br J Urol. 1996;77(6):876–80.
13. Turner-Warwick R. Complex traumatic posterior urethral strictures. J Urol. 1977;118(4):564–74. https://doi.org/10.1016/s0022-5347(17)58109-4. PMID: 916051.
14. Mouraviev VB, Santucci RA. Cadaveric anatomy of pelvic fracture urethral distraction injury: most injuries are distal to the external urinary sphincter. J Urol. 2005;173(3):869–72. https://doi.org/10.1097/01.ju.0000152252.48176.69. PMID: 15711300.
15. Andrich DE, Mundy AR. The nature of urethral injury in cases of pelvic fracture urethral trauma. J Urol. 2001;165:1492–5.
16. Bjurlin MA, Fantus RJ, Mellett MM, Goble SM. Genitourinary injuries in pelvic fracture morbidity and mortality using the National Trauma Data Bank. J Trauma. 2009;67(5):1033–9. https://doi.org/10.1097/TA.0b013e3181bb8d6c. PMID: 19901665.
17. Koraitim MM. Pelvic fracture urethral injuries: the unresolved controversy. J Urol. 1999;161(5):1433–41. PMID: 10210368.
18. Alwaal A, Zaid UB, Blaschko SD, Harris CR, Gaither TW, McAninch JW, Breyer BN. The incidence, causes, mechanism, risk factors, classification, and diagnosis of pelvic fracture urethral injury. Arab J Urol. 2015;13(1):2–6. https://doi.org/10.1016/j.aju.2014.08.006.
19. Koraitim MM. Posttraumatic posterior urethral strictures in children: a 20-year experience. J Urol. 1997;157(2):641–5. PMID: 8996388.
20. Clark SS, Prudencio RF. Lower urinary tract injuries associated with pelvic fractures. Diagnosis and management. Surg Clin North Am. 1972;52(1):183–201. https://doi.org/10.1016/s0039-6109(16)39642-6. PMID: 5013219.
21. Iselin CE, Webster GD. The significance of the open bladder neck associated with pelvic fracture urethral distraction defects. J Urol. 1999;162(2):347–51. PMID: 10411036.
22. Rosenstein DI, Alsikafi NF. Diagnosis and classification of urethral injuries. Urol Clin North Am. 2006;33(1):73–85. https://doi.org/10.1016/j.ucl.2005.11.004, vi-vii. PMID: 16488282.
23. Pokorny M, Pontes JE, Pierce JM Jr. Urological injuries associated with pelvic trauma. J Urol. 1979;121(4):455–7. https://doi.org/10.1016/s0022-5347(17)56822-6. PMID: 439217.
24. Mundy AR, Andrich DE. Urethral trauma. Part I: introduction, history, anatomy, pathology, assessment and emergency management. BJU Int. 2011;108(3):310–27. https://doi.org/10.1111/j.1464-410X.2011.10339.x. PMID: 21771241.
25. Tile M. Pelvic ring fractures: should they be fixed? J Bone Joint Surg Br. 1988;70:1–12.
26. Andrich DE, Day AC, Mundy AR. Proposed mechanisms of lower tract injury in fractures of the pelvic ring. BJU Int. 2007;100:567–73.
27. Priyadarshi V, Gupta D, Pal DK. Lower genitourinary tract trauma caused by Cow Horn injury. J Obstet Gynaecol India. 2016;66(Suppl 1):578–82. https://doi.org/10.1007/s13224-015-0748-z. Epub 2015 Sep 8. PMID: 27651664; PMCID: PMC5016394.

29 Classification of Urethral Injury

Many grading systems have been proposed for urethral injury, but they all suffer from the lack of high-level evidence and are merely based on the authors' experience [1]. One of the oldest is the Colapinto and McCallum classification proposed in 1977, based on retrograde urethrography. It was exclusively proposed for the posterior urethra [2] (Table 29.1).

The most popular classification was proposed by Goldman et al. in 1977, which is a modification and completion of the Colapinto and McCallum classification with the addition of more anatomical descriptions [3, 4] (Table 29.2; Fig. 29.1).

The AAST classification published by Moore et al. in 1995 emphasized the importance of the anatomopathological aspect of the injury being either a simple contusion, a partial or a total disruption, and for total disruption, more severe injuries are defined by a greater than 2-cm urethral gap [5].

Table 29.1 Colapinto and McCallum classification and description of posterior urethral injury

Type I	The prostate or the urogenital diaphragm is dislocated, causing elongation and tension of the bulbomembranous urethra. There may be urethral contusion or laceration (not full thickness)
Type II	The membranous urethra is ruptured above the urogenital diaphragm, with or without prostatic injury. The bulbous urethra is intact. The rupture may be partial or complete
Type III	The membranous urethra is disrupted above and below the urogenital diaphragm. The rupture usually is complete and may be associated with a rupture of the urogenital diaphragm and/or rupture of the bulbous urethra

From Colapinto V and McCallum RW [2], with permission from Wolters Kluwer Health

S. A. AL-Mamari, *Urogenital Trauma: A Practical Guide*,
https://doi.org/10.1007/978-981-99-6171-9_29

Table 29.2 Urethral trauma grading by Goldman SM et al. [3], with permission from Wolters Kluwer Health

I	Posterior urethra intact but stretched
II	Partial or complete pure posterior injury with a tear of the membranous urethra above the urogenital diaphragm
III	Partial or complete combined anterior/posterior urethral injury with disruption of the urogenital diaphragm
IV	Bladder neck injury with extension into the urethra An injury of the base of the bladder with periurethral extravasation simulating a true type IV urethral injury is called type IVA injury
V	Partial or complete pure anterior urethral injury

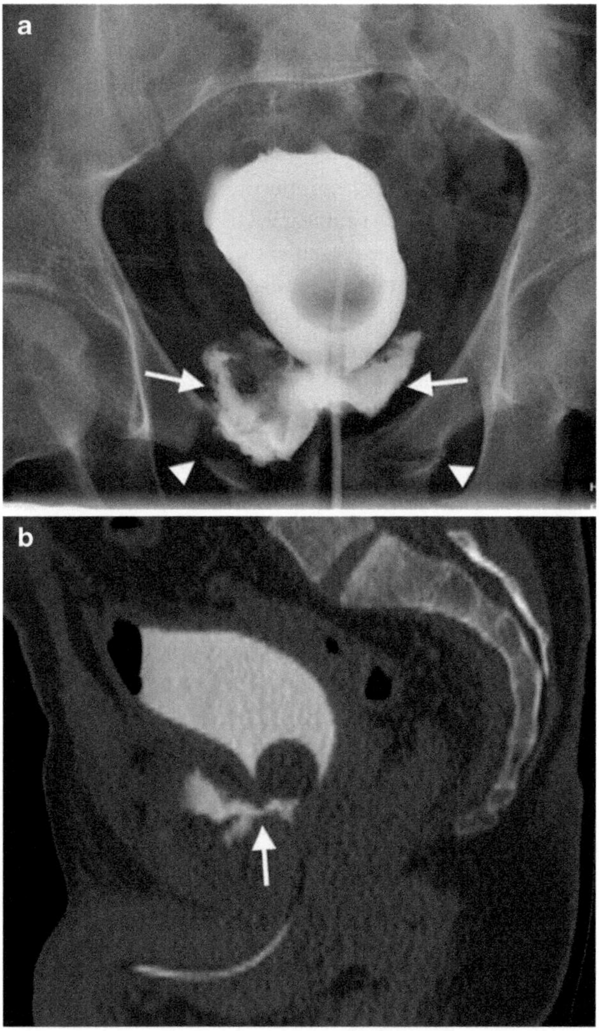

Fig. 29.1 Type IV urethral injury. (**a**) Retrograde cystographic image obtained few days after admission shows contrast leakage around the prostatic urethra (arrow). Also, note bilateral superior pubic rami fracture (arrowhead). (**b**) Sagittal CT cystographic image shows bladder neck laceration with extension to the proximal urethra as well as contrast extravasation (arrow). (From Wongwaisayawan S et al. [4], with permission from Springer Nature)

Goldman's classification has been endorsed by the WHO consensus committee in 2004 because of its predictive value for incontinence [6]. However, the same committee suggested the following simplification:

(a) Anterior urethra: (1) partial disruption, (2) complete disruption
(b) Posterior urethra: (3) posterior urethra stretched but intact, (4) partial disruption, (5) complete disruption, (6) complex (involves bladder neck/rectum)

In 2001 Al Rifaei et al. proposed a new functional and anatomical classification of urethral injury secondary to pelvic fracture adding an emphasis on the sphincteric mechanism [7] (Table 29.3).

The multiplicity of these classifications reflects the lack of consensus as none is perfect and universally accepted. Moreover, they don't clearly provide an answer to the ideal technique and timing of reconstructive surgeries for PFUIs and are therefore considered by certain researchers to have only little impact on the technique selection and the surgical outcome prediction [1].

The European Association of Urology (EAU) attempted to reach a consensus by summarizing the most relevant points of the above classifications with the purpose to have direct implications for clinical management [8] (Table 29.4).

In addition to the classification of urethral injury, there is also an EAU endoscopic classification of urethral stricture, regardless of the etiology [9] (Table 29.5).

This classification has an important bearing as prior evaluation of the stricture using a small caliber ureteroscope (4.5 and 6 Fr) has shown significant benefits in the selection of the surgical approach and helps also counseling the patient about expectations and realistic results [10].

Table 29.3 Anatomical and functional classification for urethral injury secondary to pelvic fracture

Type I	Injury to the prostate	
	Type Ia	Proximal avulsion of the prostate from the bladder neck
	Type Ib	Incomplete or complete transverse trans-prostatic urethral rupture
Type II	Stretching of the membranous urethra	
Type III	Incomplete or complete pure rupture of the prostatomembranous junction (classic injury)	
Type IV	Incomplete or complete pure rupture of the bulbo-membranous urethra (infradiaphragmatic)	
Type V	Incomplete or complete variable combined urethral injuries affecting >1 level of the urethra	

From Al Rifaei M et al. [7], with permission from Taylor and Francis

Table 29.4 Classification of blunt anterior and posterior urethra with management according to injury grade

Grade	Description	Appearance	Management
I	Stretch injury	Elongation of the urethra without extravasation on urethrography	No treatment required
II	Contusion	Blood at the urethral meatus; no extravasation on urethrography	Grades II and III can be managed conservatively with suprapubic cystostomy or urethral catheterization
III	Partial disruption	Extravasation of contrast at injury site with contrast visualized in the proximal urethra or bladder	
IV	Complete disruption	Extravasation of contrast at injury site without visualization of proximal urethra or anterior urethra or bladder	Suprapubic cystostomy and delayed repair or primary endoscopic realignment in selected patients ± delayed repair
V	Complete or partial disruption of posterior urethra with associated tear of the bladder neck, rectum or vagina	Extravasation of contrast at urethral injury site ± presence of blood in the vaginal introitus in women. Extravasation of contrast at bladder neck during suprapubic cystography ± rectal or vaginal filling with contrast material	Primary open repair

From Martínez-Piñeiro L et al. [8], with permission from Elsevier

Table 29.5 EAU classification according to the degree of urethral narrowing

Category	Description	Urethral lumen (French [Fr])	Degree
0	Normal urethra on imaging	–	–
1	Subclinical strictures	Urethral narrowing but >16 Fr	Low
2	Low-grade strictures	11–15 Fr	
3	High-grade or significant strictures	4–10 Fr	High
4	Nearly obliterative strictures	1–3 Fr	
5	Obliterative strictures	No urethral lumen (0 Fr)	

From the EAU guidelines [9], with permission from the EAU

References

1. Elbakry A. Classification of pelvic fracture urethral injuries: Is there an effect on the type of delayed urethroplasty? Arab J Urol. 2011;9(3):191–5. https://doi.org/10.1016/j.aju.2011.06.001. Epub 2011 Aug 15. PMID: 26579295; PMCID: PMC4150576.
2. Colapinto V, McCallum RW. Injury to the male posterior urethra in fractured pelvis: a new classification. J Urol. 1977;116:575.
3. Goldman SM, Sandler CM, Corriere JN Jr, McGuire EJ. Blunt urethral trauma: a unified, anatomical mechanical classification. J Urol. 1997;157(1):85–9. https://doi.org/10.1016/s0022-5347(01)65291-1. PMID: 8976222.
4. Wongwaisayawan S, Krishna S, Sheikh A, et al. Imaging spectrum of traumatic urinary bladder and urethral injuries. Abdom Radiol (NY). 2021;46:681–91. https://doi.org/10.1007/s00261-020-02679-0.

5. Moore EE, Cogbill TH, Malangoni MA, Jurkovich GJ, Shackford SR, Champion HR, McAninch JW. Organ injury scaling. Surg Clin North Am. 1995;75(2):293–303. https://doi.org/10.1016/s0039-6109(16)46589-8. PMID: 7899999.
6. Chapple C, Barbagli G, Jordan G, Mundy AR, Rodrigues-Netto N, Pansadoro V, McAninch JW. Consensus statement on urethral trauma. BJU Int. 2004;93(9):1195–202. https://doi.org/10.1111/j.1464-410x.2004.04805.x. PMID: 15180604.
7. Al Rifaei M, Eid NI, Al Rifaei A. Urethral injury secondary to pelvic fracture: anatomical and functional classification. Scand J Urol Nephrol. 2001;35(3):205–11. https://doi.org/10.1080/003655901750291971. PMID: 11487073.
8. Martínez-Piñeiro L, Djakovic N, Plas E, Mor Y, Santucci RA, Serafetinidis E, Turkeri LN, Hohenfellner M, European Association of Urology. EAU guidelines on urethral trauma. Eur Urol. 2010;57(5):791–803. https://doi.org/10.1016/j.eururo.2010.01.013. Epub 2010 Jan 20. PMID: 20122789.
9. EAU guidelines. edn. Presented at the EAU annual congress Amsterdam 2022. isbn:978-94-92671-16-5. https://uroweb.org/guidelines/urethral-strictures/chapter/classifications
10. Shahrour W, Joshi P, Hunter CB, Batra VS, Elmansy H, Surana S, Kulkarni S. The benefits of using a small caliber ureteroscope in evaluation and management of urethral stricture. Adv Urol. 2018;2018:9137892. https://doi.org/10.1155/2018/9137892. PMID: 30584423; PMCID: PMC6280311.

Diagnosis of Urethral Injury: Symptoms, Signs, and Imaging Studies

30

30.1 Symptoms and Signs

The WHO experts' consensus has recommended considering the following signs for the diagnosis of urethral injury: blood at the urethral meatus, difficulty or inability to urinate, distended urinary bladder, butterfly bruising of the perineum, high-riding prostate on digital rectal examination (DRE), pelvic fractures with displacement of the pubic rami, and pelvic hematoma on imaging [1]. **Hematuria and/or urethral bleeding remain the best indicator of urinary tract injury, and they have an incidence of 91 to 100% in urethral trauma** [2].

In RTA, patients are likely to sustain multi-organ injuries and attention will naturally be immediately diverted to the most life-threatening injury (major vessels laceration, ruptured kidney, liver or spleen, hollow viscus). Stabilization of any fracture comes second, but when the pelvic arch is involved, attention should immediately be brought to the integrity of the urinary bladder and the urethra. The history of urination since the time of the accident should be elicited. The bladder should be palpated for fullness and the external organs and the perineal region should be examined for any painful swelling and skin discoloration (urinary extravasation, hematoma). A digital rectal examination (DRE) should be performed as well as a vaginal examination in females looking for associated rectal or vaginal injury. **When the patient confirms being able to void, either clear urine or blood-stained, he/she should be catheterized. However, if he/she is not able to void and there is fresh blood coming out through the external meatus, a severe urethral injury should be suspected regardless of the importance of the bleeding, and therefore catheterization must be avoided. Blood at the external meatus is a very reliable sign of severe urethral injury** despite there being a possibility of fallacious overdiagnosis in presence of a simple mucosal contusion.

A frequent pitfall is when the examiner fails to palpate the prostate on DRE and thinks it has been displaced upward. There might just be a boggy hematoma that prevents this examination combined with the poor cooperativeness of the patient

S. A. AL-Mamari, *Urogenital Trauma: A Practical Guide*,
https://doi.org/10.1007/978-981-99-6171-9_30

Table 30.1 Clinical features associated with urethral injuries post blunt trauma

Documented clinical variable	*N*	Sensitivity (%)
Blood at the urethral meatus	10	37
Perineal hematoma	12	44.4
High-riding prostate	4	14.8
At least one of the above	18	66.7
Pubic symphysis disruption	25	92.5
Pubic symphysis disruption or clinical sign	27	100

From Lückhoff C et al. [3], with permission from Elsevier

due to pain. **However, the palpation of a free-floating prostate is almost pathognomonic of complete urethral rupture** but remains a challenging finding taking into account the tenderness and the pelvic hematoma. Nonetheless, it is noteworthy to keep in mind that palpation of a high-riding prostate is always a reliable indicator of an injured urethra, and the posterior urethra might be significantly stretched without disruption, allowing the prostate to be pushed cranially [2, 3].

The presence of any of the traditional signs of urethral injury, namely blood at the urethral meatus, perineal hematoma, and high-riding prostate, has been shown to have a sensitivity of 66.7% in the prediction of urethral injury. The presence of pubic symphysis disruption had a prediction sensitivity as higher as 92.5%, and when considering the presence of a pubic symphysis disruption or any of the above clinical signs, the sensitivity rises to 100% [3] (Table 30.1).

In the pediatric population, there might be a butterfly hematoma (bruising) at the superficial perineum associated with injuries to the urethra distal to the urogenital diaphragm. Scrotal or labial swelling in boys and girls, respectively, are also possible following the collection of extravasated fluids after the rupture of Scarpa's fascia and Dartos fascia in severe pelvic fractures [4].

Unlike the posterior urethral disruptions which are often associated with other organs' trauma of pelvic fractures, blunt anterior urethral trauma is generally isolated or just associated with cavernosal injury. Moreover, this injury might be so mild that the patients neglect it, as they have no immediate symptoms; and the majority of them will seek medical help only when a stricture develops and causes voiding difficulty, after several months or years [5, 6].

30.2 Imaging Investigations

Computed Tomography (CT) is routinely used as a first initial imaging modality in polytrauma patients, but **the best radiological means to diagnose a urethral injury is retrograde urethrography (RUG) either in an acute or chronic setting.** This will demonstrate a normal urethra, extravasation with some contrast entering the bladder (partial rupture), extravasation of all the contrast with the proximal tract not visualized (complete rupture), or a narrow segment (stricture) with or without a complete obstruction of the urethral lumen.

If the management consists of an initial suprapubic catheter insertion and delayed final treatment, a combined RUG and antegrade cystourethrography should be performed to define the length of the urethral gap before undertaking the definitive reconstructive surgery. A flexible ureteroscope can also be introduced through the SPC site to examine the bladder neck and assess its competence for medico-legal purposes as re-establishment of a patent urethral channel might unmask occult incontinence caused by sphincter damage at the time of the trauma [7].

1. *Urethrographic approaches*: Urethrography can be performed through an ascending (retrograde technique), a descending (antegrade technique), or a combination of the two.

   The standard technique includes the following steps [8, 9]:

   (a) *Retrograde or ascending urethrography* (Figs. 30.1a, b and 30.2a–e).
   - Disinfection of the external meatus with the patient in a supine position.
   - Insertion of a 6–8 Fr Foley catheter, or a hysterosalpingographic catheter in the external meatus and inflation of its balloon with 1–2 mL of saline

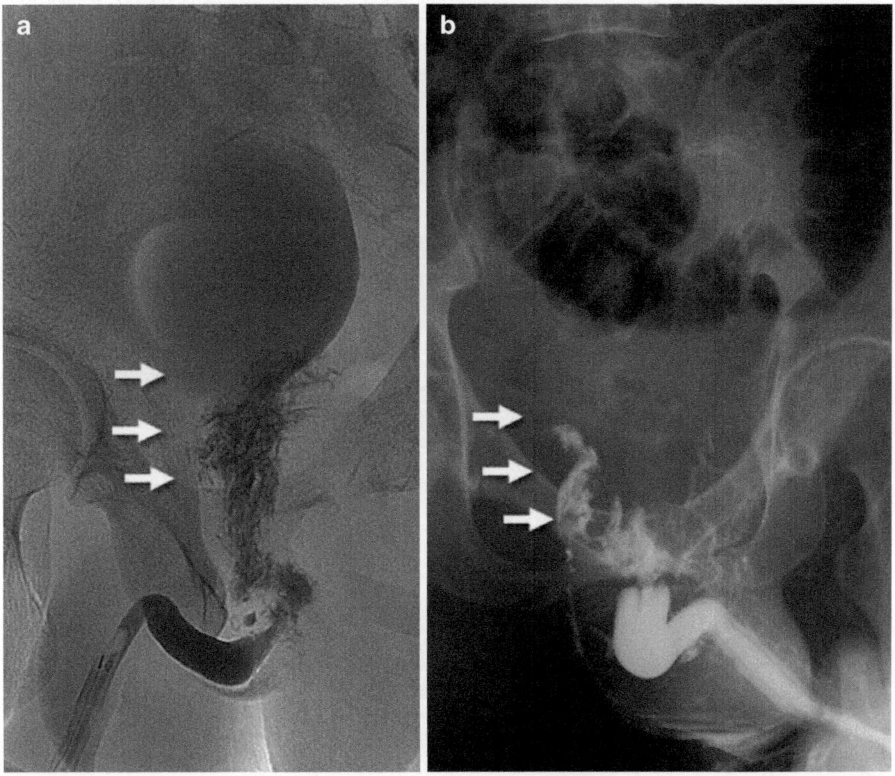

Fig. 30.1 Retrograde urethrography immediately after trauma in (**a**) a patient with partial disruption and (**b**) a patient with complete disruption. Arrows indicate contrast medium extravasated from disrupted sites. (From Horiguchi A [9] with permission John Wiley and Sons)

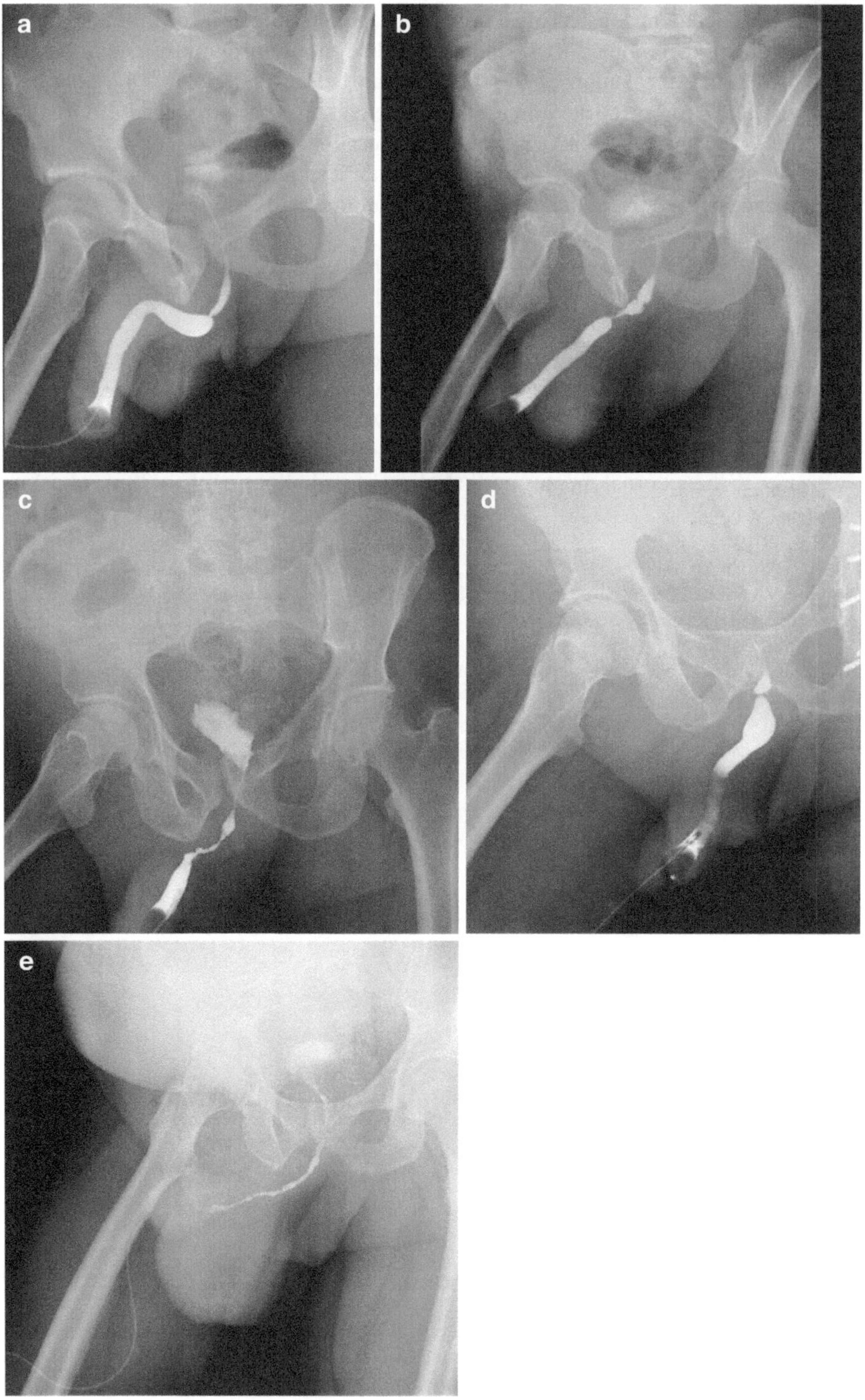
a
b
c
d
e

Fig. 30.2 (**a**–**e**) Delayed retrograde urethrography performed in five different patients: (**a**) Very short bulbar urethra. (**b**) Two bulbar strictures that collectively measure 3 cm long. (**c**) Long bulbar stricture. (**d**) Residual membranous urethral stricture after PFUI in RTA treated initially with pelvic fixation and SPC. (**e**) Panurethral stricture. (Courtesy Ashraf Abdelsalam Al Ozeni, Urology, The Royal Hospital, Muscat, Oman)

solution at the fossa navicularis to prevent reflux and leak of the contrast out the external meatus.

- Rotate the fluoroscopic C-arm 30° left or right anterior oblique position to demonstrate the full urethra.
- Place the penis laterally over the thigh, and slowly inject 20–30 mL of an iodinated contrast agent with fluoroscopic recording. Continue injecting until the contrast material is seen flowing past the external urethral sphincter and entering the bladder. **Continuous pressure is advised to overcome the external sphincter spasm that tends to prevent the filling of the membranous and prostatic urethra**.

Retrograde or ascending urethrography is contraindicated in patients with allergy or hypersensitivity to the contrast medium, urinary infection, and recent urethral instrumentation. Its complications are very rare and include anaphylaxis, urinary tract infection, extravasation, urethro-venous intravasation, and possible sepsis. The urethro-venous intravasation results from a forceful push of contrast against an obstructed urethra resulting in mucosal tear and a contrast escape into the penile venous plexus [10–12] (Fig. 30.3a, b). A case of Fournier's gangrene has been described after retrograde urethrography and extravasation [13].

(b) *Antegrade or descending urethrography* [8].

- Adequately fill the bladder with 350–400 mL of the contrast agent through the SPC.
- Instruct male patients to micturate into a bottle while in an oblique standing position.

The expression **"Pie-in-the-sky bladder"** was first used by Turner-Warwick referring to the radiological image of an upward-pushed bladder on antegrade or retrograde urethrocystography [14–16] (Fig. 30.4). He did mention at the same time that the bladder dislocation is due to the intervening pelvic hematoma and advocated an observation over months to allow shrinking of the hematoma and descent of the bladder neck toward the urethra. With this expectant management, an initial gap of 10–15 cm might reduce to 3–4 cm after 1 year.

Well before Turner-Warwick coined the above expression, Prather and Kaiser invented the expression **"tear-drop bladder"** in 1950, which is a synonym of **"pear-shaped"** bladder deformity [17]. The bladder appears vertically elongated due to extrinsic compression, either as the consequence of a pelvic hematoma or of other entities such as pelvic lipomatosis, inferior vena cava occlusion, lymphoceles, enlarged pelvic lymph nodes [18, 19] (Fig. 30.5).

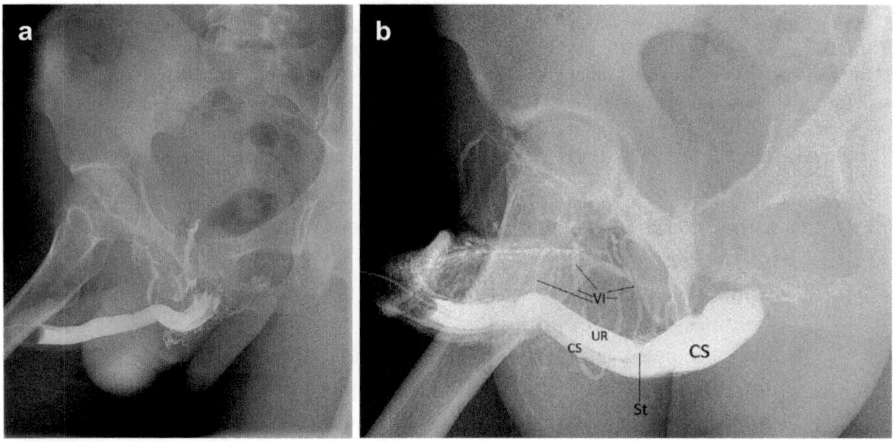

Fig. 30.3 (**a**) Retrograde urethrography in a 37-year-old man showing an obstructing bulbar urethral stricture with contrast intravasation in the corpus spongiosum, periurethral, circumflex, and pelvic (pudendal) venous plexus. (Courtesy Qais Al Hooti, Urology, The Royal Hospital, Muscat, Oman). (**b**) Another retrograde urethrography in a 26-year old man with severe stricture at the bulbar urethra demonstrating extensive intravasation into the corpus spongiosum and periurethral, cicumflex, and pelvis veins. *St* Stricture, *UR* Urethra distal to the stricture, *CS* Corpus spongiosum (superposed with proximal urethra), *VI* Venous intravasations

Combination of an antegrade with a retrograde urethrogram

The combination of a suprapubic antegrade cystourethrography with an ascending urethrogram is sometimes referred to by the funny name "**up-and-downogram.**" It is the investigation of choice in assessing the site, the severity, and the length (gap) of urethral injuries, and should be performed within a week from the time of injury if one considers a delayed primary repair, or at 3 months when a deferred or late repair is contemplated [1] (Fig. 30.6)

(c) *Pericatheter Urethrography*

In patients who have already an indwelling urethral catheter, this should be kept in position as long as the entire urethral integrity is not ascertained. Therefore, one should perform the **pericatheter ascending technique** whereby the contrast is instilled at the external meatus through a small-gauge pediatric catheter (4–6 Fr), or a small-bore (4–6 Fr) feeding tube, or a 20-gauge (1.1 mm) 1-inch (25 mm) long angiocatheter alongside the indwelling catheter [8, 20] (Figs. 30.7, 30.8, and 30.9). Once the bladder is filled with contrast, the **descending pericatheter urethrography** is simply performed by removing the small-gauge catheter, deflating or pushing the indwelling catheter balloon into the dome of the bladder, and asking the patient to void around the indwelling catheter [8, 20].

2. *Sonourethrography*

Ultrasonographic studies are possible by distending the urethra with saline or lubricant jelly and using ultra-high-frequency linear probes along the penile and perineal tract [21]. Sonourethrography showed great accuracy in measuring

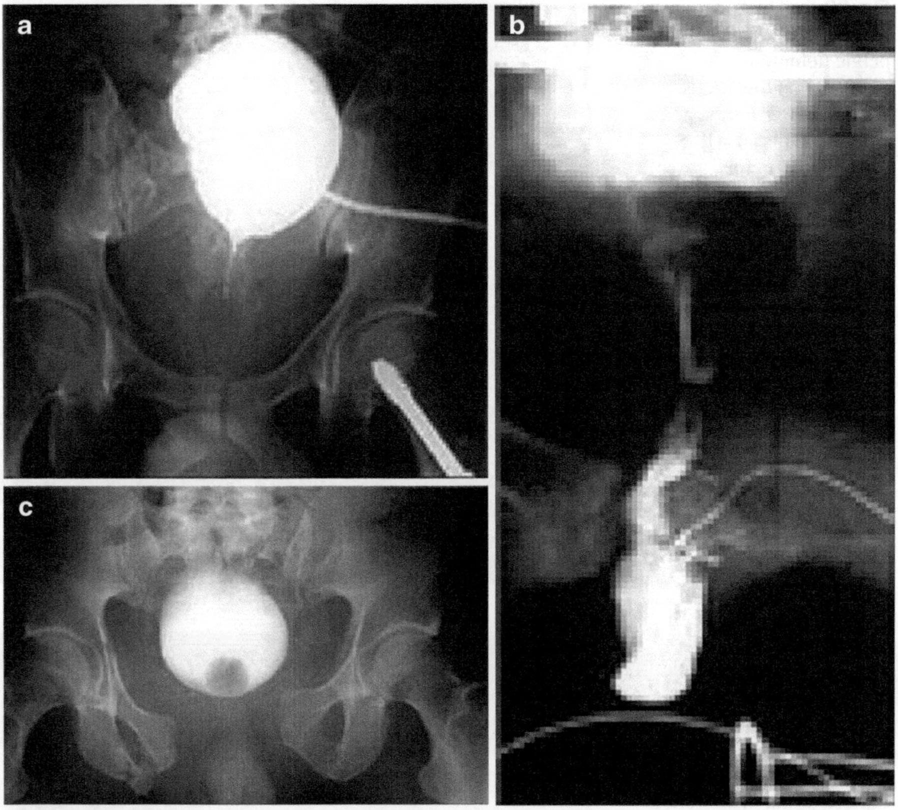

Fig. 30.4 (**a**) Cystography through SPC showing a high-riding or "Pie-in-the-sky" bladder caused by a large hematoma in the Retzius space. (**b**) Stretched supra-membranous urethra, being displaced posteriorly and superiorly and compressed laterally. (**c**) Projectional bladder displacement occurring with displacement of the anterior pelvic ring. (From Andrich DE et al. [15], with permission from John Wiley and Sons)

stricture length in the bulbar urethra, in diagnosing spongiofibrosis (shown as a lack of distensibility during retrograde instillation of saline solution), and also in detecting incidental findings such as calculi, false passage, etc. [22].

3. *Magnetic Resonance Imaging (MRI)*

   MRI can define the urethral gap very accurately and will add additional information about the direction and extent of prostatic displacement, the density of urethral and periurethral fibrosis (spongiofibrosis), the presence of paraurethral false tracks, an eventual avulsion of the corpus cavernosum as a possible cause of impotence for some patients, the presence of periurethral cavity formation, the eventual protrusion of the rectum between the urethral ends, and the presence of periurethral fistula [9, 23, 24] (Fig. 30.10).

Unfortunately, the routine use of MRI is hindered by its cost and unavailability in many rural and regional hospitals.

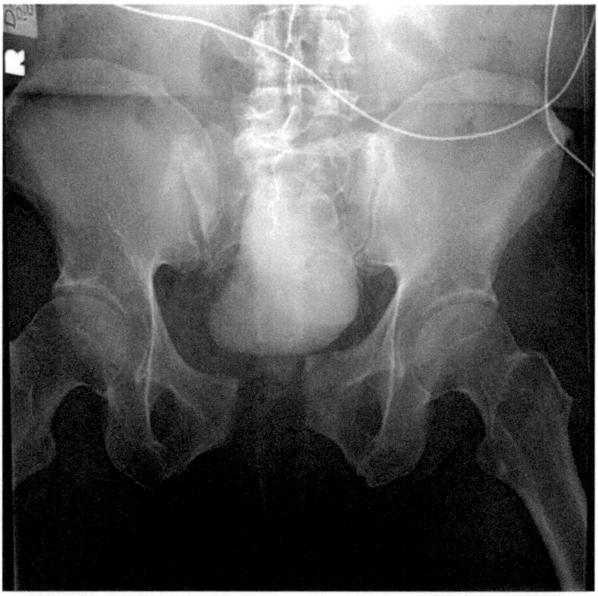

Fig. 30.5 The "pear-shaped" bladder, a result of pelvic hematoma, is opacified on this image obtained after intravenous contrast material administration for computed tomography. Note the diastasis of the symphysis pubis and right sacroiliac joint. (From Triffo W.J et al. [19], with permission from Springer Nature)

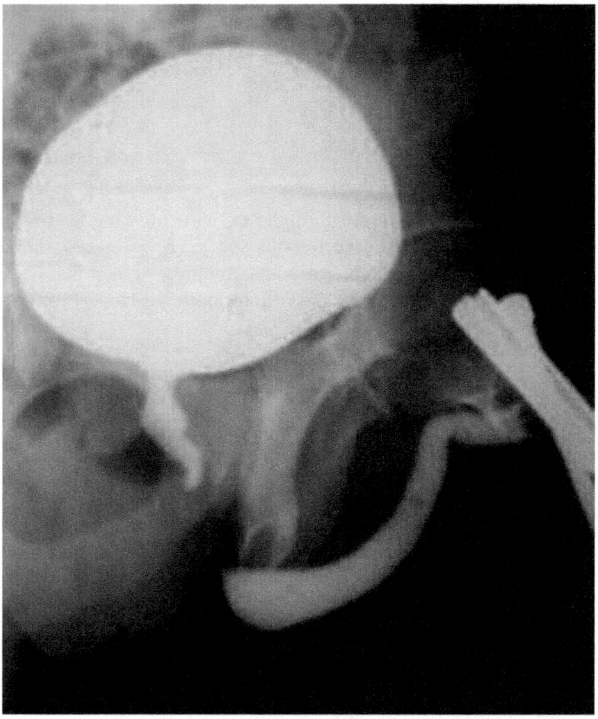

Fig. 30.6 Combined antegrade and retrograde urethrogram ("up-and-downogram") in a post-RTA patient with PFUI showing a complete rupture of the membranous urethra with significant gapping. (Courtesy Kurian George, Retiree from the Urology Department, The Royal Hospital, Muscat, Oman)

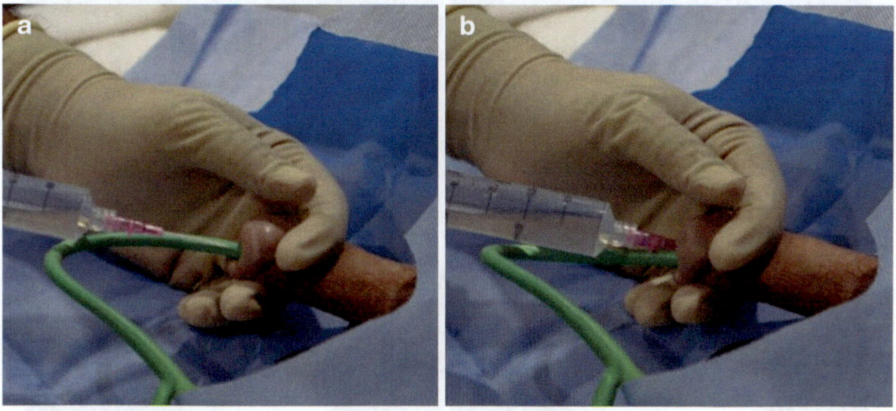

Fig. 30.7 (**a**, **b**) Insertion of angiocatheter alongside Foley catheter for pericatheter retrograde urethrography. (From Sussman RD et al. [20], with permission from Springer Nature)

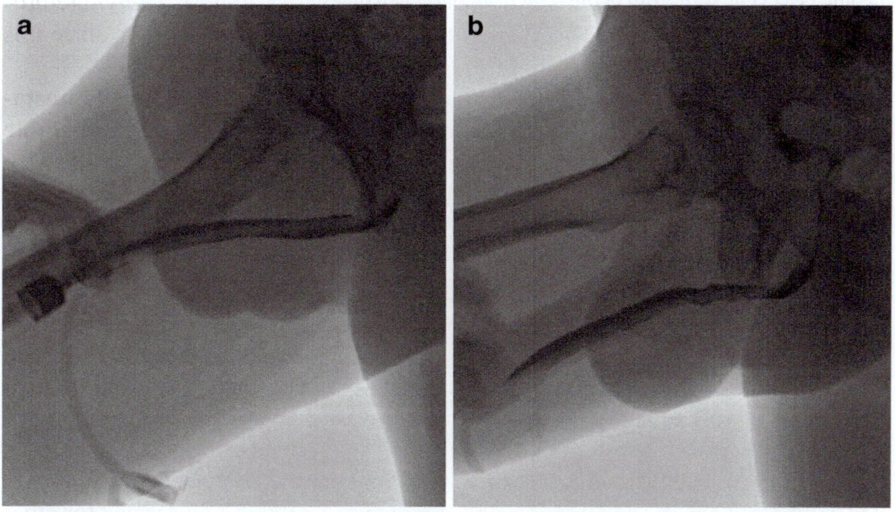

Fig. 30.8 Fluoroscopic results of pericatheter RUG: (**a**) early filling with minimal leakage from urethral meatus, (**b**) late filling with contrast alongside catheter to level of bladder without obvious extravasation. (From Sussman RD et al. [20], with permission from Springer Nature)

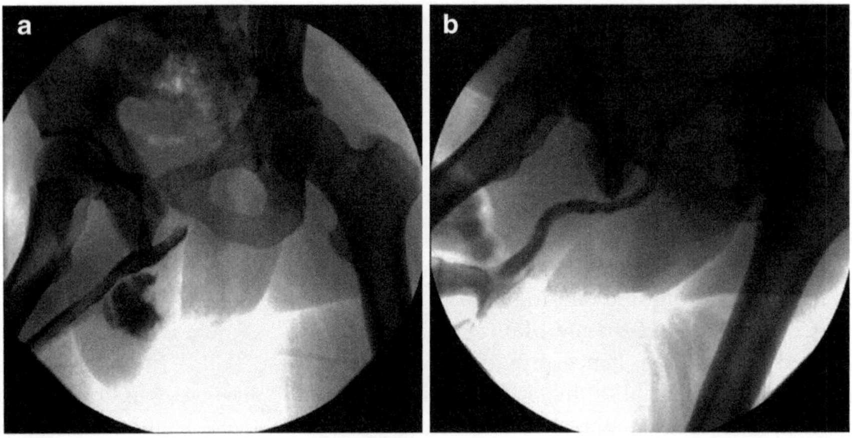

Fig. 30.9 Fluoroscopic results of pericatheter RUG: (**a**) early filling with gross extravasation, (**b**) subsequent image of the same patient after 2 weeks with resolution of extravasation. (From Sussman RD et al. [20], with permission from Springer Nature)

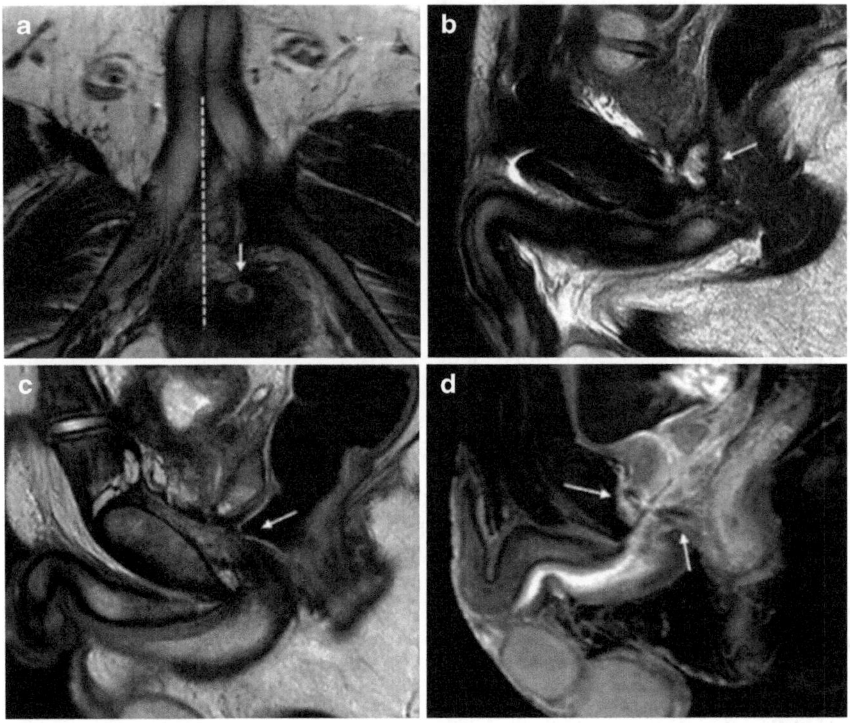

Fig. 30.10 Representative preoperative MRI findings in patients with urethral stenosis after PFUI. (**a**) Lateral displacement of the proximal urethral end (arrow) from the midline (dotted line) in the axial T2-weighted image, (**b**) cavity formation just behind the proximal urethral end (arrow) in the sagittal T2-weighted image, (**c**) bulging of the rectum into the urethral gap (arrow) in the sagittal T2-weighted image. (**d**) Periurethral fistulas (arrow) in contrast-enhanced T1-weighted image. (From Horiguchi A [9], with permission from John Wiley and Sons)

References

1. Chapple C, Barbagli G, Jordan G, Mundy AR, Rodrigues-Netto N, Pansadoro V, McAninch JW. Consensus statement on urethral trauma. BJU Int. 2004;93(9):1195–202. https://doi.org/10.1111/j.1464-410x.2004.04805.x. PMID: 15180604.
2. Koraitim MM. Pelvic fracture urethral injuries: the unresolved controversy. J Urol. 1999;161:1433–41.
3. Lückhoff C, Mitra B, Cameron PA, Fitzgerald M, Royce P. The diagnosis of acute urethral trauma. Injury. 2011;42(9):913–6. https://doi.org/10.1016/j.injury.2010.08.007. Epub 2010 Aug 24. PMID: 20739022.
4. Pichler R, Fritsch H, Skradski V, Horninger W, Schlenck B, Rehder P, Oswald J. Diagnosis and management of pediatric urethral injuries. Urol Int. 2012;89:136–42. https://doi.org/10.1159/000336291.
5. Pierce JM Jr. Disruptions of the anterior urethra. Urol Clin North Am. 1989;16(2):329–34. PMID: 2652858.
6. Park S, McAninch JW. Straddle injuries to the bulbar urethra: management and outcomes in 78 patients. J Urol. 2004;171:722–5.
7. Zaid UB, Bayne DB, Harris CR, et al. Penetrating trauma to the ureter, bladder, and urethra. Curr Trauma Rep. 2015;1:119–24. https://doi.org/10.1007/s40719-015-0015-x.
8. Ingram MD, Watson SG, Skippage PL, Patel U. Urethral injuries after pelvic trauma: evaluation with urethrography. Radiographics. 2008;28(6):1631–43. https://doi.org/10.1148/rg.286085501. PMID: 18936026.
9. Horiguchi A. Management of male pelvic fracture urethral injuries: review and current topics. Int J Urol. 2019;26(6):596–607. https://doi.org/10.1111/iju.13947. Epub 2019 Mar 20. PMID: 30895658.
10. Gupta SK, Kaur B, Shulka RC. Urethro-venous intravasation during retrograde urethrography (report of 5 cases). J Postgrad Med. 1991;37(2):102–4, 104A–104B. PMID: 1802991.
11. Bansal A, Kumar M, Goel S, Aeron R. Urethro-venous intravasation: a rare complication of retrograde urethrogram. BMJ Case Rep. 2016;2016:bcr2016215206. https://doi.org/10.1136/bcr-2016-215206. PMID: 27045054; PMCID: PMC4840624.
12. Sharma S, Agarwal MM, Mete UK. Retrograde urethrogram or a venogram? Be careful next time. Indian J Surg. 2014;76:411–2. https://doi.org/10.1007/s12262-012-0801-4.
13. Kanodia S, Prakash SH, Tejaswi KV, Puthalath RT, Pai N. Fournier's gangrene following retrograde urethrography: a rare complication. Int Surg J. 2020;7(2):567. https://doi.org/10.18203/2349-2902.isj20200044.
14. Turner-Warwick R. Complex traumatic posterior urethral strictures. J Urol. 1977;118(4):564–74. https://doi.org/10.1016/s0022-5347(17)58109-4. PMID: 916051.
15. Andrich DE, Day AC, Mundy AR. Proposed mechanisms of lower urinary tract injury in fractures of the pelvic ring. BJU Int. 2007;100(3):567–73. https://doi.org/10.1111/j.1464-410X.2007.07020.x. Epub 2007 Jul 3. PMID: 17608826.
16. Barratt RC, Bernard J, Mundy AR, Greenwell TJ. Pelvic fracture urethral injury in males-mechanisms of injury, management options and outcomes. Transl Androl Urol. 2018;7(Suppl 1):S29–62. https://doi.org/10.21037/tau.2017.12.35. PMID: 29644168; PMCID: PMC5881191.
17. Prather GC, Kaiser TF. The bladder in fracture of the bony pelvis; the significance of a "tear drop bladder" as shown by cystogram. J Urol. 1950;63(6):1019–30. https://doi.org/10.1016/s0022-5347(17)68860-8. PMID: 15422713.
18. Ambos MA, Bosniak MA, Lefleur RS, Madayag MA. Radiology. 1977;122(1):85–8.
19. Triffo WJ, Dyer RB. The "pear-shaped" bladder. Abdom Imaging. 2015;40:2912–3. https://doi.org/10.1007/s00261-015-0470-4.
20. Sussman RD, Hill FC, Koch GE, et al. Novel pericatheter retrograde urethrogram technique is a viable method for postoperative urethroplasty imaging. Int Urol Nephrol. 2017;49:2157–65. https://doi.org/10.1007/s11255-017-1701-0.

21. Pavlica P, Barozzi L, Menchi I. Imaging of male urethra. Eur Radiol. 2003;13(7):1583–96. https://doi.org/10.1007/s00330-002-1758-7. Epub 2002 Dec 19. PMID: 12835971.
22. Morey AF, McAninch JW. Sonographic staging of anterior urethral strictures. J Urol. 2000;163(4):1070–5. PMID: 10737469.
23. Koraitim MM, Reda IS. Role of magnetic resonance imaging in assessment of posterior urethral distraction defects. Urology. 2007;70(3):403–6. https://doi.org/10.1016/j.urology.2007.04.039. PMID: 17905082.
24. Horiguchi A, Edo H, Shinchi M, Ojima K, Hirano Y, Ito K, Shinmoto H. Role of magnetic resonance imaging in the management of male pelvic fracture urethral injury. Int J Urol. 2022;29:919. https://doi.org/10.1111/iju.14779. Epub ahead of print. PMID: 34986514.

31 Treatment of Urethral Injury. I: The Posterior Urethra

Before embarking on a very long journey in what looks like the Amazonian forest, it is important to clarify the exact meaning of certain concepts used in this chapter. The WHO experts' consensus recommends the following terminology be used with regard to the timing of the surgical intervention: "**immediate treatment**" when the intervention is undertaken within minutes or hours of the injury, "**delayed primary treatment**" when it is performed in 2–14 days, and "**deferred treatment**" for surgery taking place after 3 months or more [1].

The preservation of the integrity of the bladder neck is of paramount importance because urinary continence after posterior urethroplasty mainly depends on the bladder reconstruction and to a lesser extent on the preserved external sphincter which is damaged most of the time [2, 3]. A urodynamic study to assess the sphincteric and detrusor function may be necessary before posterior urethroplasty but will be possible only if there is continuity of the urethral tract. The competence of the bladder neck not only depends on its anatomical and physiological integrity but also on the stability of the detrusor. It is important to remember that the functional length of the bladder neck mechanism extends well beyond its mere anatomical location encompassing the proximal half of the posterior urethra, up to the level of the verumontanum. The bladder neck function is difficult to study in the absence of urethral patency, but one can make out a favorable impression through the cystographic observation of its closure at rest and its opening when the patient tries to void [2]. Herein it was shown that incontinent patients have a significantly greater average bladder neck and prostatic urethral opening on the cystourethrogram compared to continent patients with 1.68 cm and 0.9 cm, respectively [4].

While only a small number of urologists have enough experience to perform reconstructive procedures of the injured urethra, it is important for all to master the principles of its management as this will frequently be encountered in their professional practice. As mentioned in the epidemiology chapter, it should be remembered that in industrialized countries the prevalence of urethral stricture disease of all etiologies in men is estimated to be 900 per 100,000 population (0.9%), and in the

S. A. AL-Mamari, *Urogenital Trauma: A Practical Guide*, https://doi.org/10.1007/978-981-99-6171-9_31

United States alone, approximately 1.2 million patients sought medical care for this pathology between 2007 and 2012, which equals to an annual consultation of 240,000 patients [5].

31.1 Principles of Posterior Urethral Injury Treatment

The key points of a successful repair of an injured urethra, be it posterior or anterior, include control of local infections, correct epithelial apposition, ensuring healthy and well-vascularized urethral ends, and the use of strong but resorbable sutures. For direct anastomosis, both ends should be spatulated and approximated without tension. In addition, for PFUIs, bladder neck competence should be preserved to palliate possible distal sphincter damage [1].

In general, the acute clinical context of patients presenting with pelvic fractures leaves a very narrow window for any direct repair of the urethral injury and all that is required is to ensure urine drainage, generally through a suprapubic catheter, while dealing with other life-threatening organ damages and endeavoring to stabilize the pelvis. Even when the patient is stable and the urologist is offered a chance to operate on these patients, it is important to remember that immediate open repair of posterior urethral injuries is not advisable for low-volume surgeons and institutions as it is hindered by great difficulties in the identification and realignment* of the anatomical planes because of hematoma and edema. These obstacles are associated with an increased incidence of bleeding, immediate failures, and delayed complications such as strictures, incontinence, and impotence. **As a rule of thumb, in the majority of cases, it is advised to defer the repair for 3–6 months and refer the patient to expert surgeons.**

*This is an open realignment and should not be confused with the so-called railroading procedure, which is a closed or endoscopic realignment.

In a review of 538 patients from 19 reported series, Webster et al. compared the results of SPC alone with those of early urethral surgical realignment and revealed significantly favorable outcomes in patients who had an SPC with delayed surgery: For SPC and delayed repair, the rates of impotence and incontinence were 11.6% and 1.7%, respectively, while these rates were 44% and 20%, respectively, for immediate repair, which had also a high rate of strictures (69%) [6]. Nevertheless, the dogma of "nothing other than SPC" has been revisited by Koraitim, who compared the outcome of **SPC (with delayed or deferred repair)** with **primary realignment** and **primary suturing**. He found that **SPC alone** exposed to stricture in almost all the cases (97%), that **primary realignment** decreased the incidence of stricture to 53%, but exposed to a high impotence rate of 36% and that **primary suturing** similarly decreased the incidence of stricture (49%) but has the drawback to expose to an unacceptably high rate of impotence (56%) and incontinence (21%) [7]. This review suggested to consider SPC alone only for incomplete urethral ruptures or complete ruptures with slight distraction, for critically unstable patients, or when there is no sufficient surgical expertise available in the operating team. It results from this study that primary realignment was advised whenever there is a wide separation between the urethral ends, or associated bladder neck or rectal injuries. **Nonetheless, this study remains consistent with the old ones as it strongly disapproved of the primary suturing of the urethra** [7].

Realignment of the injured posterior urethra can be achieved using **railroading techniques,** also referred to as **primary endoscopic realignment (PER).** This closed approach has also been suggested by other investigators in stable patients to be the preferred option as it reduced by over 50% the risk of subsequent stricture urethra inherent to SPC placement and delayed or deferred repair, and yielded an acceptable rate of impotence and incontinence [8]. Despite the primary endoscopic realignment can reduce the risk of developing urethra stenosis, it harbors the risk of aggravating it when performed in poorly selected patients or by inexperienced surgeons, or in centers where facilities for endoscopy/fluoroscopy are lacking [9].

The cost-effectiveness of these procedures has been studied showing that **primary endoscopic realignment (PER)** costs a total average of $11,043 while a **suprapubic tube with elective bulbomembranous urethroplasty** costs $9743, allowing saving $1300 per patient. The same study showed that the cost-effectiveness of primary endoscopic realignment would be better only in the hypothesis of having a success rate of 40% or higher while having at the same time a success rate of SPC with elective bulbomembranous urethroplasty inferior to 78% [10]. When considering the costs for a 2-year period or longer, PER was proved the most cost-effective method being preferred over supra-pubic tube placement. **It was shown that PER followed by a single direct vision internal urethrotomy (DVIU) if needed, then eventually urethroplasty if the first two have failed had the best average cost-effectiveness with the value of $17,493 per unobstructed voider**. Delaying urethroplasty and preferring multiple repeated DVIU after PER greatly increased the costs reaching $86,280 per unobstructed voider after a second DVIU and as high as $172,205 after a third DVIU [11].

It should be understood here that the mere DVIU is not per se that costly, but rather exposes to an increased risk of failure of a subsequent urethroplasty. **This study suggested considering PER as the first-line management of PFUIs. And when PER fails, a single DVIU may be attempted provided the presumed success rate is >32%. Otherwise, urethroplasty should be immediately considered after any PER failure to improve cost-effectiveness.**

This algorithm is supported by a large United Kingdom study which showed the following costs [12]:

- urethrotomy/urethral dilation: 2250 pounds sterling (3375 dollars),
- simple 1-stage urethroplasty: 5015 pounds sterling (7522.50 dollars),
- complex 1-stage urethroplasty: 5335 pounds sterling (8002.50 dollars), and
- two-stage urethroplasty: 10,370 pounds sterling (15,555 dollars).

However, when considering that 47.6% of patients treated by endoscopic measures required a mean of 3.13 times of endoscopic retreatment, while also needing a biweekly clean self-dilatation, the total cost per patient jumped to 6113 pounds sterling (9170 dollars), exceeding the cost of a simple or complex 1-stage urethroplasty. This further supported the strategy of urethrotomy or urethral dilation as first-line treatment, followed directly by urethroplasty for any recurrence, yielding an average total cost per patient of 5866 pounds sterling (8799 dollars) [5, 12].

For female PFUIs (remember: females have no anterior urethra), a systematic review and metanalysis showed that 53% of cases were managed with immediate repair, a minority of whom (20%) underwent primary realignment while the majority (80%) were treated with an anastomotic repair. The remaining 47% were offered a delayed repair [13]. This review showed the highest rates of urethral stenosis and fistula after primary realignment, and despite the urethral integrity appeared to be similar after both primary and delayed anastomosis, the latter approach yielded a significantly higher rate of incontinence and vaginal stenosis, as patients were likely to undergo more extensive reconstructive surgery than those operated primarily. With the reservation of dealing with a very low-quality available literature, **this study concluded that female PFUIs should be managed with a primary anastomotic repair of urethral distraction defect via a vaginal approach in hemodynamically stable patients.**

Flaps have also been successfully used to correct female urethral stricture, either a pedicled flap from the labia minora [14], or pedicled flap from the vaginal vestibule [15], or free graft from the vaginal wall or the buccal mucosa [16].

31.2 Surgical Approaches

Repair of posterior urethral injury is one of the most challenging enterprises of the whole urological surgery due to the "underground" anatomical position and delicacy of the involved structures with extensive surrounding fibrosis, the propensity of bleeding, the risk of failure, the risk of functional complications (urinary incontinence and sexual impotence), either from the injury itself or from the procedure, the risk of lower limbs deep venous thrombosis and neurapraxia due to prolonged exaggerated lithotripsy position.

In a review of 145 cases of PFUI, Koraitim reported the following technical options: optical (internal) urethrotomy in 8%, urethroscrotal inlay in 16%, perineal anastomotic urethroplasty in 54%, and transpubic urethroplasty in 22% of cases [17]. In another review of 121 PFUI patients, the same author found three independent predictive factors to guide the choice of the appropriate surgical approach: **the ratio urethral gap/ bulbar urethral length (the so-called gapometry-urethrometry or G/U index), the urethral gap length, and the prostatic displacement (lateral vs. upward diastasis)** [18]. Based on these factors, a decision can be made to perform either a simple perineal operation or a complex perineal, or a combined perineo-abdominal procedure. A G/U index inferior to 0.35 was associated with a 50 times greater likelihood to undergo correction with a simple perineal operation compared to a G/U index superior to 0.35. A urethral gap inferior to 2.5 cm was associated with a simple approach. However, this factor was not always a reliable predictor. A lateral displacement of the prostate, despite generally limited to several mm only, was invariably associated with dense adhesions and fixation of the prostate in the abnormal position, calling for a tedious retropubic dissection and the need for omental wrapping through a peritoneo-abdominal transpubic approach. These findings were endorsed by the joint **"Société Internationale d'Urologie—International Consultation on Urological Diseases" (SIU-ICUD)** in their recommendations [19]. **Children are more likely to undergo more complex procedures than adults** because they have almost equal urethral gaps while having significantly shorter bulbar urethral length than adults, resulting therefore in a higher G/U index [20].

31.3 Direct Vision Internal Urethrotomy (DVIU) or Optical Urethrotomy

This is the simplest initial technique in cases of partial injury of the urethra and preservation of the continuity, where there is dense short fibrosis uniting the two ends and a persistent opening in the lumen. This procedure is performed using a cold knife and incising the stricture at 12 o'clock and an antegrade suprapubic approach can be necessary to complete it. The success rate in well-selected patients varies from 58 to 92% after a 3-year follow-up, with a 10-month median time to recurrence [17, 21].

Urethrotomy performed for urethral trauma generally has only short-term results and should be combined with intermittent self-dilatation; therefore, its role remains very limited as a definitive treatment [1]. Moreover, it should be borne in mind that when this procedure is repeated, not only does its failure rate increase but also the fibrotic segment becomes longer complicating further definitive treatment (urethroplasty) [9].

31.4 Urethroscrotal Inlay Procedure

This technique yields a high failure rate reaching 57% in one series [17]. It involves the use of substitution tissues (scrotal skin grafts) to cover the fibrotic urethral segment without completely removing it, and may prove very useful in patients with excessively long gaps [9].

31.5 Excision of the Fibrotic Segment and End-to-End Reanastomosis

Before developing this topic, let us remember the advice of R. Turner-Warwick which is more valid than ever 45 years later: ***"Posterior urethroplasty should be regarded as a specialist procedure. It can be made to appear beguilingly simple but it cannot be recommended for occasional or general use"*** [2]. This is particularly true in low-volume centers or in low and middle-income countries where an international partnership is highly recommended to improve the outcome [22].

Table 31.1 Postoperative results in 145 posterior urethral strictures

	Number (%)		
	Successful	Failure	Totals
Optical urethrotomy	7 (58)	5 (42)	12
Urethroscrotal inlay	10 (43)	13 (57)	23
Perineal anastomosis	74 (95)	4 (5)	78
Transpubic anastomosis	31 (97)	1 (3)	32

From Koraitim MM [17], with permission from Wolters Kluwer Health

Only after heeding this caveat can we safely state that **excision-anastomosis is the gold standard of posterior urethral rupture with distraction**, accomplishing a success rate ranging between 90 and 98% either with the perineal or with the transpubic approach [17, 23, 24] (Table 31.1).

The technique of posterior urethral reconstruction in PFUIs was pioneered by Turner-Warwick who preconized **three key principles** to ensure a successful outcome of the repair: **complete excision of scarred tissues, lateral fixation of healthy mucosa of the two urethral ends, and creation of a tension-free anastomosis** [2, 9]. This approach was validated, reemphasized, and developed by subsequent surgeons and investigators [23–25]. However, Mundy and Andrich proposed to use the term **bulbomembranous anastomosis (BMA)** rather than **bulboprostatic anastomosis (BPA)** because, contrary to the old belief, the injury is not a prostatic avulsion from the membranous urethra, but is rather located at the bulbomembranous junction in most of the patients [26].

The techniques described below as well as the ancillary steps to help approximate the ureteral ends cannot be reliably predicted by pre-operative imaging, and the decision to opt for one or another is mainly taken during the procedure once the surgeon faces the "battlefield" reality [18, 27].

The procedure starts with the patient in a normal or exaggerated lithotomy position, disinfected, and draped. The surgical steps are [2, 9, 23, 24, 27–30]:

31.5.1 Perineal Approach

(a) Midline or curved perineal incision of the skin and the bulbospongiosus muscles.
(b) Circumferential mobilization of the bulbar urethra from the penoscrotal junction proximally to the disrupted area distally. This step aims to use the elasticity of the healthy bulbar urethra and stretch it and is considered as the first ancillary technique to overcome the gap*.
(c) Detachment of the bulbar urethra from the perineal body and transection of the strictured segment below the gap. The introduction of the non-dominant index finger in the rectum might help guide this step [29]. This dissection generally

sacrifices the bulbar arteries with the risk of compromising the spongiosal blood flow and healing of the anastomotic area. Herein a novel bulbar artery-sparing technique has been proposed with excellent initial results in a small series [31].

(d) Incision of the apex of the prostate over a sound (such as the Van Buren's or the Béniqué's sound) antegradely pushed through the suprapubic tract and the bladder neck indicating the site of the proximal urethral end*.
(e) Retrograde piecemeal resection of the sclerosed prostatic apex up to a healthy mucosa.
(f) Spatulation of the two urethral ends and lateral mucosa fixation using 4–6 sutures of 4/0 resorbable material (PDS).
(g) Distal mobilization of the bulbar urethra from the perineal membrane up to the penoscrotal junction.
(h) Insertion of a Foley's catheter (8–12 Fr for children, 14–16 Fr for adults).
(i) Tension-free end-to-end mucosa-to-mucosa bulboprostatic anastomosis performed with 6–8 sutures of 4/0 resorbable material (PDS, Vicryl) over the Foley's catheter.
(j) Fixation of the bulbar urethra to the perineal fascia with resorbable materials to further release the tension.
(k) Closure of the bulbospongiosus muscles over the bulbar urethra by resorbable materials.
(l) Leaving a drain for 2–3 days.
(m) Keeping the suprapubic catheter as a safety urinary drainage until removal of the urethral catheter after 2–4 weeks and ascertaining the patency of the urethra. SPC shall then be clamped for 1–2 days and removed if the patient passes urine comfortably.

* There are **four ancillary steps** used to approximate the ureteral ends. These steps were first described by Webster and Ramon as **transperineal progression approach**, with the idea to stop at the step which allows satisfactory results [9, 23, 28].

First step: bulbar urethra circumferential mobilization (see above).

After this step, there are three other ancillary techniques used to overcome difficult scenarios where the proximal urethral end cannot be found despite the use of a sound, or an anastomotic tension is expected due to a very long urethral gap:

Second step: corporal splitting at the level of the triangular ligament and lateral retraction to develop the intercrural space.

Third step: partial (wedge) resection of the inferior pubic arch.

Fourth step: rerouting the urethra around one penile crus.

A simple perineal approach is defined by the use of the first two steps alone, while an elaborated perineal approach includes steps 3 and 4 (Fig. 31.1).

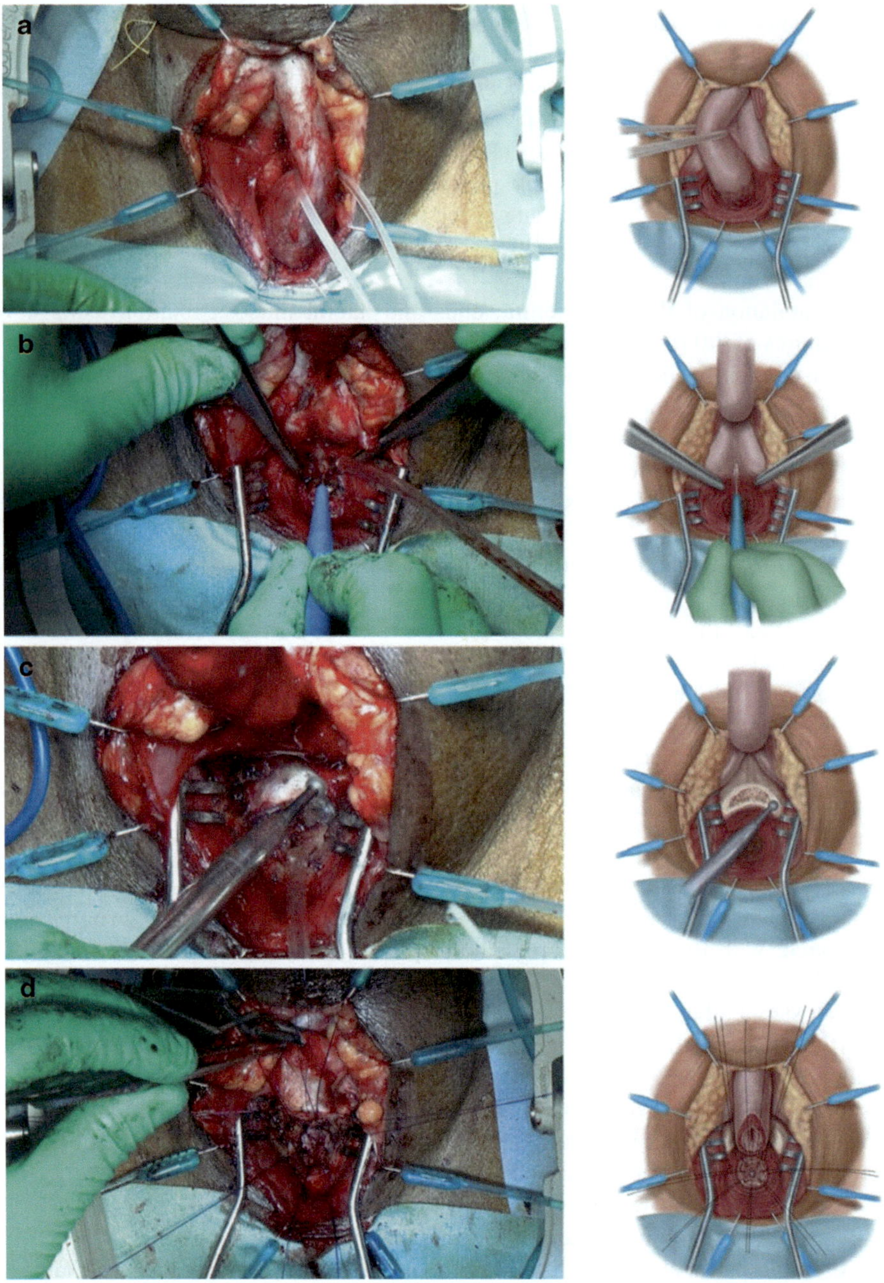

Fig. 31.1 Images and scheme of operative procedures of delayed urethroplasty. (**a**) The bulbar urethra is circumferentially mobilized from the penoscrotal junction distally and proximally. (**b**) Corporal bodies are split and (**c**) the inferior pubis is resected in steps if the proximal urethral end cannot be found or urethral tension is observed. (**d**) After complete removal of the covering fibrotic scar, eight interrupted anastomotic sutures are placed to reapproximate the urethral mucosa. (From Horiguchi A [9], with permission from John Wiley and Sons)

31.5.2 Abdomino-perineal or Perineo-transpubic Approach

This approach is seldom needed but is necessary when adequate access to the proximal urethral end cannot be achieved despite the use of all the above four ancillary steps. Statistically, this extreme scenario is mostly encountered in children, in re-do cases after initial perineal urethroplasties, in complex cases associated with recto-urethral fistula, false passage, etc. [9, 24, 29, 30] (Figs. 31.2 and 31.3).

The steps are:

(a) Extended sub-umbilical midline incision up to the root of the penis below the symphysis pubis
(b) Dissection of the retropubic space
(c) Exposure of the posterior and lower surface of the symphysis as well as the prostatic apex
(d) Disconnection of the attachments of the rectus abdominis muscles from the outer surface of the pubis using a periosteal elevator
(e) Removal of a wedge-shaped piece of bone from the superior surface of the pubis using an osteotome
(f) Exposure and dissection of the prostate from the extensive scar tissue

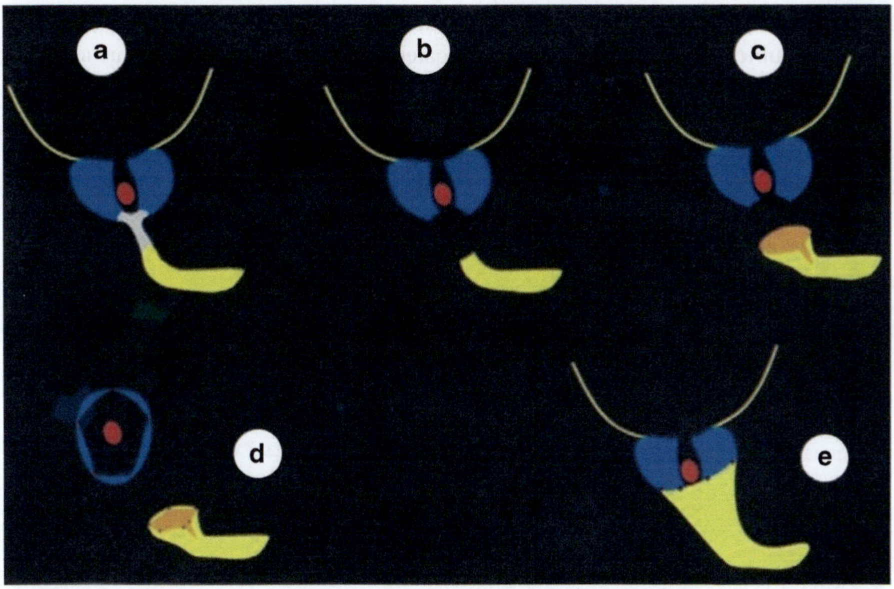

Fig. 31.2 Anastomotic posterior urethroplasty. (**a**) Bulbar urethra (yellow) and strictured segment (grey) are dissected in continuity to the apex of the prostate (blue); (**b**) complete excision of scarred tissue including prostatic apex to a level just short of verumontanum (red); (**c**) spatulation of two urethral ends. (**d**) Fixation of the mucosa of the bulbar and prostatic urethral ends; (**e**) wide-caliber bulboprostatic anastomosis. (From Koraitim MM [24], with permission from Wolters Kluwer Health)

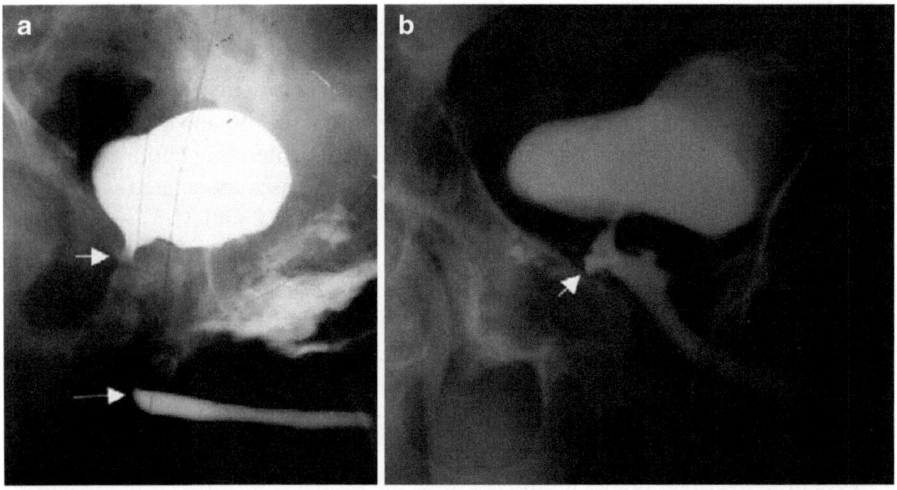

Fig. 31.3 (**a**) Combined antegrade and retrograde urethrogram shows a long gap between two distracted ends of the prostatic (short arrow) and bulbar (long arrow) urethra. Transpubic urethroplasty was performed on April 30, 1985. (**b**) Retrograde urethrogram of the same patient on March 16, 2002. Note the shorter course of the anterior urethra to the prostate and wide bulboprostatic anastomosis (arrow). (From Koraitim MM [24], with permission from Wolters Kluwer Health)

(g) Re-routing the mobilized urethra around the left penile crus to take a shorter transpubic path to the upwardly dislocated prostate.
(h) Anastomosing the urethra to the prostate and wrapping the site by an omental pedicle
(i) Insertion of a suprapubic catheter and closure of the abdomen after leaving a drain in the Retzius space

During an abdominal approach, a posterior pubectomy might be required, especially in children [29] (Fig. 31.4).

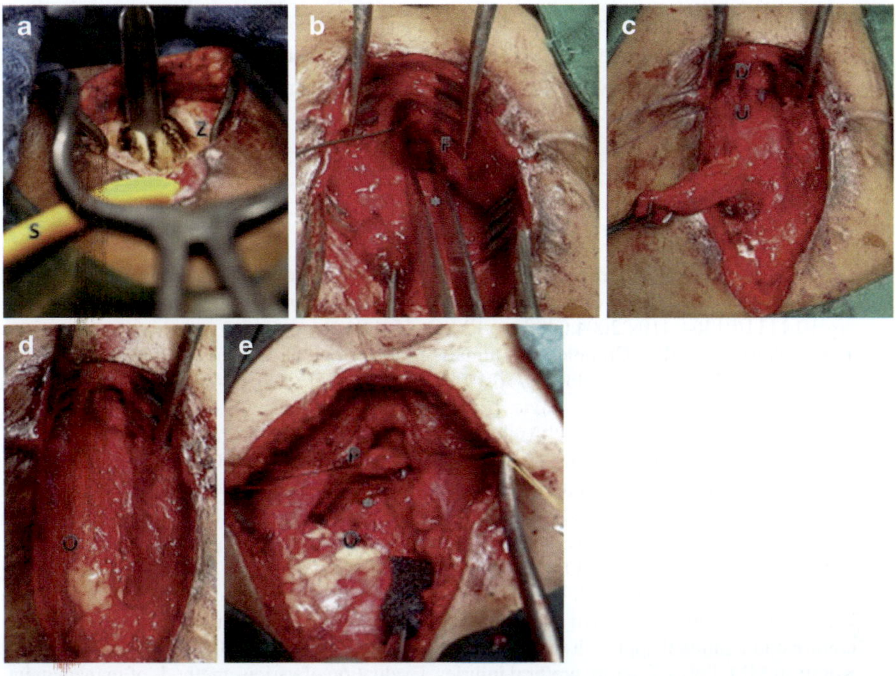

Fig. 31.4 (**a**) A transabdominal view of a posterior pubectomy (Z, posterior pubic bone; S, the suprapubic catheter). (**b**) A transabdominal view of forceps highlighting the UVF (F) (∗, bladder). (**c**) The anastomosis of the proximal (U) and distal urethra (**d**), showing a Babcock clamp on the suprapubic tract. (**d**) The omental wrap (O) interposition. (**e**) The transpubic approach in a young boy (∗ bladder, *O* omentum, *P* prostate). (From Kulkarni SB et al. [29], with permission from the Arab Association of Urology (AAU) and Taylor & Francis Group)

31.6 Urethral Stenting

Stents are contraindicated in PFUI patients with stenosis as they yield the highest risk of failure and stenosis aggravation [1, 9].

31.7 Results of Posterior Urethra Repair

In a recent study from a high-volume center in India, Kulkarni et al. reported on a series of 308 PFUIs, including 126 with earlier multiple failed surgeries [29]. **They found that the most frequent causes of initial failure were insufficient mobilization of the bulbar urethra, followed by inadequate excision of the scar and the non-performance of inferior pubectomy** which was required in >60% of patients in their series, a greater rate than that from western series, probably due to anthropometric differences. They also found that young boys aged ≤12 years were more likely to require a perineal abdominal approach with posterior pubectomy than the adult population with occurrences of 31% and 9%, respectively, confirming Koraitim's predictions based on G/U index (see reference [20]). Overall, the success rates of Kulkarni's series were 81% and 77% for primary and repeat cases, respectively [29].

References

1. Chapple C, Barbagli G, Jordan G, Mundy AR, Rodrigues-Netto N, Pansadoro V, McAninch JW. Consensus statement on urethral trauma. BJU Int. 2004;93(9):1195–202. https://doi.org/10.1111/j.1464-410x.2004.04805.x. PMID: 15180604.
2. Turner-Warwick R. Complex traumatic posterior urethral strictures. J Urol. 1977;118(4):564–74. https://doi.org/10.1016/s0022-5347(17)58109-4. PMID: 916051.
3. Elbakry A. Classification of pelvic fracture urethral injuries: is there an effect on the type of delayed urethroplasty? Arab J Urol. 2011;9(3):191–5. https://doi.org/10.1016/j.aju.2011.06.001. Epub 2011 Aug 15. PMID: 26579295; PMCID: PMC4150576.
4. Iselin CE, Webster GD. The significance of the open bladder neck associated with pelvic fracture urethral distraction defects. J Urol. 1999;162(2):347–51. PMID: 10411036.
5. Osterberg EC, Murphy G, Harris CR, Breyer BN. Cost-effective strategies for the management and treatment of urethral stricture disease. Urol Clin North Am. 2017;44(1):11–7. https://doi.org/10.1016/j.ucl.2016.08.002. PMID: 27908365.
6. Webster GD, Mathes GL, Selli C. Prostatomembranous urethral injuries. A review of the literature and a rational approach to their management. J Urol. 1983;130:898–902.
7. Koraitim MM. Pelvic fracture urethral injuries. Evaluation of various methods of management. J Urol. 1996;156:1288–91.
8. Shrinivas RP, Dubey D. Primary urethral realignment should be the preferred option for the initial management of posterior urethral injuries. Indian J Urol. 2010;26(2):310–3. https://doi.org/10.4103/0970-1591.65416. PMID: 20877620; PMCID: PMC2938566.
9. Horiguchi A. Management of male pelvic fracture urethral injuries: review and current topics. Int J Urol. 2019;26(6):596–607. https://doi.org/10.1111/iju.13947. Epub 2019 Mar 20. PMID: 30895658.
10. Tausch TJ, Lotan Y, Zhao L, Morey AF. Decision analysis model comparing cost of management strategies for pelvic fracture urethral injuries. Urol Pract. 2016;4:285. https://doi.org/10.1016/j.urpr.2016.07.004.
11. Johnsen NV, Penson DF, Reynolds WS, Milam DF, Dmochowski RR, Kaufman MR. Cost-effective management of pelvic fracture urethral injuries. World J Urol. 2017;35(10):1617–23. https://doi.org/10.1007/s00345-017-2022-8. Epub 2017 Feb 22. PMID: 28229209.
12. Greenwell TJ, Castle C, Andrich DE, MacDonald JT, Nicol DL, Mundy AR. Repeat urethrotomy and dilation for the treatment of urethral stricture are neither clinically effective nor cost-effective. J Urol. 2004;172(1):275–7. https://doi.org/10.1097/01.ju.0000132156.76403.8f. PMID: 15201793.
13. Patel DN, Fok CS, Webster GD, Anger JT. Female urethral injuries associated with pelvic fracture: a systematic review of the literature. BJU Int. 2017;120(6):766–73. https://doi.org/10.1111/bju.13989. Epub 2017 Sep 7. PMID: 28805298.
14. Tanello M, Frego E, Simeone C, Cosciani CS. Use of pedicle flap from the labia minora for the repair of female urethral strictures. Urol Int. 2002;69(2):95–8. https://doi.org/10.1159/000065554. PMID: 12187036.
15. Montorsi F, Salonia A, Centemero A, Guazzoni G, Nava L, Da Pozzo LF, Cestari A, Colombo R, Barbagli G, Rigatti P. Vestibular flap urethroplasty for strictures of the female urethra. Impact on symptoms and flow patterns. Urol Int. 2002;69(1):12–6. https://doi.org/10.1159/000064353. PMID: 12119432.

16. Tsivian A, Sidi AA. Dorsal graft urethroplasty for female urethral stricture. J Urol. 2006;176(2):611–3; discussion 613. PMID: 16813901. https://doi.org/10.1016/j.juro.2006.03.055.
17. Koraitim MM. The lessons of 145 posttraumatic posterior urethral strictures treated in 17 years. J Urol. 1995;153(1):63–6. https://doi.org/10.1097/00005392-199501000-00024. PMID: 7966793.
18. Koraitim MM. Predictors of surgical approach to repair pelvic fracture urethral distraction defects. J Urol. 2009;182:1435–9.
19. Gómez RG, Mundy T, Dubey D, El-Kassaby AW, Firdaoessaleh KR, Santucci R. SIU/ICUD consultation on urethral strictures: pelvic fracture urethral injuries. Urology. 2014;83(3 Suppl):S48–58. https://doi.org/10.1016/j.urology.2013.09.023. Epub 2013 Nov 8. PMID: 24210734.
20. Koraitim MM. Gapometry and anterior urethrometry in the repair of posterior urethral defects. J Urol. 2008;179:1879–81.
21. Al Taweel W, Seyam R. Visual internal urethrotomy for adult male urethral stricture has poor long-term results. Adv Urol. 2015;2015:656459. https://doi.org/10.1155/2015/656459. Epub 2015 Oct 1. PMID: 26494995; PMCID: PMC4606400.
22. Haider M, Jalloh M, Yin J, Diallo A, Puttkammer N, Gueye S, Niang L, Wessells H, McCammon K. The role of international partnerships in improving urethral reconstruction in low- and middle-income countries. World J Urol. 2020;38(12):3003–11. https://doi.org/10.1007/s00345-019-02819-2. Epub 2019 Jun 8. PMID: 31177304; PMCID: PMC7716901.
23. Webster GD, Ramon J. Repair of pelvic fracture posterior urethral defects using an elaborated perineal approach: experience with 74 cases. J Urol. 1991;145(4):744–8. https://doi.org/10.1016/s0022-5347(17)38442-2. PMID: 2005693.
24. Koraitim MM. On the art of anastomotic posterior urethroplasty: a 27-year experience. J Urol. 2005;173(1):135–9. https://doi.org/10.1097/01.ju.0000146683.31101.ff. PMID: 15592055.
25. Koraitim MM. Failed posterior urethroplasty: lessons learned. Urology. 2003;62(4):719–22. https://doi.org/10.1016/s0090-4295(03)00573-9. PMID: 14550450.
26. Mundy AR, Andrich DE. Urethral trauma. Part II: types of injury and their management. BJU Int. 2011;108(5):630–50. https://doi.org/10.1111/j.1464-410X.2011.10340.x. PMID: 21854524.
27. Andrich DE, O'Malley KJ, Summerton DJ, Greenwell TJ, Mundy AR. The type of urethroplasty for a pelvic fracture urethral distraction defect cannot be predicted preoperatively. J Urol. 2003;170:464–7.
28. Barratt RC, Bernard J, Mundy AR, Greenwell TJ. Pelvic fracture urethral injury in males-mechanisms of injury, management options and outcomes. Transl Androl Urol. 2018;7(Suppl 1):S29–62. https://doi.org/10.21037/tau.2017.12.35. PMID: 29644168; PMCID: PMC5881191.
29. Kulkarni SB, Joshi PM, Hunter C, Surana S, Shahrour W, Alhajeri F. Complex posterior urethral injury. Arab J Urol. 2015;13(1):43–52. https://doi.org/10.1016/j.aju.2014.11.008. Epub 2015 Jan 20. PMID: 26019978; PMCID: PMC4435922.
30. Kulkarni SB, Surana S, Desai DJ, Orabi H, Iyer S, Kulkarni J, Dumawat A, Joshi PM. Management of complex and redo cases of pelvic fracture urethral injuries. Asian J Urol. 2018;5(2):107–17. https://doi.org/10.1016/j.ajur.2018.02.005. Epub 2018 Mar 2. PMID: 29736373; PMCID: PMC5934510.
31. Gomez RG, Campos RA, Velarde LG. Reconstruction of pelvic fracture urethral injuries with sparing of the bulbar arteries. Urology. 2016;88:207–12. https://doi.org/10.1016/j.urology.2015.09.032. Epub 2015 Nov 23. PMID: 26616094.

32 Treatment of Urethral Injury. II: The Anterior Urethra

32.1 Principles of Anterior Urethra Repair

Alike the posterior urethral injury, SPC and delayed repair is preconized for anterior injury with severe contusion and hematoma. The rationale is to allow an incomplete injury to heal, then to assess the residual stricture after 3 months with combined antegrade and retrograde urethrography [1]. However, a greater room exists here for immediate urethral repair when several conditions are present, namely a complete, anterior, penetrating, or open injury, a stable patient, a minimal hematoma, an experienced surgeon, and non-involvement of other organs [1].

If the urethral disruption is found to be too extensive during an attempt for primary anastomosis, the surgeon should avoid any obstinacy and humbly proceed to a mere debridement with marsupialization of the urethra to prepare for a delayed final repair that should be planned after a period not lesser than 3 months [1].

Contrary to the posterior urethral stricture where the result depends on complete excision of the fibrotic area with end-to-end anastomosis of the urethral healthy ends while grafts are rarely used, the anterior urethroplasty often implies the use of autologous grafts for long gaps with no need for complete excision of the strictured area, while fibrous tissue excision with end-to-end anastomosis remains a valid approach for short strictures (<2 cm).

32.2 The Surgical Techniques

32.2.1 Direct Vision Internal Urethrotomy (DVIU)

The cost-effectiveness was assessed for the management of short anterior urethral strictures (precisely 2-cm bulbar urethral strictures) by a model that included the risks of a direct vision internal urethrotomy (DVIU), namely bleeding, urinary tract infection, and the possibility of recurrence, on the one hand, and the drawbacks of a

S. A. AL-Mamari, *Urogenital Trauma: A Practical Guide*,
https://doi.org/10.1007/978-981-99-6171-9_32

primary urethral reconstruction, namely wound infections or delayed healing, the eventual complications of exaggerated lithotomy position, and the possibility of treatment failure, on the other hand. This model demonstrated a greater average total cost per patient treated with DVIU compared with immediate open urethral reconstruction, with values of $17,747 and $16,444, respectively. It predicted a favorable cost for DVIU only if the long-term risk of stricture recurrence was less than 60% [2].

32.3 Excision and End-to-End Anastomosis

A US study including approximately 3700 men who underwent urethroplasty over a 10-year period (2000–2010) showed that **excision with primary anastomosis (EPA)**, the use of buccal graft, and the use of other graft or flap urethroplasty was performed in 80.3%, 14.3%, and 5.4% of the procedures, respectively. However only 1.6% of hospitals had a volume of 20 urethroplasties or greater per year, and the popularity of buccal mucosa graft procedures was noticed to increase over time, reflecting the universal trend [3].

What is the best management of a short bulbar urethral stricture defined as ≤2 cm long: resection of the fibrotic tissue with end-to-end anastomosis or buccal mucosa graft?

Despite the tremendous efforts of the pioneers to propose the best approach to ≤2 cm bulbar urethral stricture repair, there are still controversies, especially regarding the impact of urethral transection on the degree of erectile dysfunction and penile complications. This subject was recently explored by a Scandinavian multicentric randomized study that showed an **increased rate of penile complications (reduced glans filling and a shortened penis) after transection than after buccal mucosa graft**, but none of the techniques exposed to an increased rate of erectile dysfunction (IIEF-5 score). This study also revealed a similar recurrence rate in both groups (12.9%) [4].

32.4 Non-transecting Bulbar Urethroplasty

In view of the concerns related to the urethral stricture excision and primary anastomosis (EPA), namely the fear of erectile dysfunction, a non-transecting anastomotic technique was proposed for short strictures (<2 cm) with the aim to preserve a well-vascularized underlying spongiosum [5].

32.5 Urethroplasty with Autologous Graft

In a thorough review, Barbagli et al. have raised many controversies in almost all the steps of the reconstructive surgery of the anterior urethra, namely the nature of the substitute material or flap (buccal mucosa vs penile skin), the technique itself (grafting versus flapping, grafting vs end-to-end anastomosis), the variant (dorsal vs ventral), the approach of complex injuries (definitive perineal urethrostomy vs one-stage repair), etc. [6]. A historical review and summary of the most popular techniques are proposed in the following paragraphs.

Many tissues have been used in the past for urethral grafting, including **scrotal or preputial skin**. The **bladder mucosa** was also successfully used for this purpose but its drawback is the necessity for a Pfannenstiel incision and a cystotomy for graft harvesting [7]. The preputial flap is contra-indicated in balanitis xerotica obliterans and lichen sclerosus. **Nowadays the use of buccal mucosa has supplanted all other grafts** [3, 8].

The use of **buccal mucosa graft (BMG)** was first introduced in Ophthalmology by the Austrian Stellwag von Carion in 1873 to cover conjunctival defects [9]. Sapezhko from Kyiv is credited with the first use of BMG for urethral defects in 1894 [10], well before the English Humby described the same in 1941 [11]. The popularity of this technique started in the 1990s [12, 13].

32.5.1 Buccal Mucosa Harvesting

The buccal mucosa length is proportionate to the length of the stricture and may be as short as 3 cm or as long as 17 cm. To obtain such a long graft, the team may need to harvest two or three different segments (right inner cheek, left inner cheek, inner lower labial mucosa and even lingual mucosa) [13–16] (Figs. 32.1, 32.2, 32.3, 32.4, and 32.5). One of the best mouth retractors to provide a good exposure is the **Kilner-Doughty mouth gag**.

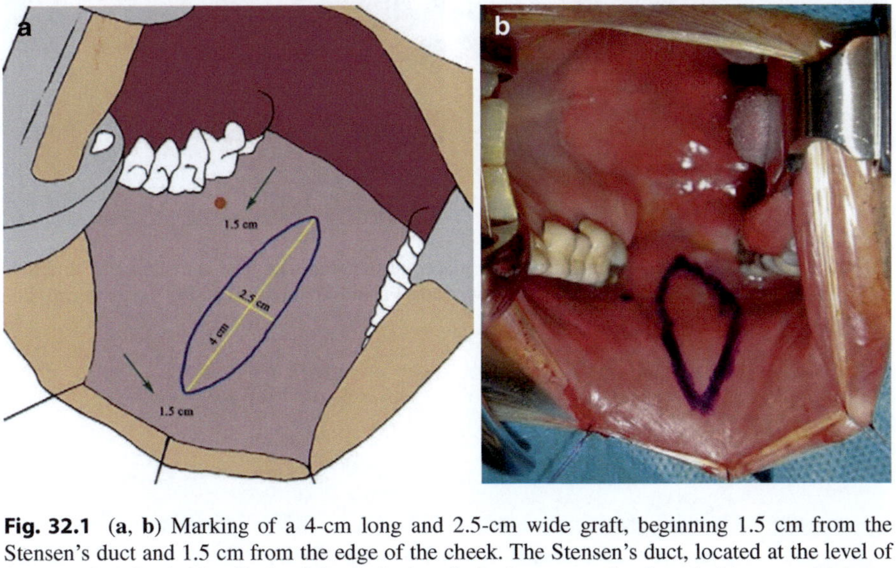

Fig. 32.1 (**a**, **b**) Marking of a 4-cm long and 2.5-cm wide graft, beginning 1.5 cm from the Stensen's duct and 1.5 cm from the edge of the cheek. The Stensen's duct, located at the level of the second molar, is identified and the desired graft size is measured and marked in an ovoid shape. (From Barbagli G et al. [15], with permission from Elsevier)

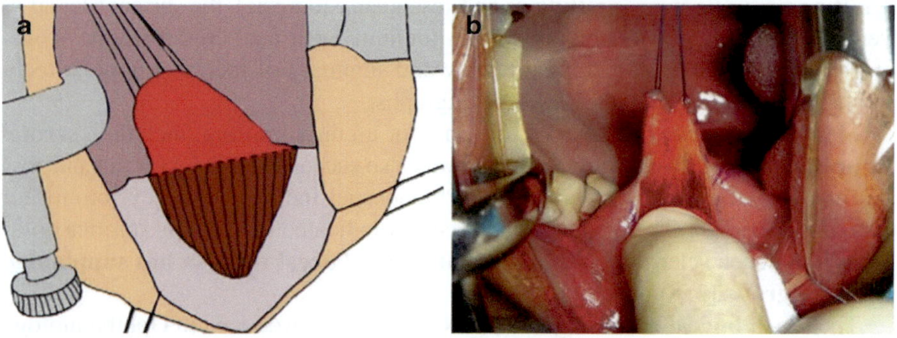

Fig. 32.2 (**a**, **b**) The graft is lifted and removed, leaving the muscular fibers intact. (From Barbagli G et al. [15], with permission from Elsevier)

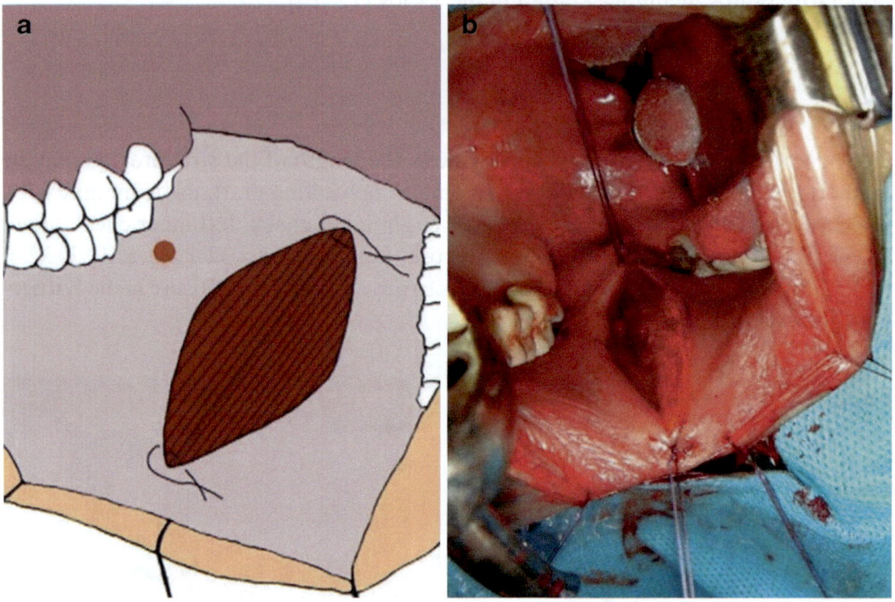

Fig. 32.3 (**a**, **b**) Optionally, two stitches are placed at the apices of the harvesting site, and then pulled, remarkably reducing the width of the wound. (From Barbagli G et al. [15], with permission from Elsevier)

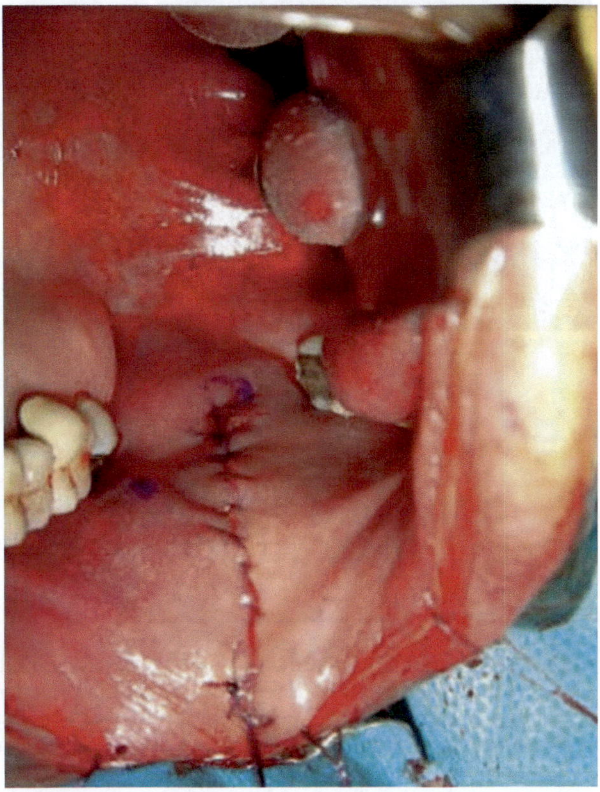

Fig. 32.4 Optionally, the donor site can be closed with interrupted or running 4-0 polyglactin sutures. When necessary, another graft can be harvested from the contralateral cheek using the same technique. (From Kulkarni SB et al. [16], with permission from the Indian Journal of Urology)

32.5.2 Buccal Graft Positioning

After harvesting the buccal mucosa, the question is now: How to position it (or any other graft) over the urethral stricture?

Monseur described a one-stage **dorsal inlay** technique in 1968 in patients with long anterior urethral strictures yielding encouraging results. His technique consisted of a dorsal incision of the fibrotic segment followed by suturing of the incisional edges to the corpora cavernosa albuginea allowing a progressive regeneration of the urothelium to completely line the urethral lumen [17]. However, this technique showed some limits when the urethral caliber was not sufficient; exposing it to stenosis, some investigators proposed to adjunct the use of pedicled penile skin graft dorsally onto the urethra [18].

Morey and McAninch proposed the **ventral onlay** technique in 1996 [13]. This technique was very attractive by its simplicity and straightforwardness; however, it was associated with a high risk of ballooning and pseudo-diverticulum formation of the ventrally positioned unsupported graft, in addition to concerns about possible vascular compromise at the ventral site [19].

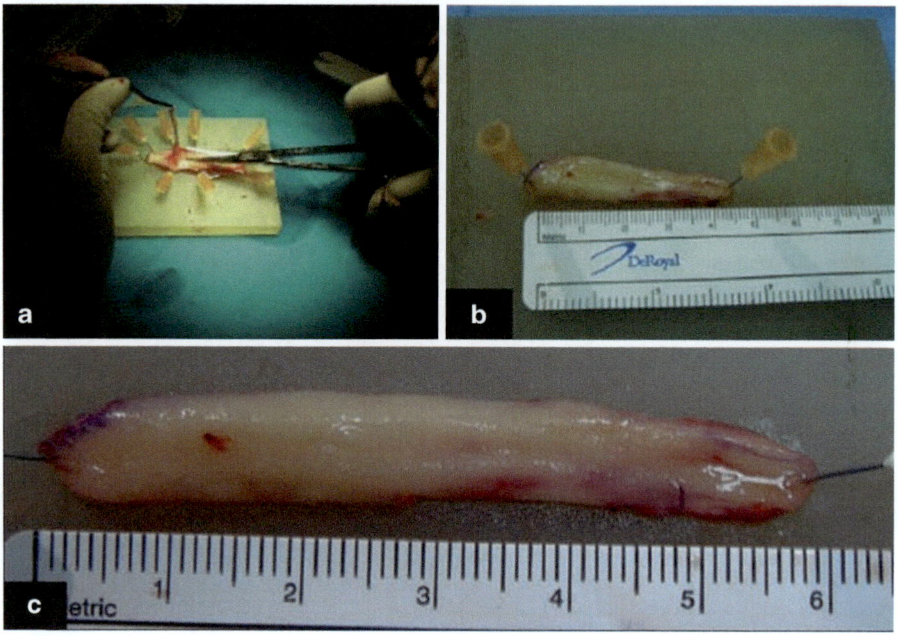

Fig. 32.5 The graft is stabilized on a silicone board using insulin needles. Once all submucosal tissue is carefully excised with iris scissors (**a**), the graft is tailored according to site, length, and stricture characteristics. While removing all the submucosal tissue, it is paramount to not excessively thin the graft, as thin grafts are more likely to heal with contracture. If the preparation of the graft is adequate, an average 4 cm long graft will stretch up to 6 cm due to the intrinsic elasticity of the mucosa (**b** and **c**). Two 6 cm long grafts (one from each cheek) are enough to repair the vast majority of penile or bulbar strictures using one-stage techniques. (From Kulkarni SB et al. [16], with permission from the Indian Journal of Urology)

Barbagli is credited for the first use of the **dorsal onlay** technique in 1998 and Asopa et al. for that of a **dorsal inlay** technique in 2001, both using penile skin (inner prepuce) or buccal mucosal graft [20, 21].

32.5.2.1 Barbagli Dorsal Onlay Technique [19, 20, 22] (Fig. 32.6)

- **Complete mobilization of the corpus spongiosum and urethra from the corpora cavernosa and 180° rotation.**
- Opening of the strictured tract along its **dorsal surface** and extension of the incision beyond the stricture proximally and distally.
- **Spreading of a fenestrated ovoid preputial free skin or buccal mucosa graft which is sutured to the corpora cavernosa (tunica albuginea) using interrupted stitches.**
- Addition of **several quilting sutures** to optimize contact between the graft and the corporeal bed and enhance the "take" of the graft.
- Making **small incisions all over the graft** to prevent hematoma or edema formation beneath it.

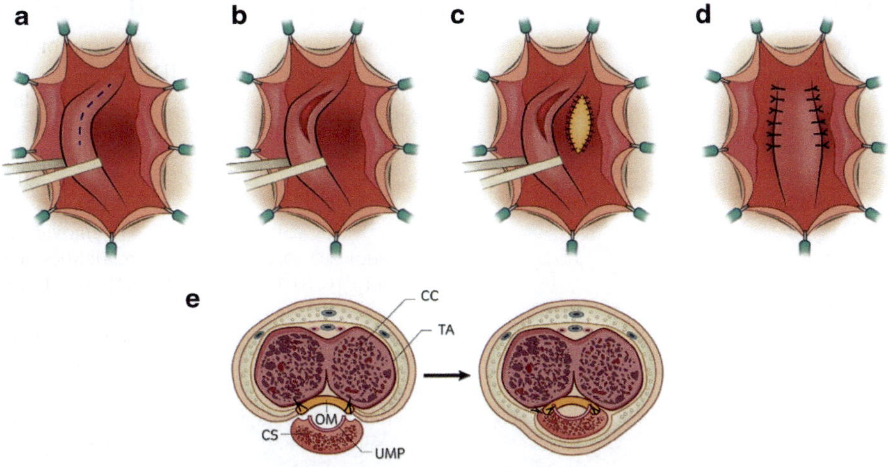

Fig. 32.6 Dorsal onlay augmentation (Barbagli technique) for bulbar urethral stricture. (**a**) The bulbar urethral is rotated, and (**b**) the dorsal urethral surface is incised along the midline to expose the entire stricture. (**c**) The oral mucosa graft is spread, fixed over the corpora cavernosa. (**d**) The bulbar urethra is rotated back, and the margin of the oral mucosa graft is sutured to the margin of the urethral mucosal plate. (**e**) Cross-sectional view of the grafted urethral lumen. *CC* corpora cavernosum, *CS* corpus spongiosum, *OM* oral mucosa, *TA* tunica albuginea, *UMP* urethral mucosal plate. (From Horiguchi A [22], with permission from John Wiley and Sons)

- Suturing of the left mucosal margin of the opened urethra to the left side of the patch graft.
- Rotation of the urethra back to its original position.
- Insertion of a 16-Fr silicone catheter.
- Suturing the edges of the stricturotomy to the graft and to the corpora cavernosa: the right urethral margin is sutured to the right side of the patch graft. This results in the graft area being entirely covered by the urethral plate.

32.5.2.2 Asopa Inlay Technique [19, 21, 22] (Fig. 32.7)

- Exposure of the urethra at the site of the stricture.
- **No attempt to mobilize the urethra or dissect the bulbospongiosus muscle and Buck's fascia.**
- **Ventral urethrostomy** carried out on the strictured area over a bougie upto 2 cm both proximally and distally into the healthy urethra.
- **Incision of the full thickness of the dorsal urethra in the mid-line** for about 1–2 cm both proximally and distally into the healthy urethra.
- Sharp dissection of the margins of the incised dorsal urethra from the tunica albuginea without lifting the two halves of the bisected urethra. This dissection creates a 1.5–2 cm-wide elliptical raw area between the bisected edges of the urethra over the tunica albuginea.
- Anchoring of the incised dorsal free margins of the urethra to the tunica albuginea with interrupted 5-0 polyglactin.

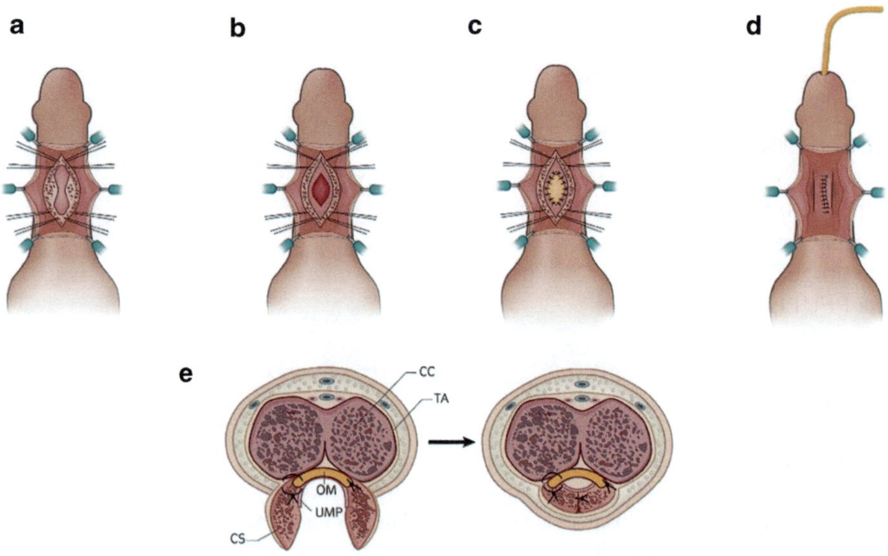

Fig. 32.7 Dorsal inlay (Asopa technique). (**a**) The urethra is left adherent to the corpora cavernosa, and is longitudinally opened ventrally extending to the distal and proximal healthy urethra. (**b**) The strictured urethral plate is longitudinally opened dorsally. (**c**) The oral graft is sutured to the margins of the urethral plate and fixed to the corpora cavernosa. (**d**) The urethra is retubularized over a urethral catheter. (**e**) Cross-sectional view of the grafted urethral lumen. *CC* corpora cavernosum, *CS* corpus spongiosum, *OM* oral mucosa, *TA* tunica albuginea, *UMP* urethral mucosal plate. (From Horiguchi A [22], with permission from John Wiley and Sons)

- Placement of full-thickness free grafts (inner prepuce or buccal mucosa) over the raw area of the incised dorsal urethra.
- Fixing the graft to the edges of the incised dorsal urethra with 5-0 resorbable sutures, and adding several quilting sutures at the underlying tunica albuginea to prevent dead space.
- Insertion of a 14- to 16-Fr silicon catheter and retubularization of the urethra by closing the ventral urethrostomy with continuous 4-0 resorbable sutures.
- Drain in situ and compressive dressing.

At first glance, it appears that the **avoidance of urethral mobilization and dissection in the Asopa or inlay technique would preserve the urethral blood supply** through circumflex and perforating vessels, and simplify the procedure. Herein a prospective randomized study comparing both techniques showed a similar success rate (86.4–88%), however, **the Asopa technique (dorsal inlay) appeared to be technically easier than the Barbagli one (dorsal onlay) with a shorter operative time (128 vs 205 min) and less blood loss (105 vs 228 mL)** [19].

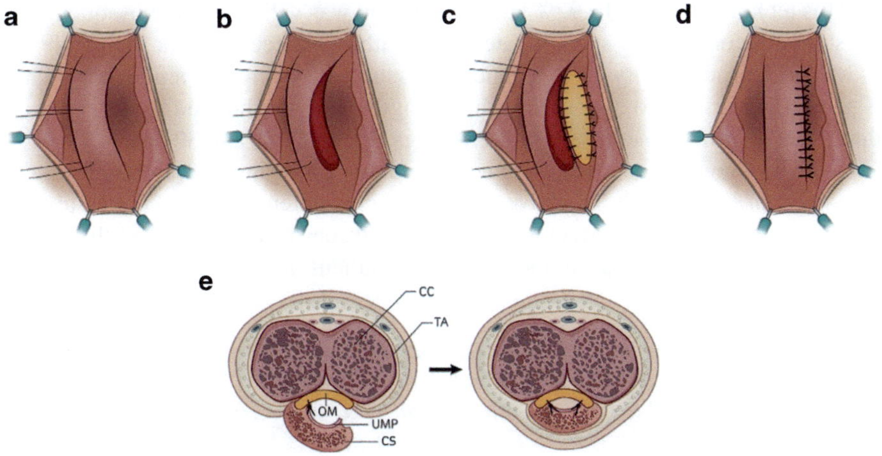

Fig. 32.8 Dorsolataral onlay (Kulkarni technique). (**a**) The urethra is mobilized from the albuginea only along the left side. (**b**) The dorsolateral side of the urethra is incised longitudinally. (**c**) The oral mucosa graft is sutured to the underlying albuginea, and the right margin of the oral graft is sutured to the left margin of the urethral plate (**d**) and on the other side. (**e**) Cross-sectional view of the grafted urethral lumen. *BF* Buck's fascia, *CC* corpora cavernosum, *CS* corpus spongiosum, *OM* oral mucosa, *TA* tunica albuginea, *UMP* urethral mucosal plate. (From Horiguchi A [22], with permission from John Wiley and Sons)

32.5.2.3 Kulkarni One-Side Dorsolateral Approach (Fig. 32.8)

In 2009, Kulkarni et al. proposed a modified technique of the Barbagli dorsal onlay buccal mucosa urethroplasty: the so-called **one-side dorsolateral approach avoiding the full circumferential mobilization of the urethra**, hence minimizing the risk of vascular compromise [23].

The steps of this technique are [22–25]:

- midline perineal incision.
- **dissection of the bulbar urethra only on one side** (left side for right-handed surgeons).
- leave the bulbospongiosus muscle and the central tendon of the perineum intact.
- **Invagination of the penis into the incision and dissection of the penile urethra on one side only.**
- rotation and dorsal incision of the urethra to expose the whole stricture.
- Deep external meatotomy at 12 o'clock position
- Fixation of the buccal mucosa graft to the dorsal aspect of the meatus using three single 5/0 resorbable sutures.
- Pushing the graft inside and fixation to the corpora cavernosa with 5/0 resorbable sutures on 2, 10, 12 o'clock positions.
- Further fixation of the graft with multiple quilting sutures.
- Insertion of a 14–16 Fr silicone Foley catheter (will be kept for one month).
- Completion of the anastomosis on the left side.

This technique yielded a 92% success rate and was validated by subsequent studies showing comparable success rates using either a buccal graft or the penile skin as well as reproducibility even in panurethral stricture where the penile invagination is particularly useful to expose the whole length of the urethra and the use of two or three buccal grafts is necessary [24–26] (Figs. 32.9, 32.10, and 32.11).

Note: In view of the abundant and eventually confusing technical information contained in the paragraphs above, the following sentence might help as a useful mnemonic to make the correct associations between the eponyms and their corresponding techniques and to memorize the salient aspects of the dorsal graft urethroplasty:

> *"**ASIN** defied the **BARON** by refusing to dance around the palm tree, then **KUONG** proposed to limit the dance to one side of the tree".*

In this sentence:

- **ASIN** stands for **As**opa + **In**lay, **BARON** stands for **Bar**bagli + **On**lay, **KUONG** stands for **K**ulkarni + **U**nilateral + **On**lay + **g**raft.
- The refusal to dance around the palm tree refers to the avoidance by Asopa's technique to mobilize the urethra all around as preconized by Barbagli et al.

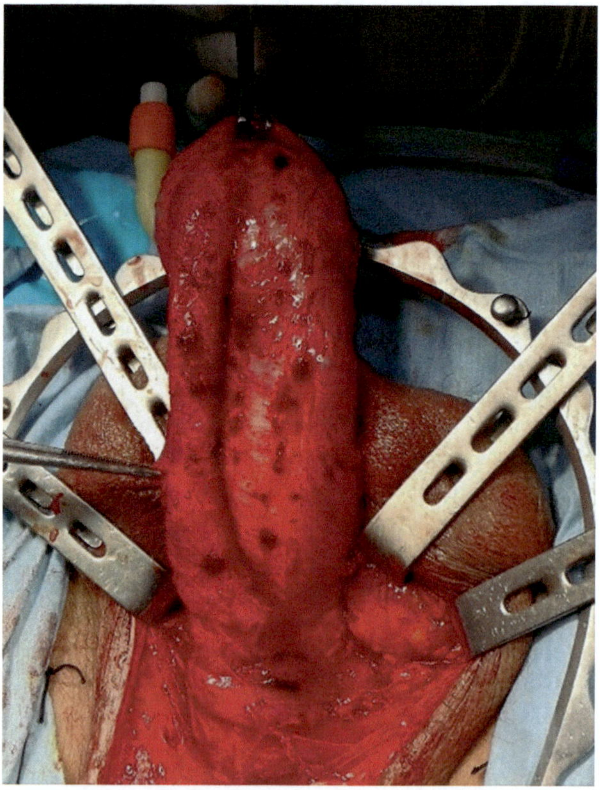

Fig. 32.9 The penis is invaginated into the incision and penile urethra is dissected only on the left side leaving the urethra attached to the corpora cavernosa on the right and preserving its neurovascular supply. (From Zumrutbas AE [25], with permission from Springer Nature)

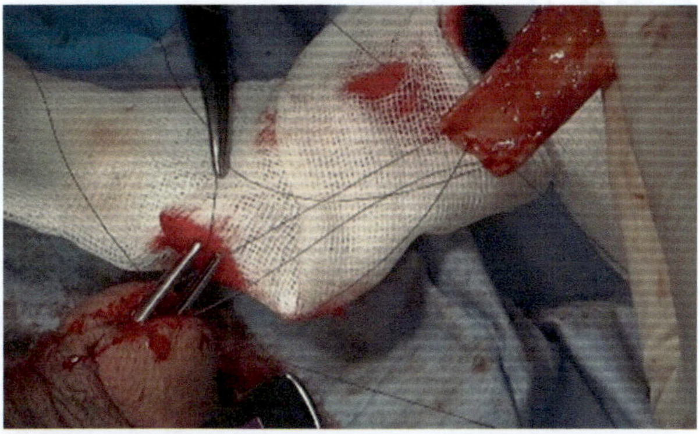

Fig. 32.10 The buccal mucosal graft is sutured to the dorsal aspect of the meatus using three single 5/0 polyglactin sutures and the graft is pushed inside through the meatus. (From Zumrutbas AE [25], with permission from Springer Nature)

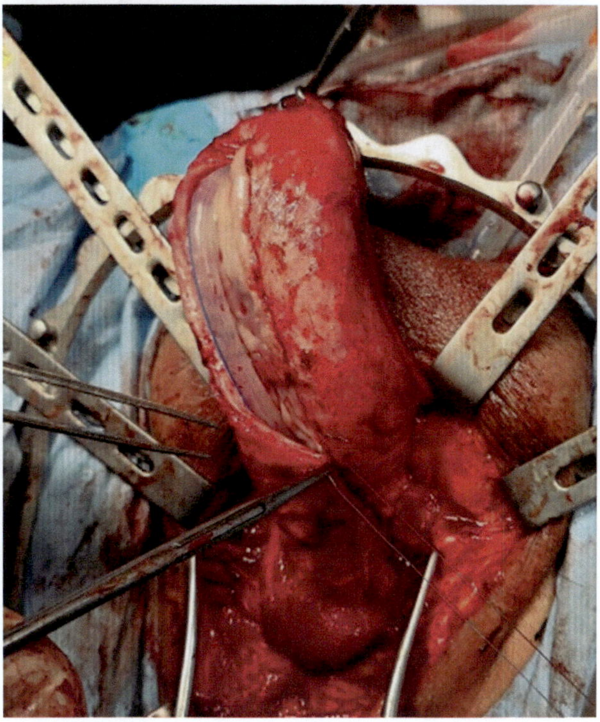

Fig. 32.11 A 14F silicone Foley catheter is inserted and anastomosis is completed on the left side. (From Zumrutbas AE [25], with permission from Springer)

- The one-side dance is the unilateral technique of Kulkarni's approach avoiding the complete mobilization of the urethra.

Note that **Asin** is a girl's first name in India. Readers from Arab countries may use **Inas** instead.

Further modification of Barbagli dorsal onlay technique includes the use of fibrine glue to fix the graft on the corpora cavernosa [27, 28] (Figs. 32.12, 32.13, and 32.14).

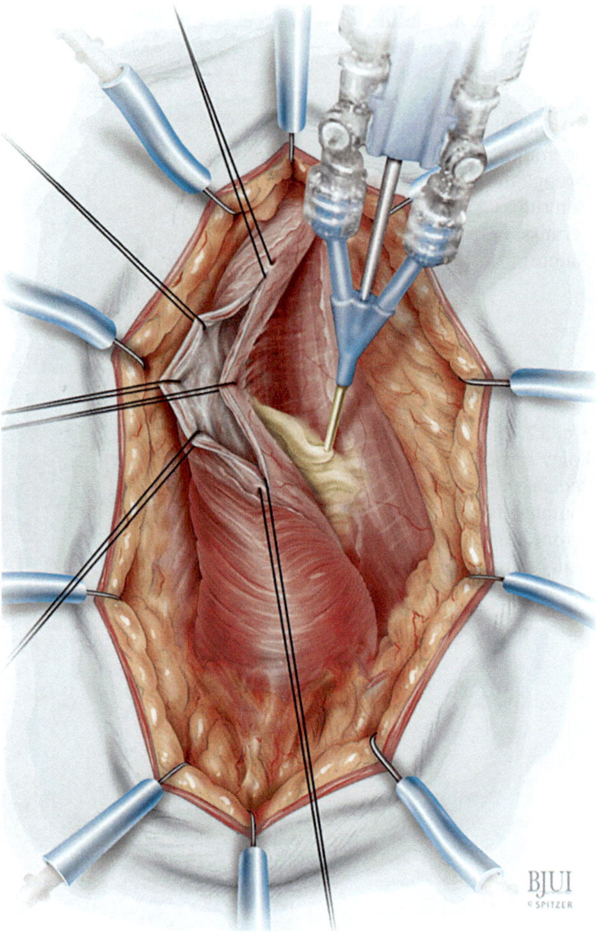

Fig. 32.12 After one-side mobilization of the urethra, a fibrin glue (2 mL) is injected over the corpora cavernosa. (From Barbagli G et al. [28], with permission from John Wiley and Sons)

When the strictured area is too narrow, one graft might not be enough to ensure adequate lumen without transecting the urethra. Herein, Palminteri et al. proposed the use of two grafts, the so-called combined dorsal plus ventral double buccal mucosa graft [29] (Figs. 32.15, 32.16, and 32.17).

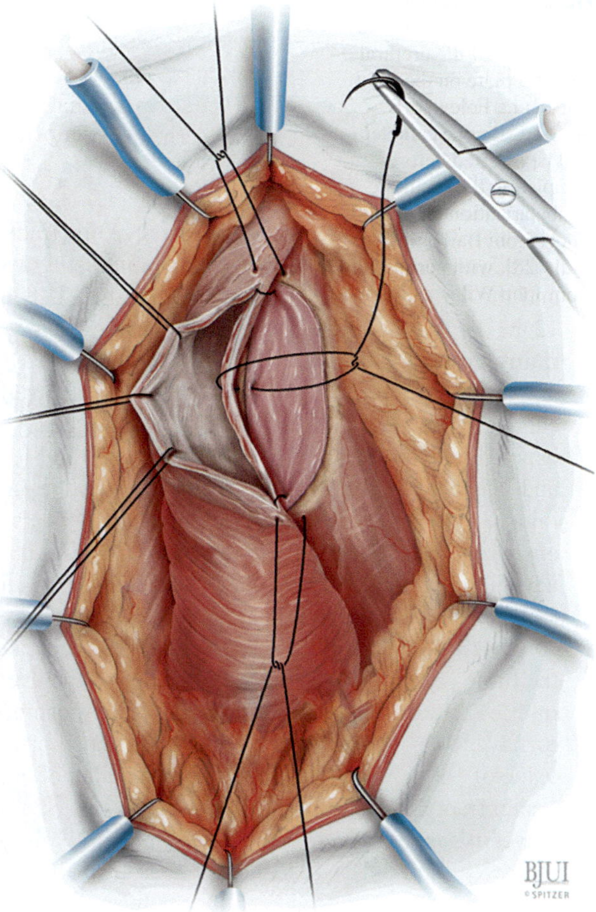

Fig. 32.13 The oral mucosal graft, trimmed to an appropriate size according to the length and width of the urethrotomy, is spread, optionally fixed over the fibrin-glue bed, and the apices of the graft are sutured to the proximal and distal apices of the urethrotomy. (From Barbagli G et al. [28], with permission from John Wiley and Sons)

Urethroplasty is rarely performed in females where the possibility for vaginal mucosa graft exists in addition to the buccal mucosa [30], and the vaginal flap can be harvested from the anterior (Blandy flap) or the lateral wall (Orandi flap) [31]*.

*The Orandi flap was first described by Ahmad Orandi in 1968 in males with anterior urethral strictures and consisted of the use of an inverted penile skin flap [32]. It is rarely used nowadays.

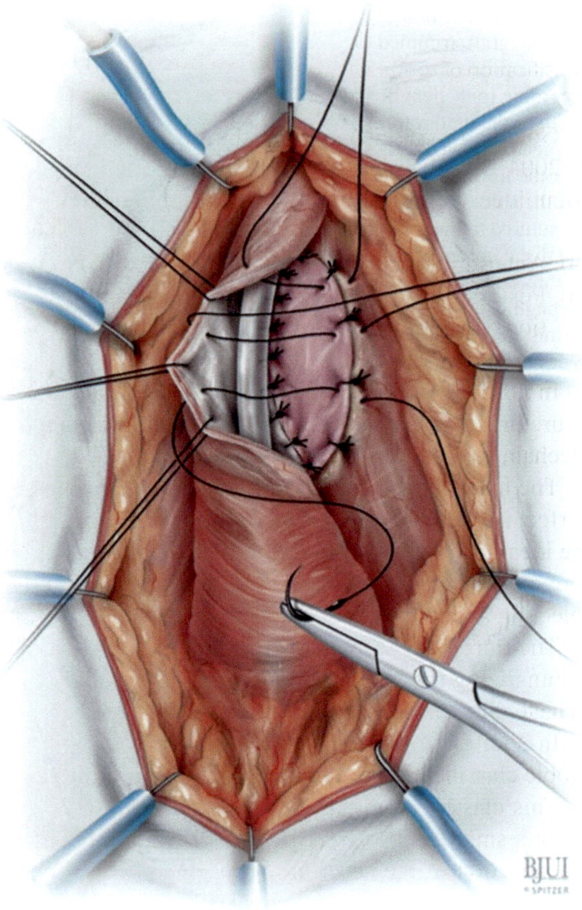

Fig. 32.14 The margin of the oral graft is sutured to the margin of the urethral mucosal plate on the right side, and a Foley 16-F grooved silicone catheter will be inserted before completing the urethral retubularization on the left side. (From Barbagli G et al. [28], with permission from John Wiley and Sons)

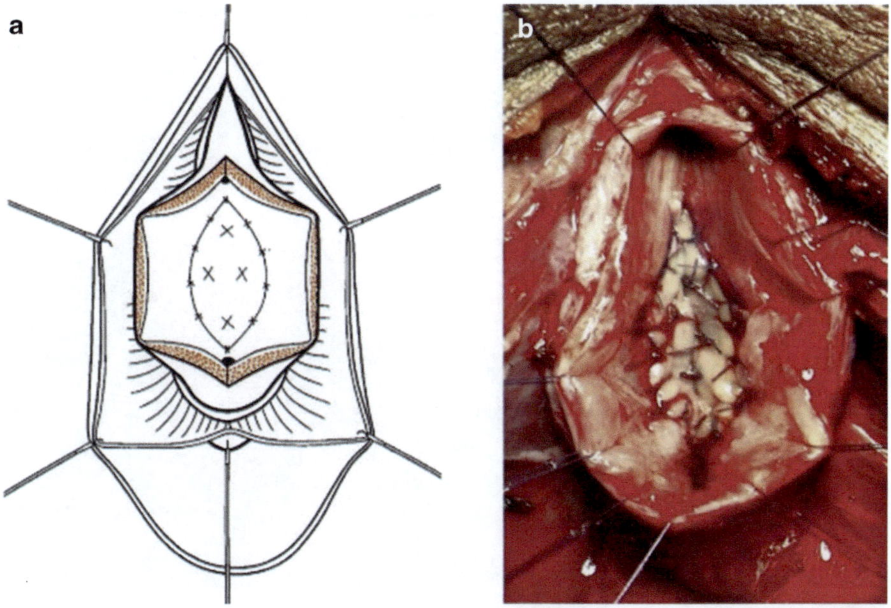

Fig. 32.15 Dorsal inlay patch augmentation. (**a** and **b**) The first buccal mucosa graft is sutured and quilted into the recipient elliptical area. (From Palminteri E et al. [29], with permission from Elsevier)

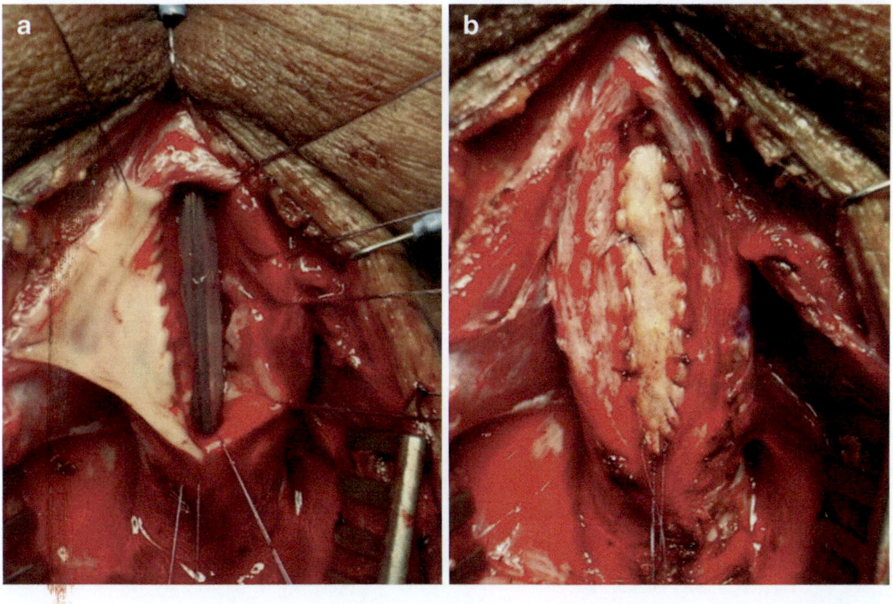

Fig. 32.16 Ventral onlay patch augmentation. (**a**) The second buccal mucosa graft is sutured laterally to the mucosal margin of the urethral plate. (**b**) The graft is rotated and sutured to the other mucosal margin. (From Palminteri E et al. [29], with permission from Elsevier)

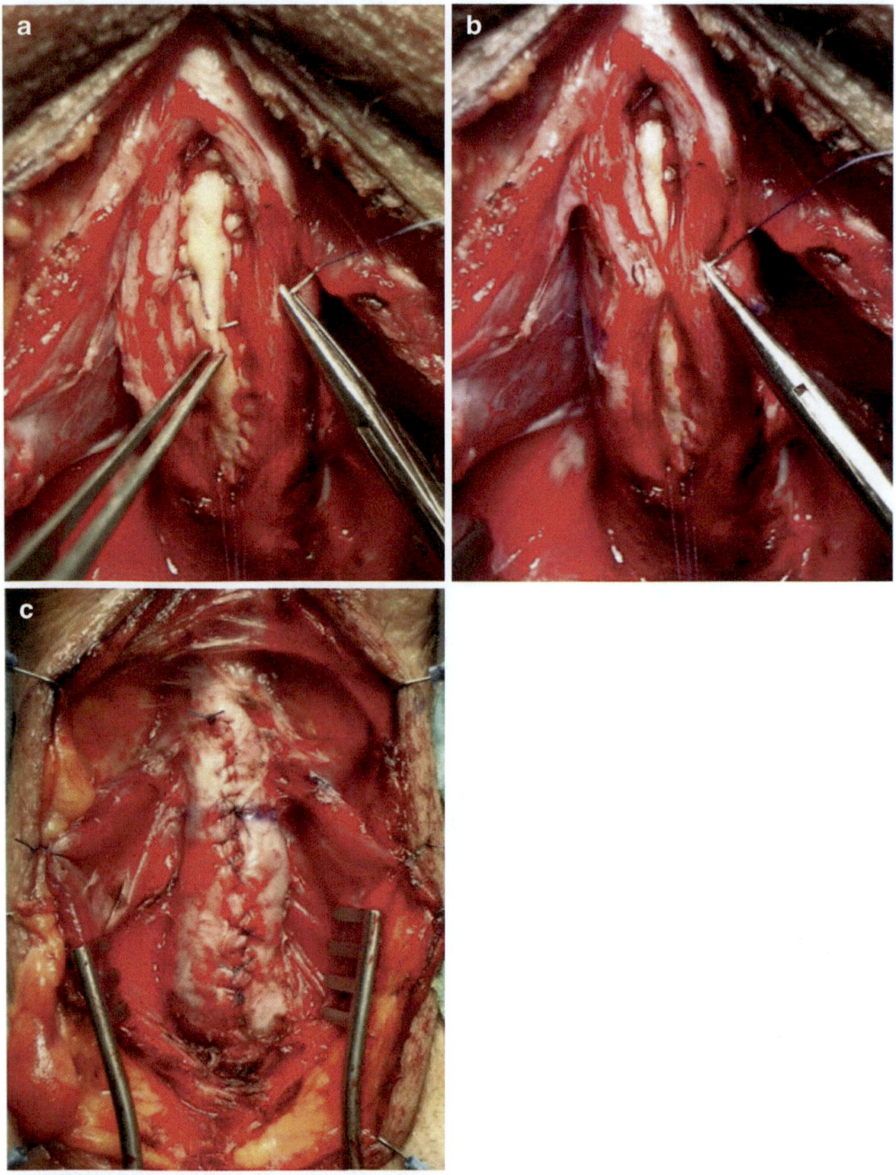

Fig. 32.17 (**a** and **b**) The inverted ventral graft is quilted by few stitches fixing the graft to the spongiosum. (**c**) Spongiosum closure over the graft. (From Palminteri E et al. [29], with permission from Elsevier)

32.6 Alternative Treatment

32.6.1 Endoscopic Realignment

Immediate endoscopic-guided urethral splinting (railroading procedure) has been advocated for stable patients with complete anterior urethral disruption. The procedure consists of a retrograde urethroscopy with or without antegrade cystoscopy under fluoroscopic guidance through suprapubic access and proceeds through the negotiation of a guidewire across the disrupted segment followed by a Foley catheter insertion. This technique proved to be safe and feasible in almost all well-selected patients and showed no recurrence in more than half of the cases [33].

32.6.1.1 Endoprosthesis

The **Urolume endoprosthesis** has been proposed as a minimally invasive treatment for recurrent bulbar urethral stricture, BPH, and detrusor-external sphincter dyssynergia in the late 1980s [34, 35]. However, subsequent researchers did not show much enthusiasm due to frequent complications, namely migration, recurrent stenosis, urethral pain, recurrent urinary tract infections, and the use of the Urolume endoprosthesis fell into desuetude [36, 37].

Recently, the randomized Robust III trial has studied the effect of a **drug-coated balloon (DCB)**, namely the **Optilume**® with a Paclitaxel coating among an adult population with stricture ≤12 Fr in diameter and ≤3 cm in length, having at least two prior endoscopic treatments, and IPSS ≥11 and maximum flow rate <15 mL per second. The study showed significant improvement at 6 months in the treated group compared to the control with values of 75% and 27% respectively [38]. Despite yielding encouraging results, the authors concluded that the Optilume® DCB should serve merely as an alternative for men who had an unsuccessful direct vision internal urethrotomy/dilation and who want to avoid or delay urethroplasty which remains the best definitive treatment.

32.6.1.2 Tissue Engineering

Various matrices have been proposed for urethral mucosa replacement including small intestinal submucosa grafts, bladder-derived matrices (collagen-based and acellular bladder matrix), acellular dermis graft, etc. However, although promising, the results are still not proportionate to the enthusiasm raised in the last decades, and 3D-bioprinting to manufacture patient-tailored designs of seeded tubular urethral constructs is still in the dreamworld, but boundless human genius has yet to say its last word [39].

The development of autologous tissue-engineered buccal mucosa has been first introduced in 2004 from a small buccal mucosa specimen (0.5 cm) [40], and its initial clinical application was tried in 2008 with encouraging results as 3 patients out of 5 had a patent urethra after a mean follow-up of 33.6 months [41].

A German pharmaceutical company (UroTiss Europe GmbH) has further developed the idea and is manufacturing an autologous tissue-engineered oral mucosa graft as **MukoCell**®. This was studied in a multicenter and prospective trial recruiting 99 patients, showing encouraging success rates in terms of improvement of peak flow rate (Qmax) of 67.3% and 58.2% at 12-month and 24-month follow-up, respectively, but the results were significantly dependent on the surgeon experience [42].

References

1. Chapple C, Barbagli G, Jordan G, Mundy AR, Rodrigues-Netto N, Pansadoros V. Consensus statement on urethral trauma. BJU Int. 2004;93:1195–202.
2. Rourke KF, Jordan GH. Primary urethral reconstruction: the cost minimized approach to the bulbous urethral stricture. J Urol. 2005;173(4):1206–10. https://doi.org/10.1097/01.ju.0000154971.05286.81. PMID: 15758749.
3. Blaschko SD, Harris CR, Zaid UB, Gaither T, Chu C, Alwaal A, McAninch JW, McCulloch CE, Breyer BN. Trends, utilization, and immediate perioperative complications of urethroplasty in the United States: data from the national inpatient sample 2000-2010. Urology. 2015;85(5):1190–4. https://doi.org/10.1016/j.urology.2015.01.008. Epub 2015 Mar 4. PMID: 25746579; PMCID: PMC4917203.
4. Nilsen OJ, Holm HV, Ekerhult TO, Lindqvist K, Grabowska B, Persson B, Sairanen J. To transect or not transect: results from the Scandinavian urethroplasty study, a multicentre randomised study of bulbar urethroplasty comparing excision and primary anastomosis versus buccal mucosal grafting. Eur Urol. 2022;81(4):375–82. https://doi.org/10.1016/j.eururo.2021.12.017. Epub 2022 Jan 8. PMID: 35012771.
5. Bugeja S, Andrich DE, Mundy AR. Non-transecting bulbar urethroplasty. Transl Androl Urol. 2015;4(1):41–50. https://doi.org/10.3978/j.issn.2223-4683.2015.01.07. PMID: 26816808; PMCID: PMC4708276.
6. Barbagli G, Sansalone S, Djinovic R, Romano G, Lazzeri M. Current controversies in reconstructive surgery of the anterior urethra: a clinical overview. Int Braz J Urol. 2012;38(3):307–16; discussion 316. PMID: 22765862. https://doi.org/10.1590/s1677-55382012000300003.
7. Ozgök Y, Ozgür Tan M, Kilciler M, Tahmaz L, Erduran D. Use of bladder mucosal graft for urethral reconstruction. Int J Urol. 2000;7(10):355–60. https://doi.org/10.1046/j.1442-2042.2000.00210.x. PMID: 11144502.
8. Gelman J, Furr J. Tissue transfer techniques in the management of urethral stricture disease: flaps and grafts. In: Martins FE, Kulkarni SB, Köhler TS, editors. Textbook of male genitourethral reconstruction. Cham: Springer; 2020. https://doi.org/10.1007/978-3-030-21447-0_7.
9. Filipas D, Wahlmann U, Hohenfellner R. History of oral mucosa. Eur Urol. 1998;34(3):165–8. https://doi.org/10.1159/000019705. PMID: 9732186.
10. Korneyev I, Ilyin D, Schultheiss D, Chapple C. The first oral mucosal graft urethroplasty was carried out in the 19th century: the pioneering experience of Kirill Sapezhko (1857-1928). Eur Urol. 2012;62(4):624–7. https://doi.org/10.1016/j.eururo.2012.06.035. Epub 2012 Jun 27. PMID: 22749735.
11. Humby G. A one-stage operation for hypospadias. Br J Surg. 1941;29:84–92.
12. el-Kasaby AW, Fath-Alla M, Noweir AM, el-Halaby MR, Zakaria W, el-Beialy MH. The use of buccal mucosa patch graft in the management of anterior urethral strictures. J Urol. 1993;149(2):276–8. https://doi.org/10.1016/s0022-5347(17)36054-8. PMID: 8426400.
13. Morey AF, McAninch JW. When and how to use buccal mucosal grafts in adult bulbar urethroplasty. Urology. 1996;48(2):194–8. https://doi.org/10.1016/S0090-4295(96)00154-9. PMID: 8753728.
14. Barbagli G, Balò S, Sansalone S, Lazzeri M. How to harvest buccal mucosa from the cheek. Afr J Urol. 2016;22(1):18–23. https://doi.org/10.1016/j.afju.2015.09.001. issn:1110-5704.

15. Barbagli G, Vallasciani S, Romano G, Fabbri F, Guazzoni G, Lazzeri M. Morbidity of oral mucosa graft harvesting from a single cheek. Eur Urol. 2010;58(1):33–41. https://doi.org/10.1016/j.eururo.2010.01.012. Epub 2010 Jan 19. PMID: 20106587.
16. Kulkarni SB, Barbagli G, Sansalone S, Joshi PM. Harvesting oral mucosa for one-stage anterior urethroplasty. Indian J Urol. 2014;30(1):117–21. https://doi.org/10.4103/0970-1591.124222. PMID: 24497698; PMCID: PMC3897044.
17. Monseur J. La reconstitution du canal de l'urètre au moyen des lames sus-urétérales et de la gouttière sous-caverneuse. J Urol Nephrol. 1968;74:755–7.
18. El-Kassaby A-W, Fath-Alla M, Maged W, Abdel-Aal A. Traitement des sténoses de l'urètre pénien par urétroplastie avec patch pédiculé dorsal : «Urétroplastie en toit». Prog Urol. 1998;8:1022–8.
19. Aldaqadossi H, El Gamal S, El-Nadey M, El Gamal O, Radwan M, Gaber M. Dorsal onlay (Barbagli technique) versus dorsal inlay (Asopa technique) buccal mucosal graft urethroplasty for anterior urethral stricture: a prospective randomized study. Int J Urol. 2014;21(2):185–8. https://doi.org/10.1111/iju.12235. Epub 2013 Aug 12. PMID: 23931150.
20. Barbagli G, Palminteri E, Rizzo M. Dorsal onlay graft urethroplasty using penile skin or buccal mucosa in adult bulbourethral strictures. J Urol. 1998;160:1307–9.
21. Asopa HS, Garg M, Singhal GG, et al. Dorsal free graft urethroplasty for urethral stricture by ventral sagittal urethrotomy approach. Urology. 2001;58:657–9.
22. Horiguchi A. Substitution urethroplasty using oral mucosa graft for male anterior urethral stricture disease: current topics and reviews. Int J Urol. 2017;24(7):493–503. https://doi.org/10.1111/iju.13356. Epub 2017 Jun 10. PMID: 28600871.
23. Kulkarni S, Barbagli G, Sansalone S, Lazzeri M. One-sided anterior urethroplasty: a new dorsal onlay graft technique. BJU Int. 2009;104(8):1150–5. https://doi.org/10.1111/j.1464-410X.2009.08590.x. Epub 2009 Apr 17. PMID: 19388990.
24. Palminteri E, Berdondini E, Lumen N, Maruccia S, Florio M, Franco G, Montanaro V, Di Pierro GB. Kulkarni dorsolateral graft urethroplasty using penile skin. Urology. 2016;90:179–83. https://doi.org/10.1016/j.urology.2015.12.014. Epub 2015 Dec 29. PMID: 26743395.
25. Zumrutbas AE, Ozlulerden Y, Celen S, Kucuker K, Aybek Z. The outcomes of Kulkarni's one-stage oral mucosa graft urethroplasty in patients with panurethral stricture: a single centre experience. World J Urol. 2020;38(1):175–81. https://doi.org/10.1007/s00345-019-02758-y. Epub 2019 Apr 8. PMID: 30963228.
26. Kulkarni S, Joshi P, Surana S, Hamouda A. Management of panurethral strictures. Afr J Urol. 2016;22(1):33–9. issn:1110-5704. https://doi.org/10.1016/j.afju.2016.01.001.
27. Barbagli G, De Stefani S, Sighinolfi MC, Annino F, Micali S, Bianchi G. Bulbar urethroplasty with dorsal onlay buccal mucosal graft and fibrin glue. Eur Urol. 2006;50:467–74.
28. Barbagli G, Sansalone S, Kulkarni SB, Romano G, Lazzeri M. Dorsal onlay oral mucosal graft bulbar urethroplasty. BJU Int. 2012;109(11):1728–41. https://doi.org/10.1111/j.1464-410X.2012.11006.x. PMID: 22564323.
29. Palminteri E, Manzoni G, Berdondini E, Di Fiore F, Testa G, Poluzzi M, Molon A. Combined dorsal plus ventral double buccal mucosa graft in bulbar urethral reconstruction. Eur Urol. 2008;53(1):81–9. https://doi.org/10.1016/j.eururo.2007.05.033. Epub 2007 Jun 8. PMID: 17583417.
30. Waterloos M, Verla W. Female urethroplasty: a practical guide emphasizing diagnosis and surgical treatment of female urethral stricture disease. Biomed Res Int. 2019;2019:6715257.
31. Navarro-Galmes MA, Hernandez-Hernandez D, Padilla-Fernandez B, Castro-Diaz DM. Female urethroplasty: anterior vaginal wall flap (Blandy flap)—simpler tends to be better. Urol Int. 2022;106(3):313–6. https://doi.org/10.1159/000515994. Epub 2021 May 6. PMID: 33957637.
32. Orandi A. One-stage urethroplasty. Br J Urol. 1968;40(6):717–9. https://doi.org/10.1111/j.1464-410x.1968.tb11872.x. PMID: 4883846.
33. Maheshwari PN, Shah HN. Immediate endoscopic management of complete iatrogenic anterior urethral injuries: a case series with long-term results. BMC Urol. 2005;5:13. https://doi.org/10.1186/1471-2490-5-13.

34. Milroy EJ, Chapple CR, Cooper JE, Eldin A, Wallsten H, Seddon AM, Rowles PM. A new treatment for urethral strictures. Lancet. 1988;1(8600):1424–7. https://doi.org/10.1016/s0140-6736(88)92238-6. PMID: 2898583.
35. Badlani GH, Press SM, Defalco A, Oesterling JE, Smith AD. Urolume endourethral prosthesis for the treatment of urethral stricture disease: long-term results of the north American multicenter urolume trial. Urology. 1995;45(5):846–56. issn:0090-4295. https://doi.org/10.1016/S0090-4295(99)80093-4.
36. Wilson TS, Lemack GE, Dmochowski RR. Urolume stents: lessons learned. J Urol. 2002;167(6):2477–80. PMID: 11992061.
37. Frankiewicz M, Karolina M, Marcin M. Diagnosis and management of urolume urethral stent complications using ultrasonography and magnetic resonance imaging. Urology. 2020;144:e4–5. https://doi.org/10.1016/j.urology.2020.06.043. Epub 2020 Jul 7. PMID: 32650016.
38. Elliott SP, Coutinho K, Robertson KJ, D'Anna R, Chevli K, Carrier S, Aube-Peterkin M, Cantrill CH, Ehlert MJ, Te AE, Dann J, DeLong JM, Brandes SB, Hagedorn JC, Levin R, Schlaifer A, DeSouza E, DiMarco D, Erickson BA, Natale R, Husmann DA, Morey A, Olsson C, Virasoro R. One-year results for the ROBUST III randomized controlled trial evaluating the Optilume® drug-coated balloon for anterior urethral strictures. J Urol. 2022;207(4):866–75. https://doi.org/10.1097/JU.0000000000002346. Epub 2021 Dec 2. PMID: 34854748.
39. Pastorek D, Culenova M, Csobonyeiova M, Skuciova V, Danisovic L, Ziaran S. Tissue engineering of the urethra: from bench to bedside. Biomedicine. 2021;9(12):1917. https://doi.org/10.3390/biomedicines9121917. PMID: 34944733; PMCID: PMC8698949.
40. Bhargava S, Chapple CR, Bullock AJ, Layton C, MacNeil S. Tissue-engineered buccal mucosa for substitution urethroplasty. BJU Int. 2004;93:807–11.
41. Bhargava S, Patterson JM, Inman RD, MacNeil S, Chapple CR. Tissue-engineered buccal mucosa urethroplasty-clinical outcomes. Eur Urol. 2008;53(6):1263–9. https://doi.org/10.1016/j.eururo.2008.01.061. Epub 2008 Feb 4. PMID: 18262717.
42. Ram-Liebig G, Barbagli G, Heidenreich A, Fahlenkamp D, Romano G, Rebmann U, Standhaft D, van Ahlen H, Schakaki S, Balsmeyer U, Spiegler M, Knispel H. Results of use of tissue-engineered autologous oral mucosa graft for urethral reconstruction: a multicenter, prospective, observational trial. EBioMedicine. 2017;23:185–92. https://doi.org/10.1016/j.ebiom.2017.08.014. Epub 2017 Aug 16. PMID: 28827035; PMCID: PMC5605371.

33 Complications of Urethral Injury

Before the first use of urinary drainage techniques such as suprapubic cystostomy and antegrade-retrograde railroading of perineal catheter into the bladder by Verguin in Toulon (France) in 1757, PFUI was always fatal due to urinary obstruction and extravasation, sepsis and uremia. The PFUI mortality recorded a significant decrease, from almost 100% in 1757, to 78% in 1907 and to 23% in 1942 because of better management of the trauma with the introduction of the following advances: Early and accurate diagnosis, adequate treatment of trauma shock, urinary drainage, debridement of devitalized tissues, and immobilization of the bony pelvis. This fatality applied also to anterior urethral injury depending on the grade [1, 2]. Further improvement has been achieved nowadays with better management of associated injuries, the introduction of antibiotics, the generalized use of blood transfusions, the improvement of techniques in the stabilization of fractures, and the creation of intensive care units, etc.

Late complications such as stricture, incontinence, and impotence are also avoided by the application of the abovementioned principles, and the early conservation of the urethral channel by a splinting catheter is of equal importance.

Nowadays the complications of urethral injuries are often intermingled with the complications of the procedures to alleviate or treat them. They consist of:

1. *In the immediate presentation*
   - hemorrhage and hypovolemic shock
   - hematoma and urinary extravasation
   - sepsis
2. *In the mid- or long term* [3]
   - Urinary incontinence
   - sexual impotence
   - urethral stricture
   - recurrent infection

S. A. AL-Mamari, *Urogenital Trauma: A Practical Guide*,
https://doi.org/10.1007/978-981-99-6171-9_33

- calculi formation: stone formation can be prevented by acidification of the urine and vesical lavage.
- chronic periurethral abscess
- chronic pubis osteomyelitis
- false passages into the bladder base or the prostate etc.
- fistulae between the urethra and the skin or neighboring hollow organs: urethro-cutaneous, urethro-vaginal, urethro-rectal fistulae, etc. (repair may require interposition of a gracilis muscle flap or a porcine small intestinal submucosal graft [4] (Fig. 33.1)
- Urethral diverticula (Fig. 33.2)

In a comprehensive review, Koraitim found the following complications in relation to the conventional treatment method of PFUI [5]:

- Primary anastomosis of the disrupted ends: incontinence 21%, impotence 56%
- Primary realignment: impotence 36%, stricture 53%
- Suprapubic cystostomy and delayed repair: impotence 19%, stricture 97%

In another study, he demonstrated that the direct effect of PFUI resulted in 40% of the patients becoming impotent, while **urethroplasty made only 4% of the potent patients become impotent**. More interestingly urethroplasty even allowed 63% of the impotent patients to regain their potency [6]. The relative innocence of urethroplasty has been further substantiated by another study that showed that

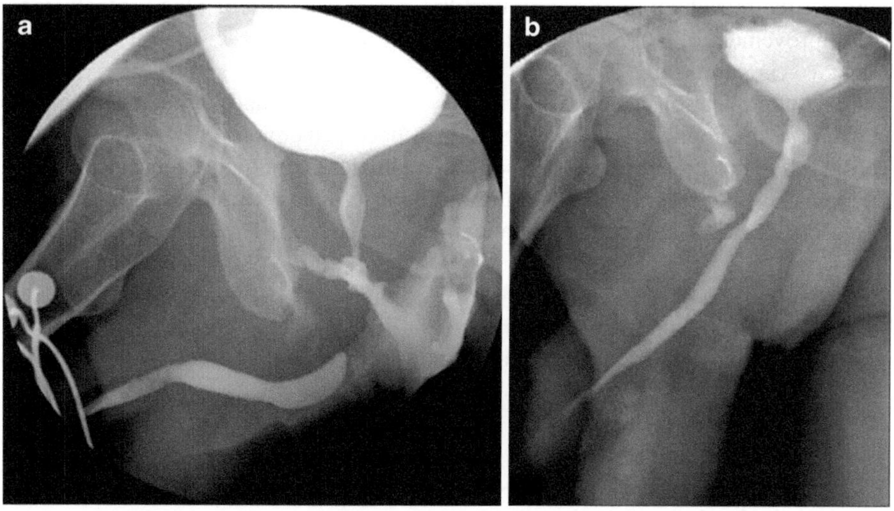

Fig. 33.1 (**a**) Cystourethrogram delineates the communication between the bulbomembranous urethra and rectum with urethral distraction defect. (**b**) Postoperative voiding cystourethrogram (after the interposition of a porcine small intestinal submucosa) showing completely healed anastomosis with the absence of contrast extravasation into the rectum. (From Rajaian S et al. [4], with permission from the *Indian Journal of Urology*)

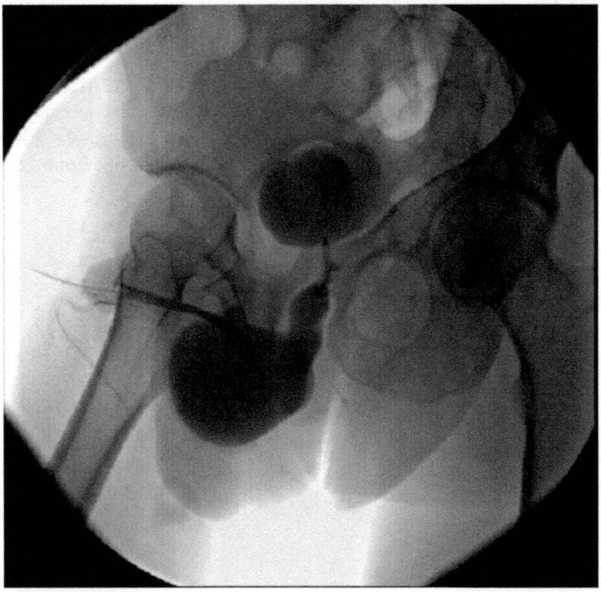

Fig. 33.2 Urethrography of a 34-year-old man with a history of road traffic accident with polytrauma and PFUI in 2011. Underwent an abdomino-perineal transpubic urethroplasty in 2012 complicated with a recto-urethro-cutaneous fistula managed with a defunctioning colostomy. Then the rectal fistula was repaired and underwent a Turner-Warwick posterior urethroplasty using scrotal invagination. This failed and a penile skin urethroplasty was performed in 2014 ending in a large diverticulum that empties by manual pressure

hazards related to this procedure occur in 6.6% of men only, mainly consisting of surgical or wound complications (5.2%), and are associated with old age, and the presence of comorbidities. Mortality following urethroplasty is exceedingly rare (0.07%) [7].

References

1. McCague EJ, Semans JH. The management of traumatic rupture of the urethra and bladder complicating fracture of the pelvis. J Urol. 1944;52:36–41.
2. Barratt RC, Bernard J, Mundy AR, Greenwell TJ. Pelvic fracture urethral injury in males-mechanisms of injury, management options and outcomes. Transl Androl Urol. 2018;7(Suppl 1):S29–62. https://doi.org/10.21037/tau.2017.12.35. PMID: 29644168; PMCID: PMC5881191.
3. Turner-Warwick R. Complex traumatic posterior urethral strictures. J Urol. 1977;118(4):564–74. https://doi.org/10.1016/s0022-5347(17)58109-4. PMID: 916051.
4. Rajaian S, Rajadoss MP, Nayak S, Kekre NS. Traumatic rectourethral fistula repair: a potential application of porcine small intestinal submucosa. Indian J Urol. 2013;29(2):148–50. https://doi.org/10.4103/0970-1591.114041. PMID: 23956521; PMCID: PMC3737675.
5. Koraitim MM. Pelvic fracture urethral injuries: the unresolved controversy. J Urol. 1999;161(5):1433–41. PMID: 10210368.

6. Koraitim MM. The lessons of 145 posttraumatic posterior urethral strictures treated in 17 years. J Urol. 1995;153(1):63–6. https://doi.org/10.1097/00005392-199501000-00024. PMID: 7966793.
7. Blaschko SD, Harris CR, Zaid UB, Gaither T, Chu C, Alwaal A, McAninch JW, McCulloch CE, Breyer BN. Trends, utilization, and immediate perioperative complications of urethroplasty in the United States: data from the national inpatient sample 2000-2010. Urology. 2015;85(5):1190–4. https://doi.org/10.1016/j.urology.2015.01.008. Epub 2015 Mar 4. PMID: 25746579; PMCID: PMC4917203.

Summary of Experts Panels' Recommendations for the Management of Urethral Injury

34

Considering the multiple controversies and the shadow areas that cover the management of urethral injuries, given the confusing grading systems, the low level of evidence of most of the publications, and the complexity and multiplicity of the described surgical approaches, a summary of the salient points of the guidelines will be of great help in order to cement the learning process of this pathological entity. In this chapter, an effort was made to combine and harmonize the recommendations enacted by various international expert panels, namely the European Association of Urology (EAU) [1], the American Urological Association (AUA) [2], the joint "Sociéte Internationale d'Urologie-International Consultation on Urological Diseases" (SIU-ICUD) [3, 4], the World Society of Emergency Surgery and the American Association for the Surgery of Trauma (WSES-AAST) [5], the Urological Society of India (USI) [6], and WHO consensuses [7].

34.1 Prevention

The EAU panel strongly recommends **training the medical and paramedical personnel in the proper technique of urethral catheterization** in order to reduce urethral trauma [1].

34.2 Investigations

– **RUG is at present the best technique for defining the site and nature of the urethral injury**. It should be performed by an experienced operator for diagnostic and staging purposes. Well-performed RUG should visualize the whole urethra, including the bladder neck when possible, to indicate the location and degree of the injury.

S. A. AL-Mamari, *Urogenital Trauma: A Practical Guide*,
https://doi.org/10.1007/978-981-99-6171-9_34

- **Clinicians should perform retrograde urethrography in patients with urethral injuries** (blood at the urethral meatus after pelvic trauma) [1–3, 5]. Alternatively, a flexible cystourethroscopic evaluation can be performed, and additionally, a vaginoscopy can be offered in female patients [1, 3, 5]

34.3 Treatment

Prompt urinary drainage (transurethral catheterization or suprapubic urinary diversion) should be performed in iatrogenic and partial blunt anterior (straddle) or posterior urethral injuries [1–6]. **If successfully inserted, the urethral catheter should be kept for 3–6 weeks** [3].

Immediate urethroplasty (<48 h) should not be performed in males with PFUI because of high morbidity [2, 3]. **However, Complete blunt anterior urethral injuries (straddle type) can be managed by immediate urethroplasty provided surgical expertise is available** [4, 6]. Otherwise, it is safer to insert a suprapubic catheter and consider referral to expert surgeons for delayed urethroplasty [7].

For uncomplicated penetrating trauma of the anterior urethra, experts recommend performing immediate direct surgical repair [2, 5].

The SIU/ICUD recommends excision and primary anastomosis (EPA) urethroplasty as the optimal treatment for short bulbar strictures in healthy men since it is reported to have a success rate of >90% for primary procedures [4, 6].

Treat pelvic fracture urethral injuries (PFUIs) in hemodynamically unstable patients by transurethral or suprapubic catheterization initially. For stable patients, early endoscopic realignment can be attempted in males with PFUI. However, if this fails, repeat endoscopic treatment should be avoided [1, 2, 5]. The WSES-AAST recommends a primary repair for penetrating injuries of the posterior urethra if the clinical conditions are favorable, an exception being made for complex pelvic fractures, where definitive surgical repair of the PFUI should be carried out only after healing of the pelvic ring [5].

For blunt anterior urethral injury: urinary drainage (urethral catheter or SPC) and attempt of endoscopic realignment before surgery and considering delayed surgical repair if failure of conservative and minimally invasive approaches [5].

Immediate surgery for urethral injury is also suggested by the WHO consensus panel in the following circumstances: the need for debridement, open injury, associated penile fracture or other injuries, and emergency procedures performed for other indications (fractures, injury to other organs) [7].

Early urethroplasty (2 days to 6 weeks) can be performed by expert surgeons for selected PFUIs patients with complete disruption who are stable, have a short urethral gap and a soft perineum, and can be put in a lithotomy position [1].

SIU-ICUD doesn't recommend early open retropubic primary suture repair or open retropubic catheter realignment because of the high morbidity but recommends immediate primary repair of the concomitant bladder, bladder neck, or rectal injuries and urethral catheter realignment of the PFUI to avoid subsequent urinary incontinence or pelvic sepsis [3]. SIU-ICUD also recommends early endoscopic and/or endourologic catheter realignment in stable patients which can be achieved by gentle simple retrograde catheterization or with the use of a flexible cystoscope and retrograde passage of a guidewire, or through the combined use of a flexible and rigid cystoscope introduced antegradely and retrogradely through a suprapubic tract [3].

Otherwise, the best management is to perform a suprapubic diversion and deferred (3–6 months) urethroplasty [1, 3, 6]. And for this delayed repair, the perineal midline progressive approach is recommended by the SIU-ICUD which warns at the same time against prolonged extended lithotomy position which should not exceed 5 h to avoid lower limbs vascular and neurological complications [3].

For females with PFUIs, an early repair (within 7 days) is recommended, rather than a simple realignment of a delayed repair [1].

34.4 Follow-Up

Patients should be monitored for complications arising from the urethral injury for **at least one year** (stricture formation, incontinence, erectile dysfunction) [2] and **urethroscopy or urethrography are the methods of choice** to evaluate the urethral repair and detect recurrent stenosis [5].

The USI recommends performing **Uroflowmetry at 3, 6, 9, and 12 months and then yearly**, to reassess the stricture urethra and considers values of >12 mL/s after a urethroplasty as optimal [6].

The SCI-ICUD recommends individualized management of post-traumatic incontinence where bladder repair should be performed, or an artificial urinary sphincter implanted, and when these procedures failed or are not feasible, continent urinary diversion should be contemplated [3]. The same expert panel suggests the early use of type 5-phosphodiesterase inhibitors to increase the chance of improvement of post-injury erectile dysfunction but recommends further evaluation of their effectiveness in this scenario [3]. For post-traumatic urethral fistula, the panel recommends ample exposure, complete excision of the tract, and interposition of a well-vascularized flap [3].

References

1. McCague EJ, Semans JH. The management of traumatic rupture of the urethra and bladder complicating fracture of the pelvis. J Urol. 1944;52:36–41.
2. Barratt RC, Bernard J, Mundy AR, Greenwell TJ. Pelvic fracture urethral injury in males-mechanisms of injury, management options and outcomes. Transl Androl Urol. 2018;7(Suppl 1):S29–62. https://doi.org/10.21037/tau.2017.12.35. PMID: 29644168; PMCID: PMC5881191.
3. Turner-Warwick R. Complex traumatic posterior urethral strictures. J Urol. 1977;118(4):564–74. https://doi.org/10.1016/s0022-5347(17)58109-4. PMID: 916051.

4. Rajaian S, Rajadoss MP, Nayak S, Kekre NS. Traumatic rectourethral fistula repair: a potential application of porcine small intestinal submucosa. Indian J Urol. 2013;29(2):148–50. https://doi.org/10.4103/0970-1591.114041. PMID: 23956521; PMCID: PMC3737675.
5. Koraitim MM. Pelvic fracture urethral injuries: the unresolved controversy. J Urol. 1999;161(5):1433–41. PMID: 10210368.
6. Koraitim MM. The lessons of 145 posttraumatic posterior urethral strictures treated in 17 years. J Urol. 1995;153(1):63–6. https://doi.org/10.1097/00005392-199501000-00024. PMID: 7966793.
7. Blaschko SD, Harris CR, Zaid UB, Gaither T, Chu C, Alwaal A, McAninch JW, McCulloch CE, Breyer BN. Trends, utilization, and immediate perioperative complications of urethroplasty in the United States: data from the national inpatient sample 2000-2010. Urology. 2015;85(5):1190–4. https://doi.org/10.1016/j.urology.2015.01.008. Epub 2015 Mar 4. PMID: 25746579; PMCID: PMC4917203.

Part V
Penile Injuries

The male organ for copulation and the shield which protects the urethra. This is the double function that one stands to lose if he doesn't take care of his penis.

Introduction to Penile Injury

Throughout history, the penis has been a source of mankind's fascination and almost always played an important role in myths, philosophy, religions, arts, science, politics, and even the economy. Its first representations can be traced up to the Paleolithic period when male organ depictions were engraved in caves and portable phalli were sculpted [1].

The penis was a subject of cult worship and veneration in ancient civilizations (Greece, Rome, etc.), the symbol of corruption and sins in ancient India and medieval Christian Europe, the object of sculpture and painting in the renaissance period, and of advanced anatomic research in the following centuries, the cause of the obsession of White explorers and settlers impressed by the size of this organ in Africans, and one of the bases of Freudian philosophy. Nowadays, it has become a lucrative business for pharmaceutical companies with the development of drugs and techniques to treat erectile impotence [2, 3].

Penile trauma is very rare. However, it creates very embarrassing situations for the patients. This can first be explained by the causes of trauma which can be more or less socially acceptable. Well beyond its social discomfort, penile injury covers a wide range of grades from a mild superficial incision up to complete severance or destruction of the organ. Fortunately, the majority of penile traumas are of mild to moderate grades with **zipper-related penis injuries (ZIRPI)** and **penile fractures (PF)** holding the top of the list, and their repairs are well mastered nowadays by most of the urology institutions with excellent results [4, 5].

The true tragedy of penile trauma occurs when this organ is amputated or irreversibly damaged. The victim becomes devirilized, hence dehumanized. From this instant, his world collapses, and he tumbles from hero to zero. He is no more the same person. He has lost his pride and perhaps also his dignity. More than anybody else, these patients need strong psychological support and solid family bonds to recover, albeit partly, from the trauma. Each word counts, each smile is important, and each solicitude and benevolent gaze counts for millions, while any awkward comment or joke could irretrievably destroy the whole chain of their psychological reconstruction. When one comprehends this drama, he/she can only fully appreciate the development of penile reconstructive and replantation techniques [6].

References

1. Angulo JC, García-Díez M. Male genital representation in paleolithic art: erection and circumcision before history. Urology. 2009;74:10–4.
2. Twisselmann B. A mind of its own: a cultural history of the penis. BMJ. 2002;325(7377):1427.
3. Friedman DM. A mind of its own: a cultural history of the penis. London: Robert Hale; 2001.
4. Rodriguez D, Li K, Apoj M, Munarriz R. Epidemiology of penile fractures in United States emergency departments: access to care disparities may lead to suboptimal outcomes. J Sex Med. 2019;16(2):248–56. https://doi.org/10.1016/j.jsxm.2018.12.009.
5. Amer T, Wilson R, Chlosta P, AlBuheissi S, Qazi H, Fraser M, Aboumarzouk OM. Penile fracture: a meta-analysis. Urol Int. 2016;96(3):315–29. https://doi.org/10.1159/000444884. Epub 2016 Mar 9.
6. Yao A, Ingargiola MJ, Lopez CD, Sanati-Mehrizy P, Burish NM, Jablonka EM, Taub PJ. Total penile reconstruction: a systematic review. J Plast Reconstr Aesthet Surg. 2018;71(6):788–806. https://doi.org/10.1016/j.bjps.2018.02.002. Epub 2018 Feb 14.

35 Anatomy of the Penis

35.1 Embryology of the Penis

In 1954, Glenister proposed the so-called *ectodermal intrusion theory of penile urethral development within the glans*, whereby the penis is formed from the surface ectoderm growing into the glans and joining the endodermal urethral plate at the junction of the penile body and the glans [1, 2]. This can explain why the most frequent location of hypospadias is at the junction between the penile shaft and the glans penis, namely at the coronal sulcus [3].

It is admitted today that the external genitalia originate from the three embryonic layers: penile skin and prepuce from the ectoderm, the erectile tissue and the stroma from the mesoderm, and the urethral plate from the endoderm [2, 4].

During organogenesis, the Y chromosome induces male differentiation through the sex-determining region Y (SRY) protein gene, which is responsible for testicular development. Cell lineage analysis has revealed the formation of two populations of progenitor cells originating at the right and left edges of the posterior hind limb buds and anterior tail of the embryo. During body wall closure, the two edges are united at the ventral midline, forming the paired genital swellings that give rise to the **genital tubercle** [5].

Both the human penis and the clitoris develop from the genital tubercle at approximately 8 weeks. The differentiation into a penis as well as the development of the scrotum is triggered by the androgens produced by the testicular Leydig cells. These cells are stimulated by a surge of luteinizing hormone (LH) produced by the pituitary gland which develops between the seventh and tenth week. The testosterone will be converted by 5-alpha-reductase to dihydrotestosterone (DHT), the active androgen responsible for the differentiation of the genital tubercle and urogenital folds into the male phallus. The development of the penis proceeds through the formation of a tubular urethra arising from the canalization of the urethral plate. In males the urethral folds or edges of the resulting wide diamond-shaped urethral groove fuse in the midline, while in females, deprived of androgens, the urethral

S. A. AL-Mamari, *Urogenital Trauma: A Practical Guide*,
https://doi.org/10.1007/978-981-99-6171-9_35

plate undergoes canalization resulting in a wide vestibular groove whose edges (vestibular folds) remain unfused. The vestibular folds ultimately form the labia minora defining the vaginal vestibule [2, 3, 6, 7].

Baskin et al. demonstrated that although the differentiation starts at the ninth week, the penis and the clitoris are still similar in size until the twelfth week when the penile size becomes clearly larger. Nonetheless, the orientation of the penis obviously projects at a 90-degree angle from the body from the ninth week, while the clitoris remains close to the body wall [2] (Fig. 35.1).

At about 13 weeks, the dorsal prepuce develops and begins to envelop the glans in both genders. Its pattern differs by 14–15 weeks where it assumes a circumferential shape in males in contrast to the females where it does not fuse ventrally [2].

As expected from the embryological origin, the developing human penis and clitoris have **similar neurovascular anatomy**, and **similar corporal bodies** that

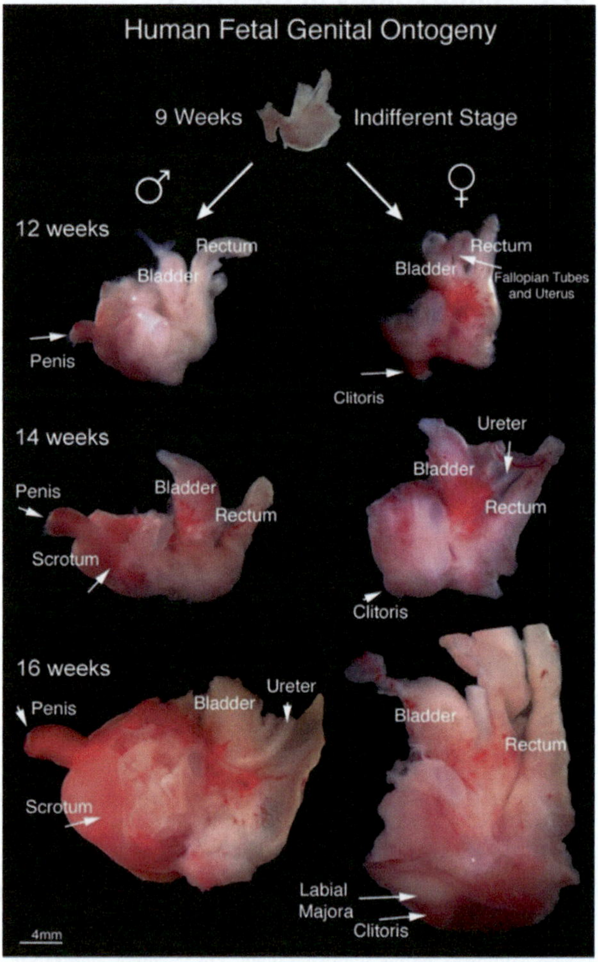

Fig. 35.1 Gross Human Fetal Pelvic Ontogeny: Gross ontogeny of the human fetal pelvis at 9 weeks of gestation (end of indifferent stage), 12 weeks, 14 weeks, and 16 weeks of gestation. Note the divergent development after 9 weeks of gestation, especially with respect to the orientation of the external genitalia with the penis clearly visible at a 90-degree angle from the body and the clitoris recessed close to the body wall. (From Baskin L et al. [2], with permission from Elsevier)

are made of thick tunica albuginea surrounding sinusoidal erectile tissue, and **analogous glans** distally which is covered by the **prepuce** in both genders. **The major difference between them is the lack of tubular urethra within the clitoris** [6].

35.2 Histology

The **tunica albuginea** is a bi-layered structure made of **an inner circular layer and an outer longitudinal one**, the latter being an incomplete coat interrupted between the 5 and 7 o'clock points where it is replaced by two triangular ligamentous structures referred to as the **ventral thickening**. There is also a **dorsal thickening** between 1 and 11 o'clock. Cadaveric studies have clarified the relationship between the perineal skeletal and smooth muscles with the tunica albuginea and showed that the ventral thickening is a continuation of the anterior fibers of the left and right bulbospongiosus muscles, and the dorsal thickening is a radiating aspect of the bilateral ischiocavernosus muscles [8]. A continuation of the outer longitudinal layer of the tunica, the **distal ligament**, forms a **central trunk** in the glans penis ensuring its rigidity and allowing it to resist the coital pressure as a penetrating ogive [8].

Another cadaveric study has demonstrated that **the tensile strength of the tunica albuginea is 1500 mmHg**, which means that any pressure above this value will produce its herniation or its fracture [9].

35.3 Gross Anatomy

35.3.1 General Aspects

The penis is the male organ for copulation. A systematic review including a final selection of 20 articles for a total of 15.521 men showed an average length of 9.16 cm, 13.24 cm, and 13.12 cm for flaccid pendulous, stretched, and erected penis respectively, and an average girth of 9.31 and 11.66 cm for flaccid and erected penis, respectively [10]. This study was inconclusive for any racial variability due to insufficient sampling and poor methodology of relevant articles, and, contrary to a general belief, no significant correlation was found between the penile size and the individual height, BMI, digits, testicular volume, foot size, and age.

The penis can be divided into three portions: The root, the shaft, and the glans.

- The **penile root** is the fixed part of the penis and consists of **cavernosal crura** attached to the pubic arch and to the urogenital diaphragm, and the **spongious bulb** adherent to the urogenital diaphragm.
- The **penile shaft** is the pendulous anterior portion that is suspended from the lower anterior surface of the symphysis pubis and its structure is formed by three cylindrical erectile bodies: **two fused dorsolateral corpora cavernosa** divided by an **incomplete septum** and covered by the **tunica albuginea**, and a smaller

corpus spongiosum lying in the ventral groove between the corpora cavernosa and containing the urethra. The **Buck's fascia** envelops all three structures. More superficially is a fine and loose areolar subcutaneous tissue, devoid of fat, referred to as **Dartos fascia**, that surrounds the deep fascia penis and contains the superficial blood vessels, nerves, and lymphatics. This fascia is the continuation of the fused two superficial fasciae of the lower abdomen, scrotum, and femoral triangles, namely **Camper's and Scarpa's fascia** [11, 12] (Fig. 35.2).

- The **penile glans** is the conical expanded end of the corpus spongiosum. It is separated from the shaft by the **corona**. At birth and in uncircumcised men, the glans is covered by a skin fold, called the **prepuce or foreskin**. As mentioned above, the prepuce covers not only the glans penis in males, but also the glans clitoris in females of humans and other primates, and paleontological studies estimated its presence for at least 65 to 100 million years [13].

35.3.2 Blood Supply

The blood supply of the penis arises from the **superficial and deep pudendal arteries, branches of the femoral artery**. During an erection, the engorgement of the corpora cavernosa and the enlargement of the glans are made of blood conveyed by branches of the pudendal artery, namely the **paired cavernosal artery**, and the

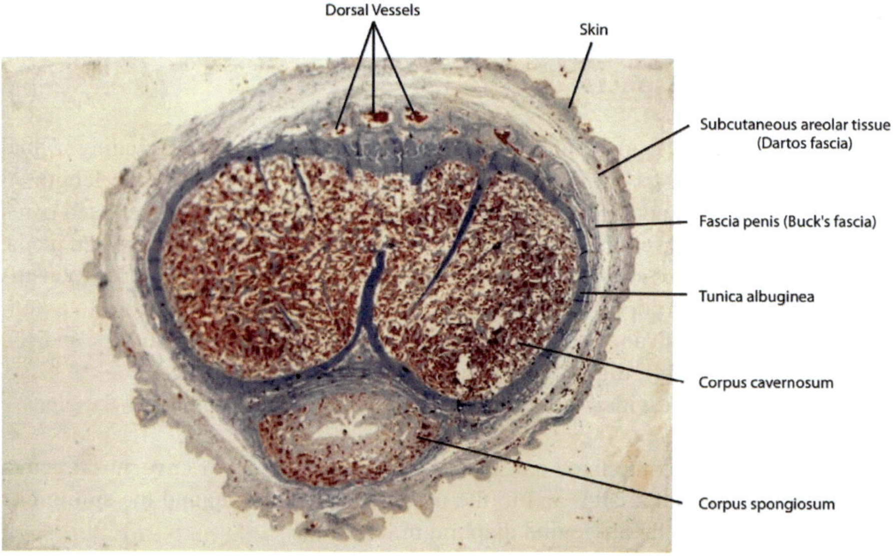

Fig. 35.2 Cross-section showing the penile layers. (From Quartey J.K [11], with permission from Springer Nature)

deep dorsal artery, respectively. In addition, there are **paired dorsal, and bulbourethral arteries** that supply the skin and the urethra with extensive anastomotic connections [14]. The venous return is ensured by multiple emissary veins from the corpora cavernosa and circumflex veins from the corpus spongiosum draining into a **single deep dorsal vein** [14].

35.3.3 Nerve Supply

- **Somatic innervation**: The dorsal skin sensation is conveyed by dorsal nerves lying within Buck's fascia, while the ventral shaft skin and the frenulum are supplied by perineal nerves, and the cavernosal nerves lying within the corpora cavernosa are responsible for sexual function. The prepuce has a particularly dense innervation network supplied by somatosensory nerves arising from both the dorsal nerve of the penis and branches of the perineal nerves. Meissner's corpuscles predominate within the somatosensory receptors and are responsible for sensing light touch. Special receptors for sensing pressure, vibratory stimuli, and pain are also present [7, 14].
- Fetal studies showed an extension of nerves from the dorsal neurovascular bundle of the prostate to form two bundles under the pubic arch which join the corporeal bodies at the proximal origin and immediately fan out along the surface of the corporeal tissue to the junction of the urethral spongiosum. From here, they extend to the 11 and 1 o'clock positions of the penile shaft and glans but remain very scarce or absent at the 12 o'clock position in the dorsal midline [14, 15].
- **Autonomic innervation**: The pelvic plexus supplies parasympathetic innervation from the sacral plexus (S2–S4) and sympathetic innervation from the thoracolumbar center (T11-L2) [7].

35.4 Congenital Penile Abnormalities

A global increase in the incidence of congenital penile anomalies (CPAs) has been observed in the 30–40 last years. An American nationwide inpatient sample showed that the incidence of CPAs has increased in the USA from 7.0/1000 newborns in 1988–1991 to 8.3/1000 in 1997–2000, **with hypospadias being the most common diagnosis (68.3%), followed by chordee (8.6%) and the combination hypospadias-chordee (5%)** [16]. Correlations were found with races (highest in whites, then Blacks, Asians, and Hispanics), and socio-economic status (higher in rich than in poor communities).

A murine study showed that the full spectrum of CPAs can be produced by disrupting androgen receptors, obtaining different effects according to the developmental stages and the specific cell types of genital tubercle: thus, earlier disruptions cause ambiguous genitalia and later events cause micropenis, and in prenatal development, they induce hypospadias and chordee [17].

- Frequent CPAs [18, 19]:
  - **Phimosis**: should not be confused with the physiologic phimosis found in 96% of newborns.
  - **Paraphimosis**
  - **Balanitis xerotica obliterans**
  - **Penile skin cysts, naevi, or vascular lesions**
  - **Congenital curvature (chordee)**: Rarely occurring without hypospadias (4–10%). Possible etiologies are skin chordee, fibrotic fascia (dartos and Buck's), corporal disproportion, and congenital short urethra [20].
  - **Isolated penile torsion**: Mild degree of isolated penile torsion occurs in 1.7–27% of newborns, but torsion of more than 45° are rare (4.3%) and those of more than 90° are extremely rare (0.7%) [20, 21].
  - **Hypospadias**: Incidence 1 in 250 boys
- Rare CPAs [22]:
  - Congenital webbed penis or penis palmatus
  - Congenital concealed penis or buried penis or Megaprepuce
  - Micropenis
  - Megaphallus
  - Intrauterine amputation of the penis
  - Epispadias: Mostly associated with bladder exstrophy, isolated in 10% of cases.
- Extremely rare abnormalities (only few cases reported in the literature):
  - Dorsal penile frenulum (only three cases reported) [22, 23]
  - Aphallia or penile agenesis: Around 100 cases are reported in the world with an estimated incidence of 1 in 10–30 million births. This anomaly is associated with an intra-uterine development of a urethra-rectal fistula allowing urine to pass by the anus [22, 24, 25] (Fig. 35.3).
  - Diphallia or double penis: Only approximately 100 cases are reported in the literature, with an incidence of one in every five to six million live births [22, 26] (Fig. 35.4).
  - Triphallia or triple penis: To date, only one case has been reported in the literature [27].

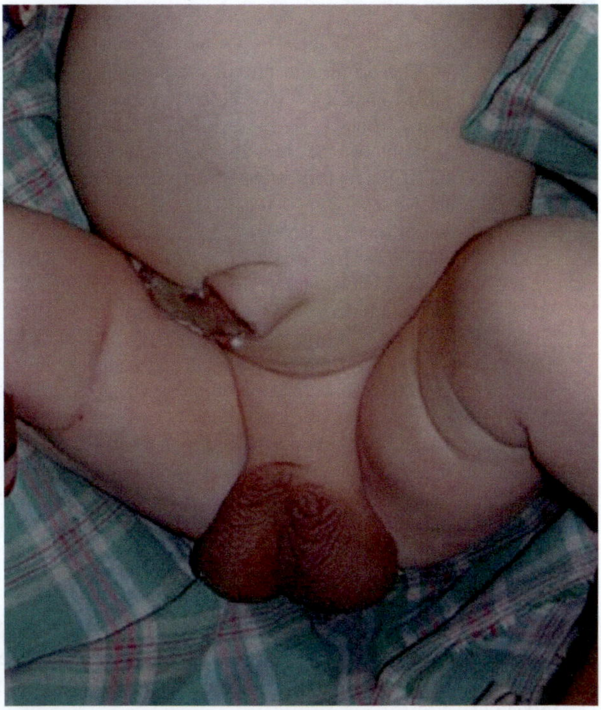

Fig. 35.3 Neonate with aphallia and normal testicle. (From Fahmy MAB [22], with permission from Springer Nature)

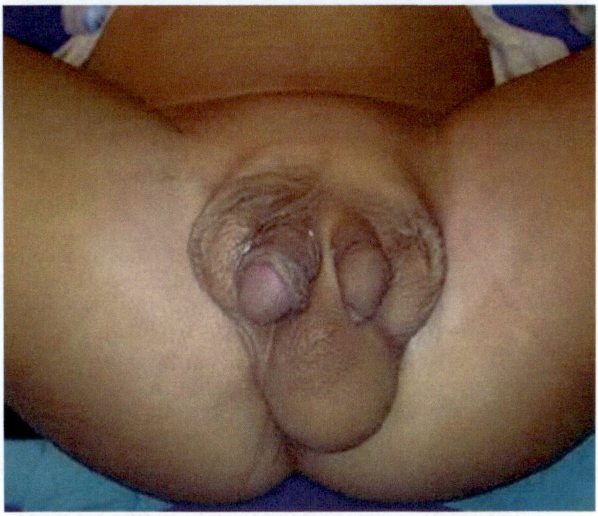

Fig. 35.4 Complete diphallia with two urethral openings and two scrotums. (From Fahmy MAB [22], with permission from Springer Nature)

References

1. Glenister TW. The origin and fate of the urethral plate in man. J Anat. 1954;88(3):413–25. PMID: 13192029; PMCID: PMC1244688.
2. Baskin L, Shen J, Sinclair A, Cao M, Liu X, Liu G, Isaacson D, Overland M, Li Y, Cunha GR. Development of the human penis and clitoris. Differentiation. 2018;103:74–85. https://doi.org/10.1016/j.diff.2018.08.001. Epub 2018 Aug 23. PMID: 30249413; PMCID: PMC6234061.
3. Baskin L. What is hypospadias? Clin Pediatr (Phila). 2017;56(5):409–18. https://doi.org/10.1177/0009922816684613. Epub 2017 Jan 12. PMID: 28081624.
4. van der Werff JF, Nievelstein RA, Brands E, Luijsterburg AJ, Vermeij-Keers C. Normal development of the male anterior urethra. Teratology. 2000;61(3):172–83. https://doi.org/10.1002/(SICI)1096-9926(200003)61:3<172::AID-TERA4>3.0.CO;2-B. PMID: 10661906.
5. Herrera AM, Cohn MJ. Embryonic origin and compartmental organization of the external genitalia. Sci Rep. 2014;4:6896. https://doi.org/10.1038/srep06896. PMID: 25372631; PMCID: PMC4894444.
6. Li Y, Sinclair A, Cao M, Shen J, Choudhry S, Botta S, Cunha G, Baskin L. Canalization of the urethral plate precedes fusion of the urethral folds during male penile urethral development: the double zipper hypothesis. J Urol. 2015;193(4):1353–9. https://doi.org/10.1016/j.juro.2014.09.108. Epub 2014 Oct 5. PMID: 25286011; PMCID: PMC4456085.
7. Hudson RG, Ebbers M. Embryology of the penis. In: Bolnick D, Koyle M, Yosha A, editors. Surgical guide to circumcision. London: Springer; 2012. https://doi.org/10.1007/978-1-4471-2858-8_3.
8. Hsu GL, Hsieh CH, Wen HS, Hsu WL, Wu CH, Fong TH, Chen SC, Tseng GF. Anatomy of the human penis: the relationship of the architecture between skeletal and smooth muscles. J Androl. 2004;25(3):426–31. https://doi.org/10.1002/j.1939-4640.2004.tb02810.x. PMID: 15064322.
9. Bitsch M, Kromann-Andersen B, Schou J, Sjøntoft E. The elasticity and the tensile strength of tunica albuginea of the corpora cavernosa. J Urol. 1990;143(3):642–5. https://doi.org/10.1016/s0022-5347(17)40047-4. PMID: 2304187.
10. Veale D, Miles S, Bramley S, Muir G, Hodsoll J. Am I normal? A systematic review and construction of nomograms for flaccid and erect penis length and circumference in up to 15,521 men. BJU Int. 2015;115(6):978–86. https://doi.org/10.1111/bju.13010. Epub 2015 Mar 2. PMID: 25487360.
11. Quartey JK. Anatomy and blood supply of the urethra and penis. In: Schreiter F, Jordan G, editors. Urethral reconstructive surgery. Berlin: Springer; 2006. https://doi.org/10.1007/3-540-29385-X_3.
12. MacKay MD, Mudreac A, Varacallo M. Anatomy, abdomen and pelvis, camper fascia. In: StatPearls [internet]. Treasure Island: StatPearls Publishing; 2022. PMID: 29489166.
13. Cold CJ, Taylor JR. The prepuce. BJU Int. 1999;83(Suppl 1):34–44. https://doi.org/10.1046/j.1464-410x.1999.0830s1034.x. PMID: 10349413.
14. Yiee JH, Baskin LS. Penile embryology and anatomy. ScientificWorldJournal. 2010;10:1174–9. https://doi.org/10.1100/tsw.2010.112. PMID: 20602076; PMCID: PMC5763683.
15. Akman Y, Liu W, Li YW, Baskin LS. Penile anatomy under the pubic arch: reconstructive implications. J Urol. 2001;166(1):225–30. PMID: 11435874.
16. Nelson CP, Park JM, Wan J, Bloom DA, Dunn RL, Wei JT. The increasing incidence of congenital penile anomalies in the United States. J Urol. 2005;174(4 Pt 2):1573–6. https://doi.org/10.1097/01.ju.0000179249.21944.7e. PMID: 16148654.
17. Zheng Z, Armfield BA, Cohn MJ. Timing of androgen receptor disruption and estrogen exposure underlies a spectrum of congenital penile anomalies. Proc Natl Acad Sci U S A. 2015;112(52):E7194–203. https://doi.org/10.1073/pnas.1515981112. Epub 2015 Nov 23. PMID: 26598695; PMCID: PMC4703017.

18. Castagnetti M, Leonard M, Guerra L, Esposito C, Cimador M. Benign penile skin anomalies in children: a primer for pediatricians. World J Pediatr. 2015;11(4):316–23. https://doi.org/10.1007/s12519-015-0015-5. Epub 2015 Mar 9. PMID: 25754752.
19. Boillot B, Teklali Y, Moog R, Droupy S. Les malformations congénitales du pénis [Penile congenital abnormalities]. Prog Urol. 2013;23(9):664–73. French. Epub 2013 Apr 4. https://doi.org/10.1016/j.purol.2013.01.022. PMID: 23830261.
20. Montag S, Palmer LS. Abnormalities of penile curvature: chordee and penile torsion. ScientificWorldJournal. 2011;11:1470–8. https://doi.org/10.1100/tsw.2011.136. PMID: 21805016; PMCID: PMC5720069.
21. Eroglu E, Gundogdu G. Isolated penile torsion in newborns. Can Urol Assoc J. 2015;9(11–12):E805–7. https://doi.org/10.5489/cuaj.2833. Epub 2015 Nov 4. PMID: 26600889; PMCID: PMC4639432.
22. Fahmy MAB. Penis. In: Rare congenital genitourinary anomalies. Berlin: Springer; 2015. https://doi.org/10.1007/978-3-662-43680-6_2.
23. Mukendi AM, Doherty SW. Dorsal penile frenulum: a rare congenital abnormality. Afr J Urol. 2019;25:1. https://doi.org/10.1186/s12301-019-0001-6.
24. Talebpour Amiri F, Nasiry Zarrin Ghabaee D, Naeimi RA, Seyedi SJ, Mousavi SA. Aphallia: report of three cases and literature review. Int J Reprod Biomed. 2016;14(4):279–84. PMID: 27351031; PMCID: PMC4918779.
25. Qiang S, Li FY, Zhou Y, Yuan Y, Li Q. Congenital absence of the penis (aphallia): a rare case report. Medicine (Baltimore). 2019;98(15):e15129. https://doi.org/10.1097/MD.0000000000015129. PMID: 30985678; PMCID: PMC6485865.
26. Mirshemirani AR, Sadeghyian N, Mohajerzadeh L, Molayee H, Ghaffari P. Diphallus: report on six cases and review of the literature. Iran J Pediatr. 2010;20(3):353–7. PMID: 23056729; PMCID: PMC3446048.
27. Jabali SS, Mohammed AA. Triphallia (triple penis), the first reported case in human. Int J Surg Case Rep. 2020;77:198–200. https://doi.org/10.1016/j.ijscr.2020.11.008. Epub 2020 Nov 4. PMID: 33166819; PMCID: PMC7652711.

36 Epidemiology of Penile Injury

Penile injuries mostly consist of circumcision mishaps in children, penile fractures in adults, and zipper entrapment at all ages. Other causes include non-sexual-related accidents, assaults, and self-inflicted injuries.

There are approximately 2000 cases of **zipper-related penis injury (ZIRPI)** reported every year in the world [1]. Since penile fracture represents the most frequent cause of penile trauma in patients seeking help in hospitals and referred to specialized Urology care, it will cover the largest place in the following discussion. The first report on penile fracture in modern medical literature was written in 1925 [2]. It mostly occurs during sexual activity and mainly affects young adults with a mean age of **36–39 years** [3–5], and its incidence varies with ethnicity and geographical regions. It has been globally estimated to be 1 in 175,000 male population but was found to reach 1.02 to 1.8 per 100,000 in the United States or to be as higher as 1.14 to 10.48 per 100,000 men in Iran [6–9] where every urologist may encounter a case of penile fracture every 3.5 months.

Apart from penile fractures, other penile injuries are extremely rare and no robust epidemiological study can be reliably made. A recent comprehensive American national database review including 753 accredited trauma centers recruited 722 patients with **penile gunshot wounds**, representing 1.7% of all GSW [10].

Cases of **genital self-mutilations** (GSM) are reported here and there in association with psychiatric instabilities. This pathological entity will be discussed separately in a special section at the end of this book. Assaults account also for an extremely low percentage of penile injuries. A noteworthy epidemic of penile amputation was observed in Thailand in the 1970s perpetrated by angry wives against philandering husbands, with an estimate of 100 such incidents between 1973 and 1980 [11].

S. A. AL-Mamari, *Urogenital Trauma: A Practical Guide*, https://doi.org/10.1007/978-981-99-6171-9_36

References

1. Leslie SW, Sajjad H, Taylor RS. Penile Zipper and ring injuries. In: StatPearls [Internet]. Treasure Island: StatPearls Publishing; 2022. PMID: 28722916.
2. Malis J. Zur Kasuistik der Fractura Penis. Arch Clin Chir. 1925;129:651–3.
3. Phillips EA, Esposito AJ, Munarriz R. Acute penile trauma and associated morbidity: 9-year experience at a tertiary care center. Andrology. 2015;3(3):632–6. https://doi.org/10.1111/andr.12043. PMID: 26013107.
4. Barros R, Hampl D, Cavalcanti AG, Favorito LA, Koifman L. Lessons learned after 20 years' experience with penile fracture. Int Braz J Urol. 2020;46(3):409–16. https://doi.org/10.1590/S1677-5538.IBJU.2019.0367. PMID: 32167705; PMCID: PMC7088490.
5. Falcone M, Garaffa G, Castiglione F, Ralph DJ. Current management of penile fracture: an up-to-date systematic review. Sex Med Rev. 2018;6(2):253–60. https://doi.org/10.1016/j.sxmr.2017.07.009. Epub 2017 Sep 2. PMID: 28874325.
6. Amer T, Wilson R, Chlosta P, AlBuheissi S, Qazi H, Fraser M, Aboumarzouk OM. Penile fracture: a meta-analysis. Urol Int. 2016;96(3):315–29. https://doi.org/10.1159/000444884. Epub 2016 Mar 9. PMID: 26953932.
7. Rodriguez D, Li K, Apoj M, Munarriz R. Epidemiology of penile fractures in United States emergency departments: access to care disparities may lead to suboptimal outcomes. J Sex Med. 2019;16(2):248–56. https://doi.org/10.1016/j.jsxm.2018.12.009. PMID: 30770071.
8. Christian-Miller N, Lenis AT, Fero KE, Madrigral J, Eleswarapu SV, Chamie K, Benharash P. Risk factors for penile fracture compared with a surgical control cohort in the United States: the role of substance abuse. Asian J Androl. 2021;23(3):236–9. https://doi.org/10.4103/aja.aja_70_20. PMID: 33243961; PMCID: PMC8152430.
9. Mirzazadeh M, Fallahkarkan M, Hosseini J. Penile fracture epidemiology, diagnosis and management in Iran: a narrative review. Transl Androl Urol. 2017;6(2):158–66. https://doi.org/10.21037/tau.2016.12.03. PMID: 28540222; PMCID: PMC5422687.
10. Maxwell BG, Chouhan JD, Lundeberg MR, Liu JJ. National patterns of injury and outcomes of gunshot wounds to the penis: a trauma quality programs retrospective cohort analysis. Acute Med Surg. 2021;8(1):e636. https://doi.org/10.1002/ams2.636. PMID: 33747534; PMCID: PMC7962619.
11. Bhanganada K, Chayavatana T, Pongnumkul C, Tonmukayakul A, Sakolsatayadorn P, Komaratat K, Wilde H. Surgical management of an epidemic of penile amputations in Siam. Am J Surg. 1983;146(3):376–82. https://doi.org/10.1016/0002-9610(83)90420-8. PMID: 6614331.

37 Etiology, Mechanism, and Anatomopathology of Penile Injury

Although rare, penile trauma produces a wide range of anatomopathological forms including open injuries (biting, stabbing, or gunshot) and blunt injuries. Open injuries comprise multiple forms of gravity from a superficial incision with or without skin loss to a total amputation of the organ. Blunt trauma mainly consists of penile fracture but includes also injuries by constricting devices, etc.

Multiple mechanisms can be associated with penile injury including stabbing, animal or human bites, burns, gunshots, constricting rings, and degloving machinery. However, **the most frequent mechanism in adults and in children is zipper-related penis injury (ZIRPI) by prepuce entrapment in uncircumcised individuals with roughly around 2000 reported cases yearly** [1]. Indeed, by premonition, the Swedish-American electrical engineer Gideon Sundback who patented the first zipper in 1917 as a "Separable Fastener" has reportedly expressed some reservations with regard to possible genital injury [1]. It is important to remember that ZIRPIs are extremely rare among circumcised males and are almost inexistent among Arabian Gulf Countries' citizens who have another reason to be spared: there is no zipper in their traditional costume.

A didactic way to study the penile injury etiology consists of the distinction between pediatric and adult causes as follows:

37.1 Pediatric Penile Injuries

ZIRPIs are probably the most common causes of penile injury in children but they are seldom reported. In the Islamic world, **circumcision complications** accounted for 67% of all pediatric penile injuries in a series of 64 boys with penile trauma [2]. However, complications occur in only 0.2% of circumcisions in the neonatal period [3], and may reach 1.7%, if performed late, and comprise a wide range from bleeding and malignant hyperthermia to disfigurement, partial or total amputation of the penis [4, 5]. In the abovementioned series from an Islamic population, less frequent

S. A. AL-Mamari, *Urogenital Trauma: A Practical Guide*,
https://doi.org/10.1007/978-981-99-6171-9_37

causes of penile injury after circumcision included mother's hair strangulation (16%), animal bite injuries (6%), bicycle accidents (6%), zipper injuries (3%), and electrical injuries (2%) [2]. The rarest causes are self-amputation and burns [6]. **Hair strangulation** also called "hair tourniquet syndrome of the penis" is caused by mother hairs and was almost exclusively reported in circumcised children in whom removal of the prepuce bares the coronal sulcus which is the most frequent site of the injury [7].

37.2 Adult Penile Injuries

Like in children, zipper entrapment is also probably the most common cause of penile injuries in uncircumcised adults. However, penile fracture related to sexual intercourse is the most frequent cause that leads the patient to the operating theater. Other causes involve penile strangulation, generally self-inflicted through the insertion of various objects such as heavy metal rings or plastic bottle-necks, etc. Another group is made of foreign bodies inserted through the urethra, which are also generally self-inflicted: wire, safety pin, etc. Penetrating injuries are also encountered: stabbing (knife, razor, etc.), gunshots, and blasts.

A 30-year single-institution retrospective study has recorded 110 patients with penetrating external genital trauma (penis and testicles), caused by gunshots, stabbing/lacerations, and bites, in 49%, 44%, and 7%, respectively, and half of the stabbing/lacerations were self-inflicted [8].

A correlation exists between conflict zones and increased occurrence of genito-urinary injuries. More specifically however, a trend toward fewer abdominal urological injuries was observed in well-equipped armies with the introduction of Kevlar body armor, while casualties involving unprotected anatomical areas such as the pelvis or external genitalia tended to increase in recent wars (Afghanistan and Iraq). This prompted the addition of a detachable genital flap on the Kevlar armor in 2004 [9] (Table 37.1).

There was an increased number of genito-urinary injuries in the US Army operations in Iraq and the majority involved the external genitalia (73.2%), including the scrotum, the testes, the penis, and/or urethra, and penile injuries alone occurred in

Table 37.1 Influence of body armor on urologic injury distribution in contemporary conflicts

Theater	Abdominal (%)	Pelvic/Genital (%)
Gulf War[a]	17	83
Bosnia	45	55
Croatia	48	52
Croatia	53	47

From Hudak SJ et al. [9], with permission from Elsevier

[a] Body armor was standard issue for all U.S. soldiers

423 US service members [10]. War-related penile injuries have also been described among Libyan and Iraqi populations as the consequence of gunshots and explosions and they involved both soldiers and civilians [11, 12].

Perhaps the largest study of penile gunshot injury is a recent comprehensive American national database review of 752 accredited trauma centers that identified 722 patients [13]. It revealed that the vast majority (90.7%) resulted from an assault, intentional self-harm, attempted suicide, or attempted homicide, while accidental injuries were very rare.

A systematic review of 86 cases of amputation has revealed that the most common cause was self-mutilation (43.9%), followed by partner violence (25.6%). Other less frequent causes were work injury (9.8%), circumcision complications (9.8%), assault (7.3%), and animal bites [14]. Indeed, hundreds of self-inflicted injuries have been reported in the medical literature and will be developed in a separate section at the end of this book due to their complex underlying etiology.

Genital electrocution has been exceptionally reported in the literature, and a new concept was introduced, the **Uromanual injury or uromanual high voltage trauma.** Its main cause is urination on a high-voltage electrical source resulting in damage to the urogenital area and upper extremities to various degrees, potentially leading to complete penile destruction and amputation (Fig. 37.1) [15]. The electricity is transmitted retrogradely by the urine from the power cable to the penis and the supporting hand(s) during micturition.

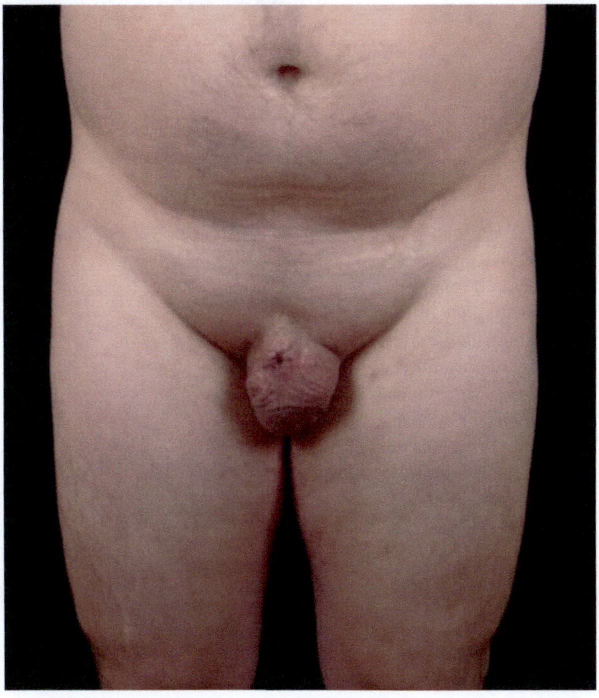

Fig. 37.1 Complete penile amputation due to uromanual high voltage trauma. (From Adamyan RT et al. [15], with permission from Wolters Kluwer)

Another peculiarity is the **penile dislocation** with inversion that resulted from a blunt pelvic trauma, with only a handful of cases reported in the literature [16–19]. The inversion may be total or partial, and the patient may present early in the acute episode, or late complaining of inability to perform sexual intercourse (Figs. 37.2, 37.3, and 37.4a, b).

Other rare events of external genital injury have occurred through inadvertent suction by a vacuum cleaner, and more exceptionally by a faulty circulation system in a swimming pool, especially with the Jacuzzi system (Fig. 37.5).

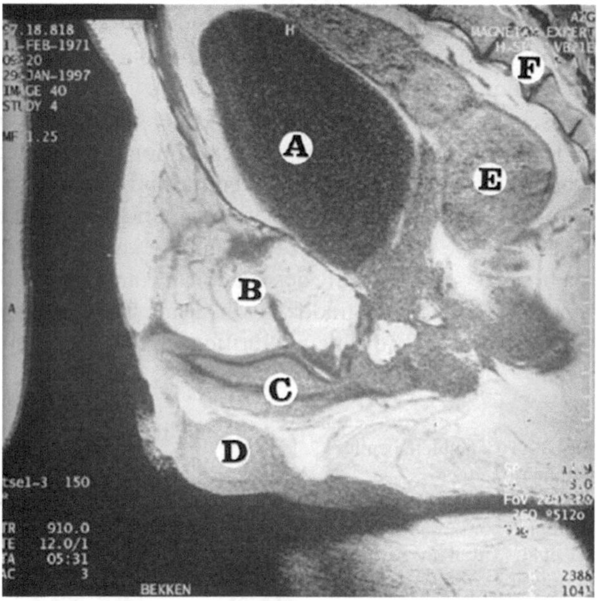

Fig. 37.2 Sagittal MRI of a 26-year-old man who sustained pelvic fracture in an RTA: (**a**) bladder; (**b**) 'herniation' of prevesical fat; (**c**) retracted corpora cavernosa; (**d**) right testicle; (**e**) bowel; and (**f**) coccyx bone. Note the absence of the pars pendulans penis. (From Simonis LA et al. [18], with permission from Springer Nature)

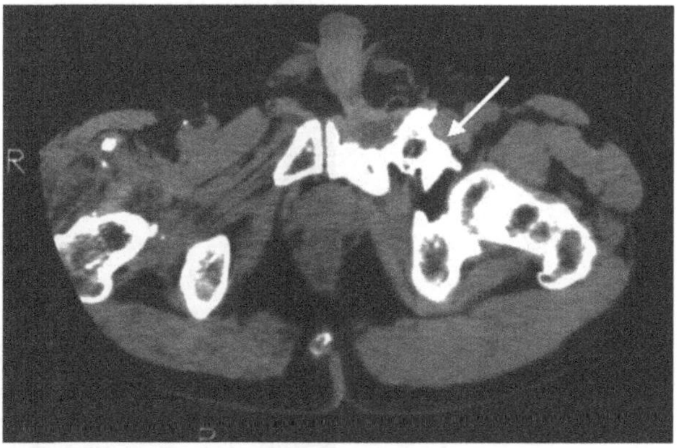

Fig. 37.3 Pelvis Computed Tomography of a 55-year-old man with a four-year history of RTA showing a fractured left pubic bone shifted inside (arrow) that was pulling the penis by its suspensory ligament. (From Masuda H et al. [19]. Copyright © 2004 Masuda et al.; licensee BioMed Central Ltd.)

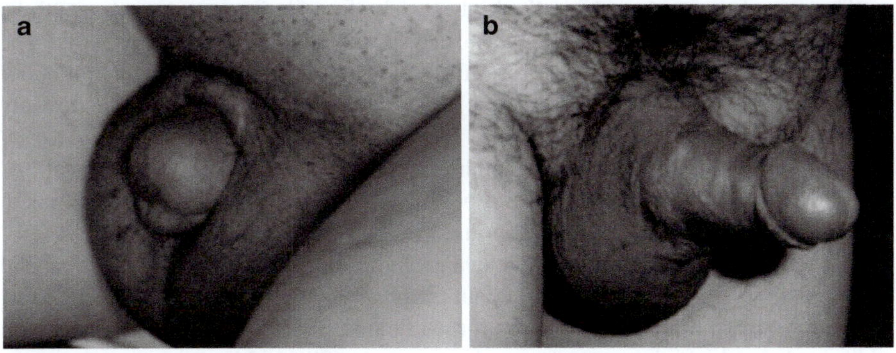

Fig. 37.4 (**a**) Preoperative view showing partially inverted penis (same patient in Fig. 37.3). (**b**) Postoperative appearance of the penis after a penile lengthening procedure including suspensory desmotomy, inverse V-Y-plasty of the dorsal skin of the penile root, and fat removal. (From Masuda H et al. [19]. Copyright © 2004 Masuda et al.; licensee BioMed Central Ltd.)

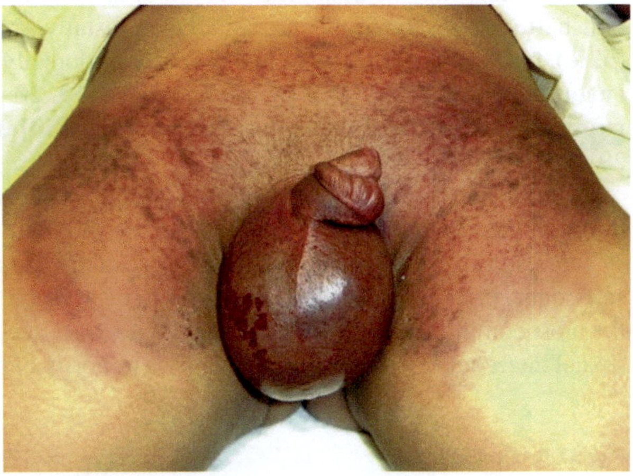

Fig. 37.5 A 13-year-old boy with extensive bruising of the scrotum, penis, lower abdominal wall and upper thighs after sustaining a suction injury by the outlet hole of a Jacuzzi system in the family swimming pool. (Courtesy Kurian George, Retiree from the Urology Department, The Royal Hospital, Muscat, Oman)

37.2.1 Specific Mechanism and Anatomopathology of Penile Fracture

Penile fracture is defined as a traumatic rupture of the tunica albuginea of the corpus cavernosum. **The tunica albuginea is 2 mm thick**. During a normal erection, the corpora cavernosa elongate and their circumference widens at the same time. Therefore, **the thickness of the tunica albuginea considerably decreases to about 0.25 mm resulting in increased susceptibility to injury once the tunica tensile strength (1500 mm Hg) is exceeded**. However, **the corpus spongiosum only elongates**, hence its tunica maintains its normal thickness and is less prone to rupture. This explains why only a minority of cases of penile fracture are associated with spongiosal rupture and urethral injury [20].

The sexual position carrying the highest risk of penile fracture was shown to be the doggy style, accounting for 40.3% in a Brazilian series of 285 patients. The "man on top" position accounted for only 12.1%, and contrary to the general belief the so-called "Position d'Andromaque" * ("woman on top") contributed to only 4.3% of all the cases [21].

*This expression is found in French literature and means "Andromache position" based on the description of the Latin Poet Martial in his Epigrams, Book XI, where he depicts the position of Hector's spouse "riding" her husband [22].

A meta-analysis including 58 relevant studies for a total of over 3 thousand patients showed that intercourse accounts for about half of the causes (48%) of penile fracture and masturbation and forced flexion for 39% [23]. Other systematic reviews showed a higher rate of sexual intercourse (80%) [24].

Unilateral cavernosal injuries are more frequent than bilateral ones with the occurrence of 69%, and 31%, respectively [20], and **the right corpus cavernosum fractures are more frequent than left** accounting for 65–71% and causing the penis to bend to the left side [25, 26]. **Most tears are transverse in orientation**, and their sizes may be as short as 0.5 cm or as long as 6 cm. 50% are located in the midshaft, others are found proximally or distally, and most of them are lateral (62%), but they can also be found ventrally or dorsally [26]. **Ureteral injuries are encountered in 10–38% of penile fractures** [19, 20, 26], but **complete urethral rupture is associated with bilateral cavernosal injuries in 100% of cases** [27–29] (Figs. 37.6, 37.7, and 37.8).

For these reasons, the **EAU** and **AUA** strongly recommend excluding urethral injury in the evaluation of any penile fracture [30, 31].

Interestingly, in the Middle East the so-called **"Taqaandan,"** a forcible manual self-squeezing and bending of the distal penis to achieve sudden detumescence, is the most common reported cause of penile fracture, accounting for 62–76.4%, while sexual intercourse was confessed only by a minority of patients (7.9–9.5%) [24, 32].

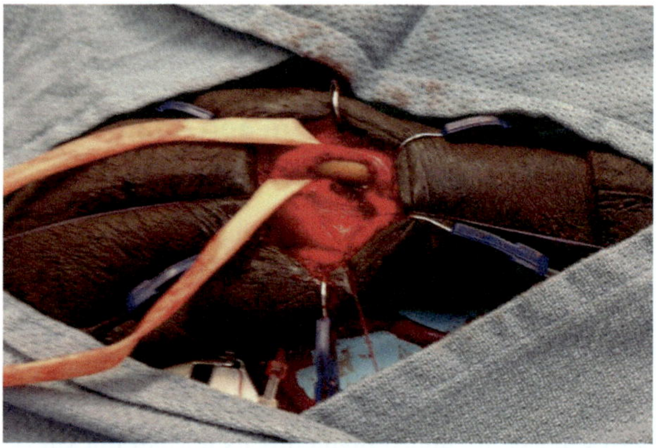

Fig. 37.6 Urethral injury at the site of a corporal tear. (From Phillips EA et al. [27], with permission from John Wiley and Sons)

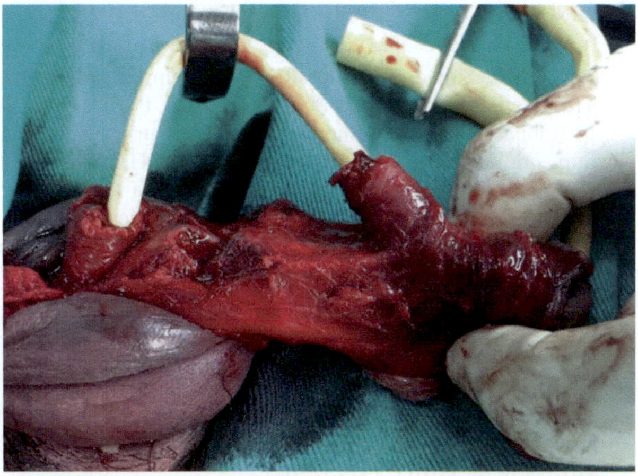

Fig. 37.7 Complete rupture of the urethra associated with bilateral injury in the corpus cavernosum. (From Barros R et al. [21]. Creative Commons Attribution License)

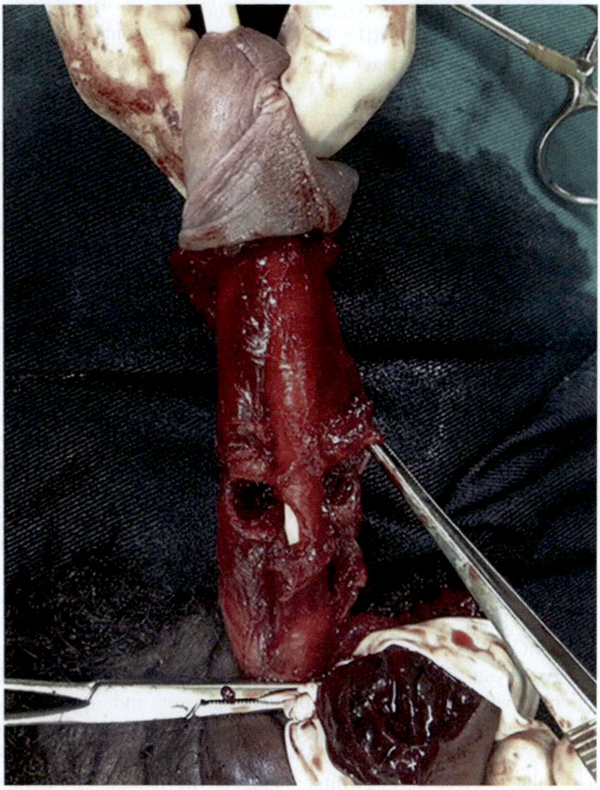

Fig. 37.8 Penile fracture with urethral injury and bilateral rupture of the corpora cavernosa. (From Barros R et al. [29], Creative Commons Attribution License)

References

1. Leslie SW, Sajjad H, Taylor RS. Penile zipper and ring injuries. In: StatPearls [Internet]. Treasure Island: StatPearls Publishing; 2022. PMID: 28722916.
2. El-Bahnasawy MS, El-Sherbiny MT. Paediatric penile trauma. BJU Int. 2002;90(1):92–6. https://doi.org/10.1046/j.1464-410x.2002.02741.x. PMID: 12081778.
3. Gee WF, Ansell JS. Neonatal circumcision: a ten-year overview: with comparison of the Gomco clamp and the Plastibell device. Pediatrics. 1976;58(6):824–7. PMID: 995507.
4. Wiswell TE, Tencer HL, Welch CA, Chamberlain JL. Circumcision in children beyond the neonatal period. Pediatrics. 1993;92(6):791–3. PMID: 8233738.
5. Kim JH, Park JY, Song YS. Traumatic penile injury: from circumcision injury to penile amputation. Biomed Res Int. 2014;2014:375285. https://doi.org/10.1155/2014/375285. Epub 2014 Aug 28. PMID: 25250318; PMCID: PMC4164514.
6. Djordjevic ML, Bumbasirevic MZ, Krstic Z, Bizic MR, Stojanovic BZ, Miocinovic R, Santucci RA. Severe penile injuries in children and adolescents: reconstruction modalities and outcomes. Urology. 2014;83(2):465–70. https://doi.org/10.1016/j.urology.2013.10.015. Epub 2013 Nov 22. PMID: 24275276.
7. Özçift B, Ağras K. Hair tourniquet syndrome of penis: a rare situation in boys with serious complications if not recognized. Turk J Urol. 2018;45(4):322–4. https://doi.org/10.5152/tud.2018.36699. PMID: 31291190; PMCID: PMC6619851.
8. Phonsombat S, Master VA, McAninch JW. Penetrating external genital trauma: a 30-year single institution experience. J Urol. 2008;180(1):192–5; discussion 195–6. Epub 2008 May 21. PMID: 18499189. https://doi.org/10.1016/j.juro.2008.03.041.
9. Hudak SJ, Morey AF, Rozanski TA, Fox CW Jr. Battlefield urogenital injuries: changing patterns during the past century. Urology. 2005;65(6):1041–6. https://doi.org/10.1016/j.urology.2004.11.031. PMID: 15913731.
10. Janak JC, Orman JA, Soderdahl DW, Hudak SJ. Epidemiology of genitourinary injuries among male U.S. service members deployed to Iraq and Afghanistan: early findings from the trauma outcomes and urogenital health (TOUGH) project. J Urol. 2017;197(2):414–9. https://doi.org/10.1016/j.juro.2016.08.005. Epub 2016 Aug 6. PMID: 27506692.
11. Etabbal AM, Hussain FF, Benkhadoura MO, Banni AM. War-related penile injuries in Libya: single-institution experience. Arab J Urol. 2018;16(2):250–6. https://doi.org/10.1016/j.aju.2018.01.005. PMID: 29892491; PMCID: PMC5992784.
12. Al-Azzawi IS, Koraitim MM. Urethral and penile war injuries: the experience from civil violence in Iraq. Arab J Urol. 2014;12(2):149–54. https://doi.org/10.1016/j.aju.2013.11.002. Epub 2014 Jan 23. PMID: 26019940; PMCID: PMC4434606.
13. Tiftikcioglu YO, Erenoglu CM, Lineaweaver WC. A systematic review of penile replantations: may it guide us in penile allotransplantation? Turk J Plast Surg [serial online]. 2018 [cited 2022 Oct 27];26:97–102. http://www.turkjplastsurg.org/text.asp?2018/26/3/97/235785
14. Maxwell BG, Chouhan JD, Lundeberg MR, Liu JJ. National patterns of injury and outcomes of gunshot wounds to the penis: a trauma quality programs retrospective cohort analysis. Acute Med Surg. 2021;8(1):e636. https://doi.org/10.1002/ams2.636. PMID: 33747534; PMCID: PMC7962619.
15. Adamyan RT, Aleshina ON, Abdeeva EI, Sinelnikov MY. Reconstructive surgery for high-voltage injury of genitoperineal area and upper extremities: the uromanual trauma concept. Plast Reconstr Surg Glob Open. 2021;9(10):e3842. https://doi.org/10.1097/GOX.0000000000003842. PMID: 34616643; PMCID: PMC8489895.
16. Sahadev R, Jadhav V, Munianjanappa NB, Shankar G. Penile dislocation with inversion: a rare complication of blunt pelvic injury. J Indian Assoc Pediatr Surg. 2018;23(2):90–2. https://doi.org/10.4103/jiaps.JIAPS_71_17. PMID: 29681700; PMCID: PMC5898211.
17. Palagonia E, Castellani D, Ronchi P, Dell'Atti L, Galosi AB. Hidden penis: a rare case of delayed complication after a pelvic blunt trauma. Transl Androl Urol. 2021;10(8):3524–8. https://doi.org/10.21037/tau-21-333. PMID: 34532276; PMCID: PMC8421820.

18. Simonis LA, Borovets S, Van Driel MF, Ten Duis HJ, Mensink HJ. Erectile dysfunction due to a 'hidden' penis after pelvic trauma. Int J Impot Res. 1999;11(1):53–5. https://doi.org/10.1038/sj.ijir.3900362. PMID: 10098955.
19. Masuda H, Azuma H, Segawa N, Iwamoto Y, Inamoto T, Takasaki N, Katsuoka Y. Surgical correction of buried penis after traffic accident—a case report. BMC Urol. 2004;4:6. https://doi.org/10.1186/1471-2490-4-6. PMID: 15182380; PMCID: PMC434514.
20. Maruschke M, Lehr C, Hakenberg OW. Traumatic penile injuries—mechanisms and treatment. Urol Int. 2008;81(3):367–9. https://doi.org/10.1159/000151421. Epub 2008 Oct 16. PMID: 18931560.
21. Barros R, Hampl D, Cavalcanti AG, Favorito LA, Koifman L. Lessons learned after 20 years' experience with penile fracture. Int Braz J Urol. 2020;46(3):409–16. https://doi.org/10.1590/S1677-5538.IBJU.2019.0367. PMID: 32167705; PMCID: PMC7088490.
22. http://remacle.org/bloodwolf/satire/Martial/livre11.htm
23. Amer T, Wilson R, Chlosta P, AlBuheissi S, Qazi H, Fraser M, Aboumarzouk OM. Penile fracture: a meta-analysis. Urol Int. 2016;96(3):315–29. https://doi.org/10.1159/000444884. Epub 2016 Mar 9. PMID: 26953932.
24. Falcone M, Garaffa G, Castiglione F, Ralph DJ. Current management of penile fracture: an up-to-date systematic review. Sex Med Rev. 2018;6(2):253–60. https://doi.org/10.1016/j.sxmr.2017.07.009. Epub 2017 Sep 2. PMID: 28874325.
25. Zargooshi J. Sexual function and tunica albuginea wound healing following penile fracture: an 18-year follow-up study of 352 patients from Kermanshah, Iran. J Sex Med. 2009;6(4):1141–50. https://doi.org/10.1111/j.1743-6109.2008.01117.x. Epub 2008 Dec 4. PMID: 19138357.
26. Hughes S, Elbaroni W, O'Donoghue J, Williams M. Atypical presentation of a vertical penile fracture. BMJ Case Rep. 2021;14(6):e243353. https://doi.org/10.1136/bcr-2021-243353. PMID: 34187802; PMCID: PMC8245442.
27. Phillips EA, Esposito AJ, Munarriz R. Acute penile trauma and associated morbidity: 9-year experience at a tertiary care center. Andrology. 2015;3(3):632–6. https://doi.org/10.1111/andr.12043. PMID: 26013107.
28. Young E, Ashrafi AN, Kahokehr AA. Tri-tubular penile fracture: a case of complete rupture of urethra and bilateral corpus cavernosa. IJU Case Rep. 2021;4(3):143–5. https://doi.org/10.1002/iju5.12264. PMID: 33977241; PMCID: PMC8088889.
29. Barros R, Ribeiro JGA, da Silva HAM, de Sá FR, Júnior AMF, Favorito LA. Urethral injury in penile fracture: a narrative review. Int Braz J Urol. 2020;46(2):152–7. https://doi.org/10.1590/S1677-5538.IBJU.2020.99.02. PMID: 31961620; PMCID: PMC7025847.
30. EAU guidelines. Edn. Presented at the EAU annual congress Amsterdam March 2022. isbn:978-94-92671-16-5. https://d56bochluxqnz.cloudfront.net/documents/full-guideline/EAU-Guidelines-on-Urological-Trauma-2022_2022-03-24-104100_fwda.pdf
31. Morey AF, Brandes S, Dugi DD 3rd, et al. Urotrauma: AUA guideline. J Urol. 2014;192:327. https://www.auanet.org/guidelines-and-quality/guidelines/urotrauma-guideline
32. el-Sherif AE, Dauleh M, Allowneh N, Vijayan P. Management of fracture of the penis in Qatar. Br J Urol. 1991;68(6):622–5. https://doi.org/10.1111/j.1464-410x.1991.tb15427.x. PMID: 1773294.

Symptoms, Signs, Diagnostic Means, Differential Diagnosis, and Grading of Penile Injury

38

38.1 Symptoms and Signs

Once again, as open penile injury or constricting devices are readily observed in physical examination, more attention will be given to penile fracture in this discussion. The diagnosis of a penile fracture can be made from the **classic clinical triad** of an **audible crack** during sexual activity, **detumescence**, and the appearance of **hematoma** [1].

Hematoma is present in all cases*, and in the majority of patients, there is detumescence (82.6%), a history of a snapping sound (76.3%), and pain (66.3%). Urethral bleeding is rare (12.8%) and urinary retention is exceptionally observed, both of these signs being correlated with some degree of urethral injury [2, 3].

* We have encountered an exceptional case in our practice that presented with sudden onset of bleeding per urethra and mild pain immediately after a sexual intercourse. The 38-year old patient did not have any obvious penile hematoma (Fig. 38.1a) and there was no palpable defect on palpation. Based on the suspicious history, an ultrasonography was requested, revealing a defect on the ventral aspect of the right corpus cavernosum at the mid penile shaft (Fig. 38.1b). On exploration, no hematoma was seen on either aspect (dorsally and ventrally) (Fig. 38.1c, d). After mobilizing the urethra from the ventral aspect of the corpora, a 2-cm tear was noted at the dorsal urethra (UC: Urethral catheter) and another 2-cm tear was noted at the ventral aspect of the right corpus cavernosum (CT: Cavernosal tear) (Fig. 38.1e). The absence of a noticeable hematoma in this case can be explained by the perfect apposition of the two tears (closely facing each other) allowing direct outside drainage of the blood from the corpus through the urethra.

If Buck's fascia remains intact, the presence of hematoma remains circumscribed resulting in the characteristic **"aubergine or eggplant deformity"** [4–7] (Fig. 38.2). When the **Buck's fascia** ruptures, the eggplant deformity remains present, but it

S. A. AL-Mamari, *Urogenital Trauma: A Practical Guide*,
https://doi.org/10.1007/978-981-99-6171-9_38

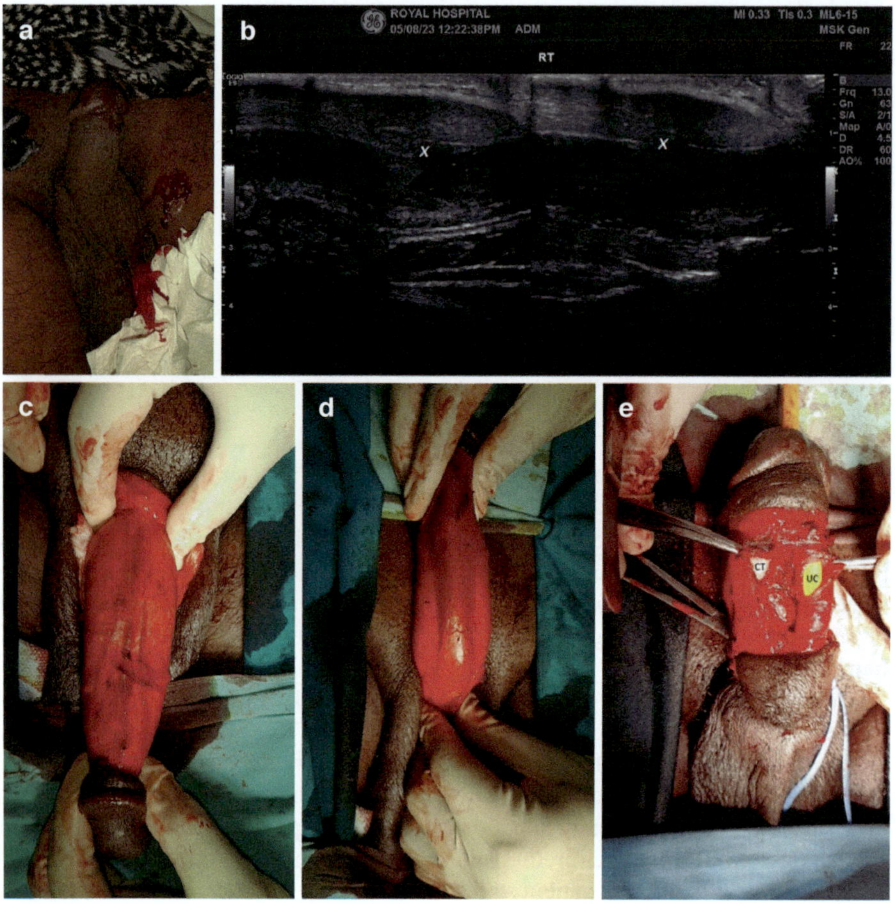

Fig. 38.1 (**a**) Urethral bleeding with no visible hematoma. (**b**) Ultrasonography showing a focal defect (*x*) at the ventral aspect of the right corpus cavernosum in the mid-distal shaft of the penis. (**c**) Dorsally intact corpora cavernosa seen after penile degloving, no hematoma seen. (**d**) No obvious hematoma seen ventrally. (**e**) Both tears of the right corpus cavernosum (*CT* Cavernosal tear) and the urethra (*UC* Urethral catheter) seen after mobilization of the ureter

might sometimes be less marked since the hematoma would spread through the **Dartos fascia** plane toward the pubic and scrotal regions (Fig. 38.3).

Many authors believe that there is no need for radiological investigations of penile fracture as the history and clinical presentation are sufficient for making the diagnosis [8]. Indeed, the typical history, signs, and symptoms are enough clues to make a correct decision in almost all cases and proceed to surgical exploration and repair. Herein, explorations of penile fracture based solely on clinical evaluation in an Iranian University Hospital confirmed the diagnosis in 97% of patients, and the three-percent error was attributed to inexperienced Junior residents who confused penile fracture with penile venous injury [9].

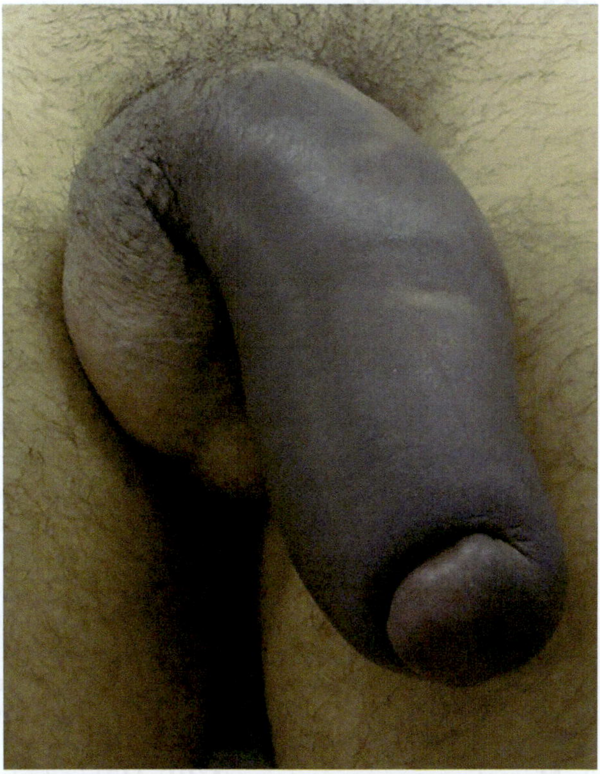

Fig. 38.2 Typical eggplant aspect in a patient with penile fracture and urethral injury. (From Barros R et al. [7], Creative Commons Attribution License)

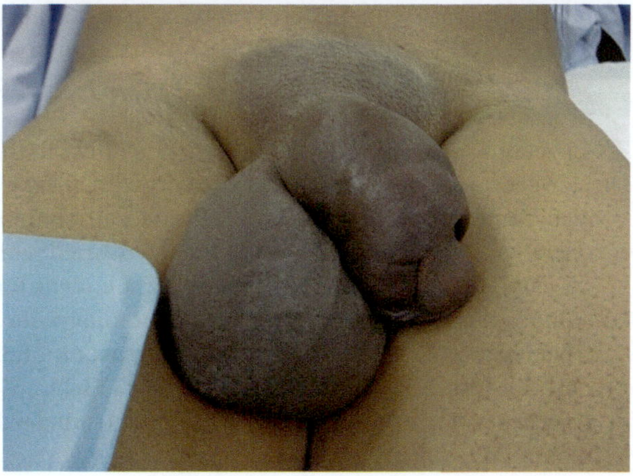

Fig. 38.3 Penile fracture. Penile eggplant deformity with hematoma expanding to the scrotal and pubic regions. (Courtesy Kurian George, Retiree from the Urology Department, The Royal Hospital, Muscat, Oman)

38.2 Imaging Means

As mentioned above, history and clinical examination are the cornerstones in making the diagnosis of penile fracture and imaging means are seldom required. However, in reality, there might well be some presentations susceptible to confuse even experienced practitioners (see the paragraph on differential diagnosis below), calling for radiological investigations. Therefore, many other authors suggest the use of various image modalities to confirm the diagnosis and the site of penile fractures, such as ultrasonography, cavernosography, retrograde urethrography, and MRI [1, 8].

1. **Ultrasonography**: The detection rate of penile fractures using **Ultrasonography** has been found to be 88% which is an interesting value considering the low cost and the rapid completion of this study [10]. **Ultrasonography with a 7.50 to 12 MHz linear probe is regarded as the preferred imaging modality by many authors**, being non-invasive contrary to cavernosography, not expensive and less time consuming than MRI, and readily available in all the modern medical centers. It can be performed in the Emergency Department and provides in expert hands an accurate diagnosis, extent, and location of the tunica rupture, and was even proposed by some investigators as a reliable means to grade the injury [11, 12]. **The use of ultrasonography is also supported by expert panels in equivocal signs and symptoms of penile fracture** and has the additional advantage to locate the tunical tear and help plan an adequate surgical approach [3, 13].
2. **Magnetic resonance imaging (MRI)**: MRI accurately detects a discontinuity of the tunica albuginea and also demonstrates the eventual presence of associated injuries to adjacent structures (corpus spongiosum, urethra) [14]. It was shown to have 100% sensitivity, 77.8–87.5% specificity, a high negative predictive value of 100%, and a positive predictive value of 90.5–96.7% in the diagnosis of penile fracture [10, 15, 16].
3. **Cavernosography:** This investigation is rarely used, being considered invasive. However, with the exclusion of patients with allergy or hypersensitivity to iodinated contrast media, it is a rather safe and simple procedure performed preoperatively by injecting **15–30 cc of diluted contrast material** through a 25-gauge butterfly needle **into the dorsolateral uninvolved corpus cavernosum**, under fluoroscopic guidance. The diagnosis of penile fracture is made when there is **extravasation of the contrast and hematoma is seen as a filling defect adjacent to the leak** [17–19] (Fig. 38.4).
4. **Urethrocystography**: This study might be indicated only if there is a suspicion of urethral injury.

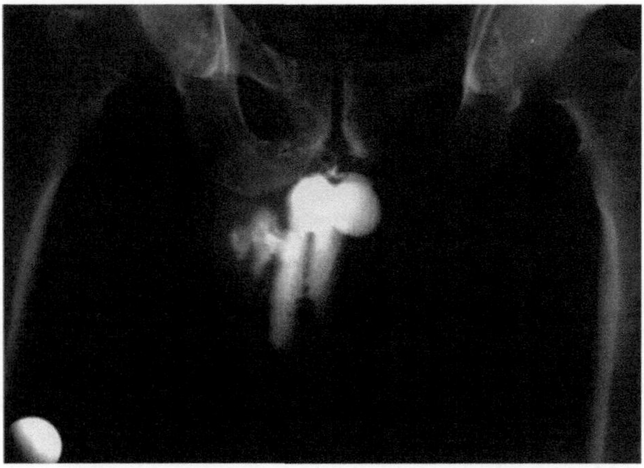

Fig. 38.4 Cavernosography film showing massive extravasation and depicting the extent of a right-sided tunical rupture. (From Beysel M et al. [19], with permission from Elsevier)

38.3 Differential Diagnosis of Penile Fracture [18, 20, 21]

- **Deep dorsal vein rupture**: The mechanism of its occurrence is the same as for the rupture of corpora cavernosa (sexual activity, forceful bending), and its clinical presentation is almost the same (with the exception of the cracking sound). Moreover, the hematoma here remains contained beneath Buck's fascia and within the penile shaft like for penile fracture.
- **Superficial dorsal vein rupture**: Here the hematoma spreads through the subcutaneous tissue of the external genitalia, and the ecchymosis may extend up to the scrotal wall.
- **Dorsal artery injuries**
- **Dartos bleeding**
- **Penile suspensory ligament injuries**
- **Isolated urethral injury** [22].

In a retrospective series, isolated vascular injuries were the sole findings in 18% of patients who presented with acute penile pain, swelling, and blueish discoloration following coitus [1].

38.4 Grading of Penile Injury

The American Association for the Surgery of Trauma (AAST) has proposed the following scale for penile injury [23] (Table 38.1).

Other more specific classifications have been proposed, either limited to the description of the penile fracture using ultrasonography [12] (Table 38.2), describing lesions related to penile constricting ring injuries [24, 25] (Table 38.3), or describing avulsion injuries of the external genitalia according to the location of the native urethra at presentation [26] (Table 38.4; Fig. 38.5).

Table 38.1 Penile injury scale

Grade[a]	Description of injury	AIS-90
I	Cutaneous laceration/contusion	1
II	Buck's fascia (cavernosum) laceration without tissue loss	1
III	Cutaneous avulsion Laceration through glans/meatus Cavernosal or urethral defect <2 cm	3
IV	Partial penectomy Cavernosal or urethral defect >2 cm	3
V	Total penectomy	3

From Moore EE, et al. [23], with permission from Wolters Kluwer Health
[a] Advance one grade for multiple injuries up to grade III

Table 38.2 Ultrasonographic grading criteria for penile fractures

Grade	Description of injury
0	Normal tunica albuginea
I	Defect in tunica albuginea. Defect in corpora Cavernosa
II	Perialbugineal and Cavernosal hematoma
III	Hematoma of deep fascia. Involvement of Corpus spongiosum
IV	Urethral injury. Vascular malformation

From Shukla et al. [12], with permission from JCDR Research and Publications Private Limited

Table 38.3 Grading of penile strangulation injury

Grade	Description of the injury
Grade 1	Oedema of distal penis. No evidence of skin ulceration or urethral injury
Grade 2	Injury to skin and constriction of corpus spongiosum but no evidence of urethral injury. Distal penile oedema with decreased penile sensation
Grade 3	Injury to skin and urethra but no urethral fistula. Loss of distal penile sensation
Grade 4	Complete division of corpus spongiosum leading to urethral fistula and constriction of corpus cavernosum with loss of distal penile sensation
Grade 5	Gangrene, necrosis, or complete amputation of the distal penis

From Bhat AL et al. [25], with permission from John Wiley and Sons

Table 38.4 Grading of penile avulsion

Type	Description
Type I	Meatus was at the corporal stump
Type II	Loss of corpora with preservation of the crura leaving the meatus near the pubic symphysis
Type III	Perineal urethrostomy
Type IV	Urinary diversion via a supra-pubic catheter is required

Adapted from Rashid et al. [26], with permission from Elsevier

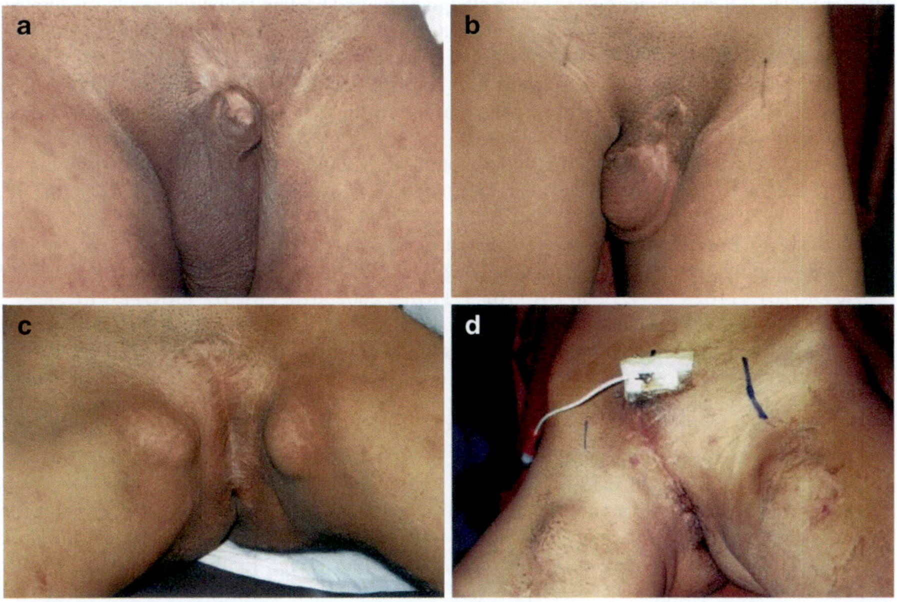

Fig. 38.5 Penile injury types: (**a**) Type I avulsion injury; (**b**) Type II avulsion injury; (**c**) Type III avulsion injury; (**d**) Type IV avulsion injury. (From Rashid et al. [26], with permission from Elsevier)

References

1. Phillips EA, Esposito AJ, Munarriz R. Acute penile trauma and associated morbidity: 9-year experience at a tertiary care center. Andrology. 2015;3(3):632–6. https://doi.org/10.1111/andr.12043. PMID: 26013107.
2. Barros R, Hampl D, Cavalcanti AG, Favorito LA, Koifman L. Lessons learned after 20 years' experience with penile fracture. Int Braz J Urol. 2020;46(3):409–16. https://doi.org/10.1590/S1677-5538.IBJU.2019.0367. PMID: 32167705; PMCID: PMC7088490.
3. Morey AF, Brandes S, Dugi DD 3rd, et al. Urotrauma: AUA guideline. J Urol. 2014;192:327. https://www.auanet.org/guidelines-and-quality/guidelines/urotrauma-guideline
4. Mirzazadeh M, Fallahkarkan M, Hosseini J. Penile fracture epidemiology, diagnosis and management in Iran: a narrative review. Transl Androl Urol. 2017;6(2):158–66. https://doi.org/10.21037/tau.2016.12.03. PMID: 28540222; PMCID: PMC5422687.
5. Krishna Reddy SV, Shaik AB, Sreenivas K. Penile injuries: a 10-year experience. Can Urol Assoc J. 2014;8(9–10):E626–31. https://doi.org/10.5489/cuaj.1821. PMID: 25295134; PMCID: PMC4164551.
6. Atreya A, Baral S. Penile fracture: a case report from Nepal. Clin Case Rep. 2021;9:e04786. https://doi.org/10.1002/ccr3.4786.
7. Barros R, Ribeiro JGA, da Silva HAM, de Sá FR, Júnior AMF, Favorito LA. Urethral injury in penile fracture: a narrative review. Int Braz J Urol. 2020;46(2):152–7. https://doi.org/10.1590/S1677-5538.IBJU.2020.99.02. PMID: 31961620; PMCID: PMC7025847.
8. Amer T, Wilson R, Chlosta P, AlBuheissi S, Qazi H, Fraser M, Aboumarzouk OM. Penile fracture: a meta-analysis. Urol Int. 2016;96(3):315–29. https://doi.org/10.1159/000444884. Epub 2016 Mar 9. PMID: 26953932.

9. Zargooshi J. Sexual function and tunica albuginea wound healing following penile fracture: an 18-year follow-up study of 352 patients from Kermanshah, Iran. J Sex Med. 2009;6(4):1141–50. https://doi.org/10.1111/j.1743-6109.2008.01117.x. Epub 2008 Dec 4. PMID: 19138357.
10. Zare Mehrjardi M, Darabi M, Bagheri SM, Kamali K, Bijan B. The role of ultrasound (US) and magnetic resonance imaging (MRI) in penile fracture mapping for modified surgical repair. Int Urol Nephrol. 2017;49:937–45.
11. Gupta N, Goyal P, Sharma K, Bansal I, Gupta S, Li S, Zinn K, Kumar Y. Penile fracture: role of ultrasound. Transl Androl Urol. 2017;6(3):580–4. https://doi.org/10.21037/tau.2017.03.38. PMID: 28725601; PMCID: PMC5503951.
12. Shukla AK, Bhagavan BC, Sanjay SC, Krishnappa N, Sahadev R, V S. Role of ultraosonography in grading of penile fractures. J Clin Diagn Res. 2015;9(4):TC1–3. https://doi.org/10.7860/JCDR/2015/11628.5754. Epub 2015 Apr 1. PMID: 26023616; PMCID: PMC4437132.
13. Rees RW, Brown G, Dorkin T, Lucky M, Pearcy R, Shabbir M, Shukla CJ, Summerton DJ, Muneer A, BAUS Section of Andrology and Genitourethral Surgery (AGUS). British Association of Urological Surgeons (BAUS) consensus document for the management of male genital emergencies—penile fracture. BJU Int. 2018;122(1):26–8. https://doi.org/10.1111/bju.14167. Epub 2018 Apr 2. PMID: 29438589.
14. Choi M-H, Kim B, Ryu J-A, Lee SW, Lee KS. MR imaging of acute penile fracture. Radiographics. 2000;20(5):1397–405.
15. Saglam E, Tarhan F, Hamarat MB, Can U, Coskun A, Camur E, Sarica K. Efficacy of magnetic resonance imaging for diagnosis of penile fracture: a controlled study. Investig Clin Urol. 2017;58(4):255–60. https://doi.org/10.4111/icu.2017.58.4.255. Epub 2017 Jun 2. PMID: 28681035; PMCID: PMC5494349.
16. Sokolakis I, Schubert T, Oelschlaeger M, Krebs M, Gschwend JE, Holzapfel K, et al. The role of magnetic resonance imaging in the diagnosis of penile fracture in real-life emergency settings: comparative analysis with intraoperative findings. J Urol. 2019;202(3):552–7. 101097JU0000000000000211
17. Dever DP, Saraf PG, Catanese RP, Feinstein MJ, Davis RS. Penile fracture: operative management and cavernosography. Urology. 1983;22(4):394–6. https://doi.org/10.1016/0090-4295(83)90418-1. PMID: 6636395.
18. Karadeniz T, Topsakal M, Ariman A, Erton H, Basak D. Penile fracture: differential diagnosis, management and outcome. Br J Urol. 1996;77(2):279–81. https://doi.org/10.1046/j.1464-410x.1996.86420.x. PMID: 8800899.
19. Beysel M, Tekin A, Gürdal M, Yücebaş E, Sengör F. Evaluation and treatment of penile fractures: accuracy of clinical diagnosis and the value of corpus cavernosography. Urology. 2002;60(3):492–6. https://doi.org/10.1016/s0090-4295(02)01813-7. PMID: 12350495.
20. Kurkar A, Elderwy AA, Orabi H. False fracture of the penis: different pathology but similar clinical presentation and management. Urol Ann. 2014;6(1):23–6. https://doi.org/10.4103/0974-7796.127015. PMID: 24669117; PMCID: PMC3963338.
21. Feki W, Derouiche A, Belhaj K, Ouni A, Ben Mouelhi S, Ben Slama MR, Ayed M, Chebil M. False penile fracture: report of 16 cases. Int J Impot Res. 2007;19(5):471–3. https://doi.org/10.1038/sj.ijir.3901574. Epub 2007 Jun 7. PMID: 17554393.
22. Wong KW, Ho BSH, Ip CH, Yiu MK. Isolated penile urethral injury: a rare case following male coital trauma. Asian J Urol. 2015;2(3):175–8. https://doi.org/10.1016/j.ajur.2015.06.006. Epub 2015 Jul 6. PMID: 29264140; PMCID: PMC5730709.
23. Moore EE, Malangoni MA, Cogbill TH, Peterson NE, Champion HR, Jurkovich GJ, Shackford SR. Organ injury scaling VII: cervical vascular, peripheral vascular, adrenal, penis, testis, and scrotum. J Trauma. 1996;41(3):523–4. https://doi.org/10.1097/00005373-199609000-00023. PMID: 8810974.

24. Dawood O, Tabibi S, Fiuk J, Patel N, El-Zawahry A. Penile ring entrapment—a true urologic emergency: grading, approach, and management. Urol Ann. 2020;12(1):15–8. https://doi.org/10.4103/UA.UA_16_19. Epub 2019 Nov 7. PMID: 32015611; PMCID: PMC6978966.
25. Bhat AL, Kumar A, Mathur SC, Gangwal KC. Penile strangulation. Br J Urol. 1991;68(6):618–21. https://doi.org/10.1111/j.1464-410x.1991.tb15426.x. PMID: 1773293.
26. Rashid M, Sarwar SU. Avulsion injuries of the male external genitalia: classification and reconstruction with the customised radial forearm free flap. Br J Plast Surg. 2005;58(5):585–92. https://doi.org/10.1016/j.bjps.2004.12.014. PMID: 15927151.

Treatment of Penile Injury. I: Minor and Intermediate Surgeries

39

The treatment of penile trauma is a vast topic that linearly correlates with the anatomopathology and the severity of the injury. It may just be a minor or intermediate intervention such as superficial wound suturing, zipper or constricting ring removal, and repair of a penile fracture, but may also consist of complex procedures such as penile replantation, reconstruction, or transplantation.

39.1 Management of Zipper Entrapment

As already mentioned in the chapter on etiology, zipper accident is the most frequent cause of penile injury, and for obvious reasons, it affects mostly uncircumcised children and adults.

Zippers can be removed through various methods. The most rapid and easiest one is lubrication and manual disengagement. Sometimes it may be necessary to saw the median bar with a hacksaw, scissor, or bone cutter, or to disassemble the fastener by cutting the zipper teeth [1–5]. Also, the insertion of a small-size screwdriver between the outer and inner faceplates of the zipper and twisting it toward the median bar may widen the faceplates and disengage the prepuce (Fig. 39.1a, b) [6]. Of course, the screwdriver should be inserted into the opposite side of the prepuce.

When these non-surgical methods are not successful, minimal surgery will be required consisting of the excision of the entrapped skin. As a last resort, circumcision can be required.

S. A. AL-Mamari, *Urogenital Trauma: A Practical Guide*,
https://doi.org/10.1007/978-981-99-6171-9_39

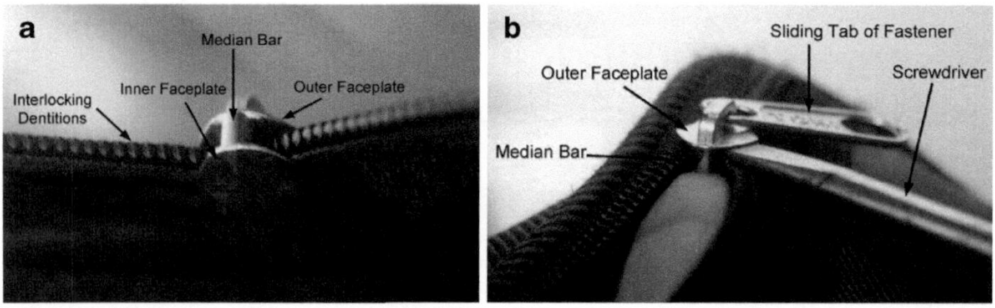

Fig. 39.1 (**a**) Macrophotography showing the structural anatomy of zip fastener from its inner aspect. The outer and inner faceplates along with the median bar form the fastener. (**b**) Macrophotography showing the position of screwdriver between the two faceplates. It should be twisted toward the median bar (anticlockwise with reference to the figure). (From Raveenthiran V [6], with permission from Wolters Kluwer Health)

39.2 Removal of a Penile Ring

The constricting ring can be metallic (wedding rings, nuts), elastic (rubber bands, bottlenecks), or made of thread or hair. The elastic rings, threads, and hairs are easily sectioned using fine scissors. The metallic rings can be removed through two methods [2, 7]:

- The easiest and fastest one is lubricating and sliding the ring off the penis
- Cutting the ring off is indicated after failure of sliding.

When the above two methods have failed, one has to proceed to surgery consisting of lateral corporotomy to reduce the edema and facilitate the first step, i.e. lubrication and sliding of the ring [8]. Penile amputation and cystotomy or perineal urethrostomy can be necessary for late presentation of a penile ring with gangrene [9].

39.3 Management of Penile Fracture

A retrospective analysis comparing interventional and conservative approaches to penile fracture showed erectile dysfunction in 11.4% and 33.3% of cases, respectively, after a mean follow-up of 19 months. Additionally, 50% of the patients treated conservatively developed penile deviation [10]. All expert panels (EAU, AUA, BAUS) strongly recommend surgically treating any penile fracture by repairing the tunica albuginea and eventual urethral injury [11–13].

Regarding the timing of intervention, a systematic review comparing immediate and delayed repair of penile fracture did not show a significant difference for ED and tunical scars with values of 6.6% vs 4.5%, and 5.4% vs 4.5%, respectively. Nevertheless, the rate of curvature significantly favored immediate repair over the delayed approach with values of 1.8% and 4.5%, respectively, although the curvature was reported as mild and not affecting sexual function [14]. These studies are supported by a meta-analysis and other systematic reviews that reached the same conclusions: **any penile fracture is better repaired, and the intervention should be performed early, preferably within 24 h** [15, 16]. These conclusions were unequivocally endorsed by the British Association of Urological Surgeons (BAUS) [13].

39.3.1 Technique for Corporeal Repair

The patient should be given prophylaxis with a broad-spectrum antibiotic and a catheter be inserted before the procedure after ruling out a urethral injury [13, 16–18].

- **Incision**: The surgeon has a choice between two common incisions to approach the corporeal tear: a sub-coronal incision with penile degloving (the most popular), or a penoscrotal vertical incision. The first incision allows full inspection of the corpora and is useful when the exact location of the tear is not defined. It has also a cosmetic advantage as the final scar will be confused with the post-circumcision one. However, its drawback is the risk of neurovascular injury if the incision is too deep dorsally, urethral injury if too deep ventrally, or skin necrosis if too superficially and thin skin is peeled off during degloving. The advantage of the vertical incision is direct exposure to the injury site but supposes that precise information is available beforehand.
- **Repair of the corporeal tear**: Once the injury site is exposed, the hematoma is removed, and the tunical defect is identified and washed with a saline solution. The tear is most commonly sutured using interrupted resorbable 2/0 suture materials (polyglactin or polydioxanone PDS) in a watertight technique with buried knots.
- If the urethra is also injured, it should be repaired with 4/0 resorbable sutures, and stented with a catheter
- Regloving and skin closure with interrupted 2/0 or 3/0 resorbable suture (rapid vicryl).

Patients are generally discharged home the next day, advised abstinence for 4–6 weeks, and reviewed after 2 weeks in the outpatient department. Cyproterone tablets can be prescribed to reduce libido and prevent erection.

39.4 Penile Wound Repair

A simple skin incision with no tissue loss can be directly closed using interrupted 4/0 resorbable sutures. When there is isolated skin loss, a split-thickness skin grafting is a good means for reliable coverage [19]. Scrotal skin flaps (based on the anterior and posterior scrotal arteries), or commercial dermal substitutes such as Integra (bovine collagen, Integra Life Sciences Corp., Plainsboro, NJ) are good options in cases not amenable to immediate split-thickness skin grafting [19]. In order to ensure a high potency rate and minimize the occurrence of urethral stricture, low-velocity gunshot injuries with urethral rupture must be repaired layer by layer after debridement and urethral spatulation [20, 21].

A recent American national database analysis of 722 cases of gunshot penile injury revealed that penile salvage is successful in most patients, with only 13 of them (1.8%) requiring penectomy [22]. Indeed low-velocity bullets generally cause limited wounds with no complete destruction of the penis [23, 24] (Figs. 39.2 and 39.3).

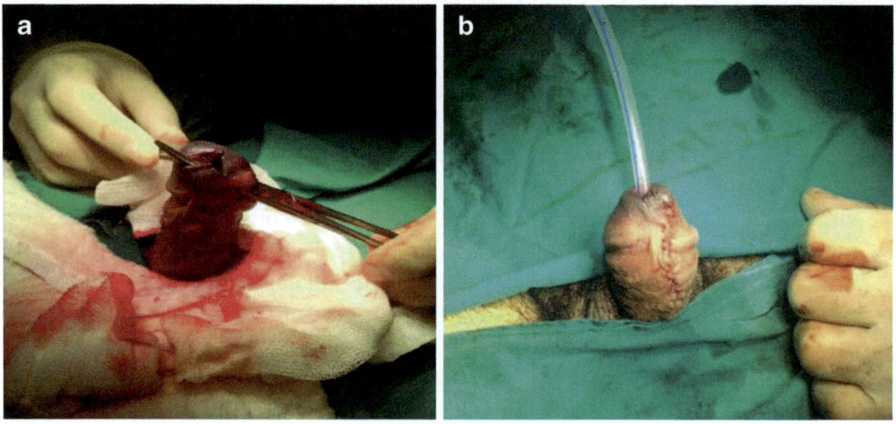

Fig. 39.2 (**a**) A forceps demonstrating the bullet path through the penile the glans penis and distal urethra. (**b**) The glans penis after reconstruction. (From Ozkan Onuk et al. [23]. Creative Commons Attribution-Share Alike 4.0 International (CC BY-SA 4.0) license)

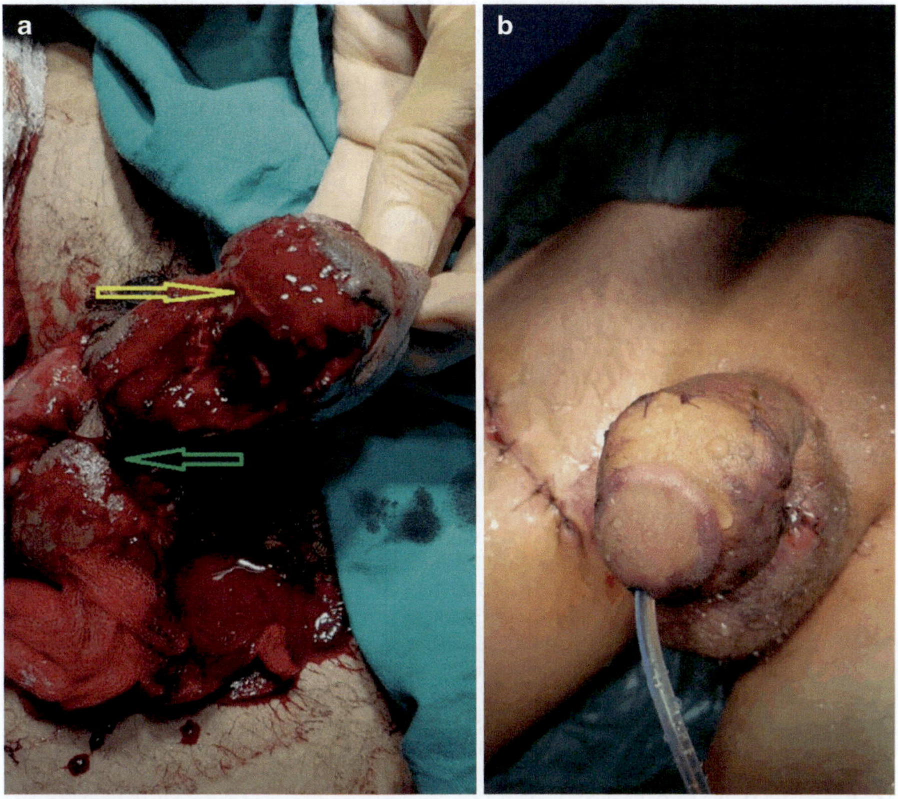

Fig. 39.3 Low-velocity penile GSW. (**a**) Perioperative view of extensive urethral and corporal disruptions (yellow arrow), and scrotal laceration (green arrow). (**b**) One-week postoperative photo showing a good cosmetic appearance of the external genitalia. (From Ghabisha S et al. [24], Creative Commons Attribution License)

References

1. Kim JH, Park JY, Song YS. Traumatic penile injury: from circumcision injury to penile amputation. Biomed Res Int. 2014;2014:375285. https://doi.org/10.1155/2014/375285. Epub 2014 Aug 28. PMID: 25250318; PMCID: PMC4164514.
2. Leslie SW, Sajjad H, Taylor RS. Penile Zipper and ring injuries. In: StatPearls [Internet]. Treasure Island: StatPearls Publishing; 2022. PMID: 28722916.
3. Nakagawa T, Toguri AG. Penile Zipper injury. Med Princ Pract. 2006;15:303–4. https://doi.org/10.1159/000092995.
4. Flowerdew R, Fishman IJ, Churchill BM. Management of penile zipper injury. J Urol. 1977;117(5):671. https://doi.org/10.1016/s0022-5347(17)58581-x. PMID: 859209.
5. Krishna Reddy SV, Shaik AB, Sreenivas K. Penile injuries: a 10-year experience. Can Urol Assoc J. 2014;8(9–10):E626–31. https://doi.org/10.5489/cuaj.1821. PMID: 25295134; PMCID: PMC4164551.

6. Raveenthiran V. Releasing of zipper-entrapped foreskin: a novel nonsurgical technique. Pediatr Emerg Care. 2007;23(7):463–4. https://doi.org/10.1097/01.pec.0000280505.37300.c1. PMID: 17666927.
7. Dawood O, Tabibi S, Fiuk J, Patel N, El-Zawahry A. Penile ring entrapment—a true urologic emergency: grading, approach, and management. Urol Ann. 2020;12(1):15–8. https://doi.org/10.4103/UA.UA_16_19. Epub 2019 Nov 7. PMID: 32015611; PMCID: PMC6978966.
8. Alkhureeb M. Case report of early release of penile strangulation by metallic rings. Int J Sci Res. 2016;5:1442–4.
9. Nuhu A, Edino ST, Agbese GO, Kallamu M. Penile gangrene due to strangulation by a metallic nut: a case report. West Afr J Med. 2009;28:340–2.
10. Yamaçake KG, Tavares A, Padovani GP, Guglielmetti GB, Cury J, Srougi M. Long-term treatment outcomes between surgical correction and conservative management for penile fracture: retrospective analysis. Korean J Urol. 2013;54(7):472–6. https://doi.org/10.4111/kju.2013.54.7.472. Epub 2013 Jul 15. PMID: 23878691; PMCID: PMC3715712.
11. EAU guidelines. Edn. presented at the EAU annual congress Amsterdam March 2022. isbn:978-94-92671-16-5. https://uroweb.org/guidelines/urological-trauma/chapter/urogenital-trauma-guidelines
12. Morey AF, Brandes S, Dugi DD 3rd, et al. Urotrauma: AUA guideline. J Urol. 2014;192:327. https://www.auanet.org/guidelines-and-quality/guidelines/urotrauma-guideline
13. Rees RW, Brown G, Dorkin T, Lucky M, Pearcy R, Shabbir M, Shukla CJ, Summerton DJ, Muneer A, BAUS Section of Andrology and Genitourethral Surgery (AGUS). British Association of Urological Surgeons (BAUS) consensus document for the management of male genital emergencies - penile fracture. BJU Int. 2018;122(1):26–8. https://doi.org/10.1111/bju.14167. Epub 2018 Apr 2. PMID: 29438589.
14. Wong NC, Dason S, Bansal RK, Davies TO, Braga LH. Can it wait? A systematic review of immediate vs. delayed surgical repair of penile fractures. Can Urol Assoc J. 2017;11(1–2):53–60. https://doi.org/10.5489/cuaj.4032. PMID: 28443146; PMCID: PMC5403677.
15. Amer T, Wilson R, Chlosta P, AlBuheissi S, Qazi H, Fraser M, Aboumarzouk OM. Penile fracture: a meta-analysis. Urol Int. 2016;96(3):315–29. https://doi.org/10.1159/000444884. Epub 2016 Mar 9. PMID: 26953932.
16. Kominsky H, Beebe S, Shah N, Jenkins LC. Surgical reconstruction for penile fracture: a systematic review. Int J Impot Res. 2020;32(1):75–80. https://doi.org/10.1038/s41443-019-0212-1. Epub 2019 Nov 4. PMID: 31685943.
17. Falcone M, Garaffa G, Castiglione F, Ralph DJ. Current management of penile fracture: an up-to-date systematic review. Sex Med Rev. 2018;6(2):253–60. https://doi.org/10.1016/j.sxmr.2017.07.009. Epub 2017 Sep 2. PMID: 28874325.
18. Kamdar C, Mooppan UM, Kim H, Gulmi FA. Penile fracture: preoperative evaluation and surgical technique for optimal patient outcome. BJU Int. 2008;102(11):1640–4; discussion 1644. Epub 2008 Aug 14. PMID: 18710448. https://doi.org/10.1111/j.1464-410X.2008.07902.x.
19. Salgado CJ, Chim H, Tang JC, Monstrey SJ, Mardini S. Penile reconstruction. Semin Plast Surg. 2011;25(3):221–8. https://doi.org/10.1055/s-0031-1281492. PMID: 22851914; PMCID: PMC3312184.
20. Hall SJ, Wagner JR, Edelstein RA, Carpinito GA. Management of gunshot injuries to the penis and anterior urethra. J Trauma. 1995;38(3):439–43. https://doi.org/10.1097/00005373-199503000-00028. PMID: 7897734.
21. Goldman C, Shaw N, du Plessis D, Myers JB, van der Merwe A, Venkatesan K. Gunshot wounds to the penis and scrotum: a narrative review of management in civilian and military settings. Transl Androl Urol. 2021;10(6):2596–608. https://doi.org/10.21037/tau-20-1175. PMID: 34295746; PMCID: PMC8261456.

22. Maxwell BG, Chouhan JD, Lundeberg MR, Liu JJ. National patterns of injury and outcomes of gunshot wounds to the penis: a trauma quality programs retrospective cohort analysis. Acute Med Surg. 2021;8(1):e636. https://doi.org/10.1002/ams2.636. PMID: 33747534; PMCID: PMC7962619.
23. Onuk O, Arslan B, Yanaral F, Hazar A, Özkan A, Gezmis C, Nuhoğlu B. Management of gunshot injury of glans penis that extends to anterior urethra: a rare case report. Haseki Tıp Bülteni. 2016;54:249–51. https://doi.org/10.4274/haseki.3125.
24. Ghabisha S, Ahmed F, Al-wageeh S, Al-shami E, Alyhari Q, Dajenah M, Mohammed F. Penetrating trauma to scrotum and penis caused by a gunshot in 17-year old man: a case report. J Emerg Med Trauma Acute Care. 2022. https://doi.org/10.5339/jemtac.2022.21.

40 Treatment of Penile Injury. II: Complex Procedures

Severe penile injuries (severance, crush, etc. are extremely rare and their management is poorly mastered by most Regional Urological surgeons and are better transferred to specialized centers where multispecialty expertise is available including plastic surgery.

40.1 Penile Replantation

Penile replantation is the best option when the penis has been sharply sectioned and the patient presents early with the amputated appendage which should be wrapped in saline-soaked gauze, then in a plastic bag and covered with ice during transport [1]. This surgery is more successful nowadays thanks to the introduction of **microsurgical** approach. But before that, pioneers have performed penile replantation using **macrosurgical** techniques, the first case was reported by Ehrich in 1929 [2]. This was followed by dozens of cases with fairly satisfactory results.

The technique consisted essentially of urethral anastomosis, repair of the corpora cavernosa and spongiosa, and skin suturing, but without neuro-vascular anastomosis. Many complications have been reported from the macrosurgical approach including a high rate of urethral stenosis, fistula formation, skin necrosis, non-recovery of sensation, and erectile dysfunction [3–5]. If the patient loses only the glans penis, a glansplasty may be all that is required. Herein no identifiable vessels are present and composite grafting, i.e. macrosurgical approach is the only possible local solution [6].

The first **microsurgical penile replantation** was performed in 1977 by two teams working independently on psychotic patients who self-amputated their genitalia: a Japanese team, Tamai et al., and an American one, Cohen et al. [7, 8]. Nowadays, the microsurgical approach should be considered the standard for this surgery [5].

S. A. AL-Mamari, *Urogenital Trauma: A Practical Guide*,
https://doi.org/10.1007/978-981-99-6171-9_40

A retrospective analysis performed in 2017, and recruiting 106 patients who underwent penile replantation from self-mutilation or trauma showed maintained full sensation in 68% of patients, adequate urinary function in 97%, and normal erection in 77%. The most common complications were skin necrosis and venous congestion in 55% and 20%, respectively. Others were urethral stricture and fistula in 11% and 6.6%, respectively. The overall patient satisfaction rate was 91.6% [9]. The majority of the patients (67%) underwent a microsurgical approach confirming the new trend. Unfortunately, this study did not differentiate the outcomes between the two techniques. This study also showed that anastomosis of the superficial dorsal artery and a larger number of coapted nerves were associated with favorable sexual, urinary, and sensation outcomes. Paradoxically, however, larger numbers of anastomosed vessels were associated with unfavorable outcomes, probably because of longer ischemic time [9].

40.1.1 Surgical Steps of Penile Replantation [3, 10]

The amputated penis is washed with saline and preserved in a plastic bag covered with ice. After a suprapubic catheter is inserted, and an I-V broad-spectrum antibiotic is given, the technique of penile replantation starts with debridement of the stump, and a silicone urethral catheter is inserted through the amputated penis and then through the stump and will act as a stabilizing stent. The operating microscope allows clear identification and safe dissection of vessels and nerves.

The replantation is performed in a progressive way where the Urologist and Plastic Surgeon work together in a stepwise manner. The operation starts ventrally and progresses through deep and dorsal structures. Hence, the urethral anastomosis is first performed by the Urologist after spatulation and using 4/0 resorbable sutures (vicryl, polydioxanone), ideally in two layers. This is followed by the challenging anastomosis of the thin and short deep (profunda) arteries performed by the Plastic Surgeon. Then the tunica albuginea of both corpora cavernosa is repaired with 5/0 resorbable (Vicryl, polydioxanone) sutures, followed by a watertight repair of the cavernosa, preferably using a continuous suture. The last structures to be anastomosed are the superficial and deep dorsal veins, the dorsal artery, and the dorsal nerves using 9/0 or 10/0 Ethilon or nylon. By the end, the fascia, the areolar tissue, and the skin are approximated with 4/0 Ethilon (Figs. 40.1 and 40.2).

Post-operatively, the patient is closely monitored for early ischemia by direct inspection every 30 min and Doppler ultrasound at short intervals or immediately whenever suspect signs are observed (coldness, change of color). He continues I-V broad-spectrum antibiotics and is started on prophylactic low-molecular weight heparins.

Sometimes the venous outflow might not be sufficient as it takes around 96 h (4 days) for graft neovascularization to be permanently established. The developing venous congestion might cause an excessive hematoma and edema resulting in skin necrosis and loss. Herein therapy with medicinal leeches (Hirudo medicinalis) was proven to be an interesting temporary measure for venous drainage [3, 11].

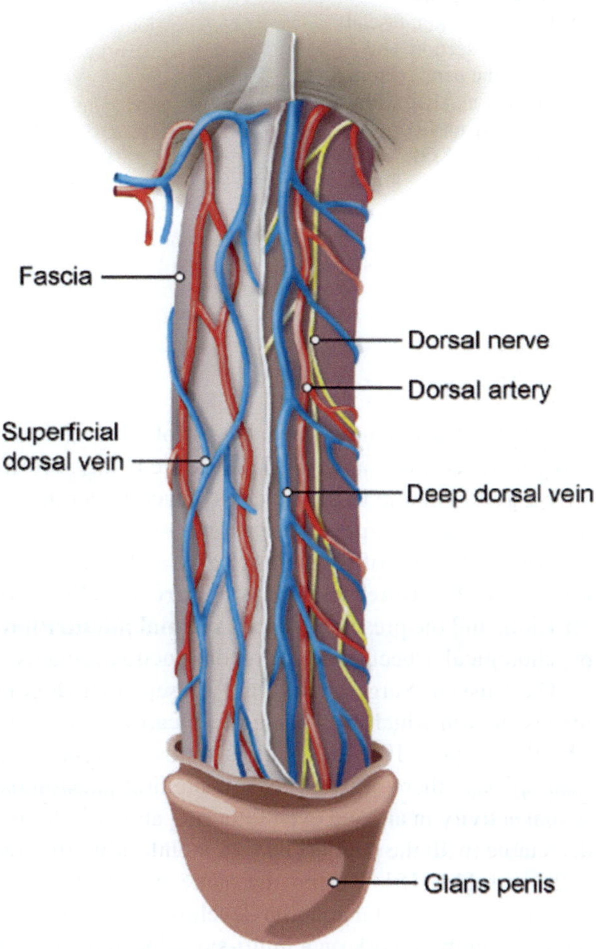

Fig. 40.1 Arteries and nerves of the penis. The skin has been removed on the left side of the illustration and the skin and superficial fascia have been removed on the right side of the illustration. (From Morrison SD et al. [9], with permission from Georg Thieme Verlag KG)

40.2 Penile Reconstruction

Penile preservation should always be attempted when there is partial amputation of the penis since total phallic reconstruction is a very complex procedure that is better left as a last resort. After a partial or subtotal loss, a penile stump of 2–3 cm might be lengthened by a conservative approach such as division of the suspensory ligament or excision of the suprapubic fat pad with a V-Y plasty of the lower abdominal skin [12, 13]. Only when a patient has lost the major part of his penis leaving no possibility for repair or preservation is phalloplasty required to replace the lost organ.

Penile reconstruction is indicated for cosmetic or functional purposes when there are congenital anomalies (microphallus, ambiguous genitalia, bladder exstrophy-epispadias complex), or when the anatomy of the penis has been disfigured or destroyed either by a natural disease (malignancy, severe Fournier's gangrene) or by

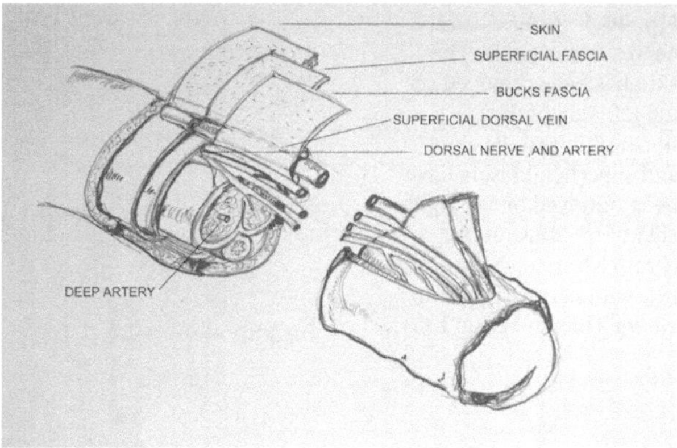

Fig. 40.2 Diagram illustrating the skin, fascial layers, cross section, and vessels of the penis. (From Biswas G et al. [10], with permission from Georg Thieme Verlag KG)

trauma, be it accidental, or the result of an assault or self-inflicted mutilation. In many instances, it is a planned procedure being performed by expert surgeons who have a good volume in the field. However, in certain circumstances, it might prove necessary as an emergency operation.

The **triple goal** of both glansplasty and phalloplasty include the creation of an **esthetic and sensate phalloid structure**, the ability to have an **erection and penetration**, and the preservation of a **normal micturition**. Besides this triple goal, the psychological aspect of penile reconstruction remains of paramount importance.

The Russian Surgeon Nikolai Aleksejevitch Bogoraz published the first penile reconstruction which was made of rib cartilage and an abdominal flap in 1936 [14, 15]. By the year 1948, he made a follow-up report of 30 patients who underwent phalloplasty: there was successful urethral anastomosis in six cases, satisfactory sexual activity in all, and even fathering ability in four of them. Skin sensitivity was detectable in all the patients by 3–4 months after the surgery and was complete after 1–2 years [14, 15]. During the same year (1948), Gilles and Harrison working together on congenital aphallia developed Bogoraz's technique and published separately a common work on a multi-staged technique of "**tube within a tube**" implying the creation of a neourethra within the neo-phallus [16, 17].

Since then, other donor sites have been used and benefited from the advent of microsurgery. The ideal site doesn't exist but the most preferable one should be hairless, sensate, thin, pliable, providing sufficient tissues to allow tubularization, and carrying a long pedicle. Gilbert and Winslow described five necessary criteria for an ideal phallic reconstruction in 1987. However, these criteria don't take into account the donor site morbidity [18, 19]:

- A single-stage reproducible procedure
- Creation of a neourethra enabling the patient to void in a standing position
- A phallus with erogenous and tactile sensibility
- Sufficient bulk allowing placement of a penile prosthesis, and henceforth a penetrative sexual intercourse
- A satisfactory aesthetic result.

Nowadays the gold standard donor site for neophalloplasty is the **radial forearm free flap (RFFF)** also called **radial artery free flap phalloplasty (RAFF)** harvested from the non-dominant upper limb [20]. RFFF has first been published by Song et al. in 1982 [21], then by Chang and Hwang in 1984 who used also a 10–11 cm segment of straight rib cartilage (from the union of eighth and ninth ribs) that was fixed to the corpora spongiosum of the penile stump [22]. Despite robbing Peter to pay Paul as it will leave a large visible scar on the patient's forearm, the RFFF is favored by many surgeons for its cosmetic penile results and urinating function. **It must be borne in mind that after harvesting a radial artery-free flap, the viability of the forearm will henceforth depend solely on the integrity of the ulnar artery. Therefore the Allen test must be performed beforehand to assess the patency of the palmar arch.**

The second most used are the suprapubic, the **fibular osteofasciocutaneous flap**, and **pedicled anterolateral thigh flaps (ALT)** which have the advantages of leaving a scar in an anatomically hidden site and having a natural skin pigmentation approaching that of the perineum. Other donor sites are less commonly used including the ulnar forearm free flap, latissimus dorsi free flap, scapular free flap, thoracodorsal artery perforator flap, bird-wing abdominal flap, upper arm flaps, and superficial circumflex iliac artery perforator flap [12, 13, 20, 23, 24]. Some authors recommended a combination of two techniques to achieve better cosmetic and functional results [25].

Designs of the neophallus are also multiple: The **tube-within-a-tube** design (the most popular), the **shaft-only** design with no included neourethra, the **composite design** (separate donor sites for the urethra and shaft), the shaft-only phalloplasty combined with the construction of a urethra using a separate graft [13, 23, 24].

The technique of RFFF can be summarized in five points [13, 19, 22, 23, 26, 27] (Figs. 40.3, 40.4, 40.5, 40.6, and 40.7a–c):

- Harvesting obliquely toward the hairless ulnar aspect of the forearm a 17 × 17 cm strip using the **tube-within-a-tube technique** (4 cm for the neourethra and 13 cm for the neophallus shaft), i.e. **two skin paddles rolled in opposite directions**, and containing a dermal vascular supply between them for the urethral skin paddle. An additional skin flap is used to create a glans-like corona.
- **Urethral anastomosis**.
- Microsurgical end-to-side or end-to-end anastomosis **between the radial artery and a branch of the femoral artery**, either the deep inferior epigastric artery, the circumflex femoris lateralis, or the profunda femoris artery.
- Microsurgical end-to-end anastomosis of the **cephalic vein** and the **deep epigastric vein** or the **greater saphenous vein**.
- Connection of the **medial cutaneous nerve** of the forearm to the **ilioinguinal or iliohypogastric nerve** for protective sensation, and connection of another nerve to the **dorsal penile nerve** for erogenous sensation.

The patients are under antibiotic prophylaxis for 2 days (Intravenous cefuroxime), the flaps are monitored hourly postoperatively to detect early ischemic

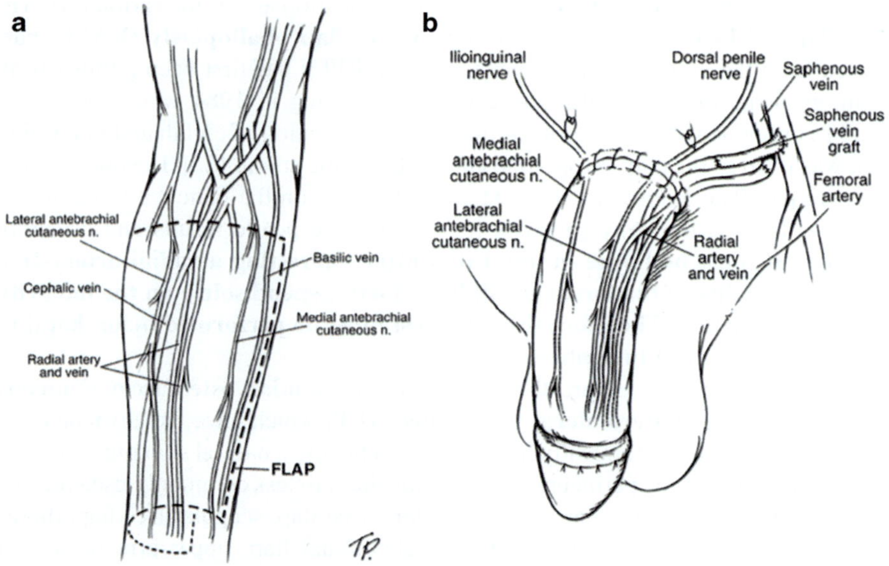

Fig. 40.3 Outline of the radial forearm free flap phalloplasty on the arm. The flap is designed to include the lateral and medial antebrachial cutaneous nerves as well as the radial artery and veins and the cephalic vein (**a**); representation of the flap following inset (**b**). (From Khavanin N and Redett RJ [19]. Creative Commons Attribution 4.0 International License)

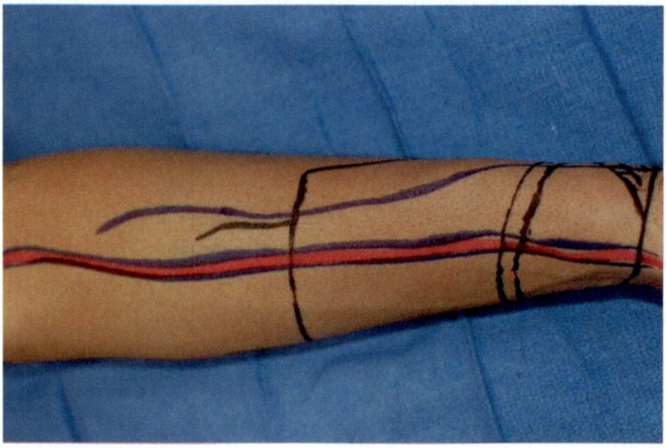

Fig. 40.4 Markings of the radial forearm free flap in situ within the forearm. The outline of the flap, including the markings for glansplasty, is made in black. The courses of the radial artery (red) along with its two venae comitantes (paired blue) and the cephalic vein (single blue) are marked out as well. (From Khavanin N and Redett RJ [19]. Creative Commons Attribution 4.0 International License)

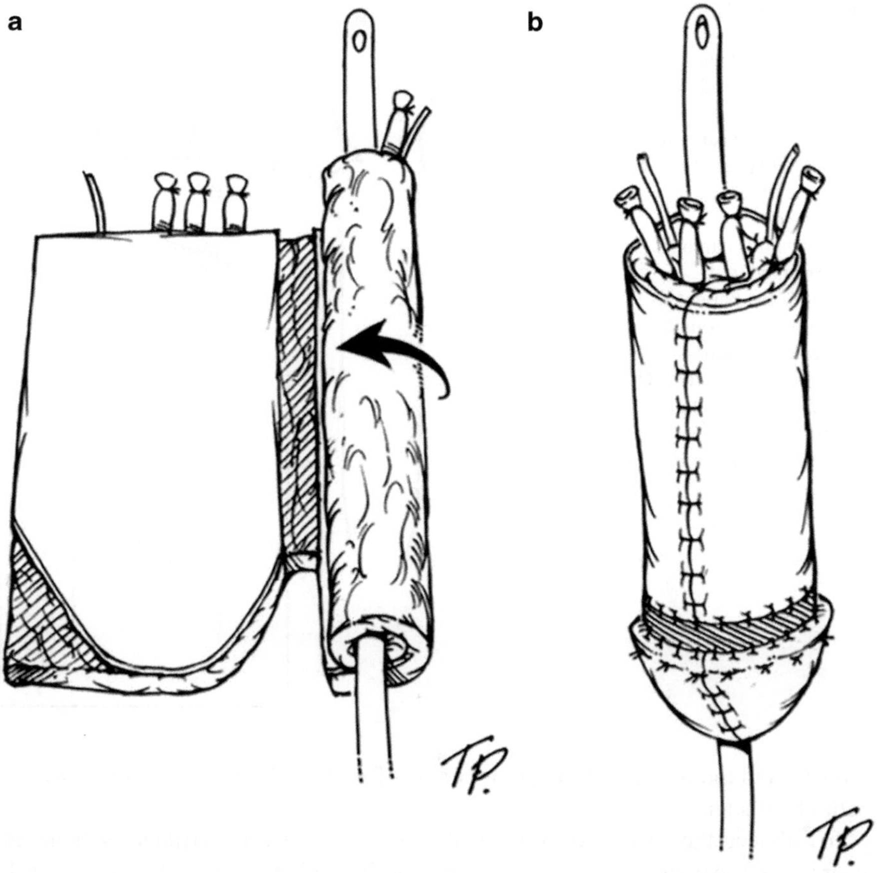

Fig. 40.5 The flap is divided into three sections prior to tubularization: the outer skin envelope of the neophallus; the de-epithelialized portion, which separates the skin and urethra; and the ulnar-sided skin paddle, which serves as the neourethra (**a**); the flap is tubularized over a 16-French Foley catheter (**b**). (From Khavanin N and Redett RJ [19]. Creative Commons Attribution 4.0 International License)

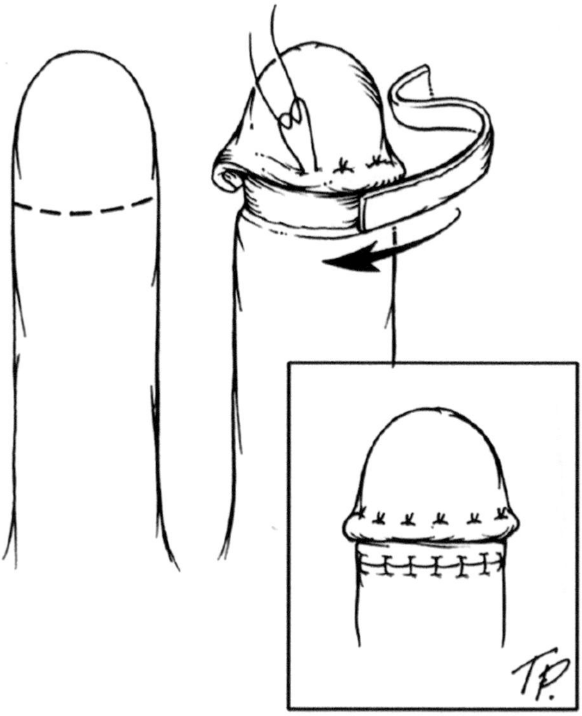

Fig. 40.6 During the glansplasty, the distal flap is de-epithelized and curled onto itself to reproduce the corona. A full-thickness skin graft is harvested from the groin and placed below. Before the return of sensation to the neophallus, this can be further refined with tattooing if the patient so wishes once the wounds have healed. (From Khavanin N and Redett RJ [19]. Creative Commons Attribution 4.0 International License)

changes, and the patients are kept on bed rest for about 10 days with an indwelling urethral catheter.

To enhance the rigidity of a neophallus that contains no cartilage or bone and ensure sexual penetration, a prosthesis is usually implanted at least 1 year after the surgery, when the patient is likely to have acquired a phallic sensation [12].

Complications of phalloplasty include hematoma, wound dehiscence, soft non-functioning phallus, infection, arterial or venous thrombosis (4% and 19%, respectively) mostly in smokers, necrosis (2–10% of cases), urethral stricture or fistula (24–42% of cases), phallic loss (1.7% of cases), etc. [12, 23, 24, 27].

When an erectile device has been implanted, further specific complications may be observed, including infection of the device, erosion, and mechanical failure, with an occurrence rate of 11.9%, 8.1%, and 22.2%, respectively [12].

Patients' satisfaction is high, being about 84–97%, with phallic sensation present in up to 86% and sexual function achievement varies between 60 and 100% [12, 23, 27].

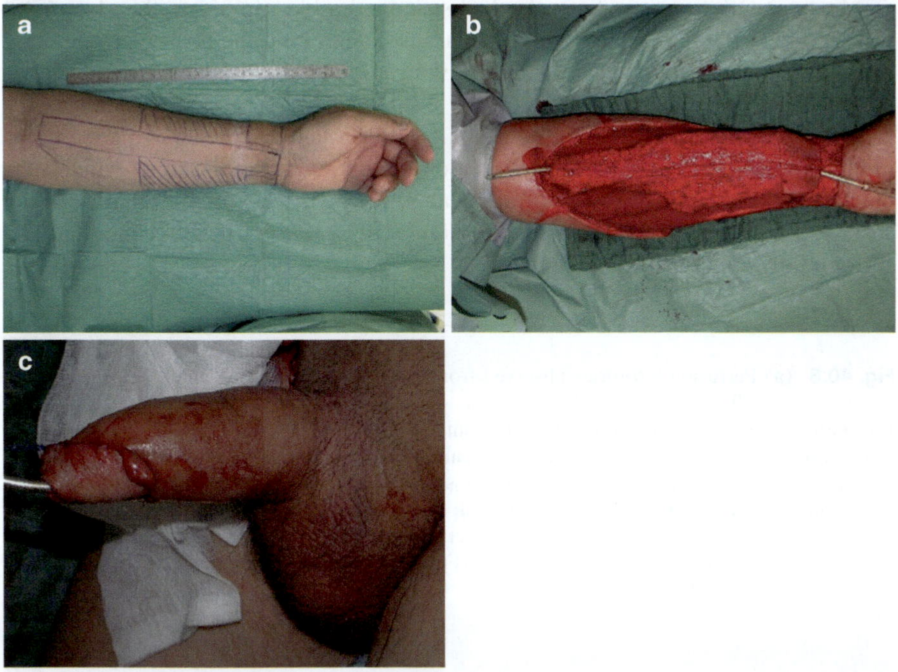

Fig. 40.7 (**a**) Flap outlined on the left forearm. The central strip will be tubed for urethral reconstruction. Skin distally (at the wrist) is planned for glans reconstruction in this patient. The stippled skin is included and then de-epithelialized to provide an augmentation effect. (**b**) The radial forearm flap tubed in-situ to form a neo-urethra, with glans distally. The fascia is sutured separately around the neo-urethra to provide a "waterproofing" layer. The radial forearm free flap donor site will be covered with a full-thickness skin graft, harvested from the left groin. (**c**) Semi-erect positioning after successful micro-anastomosis. The reconstructed glans is pink, a sign of well-vascularized free-flap tissue. (From Dabernig J et al. [26], with permission from Elsevier)

40.3 Penile Transplantation

Penile allograft transplantation is still in its infancy since the first case attempted in China in 2006 which was technically successful but the penis had to be explanted after 2 weeks reportedly due to the psychological distress of the recipient [28]. The surgery implied anastomosis of the urethra, corpus spongiosum, corpora cavernosa, and sutures of the deep dorsal vein, dorsal artery, dorsal nerve, and superficial dorsal vein.

The first successful operation was performed in South Africa in 2015 with long-term results as the patient maintained the ability to micturate and regained sexual potency (erection, orgasms, and ejaculations) [29]. This success was followed by another case in 2017 in the same institution and by the first case in the United States in 2016 [30–33].

More recently a young boy who had sustained a blast injury to the abdominal wall and perineum underwent "en-bloc" transplantation of the penis, scrotum, and lower abdominal wall in the USA in 2018 with a successful result at a 1-year follow-up [19, 33, 34].

In a cadaveric experience, Tuffaha et al. demonstrated that the three main arteries to be anastomosed in penile transplantation are the **cavernosal artery** which supplies the corpora cavernosa, the **dorsal artery** which perfuses the glans and the corpus spongiosum, and the **external pudendal artery** which perfuses the shaft and surrounding skin [35] (Fig. 40.8a–c).

Fig. 40.8 (**a**) Perfusion territories observed from the dorsal, cavernosal, and external pudendal arteries. (From Tuffaha SH et al. [35], with permission from Wolters Kluwer Health). (**b**) Illustration depicting cadaveric penile transplantation. Sup: superficial. (From Tuffaha SH et al. [35], with permission from Wolters Kluwer Health). (**c**) The recommended strategy for vascularizing penile allografts. (Left) Midshaft or distal shaft transplantation: dorsal and cavernosal arteries. (Center) Proximal shaft: dorsal, cavernosal, and external pudendal arteries with skin bridge. (Right) Proximal shaft with a surrounding defect: dorsal, cavernosal, and external pudendal arteries with additional skin to resurface the defect. (From Tuffaha SH et al. [35], with permission from Wolters Kluwer Health)

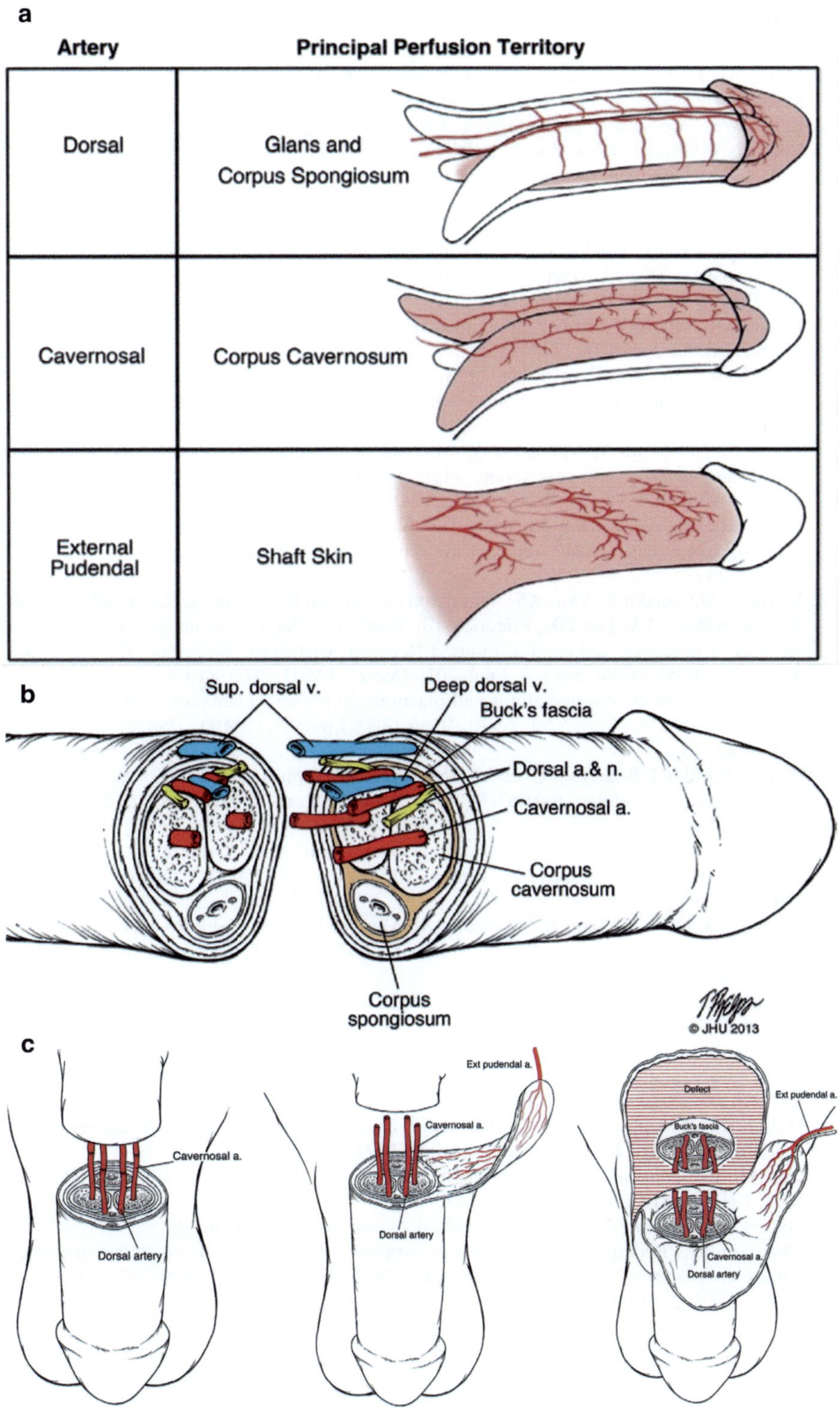
a
Artery
Principal Perfusion Territory
Dorsal
Glans and
Corpus Spongiosum
Cavernosal
Corpus Cavernosum
External
Pudendal
Shaft Skin
b
Sup. dorsal v.
Deep dorsal v.
Buck's fascia
Dorsal a.& n.
Cavernosal a.
Corpus
cavernosum
Corpus
spongiosum
© JHU 2013
c
Cavernosal a.
Dorsal artery
Ext pudendal a.
Cavernosal a.
Dorsal artery
Defect
Buck's fascia
Ext pudendal a.
Cavernosal a.
Dorsal artery

References

1. Morey AF, Brandes S, Dugi DD 3rd, et al. Urotrauma: AUA guideline. J Urol. 2014;192:327. https://www.auanet.org/guidelines-and-quality/guidelines/urotrauma-guideline
2. Ehrich WS. Two unusual penile injuries. J Urol. 1929;21:239–41.
3. Roche NA, Vermeulen BT, Blondeel PN, Stillaert FB. Technical recommendations for penile replantation based on lessons learned from penile reconstruction. J Reconstr Microsurg. 2012;28(4):247–50. https://doi.org/10.1055/s-0032-1306373. Epub 2012 Mar 7. PMID: 22399258.
4. Chou EK, Tai YT, Wu CI, Lin MS, Chen HH, Chang SC. Penile replantation, complication management, and technique refinement. Microsurgery. 2008;28(3):153–6. https://doi.org/10.1002/micr.20470. PMID: 18286649.
5. Babaei AR, Safarinejad MR. Penile replantation, science or myth? A systematic review. Urol J. 2007;4(2):62–5. PMID: 17701923.
6. Yew C, Mat Johar S, Wan Sulaiman W. Successful composite grafting of glans penis in pediatric traumatic penile amputation. Cureus. 2022;14(3):e22854. https://doi.org/10.7759/cureus.22854.
7. Tamai S, Nakamura Y, Motomiya Y. Microsurgical replantation of a completely amputated penis and scrotum: case report. Plast Reconstr Surg. 1977;60(2):287–91. https://doi.org/10.1097/00006534-197708000-00028. PMID: 887670.
8. Cohen BE, May JW Jr, Daly JS, Young HH. Successful clinical replantation of an amputated penis by microneurovascular repair. Case report. Plast Reconstr Surg. 1977;59(2):276–80. PMID: 834785.
9. Morrison SD, Shakir A, Vyas KS, Remington AC, Mogni B, Wilson SC, Grant DW, Cho DY, Rahnemai-Azar AA, Lee GK, Friedrich JB, Mardini S. Penile replantation: a retrospective analysis of outcomes and complications. J Reconstr Microsurg. 2017;33(4):227–32. https://doi.org/10.1055/s-0036-1597567. Epub 2016 Dec 21. PMID: 28002849.
10. Biswas G. Technical considerations and outcomes in penile replantation. Semin Plast Surg. 2013;27(4):205–10. https://doi.org/10.1055/s-0033-1360588. PMID: 24872770; PMCID: PMC3842340.
11. Mineo M, Jolley T, Rodriguez G. Leech therapy in penile replantation: a case of recurrent penile self-amputation. Urology. 2004;63(5):981–3. https://doi.org/10.1016/j.urology.2004.01.019. PMID: 15134999.
12. Garaffa G, Sansalone S, Ralph DJ. Penile reconstruction. Asian J Androl. 2013;15(1):16–9. https://doi.org/10.1038/aja.2012.9. Epub 2012 Mar 19. PMID: 22426595; PMCID: PMC3739136.
13. Salgado CJ, Chim H, Tang JC, Monstrey SJ, Mardini S. Penile reconstruction. Semin Plast Surg. 2011;25(3):221–8. https://doi.org/10.1055/s-0031-1281492. PMID: 22851914; PMCID: PMC3312184.
14. Bogoraz N. On complete plastic reconstruction of a penis sufficient for coitus. Sov Surg. 1936;8:303–9.
15. Schultheiss D, Gabouev AI, Jonas U. Nikolaj A. Bogoraz (1874–1952): pioneer of phalloplasty and penile implant surgery. J Sex Med. 2005;2(1):139–46. https://doi.org/10.1111/j.1743-6109.2005.20114.x. PMID: 16422917.
16. Gillies H. Congenital absence of the penis. Br J Plast Surg. 1948;1(1):8–28. https://doi.org/10.1016/s0007-1226(48)80006-8. PMID: 18874748.
17. Harrison RJ. Congenital absence of the penis with embryological considerations. Br J Plast Surg. 1948;1(1):12–28. PMID: 18874749.
18. Gilbert DA, Winslow BH. Penis construction. Semin Urol. 1987;5:262–9.
19. Khavanin N, Redett RJ. Conventional surgical techniques and emerging transplantation in complex penile reconstruction. Plast Aesthet Res. 2020;7:47. https://doi.org/10.20517/2347-9264.2020.63.

20. Yao A, Ingargiola MJ, Lopez CD, Sanati-Mehrizy P, Burish NM, Jablonka EM, Taub PJ. Total penile reconstruction: a systematic review. J Plast Reconstr Aesthet Surg. 2018;71(6):788–806. https://doi.org/10.1016/j.bjps.2018.02.002. Epub 2018 Feb 14. PMID: 29622476.
21. Song R, Gao Y, Song Y, Yu Y, Song Y. The forearm flap. Clin Plast Surg. 1982;9(1):21–6. PMID: 7094519.
22. Chang TS, Hwang WY. Forearm flap in one-stage reconstruction of the penis. Plast Reconstr Surg. 1984;74(2):251–8. https://doi.org/10.1097/00006534-198408000-00014. PMID: 6463150.
23. Ottaiano N, Pincus J, Tannenbaum J, Dawood O, Raheem O. Penile reconstruction: an up-to-date review of the literature. Arab J Urol. 2021;19(3):353–62. https://doi.org/10.1080/2090598X.2021.1957410. PMID: 34552786; PMCID: PMC8451639.
24. Sarıkaya S, Ralph DJ. Mystery and realities of phalloplasty: a systematic review. Turk J Urol. 2017;43(3):229–36. https://doi.org/10.5152/tud.2017.14554. Epub 2017 Aug 3. PMID: 28861290; PMCID: PMC5562237.
25. Ma S, Cheng K, Liu Y, Chen F. A new surgical procedure for penile reconstruction by combined free radial forearm flap and dorsalis Pedis flap. Urology. 2016;97:232–7. https://doi.org/10.1016/j.urology.2016.03.076. Epub 2016 Aug 12. PMID: 27527409.
26. Dabernig J, Shelley OP, Cuccia G, Schaff J. Urethral reconstruction using the radial forearm free flap: experience in oncologic cases and gender reassignment. Eur Urol. 2007;52(2):547–53. https://doi.org/10.1016/j.eururo.2007.01.004. Epub 2007 Jan 12. PMID: 17303320.
27. Kristinsson S, Johnson M, Ralph D. Review of penile reconstructive techniques. Int J Impot Res. 2021;33(3):243–50. https://doi.org/10.1038/s41443-020-0246-4. Epub 2020 Mar 9. PMID: 32152468.
28. Hu W, Lu J, Zhang L, Wu W, Nie H, Zhu Y, Deng Z, Zhao Y, Sheng W, Chao Q, Qiu X, Yang J, Bai Y. A preliminary report of penile transplantation. Eur Urol. 2006;50(4):851–3. https://doi.org/10.1016/j.eururo.2006.07.026. Epub 2006 Aug 8. PMID: 16930814.
29. Bateman C. World's first successful penis transplant at Tygerberg hospital. S Afr Med J. 2015;105(4):251–2. https://doi.org/10.7196/samj.9602. PMID: 26294859.
30. Carstens J. SEE: SA doctors perform second successful penis transplant. Health. 24. 2017. https://m.health24.com/News/Public-Health/see-sa-doctors-perform-second-successful-penis-transplant-20170522. Accessed 20 Jan 2019.
31. Cetrulo CL Jr, Li K, Salinas HM, Treiser MD, Schol I, Barrisford GW, McGovern FJ, Feldman AS, Grant MT, Tanrikut C, Lee JH, Ehrlichman RJ, Holzer PW, Choy GM, Liu RW, Ng ZY, Lellouch AG, Kurtz JM, Austen WG Jr, Winograd JM, Bojovic B, Eberlin KR, Rosales IA, Colvin RB, Ko DSC. Penis transplantation: first US experience. Ann Surg. 2018;267(5):983–8. https://doi.org/10.1097/SLA.0000000000002241. PMID: 28509699.
32. Ngaage LM, Elegbede A, Sugarman J, Nam AJ, Cooney CM, Cooney DS, Rasko YM, Brandacher G, Redett RJ. The Baltimore criteria for an ethical approach to penile transplantation: a clinical guideline. Transpl Int. 2020;33(5):471–82. https://doi.org/10.1111/tri.13545. Epub 2019 Dec 23. PMID: 31646681.
33. Tuffaha SH, Cooney DS, Sopko NA, Bivalacqua TJ, Lough DM, Cooney CM, Brandacher G, Lee WA, Burnett AL 2nd, Redett RJ. Penile transplantation: an emerging option for genitourinary reconstruction. Transpl Int. 2017;30(5):441–50. https://doi.org/10.1111/tri.12928. Epub 2017 Mar 5. PMID: 28130926.
34. Redett RJ 3rd, Etra JW, Brandacher G, Burnett AL, Tuffaha SH, Sacks JM, Shores JT, Bivalacqua TJ, Bonawitz S, Cooney CM, Coon D, Pustavoitau A, Rizkalla NA, Jackson AM, Javia V, Fidder SAJ, Davis-Sproul J, Brennan DC, Sander IB, Shoham S, Sopko NA, Lee WPA, Cooney DS. Total penis, scrotum, and lower abdominal wall transplantation. N Engl J Med. 2019;381(19):1876–8. https://doi.org/10.1056/NEJMc1907956. PMID: 31693813.
35. Tuffaha SH, Sacks JM, Shores JT, Brandacher G, Lee WPA, Cooney DS, Redett RJ. Using the dorsal, cavernosal, and external pudendal arteries for penile transplantation: technical considerations and perfusion territories. Plast Reconstr Surg. 2014;134(1):111e–9e. https://doi.org/10.1097/PRS.0000000000000277. PMID: 24622570.

Complications and Long-Term Sequelae of Penile Injury

41

Once again, penile fracture will take the lion's share in this discussion as it is the most frequent anatomopathological type of penile injury with the highest number of hospital attendances and surgical interventions.

A meta-analysis has shown that various complications may arise from penile fracture, either treated conservatively or surgically. **However, the occurrence rate is higher in non-surgical than in surgical approaches**, and this is true for almost all types of complications: plaques/nodules, curvature, chordee, erectile dysfunction, and pain. **The most striking difference was observed for erectile dysfunction with occurrences of 1.94% and 22% for operated and non-operated patients, respectively** [1] (Table 41.1).

There is a controversy with regard to the possible role of penile fracture in increasing the risk of Peyronie's disease. An Iranian study has shown no correlation between Peyronie's disease and penile fracture as no patient with Peyronie's disease had a history of penile trauma and no patient who sustained a penile fracture has subsequently developed Peyronie's disease after an average follow-up of 85 months [2]. However, a recent prospective observational study using an electronic microscope has revealed similar ultrastructural characteristics in post-trauma plaques and Peyronie's disease, suggesting a pernicious role of penile trauma and microtrauma in the pathogenesis of Peyronie's disease [3].

Other complications are possible due to different causes of the injury including penile ulceration and unesthetic healing and scarring scar, or even penile gangrene for constricting devices (e.g., marriage rings, metallic nut, hair, etc.) [4].

The complications of more mutilating injuries (partial or complete penile amputations) can easily be predicted as they are obvious causes of psychological disturbances in the patients arising from the loss of their virility and translated into grim consequences in their families, communities, and lives (loss of self-esteem, divorce, unsociability, loss of productivity, depression of various degrees, and suicide).

S. A. AL-Mamari, *Urogenital Trauma: A Practical Guide*,
https://doi.org/10.1007/978-981-99-6171-9_41

Table 41.1 Complications of surgically managed patients and conservatively managed patients with penile fractures

	Number	Percentage
Surgical complications		
Plaques/nodules	393	13.9
Curvature	78	2.7
Erectile dysfunction	55	1.94
Pain	40	1.40
Infection	7	0.24
Mild chordee	4	0.14
Reoperation	3	0.10
Aneurysm	2	0.07
Wound edema	1	0.04
Urinary disorder	1	0.04
Total	584	20.6
Conservative complications		
Erectile dysfunction	37	22
Curvature	23	13
Plaques/nodules	33	19.1
Pain	9	5
Chordee	7	4
Infection	4	2.3
Total	81	46

Reproduced from Amer et al. [1], with permission from Karger Publishers

Experts' panels advise anticipating these complications by initiating supportive psychological, interpersonal, and/or reproductive counseling and therapy for all patients presenting with genital trauma [5].

References

1. Amer T, Wilson R, Chlosta P, AlBuheissi S, Qazi H, Fraser M, Aboumarzouk OM. Penile fracture: a meta-analysis. Urol Int. 2016;96(3):315–29. https://doi.org/10.1159/000444884. Epub 2016 Mar 9. PMID: 26953932.
2. Zargooshi J. Trauma as the cause of Peyronie's disease: penile fracture as a model of trauma. J Urol. 2004;172(1):186–8. https://doi.org/10.1097/01.ju.0000132144.71458.86. PMID: 15201768.
3. De Rose AF, Mantica G, Bocca B, Szpytko A, Van der Merwe A, Terrone C. Supporting the role of penile trauma and micro-trauma in the etiology of Peyronie's disease. Prospective observational study using the electronic microscope to examine two types of plaques. Aging Male. 2020;23(5):740–5. https://doi.org/10.1080/13685538.2019.1586870. Epub 2019 Mar 16. PMID: 30879382.
4. Nuhu A, Edino ST, Agbese GO, Kallamu M. Penile gangrene due to strangulation by a metallic nut: a case report. West Afr J Med. 2009;28(5):340–2. https://doi.org/10.4314/wajm.v28i5.55018. PMID: 20383828.
5. Morey AF, Brandes S, Dugi DD III, et al. Urotrauma: AUA guideline. J Urol. 2014;192:327. https://www.auanet.org/guidelines-and-quality/guidelines/urotrauma-guideline.

Part VI

Scrotal and Testicular Trauma

The ancients called them "little witnesses"; however, the testicles are great actors playing a pivotal role in love life and the future of mankind.

Introduction to Scrotal and Testicular Trauma

Testicle comes from the Latin word "*testiculus*" (little witness). The first etymological theory states that it was considered a witness to male virility or manliness. Earlier than its Latin origin, it is suggested that testis comes from the Proto-Indo-European "*tris*" (three), implying that a witness is an impartial third person. A second theory states that Greeks and Romans used to place their right hands, not on a holy book, nor on the Country's constitution, nor on their hearts, but on their testicles, and swore by them before giving testimony in court. A very controversial third theory states that testicles were believed to merely play a companion role in coitus. Their presence in the scene was not for taking an active part, but only as spectators. Had the testes been able to testify, every intimate secret would have been known. The duality of the testicles might have inspired the Roman proverb "Testis unus, testis nullus" (one witness is no witness), implying that the testimony of only one person is valueless.

The antediluvian knowledge of the testicle as the source of virility and fecundity inspired Victor Medvei, the historian of endocrinology, to write: "The Oldest Key to the Endocrine Treasure Trove: The Testicles" [1]. Indeed, animal testicular extracts were taken as a medicine to treat hypogonadism and impotence from the Roman empire through the medieval Arab civilization up to modern times [2]. Conversely, male castration as a means to annihilate virility has also been reported in all ancient civilizations (Mesopotamia, Egypt, India, China, Phenicia, Greece, Rome, China, etc.) and throughout the Middle Ages up to the first half of the last century. The reasons for castration were multiple, but the most frequent were the devirilization of slaves or war captives, punishment of traitors and rapists, preparation of selected candidates for special professions (Eunuchs for harems custody, young boys to maintain their soprano or alto voices, etc.), and self-mutilation for religious devotion or delusion.

However, how the testicles play their role was unveiled only by the invention of the microscope and the first observation of spermatozoa in 1677 by the Dutch microbiologist Anthony van Leeuwenhoek (1632–1723) and the discovery and synthesis of Testosterone by three European scientists working independently, namely the Germans Ernst Laqueur and Adolf Butenandt, and the Yugoslavian Leopold Ružička in 1935 [3].

Nowadays, it is assumed that forced castration to enfeeble an individual is no longer accepted by any culture and is prohibited and punished by law. Yet the special position of the testes outside the abdomen potentially exposes them to accidental trauma. Fortunately, scrotal and testicular injuries are rare, and they seldom endanger the survival of the patient, but their dreadful aftermath lies in the risk of devirilization.

In the modern era, testicular injuries occur mostly accidentally during sports, road traffic accidents with motorcycles, or work accidents, either through a blunt or penetrating mechanism. Also, self-mutilation in psychiatric patients or transsexuals accounts for a large part of this entity. Due to its complexity, self-castration will be dealt with in detail in a separate section at the end of this book. Ultrasonography has become the first-line imaging tool to diagnose and grade a scrotal blunt trauma and some penetrating injuries, and early exploration is the recommended approach for most cases to increase the chance for testicular salvage [4–7].

Unlike the penis, testiculo-scrotal injuries cause less disfigurement because of the elasticity of the scrotum which allows its repair when partially damaged, the ease of testicular reconstruction when ruptured to some degree, and the possibility to replace the unsalvageable male gonads by size-matched silicone prostheses when necessary. These injuries also cause less functional consequences than their penile counterparts because the testes are paired organs and their endocrinological function can be replaced by exogenous androgens. However, when the trauma is bilateral or affects a solitary organ, especially in a young patient, the consequences might be dramatic.

References

1. Medvei VC. L'Envoy to the ancients. In: A history of endocrinology. Dordrecht: Springer; 1982. https://doi.org/10.1007/978-94-009-7304-6_11.
2. Nieschlag E, Nieschlag S. The history of testosterone and the testes: from antiquity to modern times. In: Hohl A, editor. Testosterone. Cham: Springer; 2017. https://doi.org/10.1007/978-3-319-46086-4_1.
3. Tomlinson JM. The testosterone story. Trends Urol Mens Health. 2012;3:34–7. https://doi.org/10.1002/tre.277.
4. EAU Guidelines. Edn. presented at the EAU annual congress Amsterdam, Mar 2022. ISBN: 978-94-92671-16-5. Available on https://uroweb.org/guidelines/urological-trauma/chapter/urogenital-trauma-guidelines.

5. Morey AF, Broghammer JA, Hollowell CMP, McKibben MJ, Souter L. Urotrauma guideline 2020: AUA guideline. J Urol. 2021;205(1):30–5. https://doi.org/10.1097/JU.0000000000001408. Epub 2020 Oct 14.
6. Lucky M, Brown G, Dorkin T, Pearcy R, Shabbir M, Shukla CJ, Rees RW, Summerton DJ, Muneer A, BAUS Section of Andrology and Genitourethral Surgery (AGUS). British Association of Urological Surgeons (BAUS) consensus document for the management of male genital emergencies—testicular trauma. BJU Int. 2018;121(6):840–4. https://doi.org/10.1111/bju.14163. Epub 2018 Apr 10.
7. Morey AF, Metro MJ, Carney KJ, Miller KS, McAninch JW. Consensus on genitourinary trauma: external genitalia. BJU Int. 2004;94(4):507–15. https://doi.org/10.1111/j.1464-410X.2004.04993.x.

42 Anatomy of the Scrotum and Testicles

42.1 Embryology

The two labioscrotal swellings appear lateral to the genital tubercle during the 4th week of gestation and migrate caudally and medially in the 9th–11th weeks of gestation merging at the 12th week of gestation to form the scrotum [1, 2].

The testicle development starts with the **genital ridge**. It originates from the **intermediate mesoderm** as paired structures near the primitive kidneys and forms by the proliferation of coelomic epithelial cells on the ventromedial aspect of the two mesonephroi. The **mesonephros** also contains two parallel structures: the **mesonephric duct (Wolffian duct)**, which contributes to the formation of the epididymis, seminal vesicles, and vas deferens after male sex determination, and the **paramesonephric duct (Müllerian duct)**, which is the female equivalent of the mesonephric duct and gives rise to the fallopian tubes, uterus, and part of the vagina after female sex determination [3, 4]. The **mesonephros** and the **genital ridge** are collectively referred to as the **urogenital ridge**.

With the secretion of **anti-Müllerian hormone (AMH)** by the fetal testis, Müllerian duct embryonic structures (e.g., Fallopian tubes, uterus, and upper vagina) regress in male fetuses. The persisting Müllerian remnants are a small appendage near the head of the epididymis called the appendix testis. The regression of Müllerian structures is paralleled by the promotion of Wolffian or mesonephric duct triggered by the secretion of testosterone by the fetal testis resulting in the development of the epididymis, vas deferens, and prostate gland [5].

By the 13th week, the lower pole of the testis and the epididymis are anchored to the internal inguinal ring by the genito-inguinal ligament, or "**gubernaculum**

S. A. AL-Mamari, *Urogenital Trauma: A Practical Guide*,
https://doi.org/10.1007/978-981-99-6171-9_42

testis,"[1] which has developed caudally to the mesonephros from a mesonephric fold under stimulation of Insulin-like peptide 3, from the sixth to the eighth week. There are two distinct phases in the testicular descent: the **transabdominal phase** which is completed by the 15th week and the **inguinoscrotal phase** which is completed by the end of the seventh month of gestation or the 35th week [7–10].

In the extra-uterine life, the gubernaculum persists as a fibrous attachment of the testes to the base of the scrotum that prevents torsion and many variations exist [11].

Many hypotheses have attempted to explain the reasons behind the testicular descent and the evolutionary origin of the scrotum; however, none of them is perfect and all are subjected to criticisms [12]:

- The classic cooling hypothesis: The testicles migrate outside the body core to lie in a cooler milieu favorable to spermatogenesis and for reducing the mutation rate in the male germ line.
- The training hypothesis: The hostile environment of the scrotum prepares the sperm to resist other stress, namely, fertilization.
- The display hypothesis: The scrotum has a sexual signaling function, being brightly colored in some mammalians.
- The galloping hypothesis: The scrotum developed in mammals that frequently gallop, leap, or jump, creating fluctuations in intraabdominal pressure that would endanger the process of spermatogenesis. Stable pressure makes the intrascrotal cavity a safer place against this risk.

42.2 Gross Anatomy

42.2.1 The Scrotum

The **scrotum** is a saccular structure located below the penis and divided into two compartments by the **scrotal septum**, each containing a testicle. It has a characteristic pleated and extensible skin that shows a vertical hyperpigmented midline referred to as the **median raphe**. It is very vascular and is covered with hairs from puberty. It is composed of skin and thin muscles deriving embryologically from the abdominal wall. It is formed by seven layers that can be remembered by the funny mnemonic "**S**ome **D**amn **E**nglishman **C**alled **I**t **T**he **T**estis": **S**kin, **D**artos fascia and smooth muscle, **E**xternal spermatic fascia, **C**remasteric fascia, **I**nternal spermatic fascia, **T**unica vaginalis, and **T**unica albuginea [13] (Fig. 42.1). **While this mnemonic is very helpful, it is important for the reader to bear in mind that the tunica albuginea is a part of the testis rather than a scrotal layer**. The first six named layers correspond to the following abdominal wall layers: skin to skin,

[1] "Gubernaculum" is a Latin word that means "steering wheel," "helm," or "rudder." It was so-named by the British Surgeon John Hunter (1728–1793) in 1762 because he thought this structure directed the descending course of the testis to the scrotum. He was the younger brother of the Anatomist, William Hunter [6].

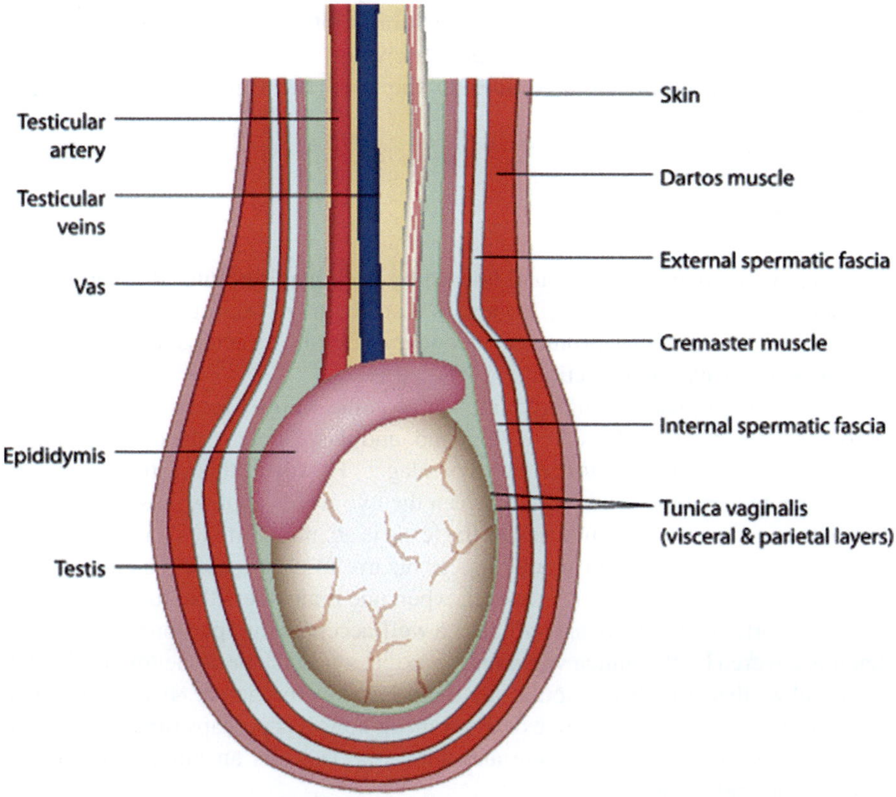

Fig. 42.1 Scrotal layers. (From Maguire et al. [13], with permission from Springer Nature)

Dartos and smooth muscle to Scarpa's fascia, external spermatic fascia to external oblique muscle, cremasteric fascia and muscle to internal oblique + transversus abdominis muscles + their aponeuroses, internal spermatic fascia to transversalis fascia, and tunica vaginalis to the peritoneum.

The scrotum has a rich arterial blood supply from both the internal and external iliac arteries with dense anastomoses. The **external iliac artery** gives rise to the **deep external pudendal artery** and then to the **anterior scrotal artery** which supplies the anterior scrotum. The **internal iliac artery** supplies the posterior scrotum through the **internal pudendal** and the **posterior scrotal artery** [14].

The scrotal venous drainage proceeds through both **superficial and deep venous networks**. The veins forming the superficial network mostly follow the arteries, with the anterior scrotum draining into the great saphenous vein through the external pudendal and the posterior scrotum draining into the internal iliac vein via the internal pudendal branches. The deep network is an aggregate from a dozen of small veins called the **pampiniform plexus** which drains the testis and epididymis [14].

The pampiniform plexus coalesces cranially to form the **gonadal or testicular vein** which empties into the renal vein on the left side and into the inferior vena cava

(IVC) on the right side. The deferential vein drains into the pelvic plexus, while the cremasteric vein ends in the inferior epigastric vein.

The scrotal lymph drainage goes to the superficial and then deep inguinal nodes.

42.2.2 The Testis

The testis is the paired male gonad housed by each hemiscrotum. It is the sperm-producing organ (spermatogenesis) and is also the most important contributor to androgen production that promotes secondary sexual characteristics in males as well as sexual drives and erection.

It has been proposed to differentiate between the words "Testis" and "Testicle" as follows: The testis is the sole male gonad, and the testicle is the combination of the testis, epididymis, and testicular appendages. However, this distinction is seldom respected, and the synonymy between the two words applies most of the time.

There is controversy about whether the testis is an intraperitoneal or an extraperitoneal organ. This statement would appear bizarre to many readers as the testis is undoubtedly extra-abdominal. However, when one remembers that the testis shares a common origin with the ovary, which is a well-accepted intraperitoneal organ, and that it is covered by the tunica vaginalis, an extension of the peritoneum, he/she will soon realize that this discussion is anything but supererogatory. It is known that some intraabdominal organs are extraperitoneal; now, it is perhaps time to acknowledge the existence of the opposite and admit the testis as an intraperitoneal and extra-abdominal organ [15].

The right testis is most frequently higher than the left counterpart, and this asymmetry has been known since old civilizations as portrayed by Ancient Greece sculptures [16]. The average testicular volume is 20 cc, and the right is slightly larger (10% more) than the left. The testis longitudinal diameter measures 4.4–5.1 cm, and its average weight is 15–19 g [5]. An Indian post-mortem study showed slight variations according to age with lower weight (17 g) in 18–20-year-old subjects, higher weight (19 g) in 41–50-year-old subjects, and again lower weight (17 g) above 60 years [17].

Functionally, the testis is a mixt gland being endocrine and exocrine. Its **Leydig cells** secrete androgens (testosterone) in the bloodstream, while its haploid germ cells develop into sperms which travel through the seminiferous tubules, epididymides, and the vasa deferentia. The mature germ cells or gametes have the unique role of perpetuating the species by "**giving rise to organisms rather than to organs**" through a combination with the opposite-sex counterparts, the ova [18].

The **Sertoli cells** are somatic or diploid cells found on the walls of the seminiferous tubules playing an important role in testis formation and spermatogenesis by facilitating the progression of germ cells to spermatozoa. Indeed, follicle-stimulating hormone **(FSH) and testosterone regulate spermatogenesis through their action on Sertoli cells** [19]. Sertoli cells also protect the germ cells by spreading around them as tentacular cells from the peripheral basement membrane of the seminiferous tubules to the lumen. Doing so, they form tight junctions between them and create the **blood–testis barrier** that protects the haploid sperms from the autoimmune response from the organism and from hazardous bloodborne substances and infections [20].

Structurally, the testis is delineated by the **tunica albuginea**, which is considered **the densest and toughest connective tissue in the body**, carrying the important mission of protecting the testis from environmental hazards. Septa from the tunica albuginea divide the testis into 200–400 wedge-shaped **lobes**, each containing 3–10 coiled **seminiferous tubules** which constitute about 90% of the testicular mass. The seminiferous tubules converge to a gathering point, the **rete testis**, located at the **testicular hilum** or **mediastinum testis**. From here, **efferent tubules** (ductuli efferentes) carry the sperms to a single tube within the **head, body, and tail of the epididymis**, which is continuous with the **vas or ductus deferens** [21] (Fig. 42.2).

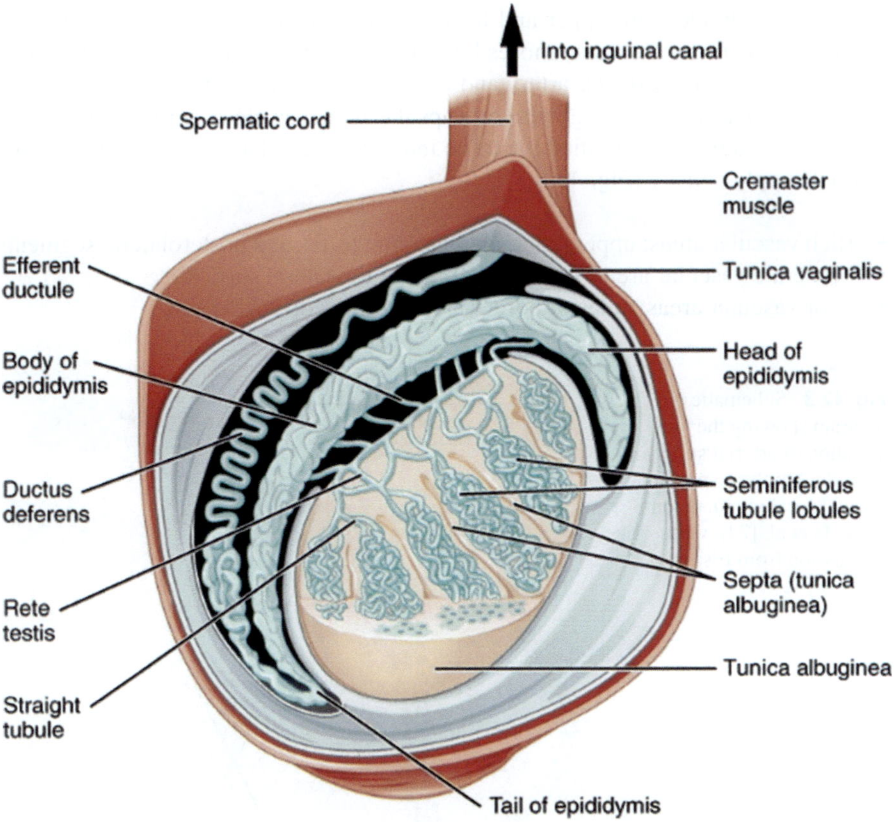

Fig. 42.2 Anatomy of the testis: This sagittal view shows the seminiferous tubules, the site of sperm production. Formed sperm are transferred to the epididymis, where they mature. They leave the epididymis during an ejaculation via the ductus deferens. (From Openstax.org books: Anatomy and physiology of the testicular reproductive system. Creative Commons Attribution license. https://openstax.org/books/anatomy-and-physiology-2e/pages/27-1-anatomy-and-physiology-of-the-testicular-reproductive-system)

The **efferent ductules** are unique because they are the sole part of the male reproductive system that is lined by an epithelium containing both absorptive cells and cells with motile cilia. On the one hand, these features allow the sperm to travel rapidly into the epididymis, and on the other hand, the potential of ductal cells in fluid reabsorption favors sperm transport, concentration, and maturation, therefore enhancing male fertility [22].

The testis has a triple arterial blood supply. The principal source is the **testicular artery**, a branch of the abdominal aorta originating at L2–L3 just below the renal arteries (remember that the embryological formation of the testes started near the kidneys), but variations exist [23]. The other two suppliers are the **cremasteric artery** arising from the inferior epigastric artery and the **deferential artery or artery to the vas** which originates from the inferior vesical artery. A cadaveric study showed that the testicular artery has a straight course in 85% and a convoluted path in 15% and mostly terminates in the upper pole of the mediastinum testis (78.8%) and divides into upper and lower polar branches in the majority of cases (69.7%) [24]. There are anastomoses between the cremasteric artery and the lower polar branch of the testicular artery and between the artery to the vas and branches of the testicular artery through several capsular branches close to the mediastinum testis. This study also classified the testis into three vascular areas according to the arterial supply density (Fig. 42.3):

- Rich vascular areas: upper polar, mediastinum testis, and posterolateral segments
- Moderate vascular areas: the middle third of the lateral surfaces
- Poor vascular areas: anterior border and anterolateral surfaces

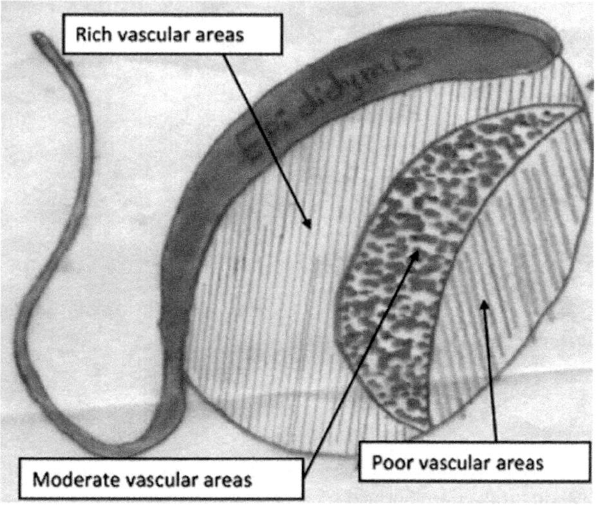

Fig. 42.3 Schematic diagram showing the variation of arterial supply according to the testicular areas (lateral view). (From Mostafa et al. [24], with permission from Elsevier)

The testicular venous return is ensured by the **pampiniform plexus**[2] which is primarily drained by the **testicular or gonadal vein**, also called the **internal spermatic vein**, and the **external pudendal vein**, a tributary of the great saphenous vein. The **cremasteric vein**, also referred to as the **external spermatic vein**, and **the vasal or deferential vein** play a minimal role and empty into the inferior epigastric vein and the pelvic plexus, respectively [14]. The testicular vein drains into the renal vein on the left side and the inferior vena cava on the right side. However, there exist some individual variations [24].

In the lower third, as many as four to six trunks of testicular vein have been described. Midway between the internal inguinal ring and the lower pole of the kidney, the testicular vein divides into medial and lateral branches to form a delta. The medial branch terminates into the left renal vein or the inferior vena cava (IVC) after communicating with the ureteral veins and the contralateral renal vein: **This cross-communication exists only in 50% of individuals and is the only site where the left and right testicular vein systems anastomose** [25]. Here again, many individual variations exist [26].

The lateral branch of the testicular vein communicates with colonic and renal capsular veins before entering the perinephric space where it terminates.

The testicular veins are valveless and subjected to reflux and possible development of varicoceles. The rationale behind varicocele ligation or embolization lies in the interruption of blood flow in these valveless veins and the promotion of the blood return through the external pudendal valved veins that drain into the great saphenous vein (the longest vein in the body), a tributary of the femoral vein. It is important to realize that the whole principle of varicocele treatment stands in this anatomical detail as any testicular vein ligation would be catastrophic to the testis (venous ischemia) if should alternative drainage be absent, or useless should it also be valveless. Noteworthy cadaveric studies have revealed that varicocelogenesis is not triggered by the sole valveless nature of the gonadal vein (if it were so, varicocele would be present in all men), and that reflux is not the primum movens but is rather secondary to a change in the pressure gradient at the junction between the testicular and the renal veins [27].

42.2.3 The Epididymis

As mentioned above, the epididymis is a comma-shaped structure that contains a single tube deriving from the efferent ductules. This tube is highly convoluted and tightly compressed, with an estimated length of about 6 m (20 ft) when straightened as reported in many old anatomical books. However, a recent study raised controversy by publishing lower values of only 30.48 cm [28]. It is made of a head lying at the upper pole of the testis, a body, and a tail which is continued by the vas deferens. The epididymis function is not just about the transportation of the sperms as this would be more effective and rapid in a shorter duct. Its main functions are the storage and maturation of sperm.

---

[2] Pampiniform comes from the Latin word "*pampinus*," tendril, and "forma," form or shape.

42.2.4 The Vas Deferens

The vas or ductus deferens originates as a continuation of the epididymal tail and has approximately a 30–45 cm length and a 2–3 mm diameter in adults. It travels within the spermatic cord through the scrotum and the inguinal canal to enter the pelvic cavity. It then crosses above the ureter and approaches its opposite, both turning downward side by side and dilating to form the **ampulla** which lies parallel and medial to the **seminal vesicles. Each ampulla fuses with the duct of the corresponding seminal vesicle to form the ejaculatory duct** which crosses the **prostate** to open into the prostatic urethra lateral to the urethral crest.

42.2.5 The Spermatic Cord

The spermatic cord's diameter is 18.6 mm (11–26 mm) [29] and travels through the inguinal canal.

It is formed by the invagination of **three** anterior abdominal wall fascial layers and serves as the connecting channel between the abdominal and scrotal cavities. The layers are as follows, from the outermost to the innermost: external spermatic fascia (from the aponeurosis of the external oblique muscle), cremasteric fascia (from the internal oblique fascia), and the internal spermatic fascia (from transversalis fascia). The cord contains the testicular artery, the vas deferens and its artery, the cremasteric artery, the pampiniform venous plexus, the deferential vein, the cremasteric vein, the genital branch of the genitofemoral nerve (supplies the cremasteric fascia and muscle), parasympathetic and sympathetic nerve fibers, and lymphatics. **The rule of "Three" helps recall these structures: three layers, three arteries, three veins, three nerves, and three other things (vas deferens, lymphatics, and the closed processus vaginalis)** [14].

Like the blood supply, lymph from the testis and epididymis recalls the embryological origins and drains into lymph nodes located in the retroperitoneum near the renal vessels' origins. Branches from the ilioinguinal nerve and the iliohypogastric nerve travel outside the cord.

42.3 Congenital Abnormalities

Congenital anomalies of the testis, epididymis, and vas deferens have been reported in 2% of normal male fetuses [30]. They include the following:

1. **Undescended testis or cryptorchidism** (from Greek words *Kryptos*, hidden, and *orchis*, testis): This is the most frequent testicular abnormality after excluding congenital hydrocele which is considered physiological up to 1 year of age. Studies have shown that the prevalence of undescended testis in boys with a birth weight of ≥2500 g has increased in several countries from around 2% to 4–8% in the last decades [31]. It is important to mention that not all mammals have descended intrascrotal testes, and authors have proposed to group them in

"four character state models": (1) testicondy (the testicles remain intraabdominal, positioned close to the kidney and the scrotum is not present, e.g., sirenians and cetaceans), (2) descended ascrotal (descended testicles but no developed scrotum), (3) descended scrotal (descended testes and fully developed scrotum), and (4) marsupial model[3] (descended testicles and well-developed scrotum, but in a prepenial position, contrary to Eutherians[4] where the scrotum is postpenial) [12].

2. **Neonatal testicular torsion**: About 150 cases have been reported in the literature and most of the cases (80%) occur before birth, justifying their presence in this paragraph as "congenital abnormalities" [33, 34].
3. **Testicular agenesis or anorchia**: Anorchia is mostly associated with agenesis of the vas deferens, and some are associated with unilateral renal agenesis [35].
4. **Vanishing testis**: This is also referred to as "**Testicular regression syndrome**," resulting from atrophy and disappearance of an initial normal testis during fetal life. It should be differentiated from testicular agenesis. It is estimated to be present in 5% of cryptorchidism [36].
5. **Polyorchidism**: A metanalysis published in 2009 revealed 140 cases of histologically confirmed polyorchidism published in the literature with the great majority being triorchidism and a predominance on the left side [37]. An exceptional case of five testicles has also been reported [38] (Fig. 42.4).
6. **Isolated epididymal agenesis**: This can be unilateral or bilateral.
7. **Agenesis of the vas deferens**: This may also be unilateral or bilateral. Congenital bilateral absence of the vas deferens (CBAVD) occurs in 1 in 1000 men and accounts for 1–2% of male infertility and for 6% of obstructive azoospermia.

   It is secondary to cystic fibrosis transmembrane conductance regulator (CFTR) gene mutation and affects nearly 95% of men with cystic fibrosis [39].
8. **Scrotal or penoscrotal transposition**: In this anomaly, the scrotum is located cephalic to the penis like in Marsupials. Fewer than 20 cases of complete penoscrotal transposition with an intact scrotum have been described in the literature [40] (Fig. 42.5).
9. **Bifid scrotum**: This is defined as a midline cleft of the scrotum and may be associated with hypospadias [41].
10. **Accessory or ectopic** scrotum [42].

---

[3] Marsupials are mammals found in Australasia, Wallacia, and the Americas. They comprise a handful of species such as kangaroos, koalas, opossums, bandicoots, wallabies, wombats, and Tasmanian devils. They do not develop a well-defined anatomical placenta but have a functional single layer of trophoblasts that produces hormones and a yolk sac. They do not have an umbilical cord, and the placentation period is shorter than for eutherians. However, this is compensated by a physiologically sophisticated and extended lactation allowing them "to exchange the umbilical cord for the teat" [32].

[4] Eutherians or placental mammals is a group of mammals comprising nearly 4000 species, including humans, monkeys, rodents, bats, elephants, whales, shrews, armadillos, dogs, cats, sheep, cattle, horses, and so on.

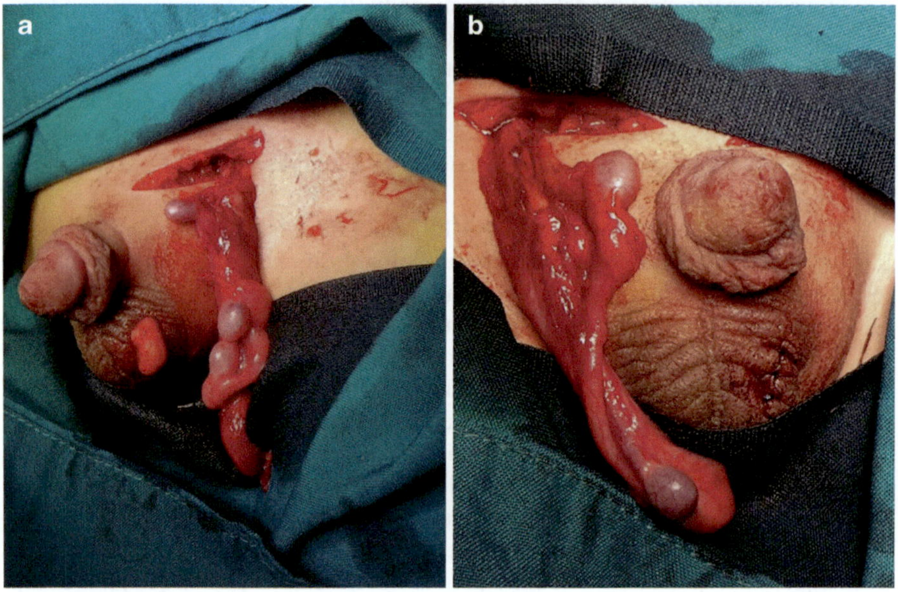

Fig. 42.4 Intraoperative view of polyorchidism in a 13-month-old boy operated for undescended testes. (**a**) Three testes seen on the left side. (**b**) Two testes seen on the right side with a very long epididymis connecting them. (From Zahirian Moghadam et al. [38], Commons Attribution 4.0 International License)

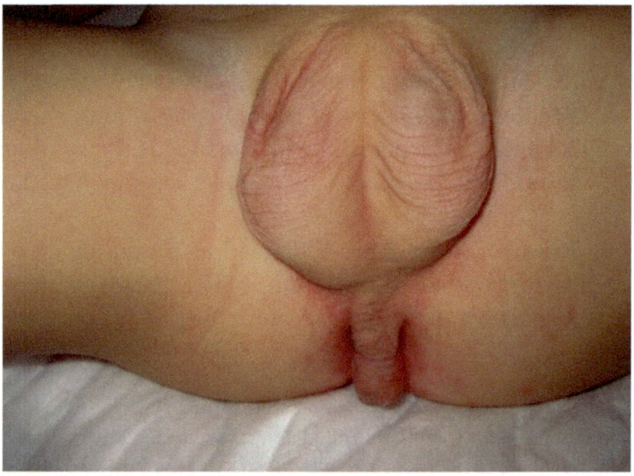

Fig. 42.5 Complete penoscrotal transposition. (From Somoza et al. [40]. Creative Commons Attribution License)

11. **Scrotal hemangioma**: Hemangiomata are benign proliferations of vascular endothelial cells. Congenital scrotal septum hemangiomas are very rare [42].
12. **Splenogonadal fusion**: This affects both sexes, but mostly the males with a male-to-female ratio of 16:1. The left testicle connects in a continuous or discontinuous fashion to splenic tissue, usually an accessory spleen. About 220 cases have been reported in the literature [43] (Fig. 42.6).

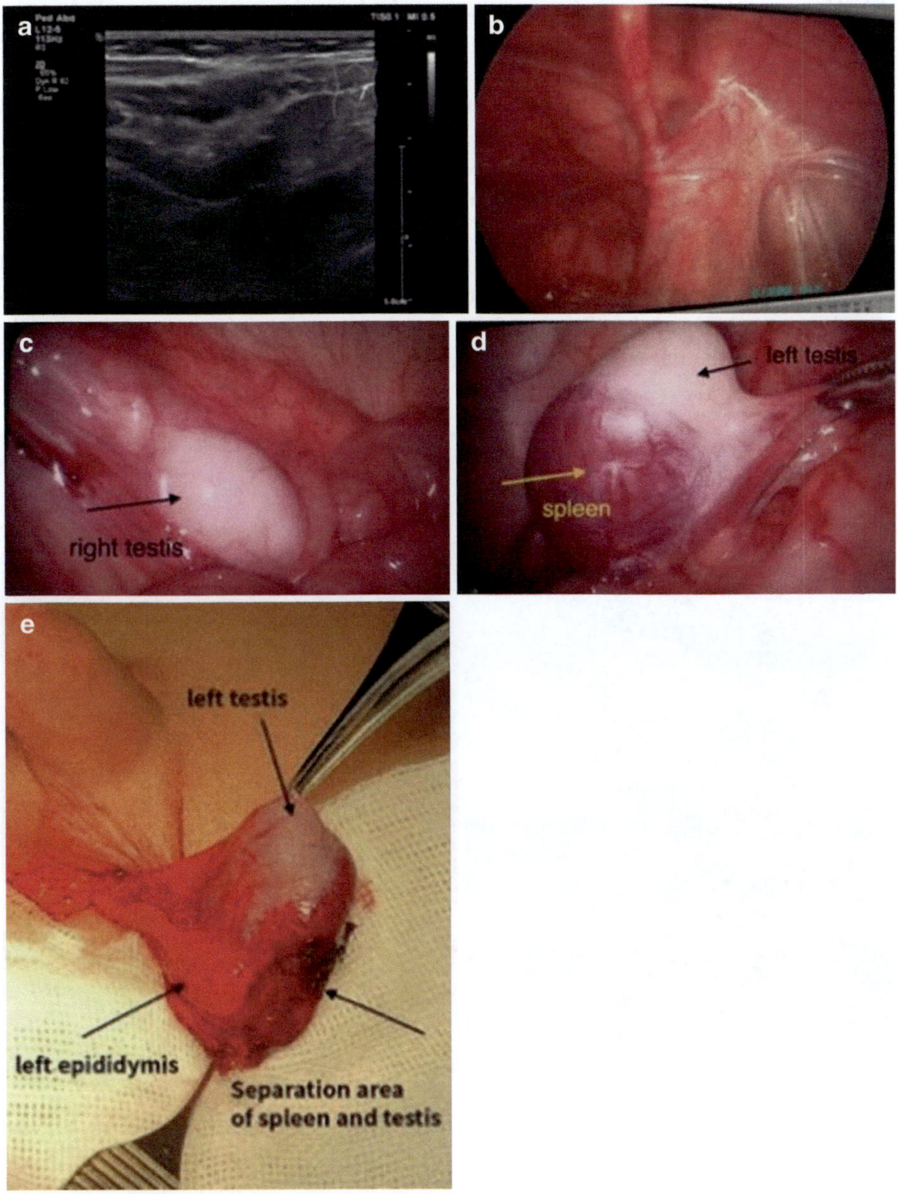

Fig. 42.6 Continuous splenogonadal fusion on the left side and undescended right testis in an 8-month-old male infant. (**a**) Pre-operative B-mode ultrasound revealed possible fusion of the left testis and the kidney; (**b**) single site laparoscopic examination revealed a closed right internal ring and the right testis in the iliac fossa, at about the same height as the junction between the iliac vessel and the right vas deferens; (**c**) single-site laparoscopic examination visualized the right testis located in the right iliac fossa, approximately 2 cm above the right internal ring, with poorly developed right spermatic vessel; (**d**) complete fusion of the spleen and the left testis in the left iliac fossa visualized by the single-site laparoscopic examination; (**e**) the left testis descended into the scrotum after being separated from the spleen. (From Chen et al. [43]. Creative Commons Attribution)

13. **Hemiscrotal agenesis**: Extremely rare. Only eight cases are reported in the English literature including some cases with heterotopic development of scrotal tissue island in the inguinal region and extra-genital abnormalities [44, 45].
14. **Scrotal agenesis**: Complete congenital agenesis has been reported in only eight cases [46, 47].
15. **Scrotoschisis**: Here the testicle eviscerates through a scrotal wall defect and lies extracorporeally. Only a dozen of cases have been reported in the literature [48, 49] (Fig. 42.7).
16. **Crossed testicular ectopia (CTE)**: This is defined by both testes being found in one hemiscrotum subsequently to a descent error. The estimated global incidence of CTE is 1:4 million, and most of the time, the right testis is abnormally located on the left side [50] (Fig. 42.8).

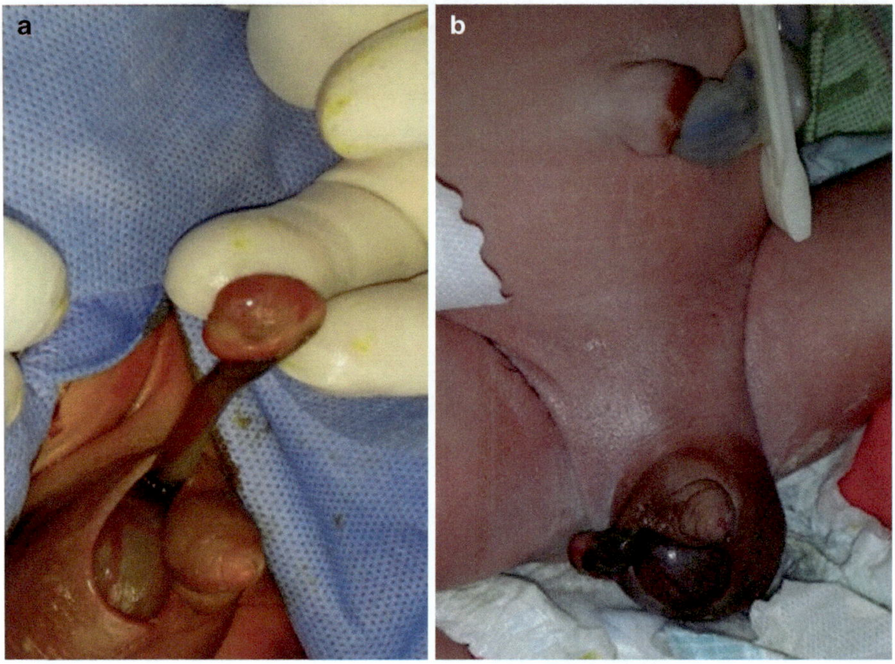

Fig. 42.7 (**a** and **b**) Congenital exposure of the right testis. (From Mohamed Mahfouz [49] with permission from Elsevier)

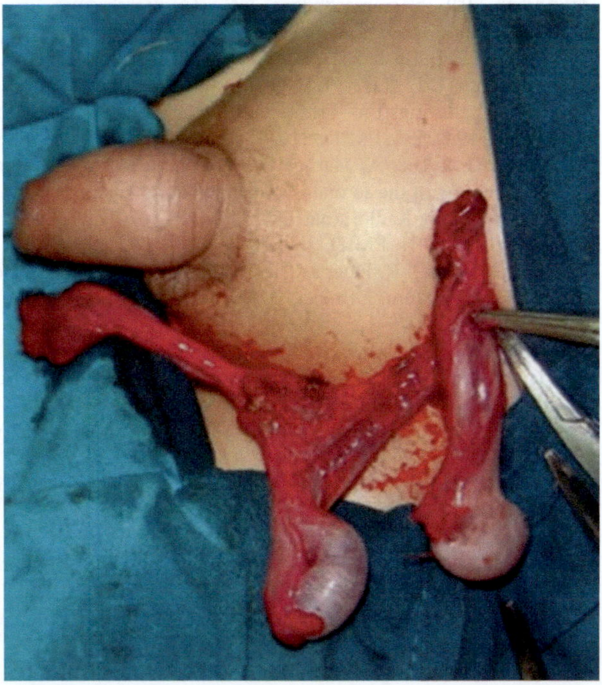

Fig. 42.8 Crossed testicular ectopia. (From Fahmy [50], with permission from Springer Nature)

References

1. Garcia RA, Sajjad H. Anatomy, abdomen and pelvis, scrotum. In: StatPearls [Internet]. Treasure Island, FL: StatPearls Publishing; 2022. PMID: 31751083.
2. van der Werff JF, Nievelstein RA, Brands E, Luijsterburg AJ, Vermeij-Keers C. Normal development of the male anterior urethra. Teratology. 2000;61(3):172–83. https://doi.org/10.1002/(SICI)1096-9926(200003)61:3<172::AID-TERA4>3.0.CO;2-B. PMID: 10661906.
3. Titi-Lartey OA, Khan YS. Embryology, testicle. In: StatPearls [Internet]. Treasure Island, FL: StatPearls Publishing; 2022. PMID: 32491695.
4. Yang Y, Workman S, Wilson M. The molecular pathways underlying early gonadal development. J Mol Endocrinol. 2018; https://doi.org/10.1530/JME-17-0314. Epub ahead of print. PMID: 30042122.
5. Silber S. Adult testis anatomy. In: Fundamentals of male infertility. Cham: Springer; 2018. https://doi.org/10.1007/978-3-319-76523-5_3.
6. Hunter J. Observations on the state of the testis in the fetus, and on the hernia congenita. In: Hunter W, editor. William Hunter medical commentaries. London: Hamilton; 1762. p. 75–90.
7. Virtanen HE, Cortes D, Rajpert-De Meyts E, Ritzén EM, Nordenskjöld A, Skakkebaek NE, Toppari J. Development and descent of the testis in relation to cryptorchidism. Acta Paediatr. 2007;96:622–7. https://doi.org/10.1111/j.1651-2227.2007.00244.x.
8. Favorito LA, Costa SF, Julio-Junior HR, Sampaio FJ. The importance of the gubernaculum in testicular migration during the human fetal period. Int Braz J Urol. 2014;40(6):722–9. https://doi.org/10.1590/S1677-5538.IBJU.2014.06.02. PMID: 25615240.

9. Amann RP, Veeramachaneni DN. Cryptorchidism in common eutherian mammals. Reproduction. 2007;133(3):541–61. https://doi.org/10.1530/REP-06-0272. PMID: 17379650.
10. Harrison SM, Bush NC, Wang Y, Mucher ZR, Lorenzo AJ, Grimsby GM, Schlomer BJ, Büllesbach EE, Baker LA. Insulin-like peptide 3 (INSL3) serum concentration during human male fetal life. Front Endocrinol (Lausanne). 2019;10:596. https://doi.org/10.3389/fendo.2019.00596. PMID: 31611843; PMCID: PMC6737488.
11. Cavalie G, Bellier A, Marnas G, Boisson B, Robert Y, Rabattu PY, Chaffanjon P. Anatomy and histology of the scrotal ligament in adults: inconsistency and variability of the gubernaculum testis. Surg Radiol Anat. 2018;40(4):365–70. https://doi.org/10.1007/s00276-017-1904-1. Epub 2017 Jul 31. PMID: 28762084.
12. Kleisner K, Ivell R, Flegr J. The evolutionary history of testicular externalization and the origin of the scrotum. J Biosci. 2010;35(1):27–37. https://doi.org/10.1007/s12038-010-0005-7. PMID: 20413907.
13. Maguire K, Sabharwal AJ. F5 acute scrotal exploration. In: Carachi R, Agarwala S, Bradnock TJ, Lim Tan H, Cascio S, editors. Basic techniques in pediatric surgery. Berlin: Springer; 2013. https://doi.org/10.1007/978-3-642-20641-2_118.
14. Patel AP. Anatomy and physiology of chronic scrotal pain. Transl Androl Urol. 2017;6(Suppl 1):S51–6. https://doi.org/10.21037/tau.2017.05.32. PMID: 28725619; PMCID: PMC5503924.
15. Pham SB, Hong MK, Teague JA, Hutson JM. Is the testis intraperitoneal? Pediatr Surg Int. 2005;21(4):231–9. https://doi.org/10.1007/s00383-005-1364-2. Epub 2005 Mar 9. PMID: 15756559.
16. McManus IC. Right-left and the scrotum in Greek sculpture. Laterality. 2004;9(2):189–99. https://doi.org/10.1080/13576500342000149. PMID: 15382717.
17. Jit I, Sanjeev. Weight of the testes in Northwest Indian adults. Am J Hum Biol. 1991;3(6):671–6. https://doi.org/10.1002/ajhb.1310030618. PMID: 28524284.
18. Wylie C. Germ cells. Cell. 1999;96(2):165–74. https://doi.org/10.1016/s0092-8674(00)80557-7. PMID: 9988212.
19. Griswold MD. The central role of Sertoli cells in spermatogenesis. Semin Cell Dev Biol. 1998;9(4):411–6. https://doi.org/10.1006/scdb.1998.0203. PMID: 9813187.
20. Mruk DD, Cheng CY. The mammalian blood-testis barrier: its biology and regulation. Endocr Rev. 2015;36(5):564–91. https://doi.org/10.1210/er.2014-1101. Epub 2015 Sep 10. Erratum in: Endocr Rev. 2015 Dec;36(6):681. Erratum in: Endocr Rev. 2016 Feb;2016(1):43. PMID: 26357922; PMCID: PMC4591527.
21. https://openstax.org/books/anatomy-and-physiology-2e/pages/27-1-anatomy-and-physiology-of-the-testicular-reproductive-system.
22. Hess RA. Efferent ductules: structure and function. In: Encyclopedia of reproduction. Elsevier; 2018. p. 270–8. https://doi.org/10.1016/B978-0-12-801238-3.64593-2.
23. Asala S, Chaudhary SC, Masumbuko-Kahamba N, Bidmos M. Anatomical variations in the human testicular blood vessels. Ann Anat. 2001;183(6):545–9. https://doi.org/10.1016/S0940-9602(01)80064-9. PMID: 11766526.
24. Mostafa T, Labib I, El-Khayat Y, El-Rahman El-Shahat A, Gadallah A. Human testicular arterial supply: gross anatomy, corrosion cast, and radiologic study. Fertil Steril. 2008;90(6):2226–30. https://doi.org/10.1016/j.fertnstert.2007.10.013. Epub 2008 Jun 13. PMID: 18555239.
25. Wishahi MM. Anatomy of the venous drainage of the human testis: testicular vein cast, microdissection and radiographic demonstration. A new anatomical concept. Eur Urol. 1991;20(2):154–60. https://doi.org/10.1159/000471687. PMID: 1752275.
26. Lechter A, Lopez G, Martinez C, Camacho J. Anatomy of the gonadal veins: a reappraisal. Surgery. 1991;109(6):735–9. PMID: 2042092.
27. Shafik A, Moftah A, Olfat S, Mohi-el-Din M, el-Sayed A. Testicular veins: anatomy and role in varicocelogenesis and other pathologic conditions. Urology. 1990;35(2):175–82. https://doi.org/10.1016/0090-4295(90)80071-t. PMID: 210.

28. Skandhan KP, Soni A, Joshi A, Avni KPS, Gupta BD. Human epididymis: structural pattern, total length and inner surface area. Urol J. 2017;84(4):215–7. https://doi.org/10.5301/uj.5000229.
29. Firoozabadi R, Stafford P, Routt M. Risk of spermatic cord injury during anterior pelvic ring and acetabular surgery: an anatomical study. Arch Bone Jt Surg. 2015;3(4):269–73. PMID: 26550592; PMCID: PMC4628634.
30. Abdelmohsen SM, Osman MA, Takrouney MH, et al. A spectrum of epididymis and vas deferens anomalies among children with cryptorchidism: a retrospective multi-center study. Ann Pediatr Surg. 2021;17:55. https://doi.org/10.1186/s43159-021-00111-w.
31. Virtanen HE, Toppari J. Epidemiology and pathogenesis of cryptorchidism. Human Reprod Update. 2008;14(1):49–58. https://doi.org/10.1093/humupd/dmm027.
32. Renfree MB. Review: Marsupials: placental mammals with a difference. Placenta. 2010;31(Suppl):S21–6. https://doi.org/10.1016/j.placenta.2009.12.023. Epub 2010 Jan 15. PMID: 20079531.
33. Abbas TO, Ali M. Bilateral neonatal testicular torsion; hidden surgical nightmare. Front Pediatr. 2018;6:318. https://doi.org/10.3389/fped.2018.00318. PMID: 30525011; PMCID: PMC6256121.
34. Riaz-Ul-Haq M, Mahdi DE, Elhassan EU. Neonatal testicular torsion; a review article. Iran J Pediatr. 2012;22(3):281–9. PMID: 23400637; PMCID: PMC3564080
35. Mercer S. Agenesis or atrophy of the testis and vas deferens. Can J Surg. 1979;22(3):245–6. PMID: 35276.
36. Pirgon Ö, Dündar BN. Vanishing testes: a literature review. J Clin Res Pediatr Endocrinol. 2012;4(3):116–20. https://doi.org/10.4274/Jcrpe.728. PMID: 22985611; PMCID: PMC3459158.
37. Bergholz R, Wenke K. Polyorchidism: a meta-analysis. J Urol. 2009;182(5):2422–7. https://doi.org/10.1016/j.juro.2009.07.063. Epub 2009 Sep 17. PMID: 19765760.
38. Zahirian Moghadam T, Mohseni Rad H, Zandian H, et al. Five testicles in the genital area of a thirteen-month-old baby: a case report. BMC Urol. 2020;20:128. https://doi.org/10.1186/s12894-020-00681-8.
39. de Souza DAS, Faucz FR, Pereira-Ferrari L, Sotomaior VS, Raskin S. Congenital bilateral absence of the vas deferens as an atypical form of cystic fibrosis: reproductive implications and genetic counseling. Andrology. 2018;6(1):127–35. https://doi.org/10.1111/andr.12450. Epub 2017 Dec 7. PMID: 29216686; PMCID: PMC5745269.
40. Somoza I, Palacios MG, Mendez R, Vela D. Complete penoscrotal transposition: a three-stage procedure. Indian J Urol. 2012;28(4):450–2. https://doi.org/10.4103/0970-1591.105775. PMID: 23450271; PMCID: PMC3579132.
41. Fahmy MAB. Bifid scrotum. In: Fahmy MAB, editor. Normal and abnormal scrotum. Cham: Springer; 2022. https://doi.org/10.1007/978-3-030-83305-3_14.
42. Kumar T, Vaughan R, Dangle PP. Hemangioma of the scrotal septum: a rare entity in infants with review of the literature. W V Med J. 2012;108(4):26–7. PMID: 22872962.
43. Chen G, Wang X, Zhao Y, et al. Splenogonadal fusion: a case report and review of the literature. BMC Urol. 2021;21:16. https://doi.org/10.1186/s12894-021-00781-z.
44. Psarris A, Dimopoulou A, Iakomidis E, Zavras N, Vaos G. Hemiscrotal agenesis: a rare congenital anomaly. J Clin Diagn Res. 2017;11(8):PD19–20. https://doi.org/10.7860/JCDR/2017/28605.10507. Epub 2017 Aug 1. PMID: 28969205; PMCID: PMC5620846.
45. Mansy M, Kotb M, Abdelmeguid Y, et al. Hemiscrotal agenesis: a novel phenotype of a rare malformation. BMC Pediatr. 2020;20:536. https://doi.org/10.1186/s12887-020-02424-y.
46. Spagnoli A, Borsellino A, Crucianelli S, Bizzarri C, Mucciolo M, Trucchi A, Ferro F. Complete scrotal agenesis: new surgical approach using self-inflating tissue expander. Urology. 2018;112:169–71. https://doi.org/10.1016/j.urology.2017.10.015. Epub 2017 Dec 6. PMID: 29080783.

47. Janoff DM, Skoog SJ. Congenital scrotal agenesis: description of a rare anomaly and management strategies. J Urol. 2005;173(2):589–91. https://doi.org/10.1097/01.ju.0000151136.56430.53. PMID: 15643265.
48. Shukla RM, Mandal KC, Roy D, Patra MP, Mukhopadhyay B. Scrotoschisis: an extremely rare congenital anomaly. J Indian Assoc Pediatr Surg. 2012;17(4):176–7. https://doi.org/10.4103/0971-9261.102342. PMID: 23243373; PMCID: PMC3518999.
49. Mahfouz M. Scrotoschisis: a rare congenital urologic anomaly. J Pediatr Surg Case Rep. 2018;32:90–2. https://doi.org/10.1016/j.epsc.2018.02.013. ISSN 2213-5766.
50. Fahmy MAB. Testis. In: Rare congenital genitourinary anomalies. Berlin: Springer; 2015. https://doi.org/10.1007/978-3-662-43680-6_5.

Epidemiology of Scrotal and Testicular Trauma

43

Located in a pendulous and extensible scrotal sac with ample space to move in all directions, the testes are relatively well protected from scrotal blunt trauma. However, a violent direct impact results in their rupture in 50% of cases.

Over 8000 adult male patients with scrotal/testicular injury were recorded in the American National Trauma Data Bank (NTDB) in the period 2007–2015 representing only 0.23% of all trauma patients. The median age of the patients was 31 years, blunt and penetrating mechanisms accounted for 44.6% and 50.5% of cases, respectively, and firearms represented 75.8% of all penetrating injuries [1]. However, these results are conflictual as other studies mention a higher rate of blunt scrotal injury accounting for up to 85% of cases of scrotal or testicular injury [2–4].

French studies showed that the most common genito-urinary organ injured in the RTA is the kidney followed by the testis representing 41–43% and 23–24% of the total, respectively. Scrotal wall injuries accounted for about 8% of the total [5, 6]. However, when refining the data for two-wheeled motorized vehicles (motorcyclists) only, the proportion of testicular injuries was predominant accounting for 41% followed by renal injury with 28% contribution, while scrotal wall injury accounted for 10% [6].

Scrotal injuries mainly occur in young people aged 15–40 years. Other data from the American NTDB suggest that patients older than 65 years are less likely to develop injuries to the penis, testes, or scrotum while being more prone to sustain bladder and urethral injury and having equal odds for renal trauma compared with younger patients [4, 7–9].

Testicular and scrotal injuries account for less than 1% of all trauma cases. However, genito-urinary tract injuries are observed in 2.2–10.3% of trauma patients admitted to emergency units, and external genitalia injuries are observed in 27.8–68.1% (roughly one-third to two-thirds) of patients with genitourinary (GU) tract injuries [10, 11].

S. A. AL-Mamari, *Urogenital Trauma: A Practical Guide*,
https://doi.org/10.1007/978-981-99-6171-9_43

Notably, 60% of all penetrating genitourinary trauma involve the external genitalia [12], and it is estimated that as many as 35% of all gunshot wounds (GSW) include external genitalia injuries of various degrees [11].

A large 30-year monocentric review recorded 110 patients with penetrating external genital trauma. Gunshot wounds (GSW) accounted for 49% of all the causes, followed by stab wounds/lacerations and bites accounting for 44% and 7%, respectively. Half of the cases were self-emasculation injuries, and testicular involvement was observed in all the above three mechanisms. Half of the patients having scrotal GSW had testicular injuries, and 35% had bilateral testicular involvement [13].

A study showed that the occurrence of blunt scrotal trauma is higher in militaries than in the general population. It involved 0.175% of nearly 400,000 soldiers, representing 1 out of 571 individuals [14]. Twenty-seven cases of scrotal injury were reported among British soldiers in Iraq and Afghanistan between 2003 and 2009, and the majority (21 cases) were caused by improvised explosive devices. Others were caused by mines, rocket-propelled grenades, and mortar rounds [15]. In wartime, civilians are sometimes more exposed than soldiers to either explosive devices or bullets [16].

References

1. Grigorian A, Livingston JK, Schubl SD, Hasjim BJ, Mayers D, Kuncir E, Barrios C, Joe V, Nahmias J. National analysis of testicular and scrotal trauma in the USA. Res Rep Urol. 2018;10:51–6. https://doi.org/10.2147/RRU.S172848. PMID: 30128306; PMCID: PMC6089605.
2. McAninch JW, Kahn RI, Jeffrey RB, Laing FC, Krieger MJ. Major traumatic and septic genital injuries. J Trauma. 1984;24(4):291–8. https://doi.org/10.1097/00005373-198404000-00002. PMID: 6368854.
3. Morey AF, Metro MJ, Carney KJ, Miller KS, McAninch JW. Consensus on genitourinary trauma: external genitalia. BJU Int. 2004;94(4):507–15. https://doi.org/10.1111/j.1464-410X.2004.04993.x. PMID: 15329102.
4. Wang Z, Yang JR, Huang YM, Wang L, Liu LF, Wei YB, Huang L, Zhu Q, Zeng MQ, Tang ZY. Diagnosis and management of testicular rupture after blunt scrotal trauma: a literature review. Int Urol Nephrol. 2016;48(12):1967–76. https://doi.org/10.1007/s11255-016-1402-0. Epub 2016 Aug 27. PMID: 27567912.
5. Terrier JE, Paparel P, Gadegbeku B, Ruffion A, Jenkins LC, N'Diaye A. Genitourinary injuries after traffic accidents: analysis of a registry of 162,690 victims. J Trauma Acute Care Surg. 2017;82(6):1087–93. https://doi.org/10.1097/TA.0000000000001448. PMID: 28328677.
6. Paparel P, N'Diaye A, Laumon B, Caillot JL, Perrin P, Ruffion A. The epidemiology of trauma of the genitourinary system after traffic accidents: analysis of a register of over 43,000 victims. BJU Int. 2006;97(2):338–41. https://doi.org/10.1111/j.1464-410X.2006.05900.x. PMID: 16430642.
7. Bjurlin MA, Goble SM, Fantus RJ, Hollowell CM. Outcomes in geriatric genitourinary trauma. J Am Coll Surg. 2011;213(3):415–21. https://doi.org/10.1016/j.jamcollsurg.2011.06.001. Epub 2011 Jul 1. PMID: 21723152.
8. Buckley JC, McAninch JW. Diagnosis and management of testicular ruptures. Urol Clin North Am. 2006;33(1):111–6, vii. https://doi.org/10.1016/j.ucl.2005.11.002. PMID: 16488285.

9. Lee SH, Bak CW, Choi MH, Lee HS, Lee MS, Yoon SJ. Trauma to male genital organs: a 10-year review of 156 patients, including 118 treated by surgery. BJU Int. 2008;101(2):211–5. https://doi.org/10.1111/j.1464-410X.2007.07265.x. Epub 2007 Oct 8. PMID: 17922859.
10. McGeady JB, Breyer BN. Current epidemiology of genitourinary trauma. Urol Clin North Am. 2013;40(3):323–34. https://doi.org/10.1016/j.ucl.2013.04.001. Epub 2013 Jun 12. PMID: 23905930; PMCID: PMC4016766
11. Plas E, Berger I. Genital trauma. In: Hohenfellner M, Santucci RA, editors. Emergencies in urology. Berlin: Springer; 2007. https://doi.org/10.1007/978-3-540-48605-3_21.
12. Goldman C, Shaw N, du Plessis D, Myers JB, van der Merwe A, Venkatesan K. Gunshot wounds to the penis and scrotum: a narrative review of management in civilian and military settings. Transl Androl Urol. 2021;10(6):2596–608. https://doi.org/10.21037/tau-20-1175. PMID: 34295746; PMCID: PMC8261456.
13. Phonsombat S, Master VA, McAninch JW. Penetrating external genital trauma: a 30-year single institution experience. J Urol. 2008;180(1):192–5; discussion 195–6. https://doi.org/10.1016/j.juro.2008.03.041. Epub 2008 May 21. PMID: 18499189.
14. Misgav Rottenstreich MC, Gofrit ON. Blunt scrotal trauma in soldiers—epidemiology and outcome. Mil Med. 2017;182(9–10):e1929–31. https://doi.org/10.7205/MILMED-D-16-00375.
15. Williams RJ, Fries CA, Midwinter M, Lambert AW. Battlefield scrotal trauma: how should it be managed in a deployed military hospital? Injury. 2013;44(9):1246–9. https://doi.org/10.1016/j.injury.2013.02.023. Epub 2013 Apr 12. PMID: 23587211.
16. Abid AF, Naoum N. Penetrating scrotal injuries: a war time experience in a civilian setup. Open Access Maced J Med Sci. 2021;9(B):1198–202. https://oamjms.eu/index.php/mjms/article/view/6888.

Etiology, Mechanism, and Anatomopathology of Scrotal and Testicular Trauma

44

44.1 Etiology and Mechanism

As mentioned in Chap. 43, the American National Trauma Data Bank (NTDB) registry showed that **blunt and penetrating (gunshot wounds and stabbing) mechanisms** account for 44.6% and 50.5% of cases, respectively, and firearms represent 75.8% of all penetrating injuries [1]. A mention was also made of conflicting results with other studies that showed a predominance of blunt over penetrating mechanisms in scrotal/testicular injury [2–4]. An attempt to explain this discrepancy is the fact that NTDB data are provided by heterogeneous participating trauma centers, including large urban trauma centers accounting for a high volume of penetrating trauma [1].

Despite its relative protective environment, the testis can rupture when subjected to sudden pressure (blow, kick, etc.) against the bony pelvis or inner thigh. Wesson reportedly found in 1956 that a 50-kg force was necessary to rupture the tunica albuginea [5]. However, this research failed to clarify Wesson's methodology. Nonetheless, this finding has been endorsed by many authors, although no further studies were performed using modern measurement technologies [4–9].

Direct impact in sports or in motor vehicle accidents accounts, respectively, for 50% and 14% of all causes of blunt testicular rupture, and because of its bigger volume and more cranial position which increase the odds of being trapped against the inner thigh, the inferior pubic ramus, or the symphysis, **the right testis is slightly more prone to injury than the left** [4, 7, 9].

Other causes of blunt testicular injuries are straddle impacts, kicking during fights, tractions, and birth injuries in breech presentation [9–11]. In a prospective study of 134 male breech infants delivered vaginally, 10 infants (7.5%) had testicular damage, and the injury appeared to be more likely to occur in infants with a birth weight of greater than or equal to 2500 g and born to primipara [11].

For penetrating injuries, besides stabbing and gunshots, less frequent causes are degloving/avulsion resulting from rapid deceleration mechanisms and human or

S. A. AL-Mamari, *Urogenital Trauma: A Practical Guide*,
https://doi.org/10.1007/978-981-99-6171-9_44

animal bites [12]. Very rarely, penetrating injuries may arise from falling astride onto perforating objects such as a metallic rod (impalement injury) (Fig. 44.1).

Patients riding motorcycles have a higher risk for scrotal/testicular trauma during a collision than bicycle riders because of the high-impact collision. **Indeed, 62% of injuries in motorcyclist victims of road traffic accidents involve external genitalia, and the testes alone are injured in 38%** [1, 13, 14]. However, even low-velocity impact sustained by cyclers hitting the handlebar or top tube can be harmful, and the most unfortunate of them can suffer severe trauma to the scrotum, testes, perineum, penis, and groin from impalement [15].

In contact sports (e.g., football, rugby, hockey, lacrosse, and wrestling cricket) and other sports involving jumping and balancing over hard objects (e.g., skateboard and pommel horse) in general and in the adolescent and pediatric population in particular, accidental scrotal kicking either by the ball or by the opponent or by falling astride on the hard supporting object is a common cause of blunt testicular trauma [16, 17].

A survey conducted in Pennsylvania in 2014 including 731 respondents of a mean age of 17.7 years revealed that 18% of all athletes sustained a testicular injury during sports and 36.4% observed the same in team members. The prevalence of

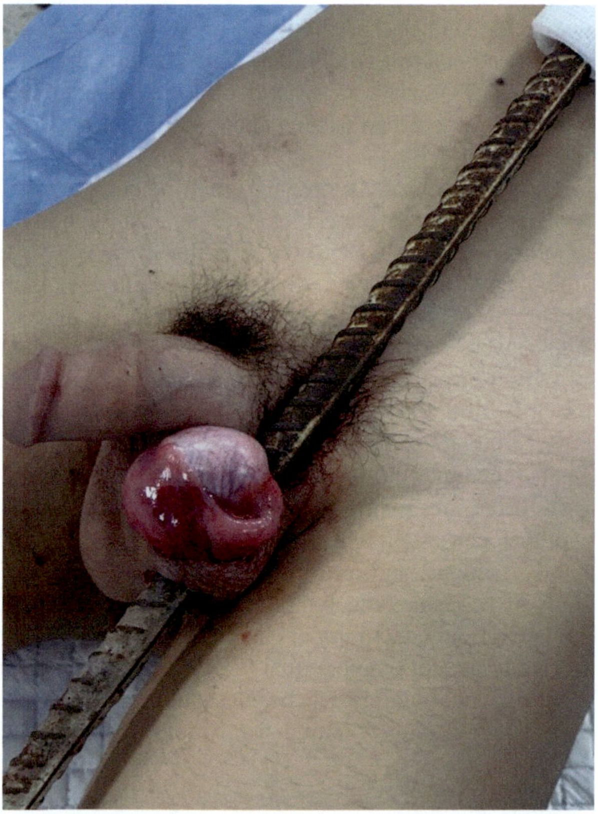

Fig. 44.1 Penetrating injury of the scrotum with left testicular evisceration in a 13-year-old boy who fell astride from height on a metallic rod in a construction area. The rod path through the scrotum was lateral to the left testis and spermatic cord, and there were no associated injuries. (Courtesy Khurram Siddiqui, Urology, Sultan Qaboos University Hospital, Muscat, Oman)

testicular injuries was the highest for lacrosse with a value of 48.5%, followed by wrestling, baseball, and American football with values of 32.8%, 21%, and 17.8%, respectively [18].

Thermal scrotal injuries (burns) have also been reported but are rarely isolated [12]. Another extremely rare mechanism is the degloving injury or avulsion caused by modern industrial machines [19]. Scrotal blast injuries are extremely rare and almost always extend to other anatomic regions [20].

44.2 Anatomopathology

Depending on the severity of the impact, **blunt** scrotal injuries may result in a simple **hematoma** of various sizes, a **hematocele**, **testicular fracture or rupture**, a **torsion**, a **dislocation**, and the spermatic cord might be injured and even avulsed when subjected to extreme traction forces. The so-called **traumatic dislocation of the testis (TDT)** is a rare event resulting from a forcible testicular push outside its normal position during blunt trauma. The most common TDT site is the superficial inguinal pouch accounting for 50% of all the cases [21]. Other possible sites are the pubic, penile, canalicular, abdominal, perineal, acetabular, and crural areas [21, 22] (Fig. 44.2).

Penetrating agents produce **superficial or deep incisions, partial or total scrotal excision, injury to the cord** (partial injury or transection), and injury to the testis of various degrees.

When there is isolated scrotal wall rupture (generally in penetrating injury), the intact testis may lie outside, i.e., eviscerate [23] (Figs. 44.1 and 44.3). The true rupture of the testis is defined by breaking or giving way of its tunica albuginea followed by a protrusion of the seminiferous tubules.

The incidence of testicular rupture associated with blunt trauma was reported to be 48% (almost half of the cases) [24]. It is important, however, to mention that this figure has been calculated from the number of patients presenting to the hospital for what they considered to be worrisome aftermath of the trauma: severe pain, swelling, and so on. In reality, the majority of testicular blunt traumas are mild, the pain disappears within minutes, and the individuals find no reason to report to a hospital. Almost every boy in the world can attest to the truth of this statement.

Based on the American NTDB registry, the majority of the patients have isolated scrotal or testicular trauma (74.5%), and 48.3% require operation [1].

Scrotal blast injuries are very rarely isolated [20], and the most common associated genitourinary (GU) injuries with scrotal and testicular trauma are corpora cavernosa and urethra injuries. Soft tissue injury to the extremities is the most common non-GU-associated injury seen in more than half of the patients [25].

Industrial injuries might have devastating consequences in the genital organs consisting of complete penoscrotal skin degloving or complete avulsion in extreme cases [19] (Fig. 44.4).

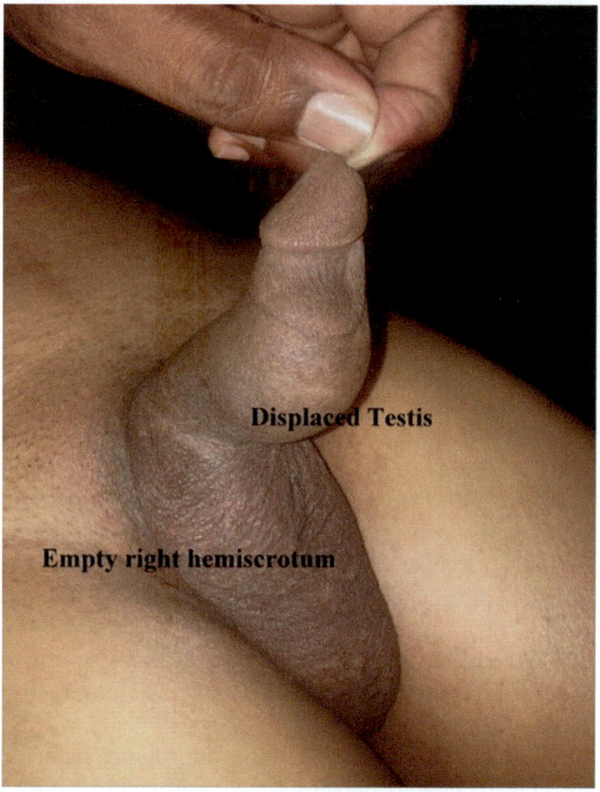

Fig. 44.2 A 45-year-old man with a history of bike accident, sustaining undisplaced pubic fracture and testicular dislocation in the penis. There is a visible swelling on the ventral aspect of penis with an empty right hemiscrotum. (From Raykar et al. [22], with permission from Springer Nature)

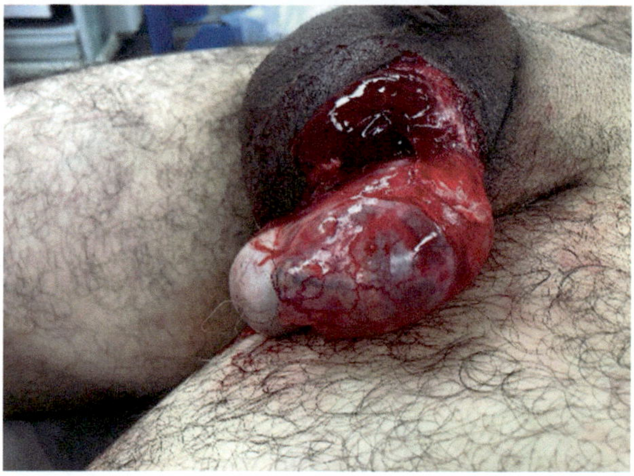

Fig. 44.3 Scrotal rupture with evisceration of the testicle and hematoma. (From Olivas et al. [23]. Creative Commons Attribution License CC-BY 4.0)

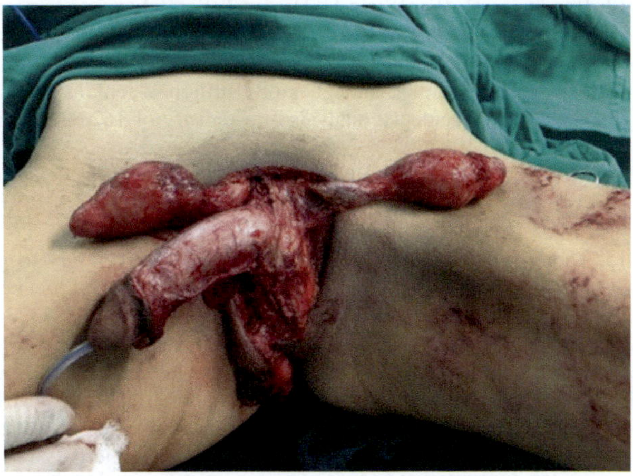

Fig. 44.4 Total degloving injury of penis and scrotum. (From Li et al. [19], with permission from Wolters Kluwer Health)

References

1. Grigorian A, Livingston JK, Schubl SD, Hasjim BJ, Mayers D, Kuncir E, Barrios C, Joe V, Nahmias J. National analysis of testicular and scrotal trauma in the USA. Res Rep Urol. 2018;10:51–6. https://doi.org/10.2147/RRU.S172848. PMID: 30128306; PMCID: PMC6089605.
2. McAninch JW, Kahn RI, Jeffrey RB, Laing FC, Krieger MJ. Major traumatic and septic genital injuries. J Trauma. 1984;24(4):291–8. https://doi.org/10.1097/00005373-198404000-00002. PMID: 6368854.
3. Morey AF, Metro MJ, Carney KJ, Miller KS, McAninch JW. Consensus on genitourinary trauma: external genitalia. BJU Int. 2004;94(4):507–15. https://doi.org/10.1111/j.1464-410X.2004.04993.x. PMID: 15329102.
4. Wang Z, Yang JR, Huang YM, Wang L, Liu LF, Wei YB, Huang L, Zhu Q, Zeng MQ, Tang ZY. Diagnosis and management of testicular rupture after blunt scrotal trauma: a literature review. Int Urol Nephrol. 2016;48(12):1967–76. https://doi.org/10.1007/s11255-016-1402-0. Epub 2016 Aug 27. PMID: 27567912.
5. Wasko R, Goldstein AG. Traumatic rupture of the testicle. J Urol. 1966;95(5):721–3. https://doi.org/10.1016/s0022-5347(17)63527-4. PMID: 5935538.
6. Blok D, Flannigan M, Jones J. Testicular rupture following blunt scrotal trauma. Case Rep Emerg Med. 2019;2019:7058728. https://doi.org/10.1155/2019/7058728. PMID: 31934468; PMCID: PMC6942712.
7. Essien F, Eagle Z, Tate J, Barber A. Testicular rupture: the other nutcracker syndrome. Clin Med Insights Case Rep. 2022;15:11795476211052416. https://doi.org/10.1177/11795476211052416.
8. Holliday TL, Robinson KS, Dorinzi N, et al. Testicular rupture: a tough nut to crack. Clin Pract Cases Emerg Med. 2017;1:221–4.
9. Dalton DM, Davis NF, O'Neill DC, Brady CM, Kiely EA, O'Brien MF. Aetiology, epidemiology and management strategies for blunt scrotal trauma. Surgeon. 2016;14(1):18–21. https://doi.org/10.1016/j.surge.2014.06.006. Epub 2014 Aug 21. PMID: 25151340.
10. Negrine R, Easter W, Fraser I, Ellis S. Neonatal testicular trauma: scrotal rupture. Arch Dis Child Fetal Neonatal Ed. 2010;95(3):F193. https://doi.org/10.1136/adc.2009.181594. PMID: 20444811.
11. Tiwary CM. Testicular injury in breech delivery: possible implications. Urology. 1989;34(4):210–2. https://doi.org/10.1016/0090-4295(89)90374-9. PMID: 2800086.

12. Randhawa H, Blankstein U, Davies T. Scrotal trauma: a case report and review of the literature. Can Urol Assoc J. 2019;13(6 Suppl 4):S67–71. https://doi.org/10.5489/cuaj.5981. PMID: 31194930; PMCID: PMC6565400.
13. Terrier JE, Paparel P, Gadegbeku B, Ruffion A, Jenkins LC, N'Diaye A. Genitourinary injuries after traffic accidents: analysis of a registry of 162,690 victims. J Trauma Acute Care Surg. 2017;82(6):1087–93.
14. McGeady JB, Breyer BN. Current epidemiology of genitourinary trauma. Urol Clin North Am. 2013;40(3):323–34. https://doi.org/10.1016/j.ucl.2013.04.001. Epub 2013 Jun 12. PMID: 23905930; PMCID: PMC4016766
15. Thompson H, Burdall O, Lakhoo K. Degloving injury to groin, scrotum and penis due to low-velocity handlebar injury. BMJ Case Rep. 2019;12(11):e231598. https://doi.org/10.1136/bcr-2019-231598. PMID: 31772130; PMCID: PMC6887373.
16. Pogorelić Z, Jurić I, Biočić M, Furlan D, Budimir D, Todorić J, Milunović KP. Management of testicular rupture after blunt trauma in children. Pediatr Surg Int. 2011;27(8):885–9. https://doi.org/10.1007/s00383-011-2873-9. Epub 2011 Mar 9. PMID: 21387107.
17. Adams RJ, Attia M, Cronan K. Report of 4 cases of testicular rupture in adolescent boys secondary to sports-related trauma. Pediatr Emerg Care. 2008;24(12):847–8. https://doi.org/10.1097/PEC.0b013e31818ea0eb. PMID: 19092565.
18. Bieniek JM, Sumfest JM. Sports-related testicular injuries and the use of protective equipment among young male athletes. Urology. 2014;84(6):1485–9. https://doi.org/10.1016/j.urology.2014.09.007. PMID: 25432843.
19. Li D, Chen F, Hu C, Zhang J, Wu J, Dongye Y, Li H. A case report of a complete penile and scrotum skin degloving injury. Plast Reconstr Surg Glob Open. 2018;6(11):e2029. https://doi.org/10.1097/GOX.0000000000002029. PMID: 30881811; PMCID: PMC6414104.
20. Dubhashi SP, Kumar A, Kadam R. Blast injury of the scrotum. J Emerg Trauma Shock. 2020;13(3):233. https://doi.org/10.4103/JETS.JETS_59_20. Epub 2020 Sep 18. PMID: 33304078; PMCID: PMC7717457.
21. Zavras N, Siatelis A, Misiakos E, Bagias G, Papachristos V, Machairas A. Testicular dislocation after scrotal trauma: a case report and brief literature review. Urol Case Rep. 2014;2(3):101–4. https://doi.org/10.1016/j.eucr.2014.02.004. PMID: 26955557; PMCID: PMC4733017.
22. Raykar R, Ratkal JM, Jadhav R, et al. Traumatic dislocation of testis into penis, what and how? Case report and review of literature. Indian J Surg. 2019;81:175–7. https://doi.org/10.1007/s12262-018-1846-9.
23. Olivas R, Uddin S, Chawla Kondal B, et al. Blunt trauma resulting in testicular evisceration: a case report. Cureus. 2021;13(3):e14019. https://doi.org/10.7759/cureus.14019.
24. Cass AS. Testicular trauma. J Urol. 1983;129(2):299–300. https://doi.org/10.1016/s0022-5347(17)52062-5. PMID: 6834494.
25. Simhan J, Rothman J, Canter D, Reyes JM, Jaffe WI, Pontari MA, Doumanian LR, Mydlo JH. Gunshot wounds to the scrotum: a large single-institutional 20-year experience. BJU Int. 2012;109(11):1704–7. https://doi.org/10.1111/j.1464-410X.2011.10631.x. Epub 2011 Oct 12. PMID: 21992688.

Symptoms, Signs, Diagnostic Means, and Grading of Scrotal and Testicular Trauma

45

45.1 Symptoms and Signs

It is a truism to say that the symptoms of scrotal and testicular injuries are obvious because this is expected to be so for any superficial organ injury. The patient presents with pain and swelling after blunt trauma or an obvious laceration and bleeding from a penetrating agent and readily gives the history of the incident. The pain might be associated with nausea and vomiting. In mild cases, there are skin abrasion and ecchymosis or a small shallow cut. In severe cases, there is a huge hematoma and severe pain suggesting a testicular rupture or a large laceration deep to the testis. In extreme cases, the testis is shattered or the patient presents with an amputated testis and/or scrotum. After a rapid history and local wound evaluation, a general evaluation must be conducted to rule out associated injuries that might or not be prioritized over the testicular-scrotal injury.

A study among Israeli soldiers with scrotal trauma showed the occurrence of the following symptoms: scrotal pain in 100%, scrotal tenderness in 71.7%, scrotal edema in 16.2%, scrotal hematoma in 4.8%, and dysuria in 10%. Additionally, there was microscopic hematuria (positive urine dipstick) in 11.8% [1].

In unilateral testicular trauma, the affected testis must be palpated very delicately to avoid harming the patient and must always be compared with the contralateral normal one. Assessment of the injured organs is made along with the evaluation of the general condition of the patient as the patient might be in shock, sepsis, or anemia. The patient's past history is also important to exclude preexisting hernia, presence or absence of both testes (e.g., previous surgery, undescended testis, hydrocele, etc.), and medical conditions (hematological disease) [2].

Information about the patient's age, marital status, and offspring is also important, especially in the management of severe bilateral testicular injury or trauma on a solitary testicle.

S. A. AL-Mamari, *Urogenital Trauma: A Practical Guide*,
https://doi.org/10.1007/978-981-99-6171-9_45

45.2 Diagnostic Means

45.2.1 Ultrasonography (US)

Ultrasonography (US) is strongly recommended by all expert panels (i.e., European association of urology (EAU), American Urological Association (AUA), British Association Of Urological Surgeons (BAUS), and Société Internationale d'Urologie (SIU)) as the **first-line** imaging modality for scrotal trauma as it helps evaluate and grade eventual testicular damage [3–6].

The advantages of US lie in its simplicity, its rapidity, its noninvasiveness, its wide distribution, and its cost-effectiveness. US allows a rapid diagnosis of eventual testicular rupture shown as a **discontinuity of the echogenic tunica albuginea**, triggering an urgent surgery which is of paramount importance for salvaging the testis. Color flow and duplex Doppler imaging are very useful for assessing testicular integrity (rupture), viability, and perfusion as well as for evaluating associated vascular injuries such as pseudoaneurysms. Determining vascular integrity is of critical importance, especially in cases of penetrating trauma and electrical burns [7, 8] (Table 45.1).

With the ability to define a loss of contour of the testicular parenchyma, abnormal heterogeneous echo pattern, adjacent hematoma, and eventual extrusion of the seminiferous tubules, US has shown a **65–93.5% specificity and a 100% sensitivity to diagnose testicular rupture** avoiding missing the diagnosis and the risk of orchidectomy for delayed diagnosis [9–13] (Figs. 45.1 and 45.2). Moreover, US also provides the diagnosis of other traumatic features such as hematocele (87% sensitivity and 89% specificity), testicular hematoma (71% sensitivity and 77% specificity), and testis avulsion (100% sensitivity and 97% specificity) [10].

Ultrasound should be requested even in cases with only mild scrotal pain and limited post-traumatic swelling in the absence of tenderness as this scenario does not exclude a testicular rupture [11] (Figs. 45.3 and 45.4a, b).

It is important, however, to notice that a study has shown lower sensitivity and specificity of ultrasound in detecting testicular trauma, with values of 70.8% and 71.2%, respectively [14]. While the experience of the radiologist definitely plays an

Table 45.1 Sonographic findings in scrotal injuries

Injury type	Sonographic findings
Hematocele	Acute: echogenic extra-testicular fluid collections with internal echoes
	Sub-acute to chronic: hypoechoic with multiple septations
Testicular hematoma	Acute: May be isoechoic to normal testicular parenchyma. May mimic a solid neoplasm
	Sub-acute to chronic: Hypoechoic to testicular parenchyma with interval decrease in size
Testicular fracture	Linear band of decreased parenchymal echogenicity
	Associated with intratesticular hematoma and segmental infarction
Testicular rupture	Heterogeneous testicular parenchyma with contour deformity
	Tunica disruption may be visible (the absence of this finding does not exclude rupture)

From Lehnert et al. [8], with permission from Springer Nature.

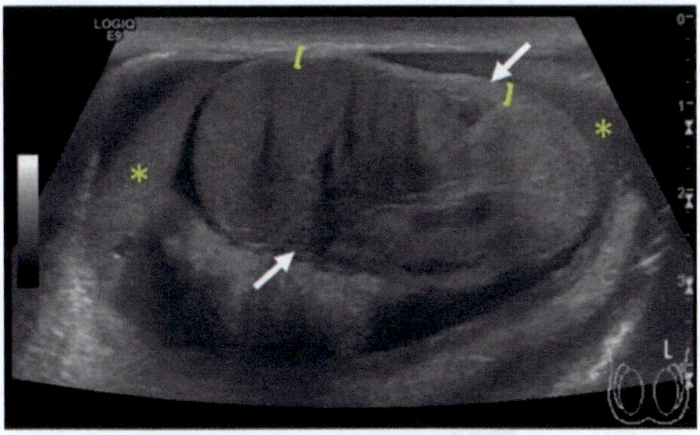

Fig. 45.1 Left testicle sagittal plane. There is abnormal tunica albuginea thickening ([ ]) without obvious disruption, a moderate-sized hematocele (asterisks), and a linear hypoechoic fracture line (between white arrows) separating a heterogeneous appearing testicular parenchyma. Normal testicular parenchyma is present to the left with an abnormal appearance testicle to the right of the fracture line, consistent with an intratesticular contusion. (From Blok et al. [13]. Creative Commons attribution license)

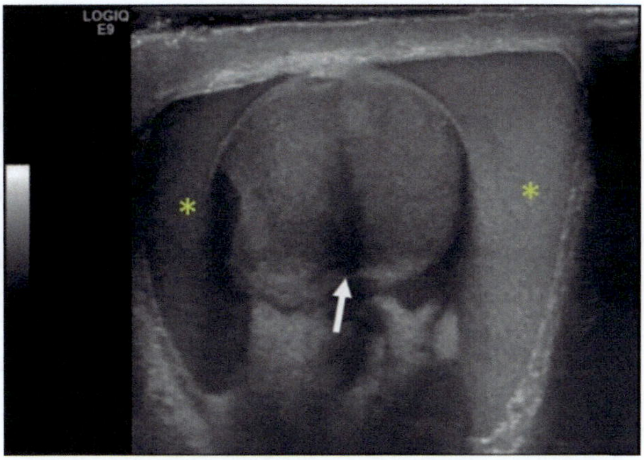

Fig. 45.2 Left testicle mid-transverse plane. Complex fluid collection with low-level echoes surrounding the left testicle consistent with a hematocele (asterisks) with hypoechoic testicular echogenicity consistent with a fracture line (arrow). (From Blok et al. [13]. Creative Commons attribution license)

important role in improving US accuracy, this study should raise attention to the fact that **the urologist should always consider early exploration in equivocal cases or those whose imaging reports deviate from the expected results in view of the history and physical examination**. Always being alert is the best strategy to avoid any delay in the management and give the best chance to the patient for testicular salvaging.

Contrast-enhanced US (CEUS) has shown interest in detecting early and minimal intratesticular changes such as mild fluid collection or hypoechoic and hypoperfused areas suggestive of minor vascular trauma and might be useful in cases where the conventional US is not conclusive [15, 16].

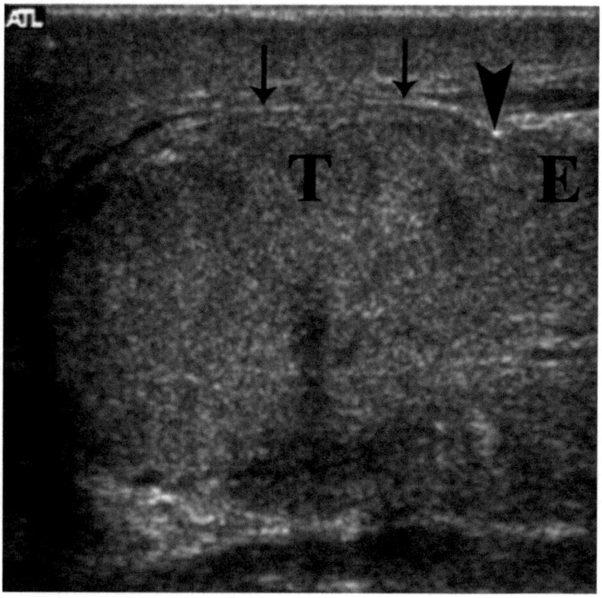

Fig. 45.3 Ultrasound scan showing ruptured testis, with interruption of the normal echoic line of tunica albuginea (arrows) at arrowhead. Extruded seminiferous tubules (E) have herniated through tunica defect. Testis (T) was markedly heterogeneous. These findings were confirmed intraoperatively and successfully repaired. (From Chandra et al. [11], with permission from Elsevier)

45.2.2 Magnetic Resonance Imaging (MRI)

Besides ultrasonography, **MRI** can also provide excellent information as **second-line** imaging means when ultrasound findings are inconclusive [17] and have a 100% accuracy in diagnosing testicular rupture [18] (Figs. 45.5a, b and 45.6a, b).

A few years ago, the Scrotal and Penile Imaging Working Group (SPI-WG) appointed by the board of the European Society of Urogenital Radiology (ESUR) elaborated recommendations for the use of scrotal MRI whereby the protocol should include T1- and T2-weighted imaging, diffusion-weighted imaging, and dynamic contrast-enhanced MRI for various indications including selected cases of trauma [17].

45.2.3 Other Diagnostic Means

Little research exists pertaining to the role of **CT scan** in diagnosing scrotal injuries, and it is generally admitted that this imaging is not the modality of choice for scrotal trauma as MRI and ultrasound provide an excellent soft tissue contrast definition and deliver no radiation to gonadal tissues [19].

Scrotoscopy has also been proposed as an aid in the diagnosis of testicular trauma by allowing direct observation of the lesion in equivocal cases. It has first been introduced by Shafik in Egypt in 1990 [20] and was initially aimed at elucidating questionable masses in the testis, epididymis, and spermatic cord. It also helped in the testicular biopsy, pampiniform plexus venography, vasography, and even in the treatment of intrascrotal lesions such as excision of testicular, epididymal, or

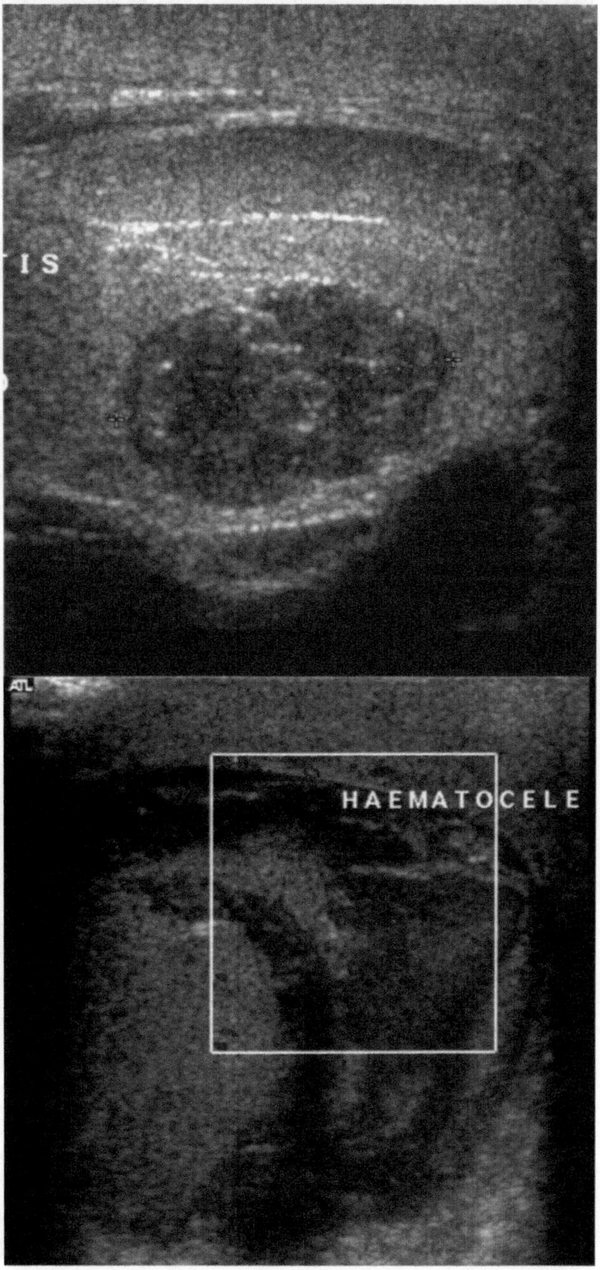

Fig. 45.4 (a, b) Ultrasound scans showing (top) intratesticular hematoma and (bottom) hematocele in two different patients. (From Chandra et al. [11], with permission from Elsevier)

cord masses and cysts, drainage of testicular abscesses or secondary hydroceles, injection of varicose veins, and vasal ligation. This minimally invasive method has gained popularity among some Chinese Urologists who proposed it to diagnose testicular rupture under epidural, spinal, general anesthesia, or even local anesthesia

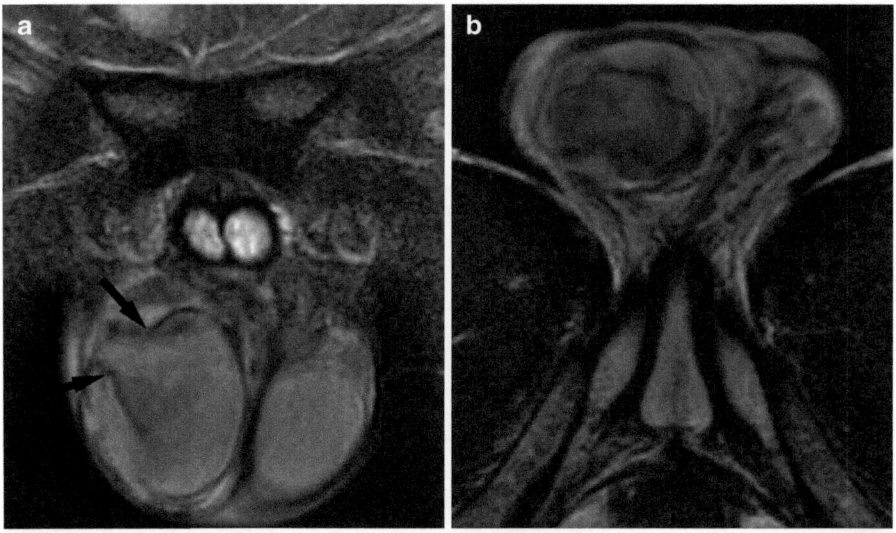

Fig. 45.5 A 22-year-old man with testicular rupture after being kicked in the right scrotum at a soccer game. (**a**) Fat-suppressed coronal T2-weighted MRI shows the corresponding rupture site (arrows) at the superolateral aspect of the right testis. (**b**) Axial T2-weighted MRI shows the contour irregularity of the right testis. (From Kim et al. [18], with permission from Wolters Kluwer Health)

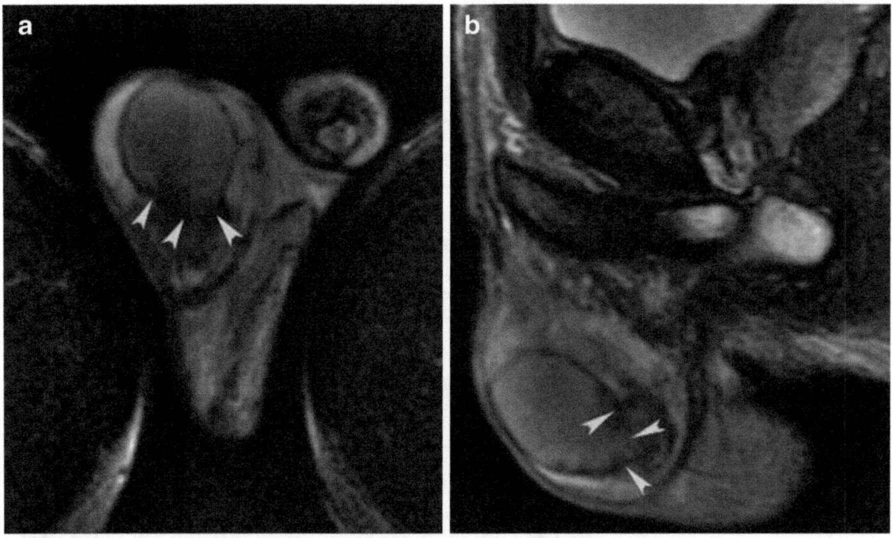

Fig. 45.6 A 22-year-old man with epididymal hematoma after being kicked in the right scrotum during Korean martial art. (**a**) Axial T2-weighted MRI shows the intact tunica albuginea (arrowheads) at the lower part of the right testis. (**b**) Sagittal T2-weighted MRI shows the continuity of the tunica albuginea (arrowheads). However, its dark signal intensity line is less prominent in the interface with the swollen epididymal tail. (From Kim et al. [18] with permission from Wolters Kluwer Health)

by infiltration of the spermatic cord [21]. However, scrotoscopy was limited only to diagnosis as an open approach had to be performed for the repair of testicular rupture. Hence, when considering it as a sole diagnostic means, it can hardly compete with ultrasound, which is less time-consuming and invasive and does not require anesthesia, although scrotoscopy would logically be expected to have 100% accuracy. Moreover, in an anesthetized patient, it takes no time to incise the scrotum and proceed to open exploration and repair with very low morbidity. One can imagine that proceeding first to a scrotoscopy before opening the scrotum would appear superfluous. Therefore, more studies are required to sculpt a comfortable seat for scrotoscopy in the armamentarium of recommended imaging means in testicular trauma.

45.3 Grading Systems

Data from physical and imaging examinations should help classify the trauma according to the AAST system published by Moore et al. in 1996 which was written separately for testicular and scrotal trauma [22] (Tables 45.2 and 45.3).

This AAST grading system was evaluated by many subsequent studies [14, 23, 24] demonstrating its usefulness in rapidly differentiating serious cases requiring urgent exploration and repair and mild cases requiring conservative management.

Table 45.2 AAST grading for testicular trauma

Grade[a]	Description of the injury	AIS-90
I	Contusion/hematoma	1
II	Subclinical laceration of tunica albuginea	1
III	Laceration of tunica albuginea with <50% parenchymal loss	2
IV	Major laceration of tunica albuginea with ≥50% parenchymal loss	2
V	Total testicular destruction or avulsion	2

From Moore et al. [22], with permission from Wolters Kluwer Health

[a]Advance one grade for bilateral lesions up to grade V

Table 45.3 AAST grading for scrotal trauma

Grade	Description of Injury	AIS-90
I	Contusion	1
II	Laceration <25% of scrotal diameter	1
III	Laceration ≥25% of scrotal diameter or stellate	2
IV	Avulsion <50%	2
V	Avulsion ≥50%	2

From Moore et al. [22], with permission from Wolters Kluwer Health

References

1. Rottenstreich M, Gofrit ON. Blunt scrotal trauma in soldiers—epidemiology and outcome. Mil Med. 2017;182(9):e1929–31. https://doi.org/10.7205/MILMED-D-16-00375. PMID: 28885957.
2. Wang Z, Yang JR, Huang YM, Wang L, Liu LF, Wei YB, Huang L, Zhu Q, Zeng MQ, Tang ZY. Diagnosis and management of testicular rupture after blunt scrotal trauma: a literature review. Int Urol Nephrol. 2016;48(12):1967–76. https://doi.org/10.1007/s11255-016-1402-0. Epub 2016 Aug 27. PMID: 27567912.
3. EAU Guidelines. Edn. Presented at the EAU Annual Congress Amsterdam March 2022. ISBN 978-94-92671-16-5. https://uroweb.org/guidelines/urological-trauma/chapter/urogenital-trauma-guidelines.
4. Morey AF, Broghammer JA, Hollowell CMP, McKibben MJ, Souter L. Urotrauma guideline 2020: AUA guideline. J Urol. 2021;205(1):30–5. https://doi.org/10.1097/JU.0000000000001408. Epub 2020 Oct 14. PMID: 33053308.
5. Lucky M, Brown G, Dorkin T, Pearcy R, Shabbir M, Shukla CJ, Rees RW, Summerton DJ, Muneer A, BAUS Section of Andrology and Genitourethral Surgery (AGUS). British Association of Urological Surgeons (BAUS) consensus document for the management of male genital emergencies—testicular trauma. BJU Int. 2018;121(6):840–4. https://doi.org/10.1111/bju.14163. Epub 2018 Apr 10. PMID: 29635819.
6. Morey AF, Metro MJ, Carney KJ, Miller KS, McAninch JW. Consensus on genitourinary trauma: external genitalia. BJU Int. 2004;94(4):507–15. https://doi.org/10.1111/j.1464-410X.2004.04993.x. PMID: 15329102.
7. Deurdulian C, Mittelstaedt CA, Chong WK, Fielding JR. US of acute scrotal trauma: optimal technique, imaging findings, and management. Radiographics. 2007;27(2):357–69. https://doi.org/10.1148/rg.272065117. PMID: 17374858.
8. Lehnert BE, Sadro C, Monroe E, Moshiri M. Lower male genitourinary trauma: a pictorial review. Emerg Radiol. 2014;21(1):67–74. https://doi.org/10.1007/s10140-013-1159-z. Epub 2013 Sep 20. PMID: 24052083.
9. Buckley JC, McAninch JW. Use of ultrasonography for the diagnosis of testicular injuries in blunt scrotal trauma. J Urol. 2006;175(1):175–8. https://doi.org/10.1016/S0022-5347(05)00048-0. PMID: 16406902.
10. Guichard G, El Ammari J, Del Coro C, Cellarier D, Loock PY, Chabannes E, Bernardini S, Bittard H, Kleinclauss F. Accuracy of ultrasonography in diagnosis of testicular rupture after blunt scrotal trauma. Urology. 2008;71(1):52–6. https://doi.org/10.1016/j.urology.2007.09.014. PMID: 18242364.
11. Chandra RV, Dowling RJ, Ulubasoglu M, Haxhimolla H, Costello AJ. Rational approach to diagnosis and management of blunt scrotal trauma. Urology. 2007;70(2):230–4. https://doi.org/10.1016/j.urology.2007.03.064. PMID: 17826476.
12. Randhawa H, Blankstein U, Davies T. Scrotal trauma: a case report and review of the literature. Can Urol Assoc J. 2019;13(6 Suppl 4):S67–71. https://doi.org/10.5489/cuaj.5981. PMID: 31194930; PMCID: PMC6565400.
13. Blok D, Flannigan M, Jones J. Testicular rupture following blunt scrotal trauma. Case Rep Emerg Med. 2019;2019:7058728. https://doi.org/10.1155/2019/7058728. PMID: 31934468; PMCID: PMC6942712.
14. Sallami S, Khouni H, Ichaoui H, Ben Atta M, Abou El Makarim S, Ben Rhouma S. Blunt scrotal trauma in adults: a multi-institution study evaluating the American Association for the Surgery of Trauma organ injury grading scale about 107 cases. Tunis Med. 2017;95(5):331–5. PMID: 29509213.
15. Lobianco R, Regine R, De Siero M, Catalano O, Caiazzo C, Ragozzino A. Contrast-enhanced sonography in blunt scrotal trauma. J Ultrasound. 2011;14(4):188–95. https://doi.org/10.1016/j.jus.2011.09.003. Epub 2011 Oct 1. PMID: 23396988; PMCID: PMC3558072.

16. Trinci M, Cirimele V, Ferrari R, Ianniello S, Galluzzo M, Miele V. Diagnostic value of contrast-enhanced ultrasound (CEUS) and comparison with color Doppler ultrasound and magnetic resonance in a case of scrotal trauma. J Ultrasound. 2020;23(2):189–94. https://doi.org/10.1007/s40477-019-00389-y. Epub 2019 Jun 5. PMID: 31168706; PMCID: PMC7242606.
17. Tsili AC, Bertolotto M, Turgut AT, Dogra V, Freeman S, Rocher L, Belfield J, Studniarek M, Ntorkou A, Derchi LE, Oyen R, Ramchandani P, Secil M, Richenberg J. MRI of the scrotum: recommendations of the ESUR Scrotal and Penile Imaging Working Group. Eur Radiol. 2018;28(1):31–43. https://doi.org/10.1007/s00330-017-4944-3. Epub 2017 Jul 11. PMID: 28698942.
18. Kim SH, Park S, Choi SH, Jeong WK, Choi JH. The efficacy of magnetic resonance imaging for the diagnosis of testicular rupture: a prospective preliminary study. J Trauma. 2009;66(1):239–42. https://doi.org/10.1097/TA.0b013e318156867f. PMID: 19131833.
19. Wang A, Stormont I, Siddiqui MM. A review of imaging modalities used in the diagnosis and management of scrotal trauma. Curr Urol Rep. 2017;18(12):98. https://doi.org/10.1007/s11934-017-0744-1. PMID: 29081016.
20. Shafik A. The scrotoscope. A new instrument for examining the scrotal contents. Br J Urol. 1990;65(2):209–10. https://doi.org/10.1111/j.1464-410x.1990.tb14702.x. PMID: 2317658.
21. Wei Y, Yang J, Hong H, Gao Y, Wu J, Wu X, Zhang R, Lin L, Li T, Yang F, Ye L, Zhu Q. Scrotoscopy exploration of testicular rupture: a pilot study. Medicine (Baltimore). 2019;98(41):e17389. https://doi.org/10.1097/MD.0000000000017389. PMID: 31593090; PMCID: PMC6799513.
22. Moore EE, Malangoni MA, Cogbill TH, Peterson NE, Champion HR, Jurkovich GJ, Shackford SR. Organ injury scaling VII: cervical vascular, peripheral vascular, adrenal, penis, testis, and scrotum. J Trauma. 1996;41(3):523–4. https://doi.org/10.1097/00005373-199609000-00023. PMID: 8810974.
23. Mohr AM, Pham AM, Lavery RF, Sifri Z, Bargman V, Livingston DH. Management of trauma to the male external genitalia: the usefulness of American Association for the Surgery of Trauma organ injury scales. J Urol. 2003;170(6 Pt 1):2311–5. https://doi.org/10.1097/01.ju.0000089241.71369.fa. PMID: 14634403.
24. Park JS, Lee SJ. Testicular injuries-efficacy of the Organ Injury Scale developed by the American Association for the Surgery of Trauma. Korean J Urol. 2007;48(1):61–5.

46 Treatment of Scrotal and Testicular Trauma: I—Minor and Intermediate Interventions

Penetrating scrotal injury poses no question about its surgical management as the wound has to be explored, debrided, and closed. In addition, common sense obliges one to question deep organ (testicles) damage during the exploration. However, the interventional approach has not always been prioritized for blunt scrotal trauma in the past. Indeed, up to half a century back, blunt testicular trauma was mainly managed conservatively. An unacceptably higher number of testicles were lost because of this approach as the intervention was decided only late after the occurrence of complications: aggravation of the hematoma and worsening of the pain, abscess, testicular ischemic necrosis, fistula, and so on. A late complication is testicular atrophy and the loss of spermatogenesis.

The 1970s marked a paradigm shift from conservative to early scrotal exploration and testicular repair in blunt trauma. This shift has been greatly supported by modern imaging techniques. Nowadays, testicular rupture is readily diagnosed with the aid of ultrasonography (US), prompting urgent repair and enhancing the testis salvage rate [1]. Early comparative studies showed a failure rate, i.e., an orchidectomy rate of 45% and 9% for delayed and early exploration, respectively [2, 3]. As per many authors, a maximum interval of 3 days from the time of trauma is the limit between an early intervention and a delayed one [1–3].

Today, all the expert panels (i.e., European association of urology (EAU), American urological association (AUA), British association of urological surgeons (BAUS), and société internationale d'urologie (SIU)) recommend prompt exploration of the injured testis whenever there is a large hematoma, obvious physical findings of testicular rupture, sonographic evidence of testicular rupture, or inconclusive US findings [4–7].

Data from the NTDB for the period 2007–2015 showed that nearly half (48.3%) of scrotal or testicular trauma victims underwent a subsequent scrotal or testicular operation, the most common procedure being either a repair of scrotal laceration or testicular rupture (37.3%), followed by unilateral orchiectomy (23.4%) [8].

Despite the progress in testicle preservation, the surgeon should always get signed consent from the patient for possible orchidectomy before taking him to the operating theater.

S. A. AL-Mamari, *Urogenital Trauma: A Practical Guide*,
https://doi.org/10.1007/978-981-99-6171-9_46

The intervention is performed under general or regional (spine) anesthesia with the patient in a supine position. He should be catheterized and a broad-spectrum IV antibiotic (Tazocin) be given before the scrotal incision which is centered on the injury side and preferably transverse. Once the tunica vaginalis is opened, clots are rapidly removed, the testis is delivered, and the tunica albuginea is meticulously inspected for any tear, and care is taken to delicately manipulate eventually extruded seminiferous tubules. Assessment of the testis vitality is carried out including ruling out possible cord injury. After debridement of necrotic tissues, the viable tunica albuginea is repaired with a continuous 4/0 resorbable suture taking care to progressively reintroduce all the viable seminiferous tubules. Once the repair is over, the testis is replaced in the scrotal cavity and the scrotal wall is closed with resorbable sutures after leaving a drain in situ [1, 9] (Fig. 46.1a, b).

A follow-up with ultrasound is performed at 3 months to evaluate the testis viability.

In the pediatric population, a study has also confirmed that early exploration (defined by the authors as less than 35 h from the trauma time) results in a high rate of testicular salvage, with no post-operative complications, shorter hospital stays (2 days), and no late sequels after a mean follow-up of nearly 5 years: sustained viability of the testis, no atrophy on Doppler ultrasound, normospermia after 6 months, and no abnormal anti-sperm antibodies [10].

When there is a significant loss of tunica albuginea and the quantity of extruded and viable seminiferous tubules is too large to be reintegrated within the capsule, a neo-capsule can be created by wrapping the tunica vaginalis around the defect and suturing its free edges to the albuginea with 3/0 resorbable materials (polyglactin) or by using a free graft of the tunica vaginalis. On the one hand, this prevents the creation of a mini-compartment syndrome, and on the other hand, it avoids unnecessary excision and loss of viable testicular tissues. This technique was proven to be superior to the use of synthetic material (polytetrafluoroethylene Gore-Tex patch graft) which is associated with a high rate of secondary infection and the need for orchidectomy [11–15] (Figs. 46.2, 46.3, and 46.4).

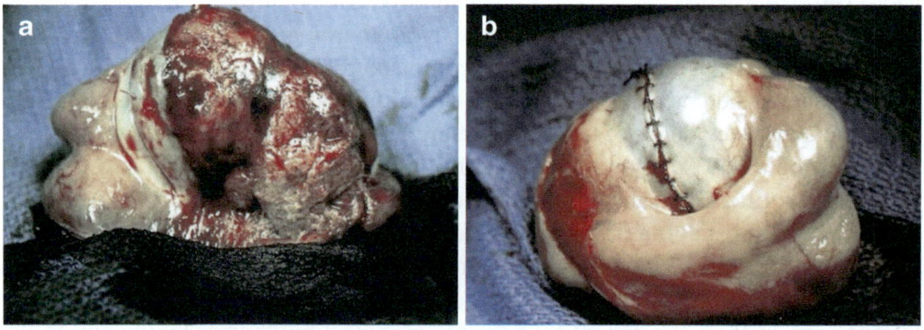

Fig. 46.1 (**a**) Intraoperative view of testicular rupture with extruded seminiferous tubules. (**b**) Testicular repair consisting of débridement and primary tunical closure. (From Buckley and McAninck [1], with permission from Wolters Kluwer Health)

Fig. 46.2 Repair of ruptured testis using tunica vaginalis. Free edges of tunica vaginalis were wrapped around the extruding seminiferous tubules and secured with 3.0 polyglactin 910 sutures. (From Molokwu et al. [13], with permission from Elsevier)

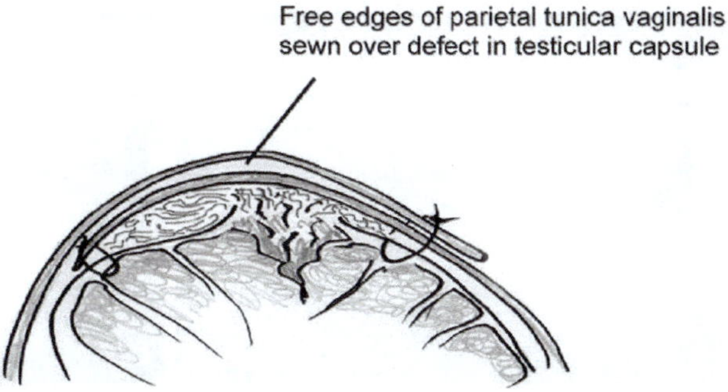

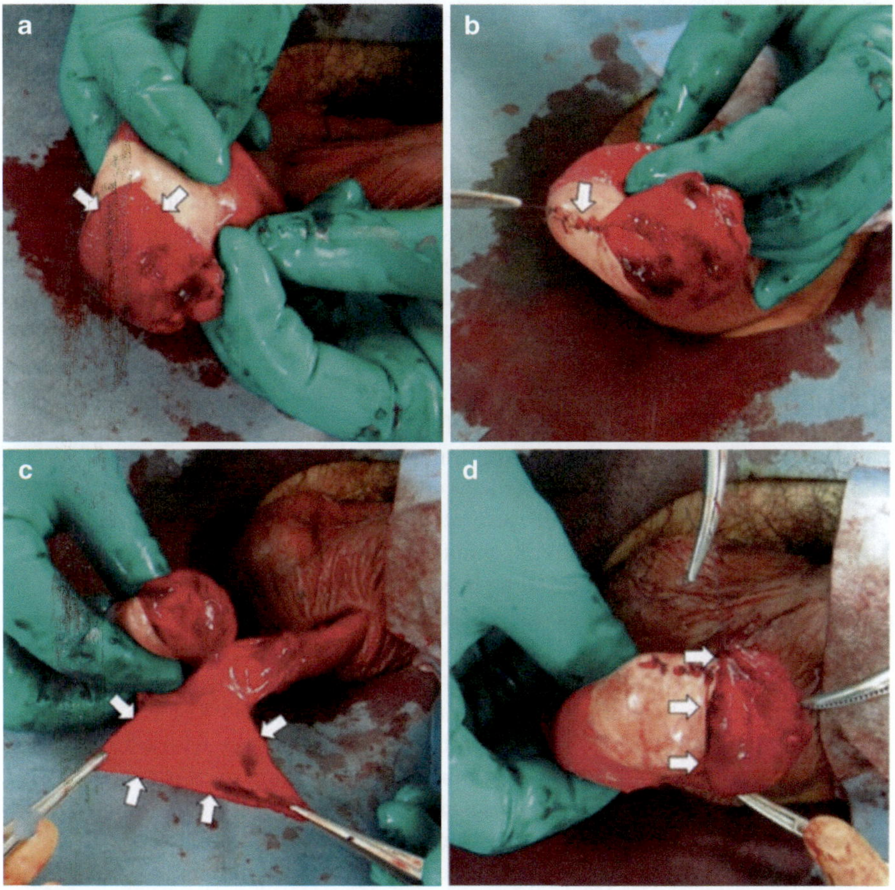

Fig. 46.3 Testicular repair using tunica vaginalis: (**a**) Ruptured tunica albuginea and prolapsed testicular contents. (**b**) Suture between the layers of the tunica albuginea. (**c**) Tunica vaginalis flap. (**d**) Suture of the tunica albuginea and testicular serosal flap. (From Yokokawa et al. [14]. Creative Commons License)

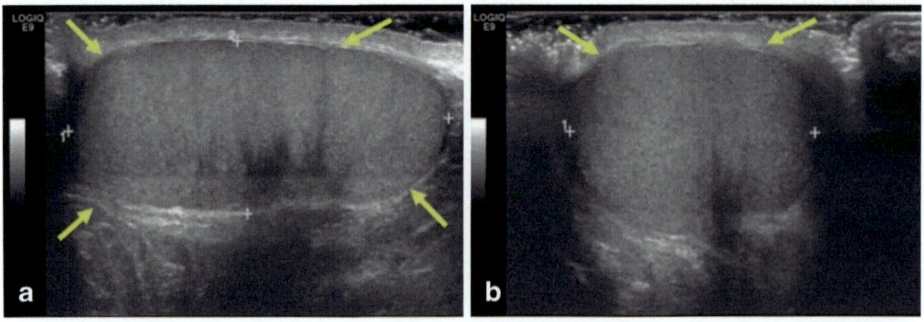

Fig. 46.4 (**a**, **b**) Post-repair using a tunica vaginalis flap: Right testicle in sagittal and transverse planes. Thin tunica albuginea uniformly surrounding testicle (yellow arrows), homogeneous testicular parenchyma echogenicity, and absent hematocele. (From Blok et al. [15]. Creative Commons attribution license)

Nevertheless, a study has reported the successful use of biosynthetic material in a small series of extensive testicular ruptures with excellent results even with penetrating wounds (gunshot) [16]. This technique might prove useful in cases where the tunica vaginalis itself has been extensively damaged by the trauma but implies strict asepsis, thorough wound debridement and wash, and the continuation of antibiotics after discharge. Extracellular matrix graft materials were also successfully tried for the reconstruction of tunica albuginea using bovine pericardium and cadaveric dermis [17].

As mentioned in the introduction, the decision to explore the scrotum should be straightforward for penetrating trauma. In a large single institutional series of 97 patients who sustained scrotal gunshot injuries, 91 (94%) of them were explored, and in almost half of these (44 patients or 48%), a testicular injury was found. In the group with testicular injury, half were repaired and half underwent orchidectomy [18]. A 30-year monocentric review mentioned an overall testicular salvage rate of 46% after penetrating trauma, and a particular 77%, 11%, and 0% salvage rate for gunshot wounds (GSWs), stab wounds, and bites, respectively [19–21] (Figs. 46.5 and 46.6).

In GSWs, the clinician should also have a low suspicion threshold for associated urethral and/or penile injury and request additional studies to rule them out [21].

An inguinal testicular dislocation can be achieved manually with a fully sedated patient or under general anesthesia. If this non-invasive approach is not successful, an inguinal exploration is indicated to gently push the testis back to the scrotal cavity, and a combined small transverse scrotal incision will be needed for testicular fixation [22]. The extremely rare case of testicular dislocation into the penis is managed with complete penile degloving and testicular relocation inside the scrotum [23] (Fig. 46.7).

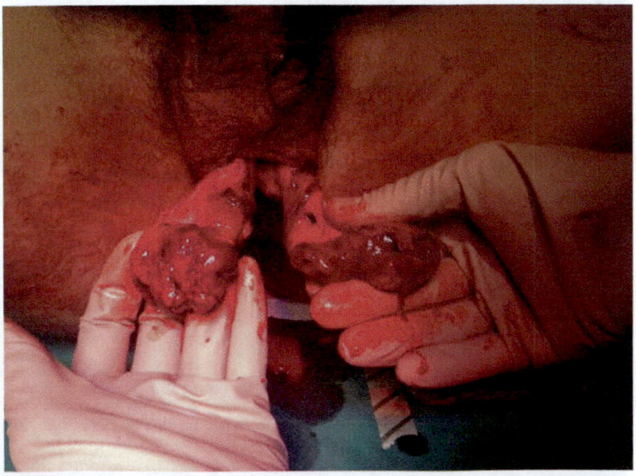

Fig. 46.5 Bilateral testicular gunshot injury: Tunica albuginea defects and bullet hole. (From Abidoğlu et al. [20], with permission from Springer)

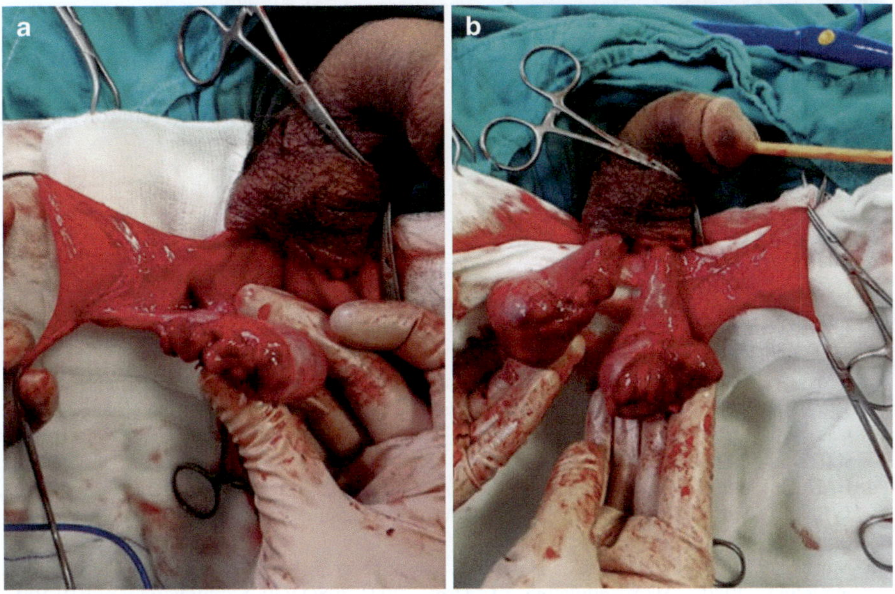

Figs. 46.6 (**a**) Repair of the right testis with tunica vaginalis flap. (**b**) Repair of the left testis with tunica vaginalis flap. (From Abidoğlu et al. [20], with permission from Springer)

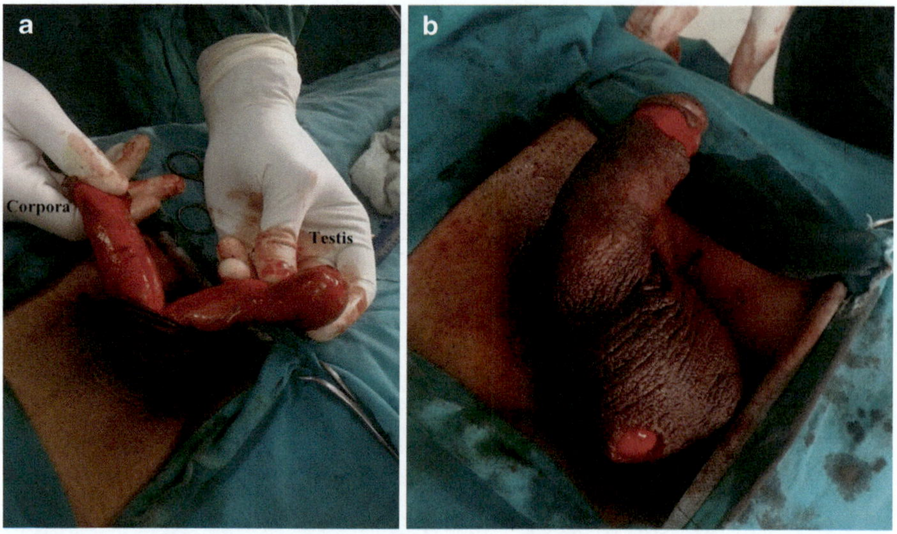

Fig. 46.7 (**a**) Operative photograph showing the exposure of a dislocated right testis into the penis through a degloving circumcoronal incision. (**b**) Operative photograph showing completed relocation of testis in the right hemiscrotum (same patient discussed in Fig. 44.1). (From Raykar et al. [23], with permission from Springer Nature)

References

1. Buckley JC, McAninch JW. Use of ultrasonography for the diagnosis of testicular injuries in blunt scrotal trauma. J Urol. 2006;175(1):175–8. https://doi.org/10.1016/S0022-5347(05)00048-0. PMID: 16406902.
2. Gross M. Rupture of the testicle: the importance of early surgical treatment. J Urol. 1969;101(2):196–7. https://doi.org/10.1016/s0022-5347(17)62310-3. PMID: 5765482.
3. Cass AS. Testicular trauma. J Urol. 1983;129(2):299–300. https://doi.org/10.1016/s0022-5347(17)52062-5. PMID: 6834494.
4. EAU Guidelines. Edn. Presented at the EAU Annual Congress Amsterdam, March 2022. ISBN 978-94-92671-16-5. https://uroweb.org/guidelines/urological-trauma/chapter/urogenital-trauma-guidelines.
5. Morey AF, Broghammer JA, Hollowell CMP, McKibben MJ, Souter L. Urotrauma guideline 2020: AUA guideline. J Urol. 2021;205(1):30–5. https://doi.org/10.1097/JU.0000000000001408. Epub 2020 Oct 14. PMID: 33053308.
6. Lucky M, Brown G, Dorkin T, Pearcy R, Shabbir M, Shukla CJ, Rees RW, Summerton DJ, Muneer A, BAUS Section of Andrology and Genitourethral Surgery (AGUS). British Association of Urological Surgeons (BAUS) consensus document for the management of male genital emergencies—testicular trauma. BJU Int. 2018;121(6):840–4. https://doi.org/10.1111/bju.14163. Epub 2018 Apr 10. PMID: 29635819.
7. Morey AF, Metro MJ, Carney KJ, Miller KS, McAninch JW. Consensus on genitourinary trauma: external genitalia. BJU Int. 2004;94(4):507–15. https://doi.org/10.1111/j.1464-410X.2004.04993.x. PMID: 15329102.

8. Grigorian A, Livingston JK, Schubl SD, Hasjim BJ, Mayers D, Kuncir E, Barrios C, Joe V, Nahmias J. National analysis of testicular and scrotal trauma in the USA. Res Rep Urol. 2018;10:51–6. https://doi.org/10.2147/RRU.S172848. PMID: 30128306; PMCID: PMC6089605.
9. Buckley JC, McAninch JW. Diagnosis and management of testicular ruptures. Urol Clin North Am. 2006;33(1):111–6, vii. https://doi.org/10.1016/j.ucl.2005.11.002. PMID: 16488285.
10. Pogorelić Z, Jurić I, Biočić M, Furlan D, Budimir D, Todorić J, Milunović KP. Management of testicular rupture after blunt trauma in children. Pediatr Surg Int. 2011;27(8):885–9. https://doi.org/10.1007/s00383-011-2873-9. Epub 2011 Mar 9. PMID: 21387107.
11. Kapoor D, Leech J, Yap W. Use of tunica vaginalis patch graft for repair of traumatic testicular rupture. Urology. 1992;40(4):374–5. https://doi.org/10.1016/0090-4295(92)90394-c. PMID: 1413362.
12. Ferguson GG, Brandes SB. Gunshot wound injury of the testis: the use of tunica vaginalis and polytetrafluoroethylene grafts for reconstruction. J Urol. 2007;178(6):2462–5. https://doi.org/10.1016/j.juro.2007.08.021. Epub 2007 Oct 15. PMID: 17937945.
13. Molokwu CN, Doull RI, Townell NH. A novel technique for repair of testicular rupture after blunt trauma. Urology. 2010;76(4):1002–3. https://doi.org/10.1016/j.urology.2010.06.011. PMID: 20932424.
14. Yokokawa S, Tabei T, Kobayashi K. Testicular rupture successfully treated with a tunica vaginalis flap. IJU Case Rep. 2020;4(2):82–5. https://doi.org/10.1002/iju5.12246. PMID: 33718811; PMCID: PMC7924093.
15. Blok D, Flannigan M, Jones J. Testicular rupture following blunt scrotal trauma. Case Rep Emerg Med. 2019;2019:7058728. https://doi.org/10.1155/2019/7058728. PMID: 31934468; PMCID: PMC6942712.
16. Doan PN, Yip J, Wang H, Chia D, Kim LHC, Wang A. Case—Repair of extensive testicular rupture: a unique use for biosynthetic grafts. Can Urol Assoc J. 2020;14(1):E42–4. https://doi.org/10.5489/cuaj.6052. Epub 2019 Jun 17. PMID: 31670646; PMCID: PMC6955173
17. Marchalik D, Triest JA, Wright HC, Bandi G. Use of "off the shelf" extracellular matrix graft materials for repair of testicular rupture: a novel technique. Urology. 2014;84(3):719–21. https://doi.org/10.1016/j.urology.2014.05.026. PMID: 25168558.
18. Simhan J, Rothman J, Canter D, Reyes JM, Jaffe WI, Pontari MA, Doumanian LR, Mydlo JH. Gunshot wounds to the scrotum: a large single-institutional 20-year experience. BJU Int. 2012;109(11):1704–7. https://doi.org/10.1111/j.1464-410X.2011.10631.x. Epub 2011 Oct 12. PMID: 21992688.
19. Phonsombat S, Master VA, McAninch JW. Penetrating external genital trauma: a 30-year single institution experience. J Urol. 2008;180(1):192–5; discussion 195–6. https://doi.org/10.1016/j.juro.2008.03.041. Epub 2008 May 21. PMID: 18499189.
20. Abidoğlu S, Karagözlü Akgül A. Close range gun shot injury bilateral ruptured testis repair using tunica vaginalis flap. Indian J Surg. 2022;84:824–7. https://doi.org/10.1007/s12262-021-03043-2.
21. Goldman C, Shaw N, du Plessis D, Myers JB, van der Merwe A, Venkatesan K. Gunshot wounds to the penis and scrotum: a narrative review of management in civilian and military settings. Transl Androl Urol. 2021;10(6):2596–608. https://doi.org/10.21037/tau-20-1175. PMID: 34295746; PMCID: PMC8261456.
22. Zavras N, Siatelis A, Misiakos E, Bagias G, Papachristos V, Machairas A. Testicular dislocation after scrotal trauma: a case report and brief literature review. Urol Case Rep. 2014;2(3):101–4. https://doi.org/10.1016/j.eucr.2014.02.004. PMID: 26955557; PMCID: PMC4733017.
23. Raykar R, Ratkal JM, Jadhav R, et al. Traumatic dislocation of testis into penis, what and how? Case report and review of literature. Indian J Surg. 2019;81:175–7. https://doi.org/10.1007/s12262-018-1846-9.

Treatment of Testicular Trauma: II—Complex Interventions

47

47.1 Replantation of an Amputated Testis

Many cases of testicular amputations occur as a consequence of self-mutilation, and this aspect will be developed in a special section at the end of this book. Many others are reported following an assault, road traffic accident (RTA), or industrial accident. A shattered or badly crushed testis is generally nonviable and should be discarded. However, when a sharp instrument (e.g., knife, scissors, razor, etc.) has penetrated the upper scrotum and severed the spermatic cord, the testis can still be viable if the patient presents within 4–6 h. It should be mentioned that unilateral injury exceptionally justifies a fastidious microsurgical replantation taking into account the very small diameters of involved vessels, the necessity for specialized centers, and the uncertainty of success. But when dealing with a solitary testis or bilateral testes amputation in a young patient victim of accident or assault, all local and regional competencies should be solicited to optimize the future chances of the unfortunate patient to live a normal marital life and prevent psychological drama.

Evins et al. reported the first attempt to replant testes in 1977 in a paranoic patient who had self-emasculated. They filleted and positioned them into bilateral subcutaneous thigh pockets. However, subsequent follow-up with biopsy showed nonfunctional gonadal tissues [1]. Nonetheless, the idea of locating a testis into a thigh pocket is meaningful when the testis has kept its pedicle, i.e., an intact spermatic cord and vessels. Indeed, this technique is frequently performed after creating a tunnel from the inguinal area and is indicated when there is a traumatic avulsion of the scrotum or after debridement of an extensive Fournier's gangrene [2–4].

The first successful testicular microvascular replantation was reported by Rodríguez Costa et al. from Spain in 1978 on a 3-year-old boy [5]. Then a successful microvascular testicular autotransplantation was reported by Giuliani et al. on two patients with cryptorchidism in Genoa (Italy) in 1981 [6]. Shioshvili from Tbilisi (Georgia, old Union Of Soviet Socialist Republics (USSR)) successfully performed a microvascular testicular replantation in 1987 on a 19-year schizophrenic patient

S. A. AL-Mamari, *Urogenital Trauma: A Practical Guide*,
https://doi.org/10.1007/978-981-99-6171-9_47

who self-amputated the right testis [7]. And just a year later, Xu et al. reported a similar technique showing normal follicle-stimulating hormone levels, normal seminiferous tubules, germ cells, and Leydig cells on biopsy at 4 months [8]. Since then, a handful of encouraging cases have been reported in the literature [9, 10].

A very recent review published in 2022 has listed a total of 13 cases of testis replantation in the English literature, most of them being subsequent to self-mutilation in psychiatric patients [11]. In one situation, testis replantation was the ultimate and forced solution to correct a horrible medical error consisting of a wrong side orchidectomy for a right testicular tumor in a 25-year-old man. After noticing the error, the tumor-bearing (right) testis was also totally removed as a partial approach was not an option and the left testis was salvaged with microsurgical replantation after an urgent referral to a specialized center [11].

Technique of Testicular Reimplantation
The amputated testis must be kept in moist gaze, covered with ice, and thoroughly washed and debrided on arrival. The intervention is performed under general anesthesia. The vessels are flushed with diluted heparin and anastomosed directly to the corresponding proximal vessels in an end-to-end fashion using 10/0 Prolene on the artery and the veins with interrupted sutures. Obviously, this procedure requires an operating microscope taking into account the very small diameter of the vessels, artery 1 mm, and vein 2–3 mm. The vas deferens is also flushed with diluted heparin and anastomosed in an end-to-end fashion using interrupted 7/0 Prolene [9].

If, for any reason, the proximal cord vessels cannot be utilized, being too small, damaged by a crushing injury, or retracted, branches of the femoral vessels can be used and the superficial inferior epigastric artery and vein offer a solution for revascularizing the severed testis [11, 12].

When the amputated testis is intact but does not have sufficient pedicle length to be replanted orthotopically or when the perineum was also seriously damaged by a dramatically mutilating trauma, it has been proposed to **temporarily implant the healthy gonad in an ectopic site (e.g., the non-dominant forearm)** where it will continue its endocrine function. Here, the testis vessels can be anastomosed to the radial artery and to one of its venae comitantes just proximal to the wrist. Later on, after stabilization of the hormonal function, which takes several months, the testis is harvested from its temporary site along with the underlying skin and a good length of the vessels (radial artery and one vena comitans) and replanted into the perineum with vascular anastomosis to the deep inferior epigastric vessels and end-to-end possible anastomosis of the proximal and distal vas deferens [13] (Figs. 47.1 and 47.2). **It is important to remember that the viability of the forearm will henceforth rely on the integrity of the ulnar artery and the Allen test is necessary to assess the patency of the palmar arch before this procedure**.

In view of the uncertainty of the results in testicular replantation, it is advisable to take a sample of seminiferous tubules and proceed to testicular sperm extraction (TESE) for cryopreservation before the surgery [10]. Indeed, sperm

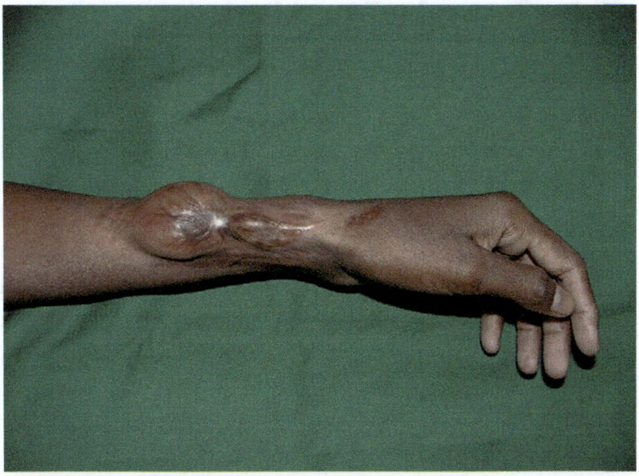

Fig. 47.1 Replanted testis in its ectopic position. (From Ramdas et al. [13], with permission from Elsevier)

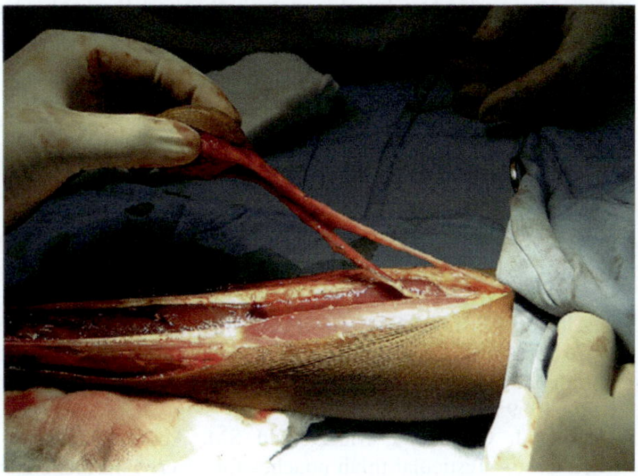

Fig. 47.2 Refabricated testicular pedicle prior to transfer. (From Ramdas et al. [13], with permission from Elsevier)

cryopreservation from an ejaculate is recommended in all other fertility-threatening conditions such as a testicular tumor, severe infection, surgery, or gonadotoxic therapy (e.g., chemotherapy and radiation therapy). **However, TESE and sperm cryopreservation are possible only in post-puberty and adult boys. They are useless in pre-pubertal boys, who have only spermatogonial stem cells (SSCs) and not mature spermatozoa**. Ongoing research is aiming at the cryopreservation of testicular tissues (rather than sperms alone) to allow a chance for the spermatogonial stem cells (SSCs) to mature and produce sperms through the new concept of "**in-vitro spermatogenesis**" [14, 15].

47.2 Testicular Transplantation

Silber reported the first experience of human testicular transplantation in 1978 in St. Louis (Missouri, USA) involving two identical adult twins, one of whom was born with anorchia. When they reached 30 years of age, one testis of the normal twin was harvested and transplanted to his anarchic brother using a microvascular technique and the results were encouraging in terms of hormonal function and spermatogenesis [16].

Since then, testicular transplantation has mostly been reported by Chinese surgeons for congenital dysplasia and acquired atrophy with good results as per the authors [17–19]. This technique is obviously hindered by many reasons: ethical, technical, practical, and so on [20]. The very purpose of this surgery can also be questioned. Is it for restoring the bodily image? Or for achieving a good androgen activity for sexual purposes? Or for fathering a child who will carry the donor's genome? A silicon prosthesis would be satisfactory for the bodily image, normal plasmatic androgen level can be achieved through injection of synthesized molecules allowing normal sexual activities, and the need for a child from another man's genome can be fulfilled by adoption.

References

1. Evins SC, Whittle T, Rous SN. Self-emasculation: review of the literature, report of a case and outline of the objectives of management. J Urol. 1977;118(5):775–6. https://doi.org/10.1016/s0022-5347(17)58190-2. PMID: 916099.
2. Allegretti E, Luca G, Arato I, Falabella G, Garolla A, Maffia R, Ricci G, Ghezzi M, Alfano C, Foresta C, Calafiore R. Full restoration of spermatogenesis and male fertility after post-traumatic ectopic testis implant. Ann Ital Chir. 2014;85:S2239253X14021860. PMID: 24535695.
3. Loloi J, Gottlieb J, MacDonald SM, Aboumohamed A, Ricci JA, Laudano M, Watts K. Case—Testicular thigh pouches for severe Fournier's gangrene: a how-to guide. Can Urol Assoc J. 2022;16(10):374–6. https://doi.org/10.5489/cuaj.7901. PMID: 35621290; PMCID: PMC9565065.
4. Okwudili OA. Temporary relocation of the testes in anteromedial thigh pouches facilitates delayed primary scrotal wound closure in Fournier gangrene with extensive loss of scrotal skin-experience with 12 cases. Ann Plast Surg. 2016;76(3):323–6. https://doi.org/10.1097/SAP.0000000000000505. PMID: 25785387.
5. Rodríguez Costa A, Romeo C, López G De Viedma A, Agra Cadarso B. Amputación testicular traumática. Reimplantación con éxito mediante microcirugía [Traumatic amputation of the testicle. Successful reimplantation using microsurgery (author's transl)]. An Esp Pediatr. 1978;11(12):865–7. Spanish. PMID: 742770.
6. Giuliani L, Carmignani G, Belgrano E, Puppo P. Autotransplantation de testicules dans la cryptorchidie abdominale. J Urol. 1981;87(5):279–81.
7. Shioshvili T. I: A case of successful replantation of testis after autohemicastration. Eur Urol. 1987;13:285–6. https://doi.org/10.1159/000472797.
8. Xu YM, Wu P, Cai PC, Cheng ZC. Replantation of the testis: report of a case. J Urol. 1988;139(3):596–8. https://doi.org/10.1016/s0022-5347(17)42539-0. PMID: 3343750.
9. Altarac S. A case of testicle replantation. J Urol. 1993;150(5 Pt 1):1507–8. https://doi.org/10.1016/s0022-5347(17)35828-7. PMID: 8411440.

10. Starmer BZ, Baird A, Lucky MA. Considerations in fertility preservation in cases of testicular trauma. BJU Int. 2018;121(3):466–71. https://doi.org/10.1111/bju.14084. Epub 2017 Dec 10. PMID: 29164757.
11. Tuncer FB, Frautschi RS, Lundy SD, Haber GP, Gastman B. First report of testicular replantation following wrong-site surgery. Urology. 2022;164:267–72. https://doi.org/10.1016/j.urology.2021.11.044. Epub 2022 Feb 1. PMID: 35114199.
12. Griffiths M, Britto J, Frame J. 5-Year follow-up of replantation of penis and testis in a child. Lancet. 2003;361(9353):263. https://doi.org/10.1016/S0140-6736(03)12302-1. PMID: 12547580.
13. Ramdas S, Thomas A, Arun Kumar S. Temporary ectopic testicular replantation, refabrication and orthotopic transfer. J Plast Reconstr Aesthet Surg. 2007;60(7):700–3. https://doi.org/10.1016/j.bjps.2007.01.074. Epub 2007 May 29. PMID: 17526441.
14. Onofre J, Baert Y, Faes K, Goossens E. Cryopreservation of testicular tissue or testicular cell suspensions: a pivotal step in fertility preservation. Hum Reprod Update. 2016;22(6):744–61. https://doi.org/10.1093/humupd/dmw029. Epub 2016 Aug 27. PMID: 27566839; PMCID: PMC5099994.
15. Kilcoyne KR, Mitchell RT. FERTILITY PRESERVATION: testicular transplantation for fertility preservation: clinical potential and current challenges. Reproduction. 2019;158(5):F1–F14. https://doi.org/10.1530/REP-18-0533. PMID: 30844751.
16. Silber SJ. Transplantation of a human testis for anorchia. Fertil Steril. 1978;30(2):181–7. PMID: 680196.
17. Zhao GX, Bai YX, Yang TS, He CQ, Chen YT, Qiao BP, Jiang HY. Homotransplantation of testis. A report of 11 cases. Chin Med J (Engl). 1993;106(12):907–10. PMID: 8143508.
18. Zhang Y, Jin FS, Li QS, Sun HZ, Zhu FQ, Zhang KQ. Testis homotransplantation: a report of 12 cases. Zhonghua Nan Ke Xue. 2008;14(3):248–50. Chinese. PMID: 18488341.
19. Zhan B, Wang L, Zhang X, Sun Y, Chen M. Homotransplantation of testis: experimental study and clinical practice (13 case reports). Transplant Proc. 1988;20(1 Suppl 1):918–21. PMID: 3347960.
20. Lee S, Mao L, Wang Y, D'Silva M, Yoo CH, Wolf P, Chung WS, Takahashi E, Chung DY, Gittes RF. Transplantation of reproductive organs. Microsurgery. 1995;16(4):191–8. https://doi.org/10.1002/micr.1920160406. PMID: 7674907.

Prevention, Complications, and Follow-Up of Scrotal and Testicular Trauma

48

In general, violent events are difficult to prevent. However, as blunt testicular trauma is associated with sports in the young population, the question of scrotal protection (athletic cup) in these activities has been raised by many researchers [1, 2]. In the army, after noticing an increase in casualties involving unprotected anatomical areas such as the pelvis or external genitalia in recent wars (Afghanistan and Iraq), it was decided to add a detachable genital flap on the Kevlar armor in 2004 [3].

Severe scrotal and testicular injuries expose the patients to the same systemic early complications as any other severe trauma. A review of the American National Trauma Data Bank (NTDB) revealed the following intra-hospital complications following testicular trauma: pneumonia (3.1%), deep vein thrombosis (2.3%), acute respiratory distress syndrome (ARDS) (1.6%), and acute kidney injury (1.6%). Other less frequent complications include urinary tract infection, pulmonary embolism, severe sepsis, myocardial infarction, unplanned intubation, and ICU admission. The mortality rate was 7.6% [4, 5].

Testicular torsion has been reported as a possible consequence of trauma with an occurrence of 4–8%. This strengthens the indication of ultrasonography and the early exploratory approach in patients presenting with scrotal pain and scrotal swelling after blunt trauma [6].

The post-testicular trauma patient should be followed up psychologically, physically, hormonally, and radiologically. His sexual life and fertility should be assessed by blood tests and semen analysis. And because of the breach in the blood–testis barrier, anti-sperm antibodies should also be assayed if technically possible. Ultrasonography should be performed at regular intervals (3–6 months) to detect testicular atrophy.

For long-term complications, short series showed that blunt trauma was found to cause testicular atrophy in as much as 13–56% of cases [7–9]. The majority of the patients (75%) had subfertile semen analysis despite having a normal hormonal status and only a very small percentage (12.5%) had anti-sperm antibodies [8]. Residual pain is another long-term complication and is observed in 10% of cases [9].

S. A. AL-Mamari. *Urogenital Trauma: A Practical Guide*,
https://doi.org/10.1007/978-981-99-6171-9_48

References

1. Dalton DM, Davis NF, O'Neill DC, Brady CM, Kiely EA, O'Brien MF. Aetiology, epidemiology and management strategies for blunt scrotal trauma. Surgeon. 2016;14(1):18–21. https://doi.org/10.1016/j.surge.2014.06.006. Epub 2014 Aug 21. PMID: 25151340.
2. Bieniek JM, Sumfest JM. Sports-related testicular injuries and the use of protective equipment among young male athletes. Urology. 2014;84(6):1485–9. https://doi.org/10.1016/j.urology.2014.09.007. PMID: 25432843.
3. Hudak SJ, Morey AF, Rozanski TA, Fox CW Jr. Battlefield urogenital injuries: changing patterns during the past century. Urology. 2005;65(6):1041–6. https://doi.org/10.1016/j.urology.2004.11.031. PMID: 15913731.
4. Grigorian A, Livingston JK, Schubl SD, Hasjim BJ, Mayers D, Kuncir E, Barrios C, Joe V, Nahmias J. National analysis of testicular and scrotal trauma in the USA. Res Rep Urol. 2018;10:51–6. https://doi.org/10.2147/RRU.S172848. PMID: 30128306; PMCID: PMC608960.
5. Vidhate S, Pathak H, Deokar R. Death of a pedestrian due to fatal scrotal trauma: a case report. Int J Med Toxicol Forensic Med. 2016;6(2(Spring)):108–11. https://doi.org/10.22037/ijmtfm.v6i2(Spring).10447.
6. Seng YJ, Moissinac K. Trauma induced testicular torsion: a reminder for the unwary. Emerg Med J. 2000;17:381–2.
7. Cross JJ, Berman LH, Elliott PG, Irving S. Scrotal trauma: a cause of testicular atrophy. Clin Radiol. 1999;54(5):317–20. https://doi.org/10.1016/s0009-9260(99)90562-7. PMID: 10362239.
8. Kukadia AN, Ercole CJ, Gleich P, Hensleigh H, Pryor JL. Testicular trauma: potential impact on reproductive function. J Urol. 1996;156(5):1643–6. https://doi.org/10.1016/s0022-5347(01)65472-7. PMID: 8863560.
9. Kleinclauss F, Martin M, Chabannes E, Bernardini S, Della Negra E, Bittard H. Traumatismes testiculaires: à propos de 56 cas. Prog Urol. 2001;11:486–91.

Part VII

Male Genital Self-Mutilation: Immersion into a Transhistorical, Ubiquitous, and Multicultural Madness

The only antidote to mental suffering is physical pain
Karl Marx (1818–1883)

Introduction to Male Genital Self-Mutilation

Male genital mutilation is an incredibly old phenomenon in which the limitless insanity and cruelty of humans are matched only by their vivid imagination and their sake of justification from their Gods. Its origins can be traced to the Egyptian, Greek, Roman, and Ancient India mythologies where deities were depicted cursing and punishing each other through castration or attempting to raise their powers by self-amputating the so-called impure and devilish organs [1].

Outside the mythology context, castration was historically a social means to enfeeble captive enemies and criminals or to prepare prepubescent boys for special activities (singer, guardian of harem). In ancient Egypt, Rome, Greece, the Ottoman empire, China, etc. castration was very frequent, and the phenomenon continued for centuries only to progressively disappear in the modern era. The consented procedures for non-psychotic persons performing "self-purification" to worship their gods have almost disappeared as a mass phenomenon in the world (**Skoptsy** in Russia) except in India where they are still present through the **Hijras** who are now recognized by the legal authorities as the third gender [2]. The Chinese counterpart of this phenomenon where the individuals were devoted to the Emperor's court has completely disappeared (**Imperial Eunuchs**) [3].

Apart from the **Hijras** and other **eunuchs** outside India, cases of **male genital self-mutilation (GSM)** are rare, being reported sporadically and their main underlying factors are psychiatric imbalances with or without religious delusions and transsexualism.

The present study is an overview of the phenomenon of male GSM, addressing its mythological and historical origins, and progressing to its modern aspects through a review of its etiological factors, anatomic pathology, management, and prognosis.

For self-orchidectomy, the treatment is based on hemostasis and scrotal closure when one or both testes have been removed. Reanastomosis of the testicular artery and vas deferens are performed exceptionally. For penile severance, in some cases, the treatment consists of **debridement of the stump** if having enough length, or **perineal urethrostomy** if the full length of the organ was lost. In other cases where the amputated penis is viable and a local competence is available, **replantation (macro or microsurgical)** is performed with variable successes. To ensure the success of surgical treatment and prevent GSM recurrence, **early psychiatric management** in acute presentation, as well as a close follow-up is of paramount importance.

Despite the scarceness of reported GSM incidents, it is likely that every urologist will encounter a case of this malady once in his/her career and it is therefore important for him/her to be mentally, scientifically, and technically prepared for its management.

This topic would have fit within the relevant sections on genital trauma (urethral, penile, scrotal, and testicular injuries). However, a decision was taken to develop it as a separate entity given its numerous particularities from etiology to the management.

References

1. Wade J. The castrated gods and their castration cults: revenge, punishment, and spiritual supremacy. Int J Transpersonal Stud. 2019;38(1).
2. Mal S. The Hijras of India: a marginal community with paradox sexual identity. Indian J Soc Psychiatry. 2018;34:79–85.
3. Cartwright M. Eunuchs in ancient China. World History Encyclopedia, 27 Jul 2017. Web. 25 Jun 2021.

Genital Self-Mutilation in Mythology 49

Ancient civilizations' mythology is strewn with conflict tales among Gods and between Gods and humans that often ended in emasculation. Further myths and legends depict self-castrating Gods or worshippers obeying some Goddess injunctions.

It is unanimously admitted that the very first genital amputations were reported from the Egyptian theogony where the God Osiris was murdered and emasculated by his brother Set. It did not take long for Osiris' son Horus to avenge his father by castrating his uncle Set. Another myth originated in Anatolia from the Hurrians-Hittites where Kumarbi overthrew his father Anu, bitted, and swallowed his genitals. In the Greek pantheon, Ouranos was castrated by one of his sons, the Titan Kronos (Saturn) avenging for having been imprisoned by the former. Following this assault, Kronos threw his father's testes into the sea, provoking a foaming that engendered Aphrodite (Venus), the Goddess of beauty and sexual love. Another case is the reciprocal emasculation of a Phrygian king and Attis, the priest, and lover of the Anatolian or Phrygian Goddess Cybele, during a fight. Following the battle, Attis died, and the Goddess Cybele ordered all the priests to honor his memory by becoming eunuchs according to one of the many contradictory versions. These eunuch priests were henceforth referred to as "Galli." In Hierapolis, the Goddess Astarte's cult was remarkably similar to that of Cybele, and historians have observed many men sacrificing their genitals during the paroxysm of their ecstasies [1, 2].

Interestingly, there is also a mythological report of self-castration by Combabus to escape from the dangerous seduction of the Assyrian Queen Stratonice. With a similar motivation, Eshmum, a Phoenician beautiful young man who was fond of hunting, castrated himself to escape from the Goddess Astronoë harassment. He died following his injury, and the Goddess brought him back to life as the God of healing.

Similar tales are found in India where the God Indra, a very sexually active deity, was cursed by the sage and ascetic Gautama Maharishi as a punishment for committing adultery with his wife Ahalya. Indra lost his male genitalia, and his body was

S. A. AL-Mamari, *Urogenital Trauma: A Practical Guide*,
https://doi.org/10.1007/978-981-99-6171-9_49

covered with a thousand vulvae, later on changed into eyes, while Ahalya was petrified. The Indian God Shiva performed self-phallectomy to demonstrate his lack of interest in sexual attraction and kept his penis as a holy object for his worshippers. The Goddess Bahuchara Mata self-ablated her breasts preferring death to dishonor when her caravan was attacked by a bandits' gang. Later, the aggressors worshiped her by self-mutilating their genitals, pioneering the **Hijra** phenomenon that is still active nowadays [1–3].

Not satisfied by attributing to Gods the origin of castration (either involuntary or voluntary and self-inflicted), humans also believed that certain animals were self-castrating. The more the merrier. Hence, old Egyptian and Roman tales stated that beavers used to cut off their testicles when chased by hunters to leave them as prey and save their lives [4]. Although this beavers' behavior has never been corroborated by observations, it is important to know that modern scientific studies have proved the existence of self-penectomy in mice [5].

References

1. Casadio G. The failing male god: emasculation, death and other accidents in the ancient Mediterranean world. Numen. 2003;50(3):231–68. www.jstor.org/stable/3270488.
2. Androutsos G, Marketos S. La castration à travers les âges. Andrologie. 1993;3(1):61–6.
3. Wade J. The castrated gods and their castration cults: revenge, punishment, and spiritual supremacy. Int J Transpers Stud. 2019;38(1). https://doi.org/10.24972/ijts.2019.38.1.31
4. Jonckheere F. L'Eunuque dans l'Égypte pharaonique. Revue d'Histoire des Sciences. 1954;7(2):139–55.
5. Hong CC, Ediger RD. Self-mutilation of the penis in C57BL/6N mice. Lab Anim. 1978;12:55–7.

Male Castration in History

50

Male genital amputation or castration has been widely performed since the dawn of time, especially in the ancient peri-Mediterranean civilizations for multiple reasons: Weakening the enemies, punishing for misconduct, preparing young boys for future specific professions (harem guardians, singers…) or for sexual objectification. Three varieties of eunuchs were recognized in antiquity: (1) *Castrati*, clean-cut, both penis and testicles were removed; (2) *Spadones*, testicles only were removed; and (3) *Thlibiae*, testicles were bruised and/or crushed [1–3]. Only ancient Subsaharan Africa, pre-Colombian America, and pre-colonial Oceania seem to be spared by this phenomenon possibly due to underreporting.

As will be discussed hereafter, all three monotheist religions (Judaism, Christianity, and Islam) strongly prohibit castration. Nonetheless, many of their respective members have been involved directly or indirectly in this phenomenon throughout human history.

50.1 Pharaonic Egypt

The existence of eunuchs in ancient Egypt serving various purposes such as women guardians, servants, scribes, priests, and singers is still subject to debate, but there appears to be evidence tending to corroborate this fact and even the existence of self-castrated individuals. Horapollon mentioned in his Hieroglyphica about Egyptians "If they want to portray a male who commits the crime of mutilating himself, they draw a beaver: because the latter, when chased (by hunters), tears off its own testicles and leaves them behind as prey" [2].

S. A. AL-Mamari, *Urogenital Trauma: A Practical Guide*,
https://doi.org/10.1007/978-981-99-6171-9_50

50.2 Mesopotamia and Persian Empire

The existence of Eunuchs in the Sumerian, Babylonian, Assyrian, and Persian empires is robustly established since the fourth Millennium in association with the cult of the Sumerian Goddess Inanna or Ishtar [4]. In the Hammurabi code (2000 BC), castration was the sanction reserved for sexual criminals.

50.3 Greece

It is believed that the concept of castration was introduced in Greece by Phoenicians who brought Eunuchs from Asian countries [5].

50.4 Roman and Byzantium Empires

Roman empire expansion resulted in the adoption of deities and religions from some conquered territories, including the cult of Cybele, considered the Great Mother of Gods. The consequence was the increased number of self-castrations for men and self-mastectomies for women during ceremonies in the honor of Cybele. There is a castration bronze clamp fished out from the Thames in London proving that the cult has been practiced even in old Roman Britain (Fig. 50.1).

By the year 81 Before Christ, the Roman General and Consul Lucius Cornelius Sulla enacted a law prohibiting this practice on Roman soil [6].

Epiphanius of Salamis reported on the history of the **Valesians**, a heretic Christian sect that advocated self-castration in the second to third century AD. Very little information is known about these insane men who were also known to forcibly castrate travelers whom they encountered or guests who visited them. They are thought to have lived in the land of Philadelphia, the old name of the Jordan Capital city Amman during the Greek and Roman periods. Disciples of this sect were not allowed to eat meat until they underwent castration [7].

Many castrates were still imported from outside the roman empire, as the demand for slaves and eunuchs especially as "*Cubicularii*" (chamberlains) did not decrease. Despite the prohibiting laws edited by successive Emperors, the phenomenon persisted up to the reign of the Christian Emperor Justinian I (527–565) who published a series of more severe and dissuasive laws stipulating that men who castrate others would be punished by the mutilation of their genitals, will be sent to exile, and their property would be confiscated. And women who perform castration will be permanently banished and their properties will be confiscated [6]. Certain Eunuchs occupied remarkably high functions in the roman administration, the so-called *Praepositus sacri cubiculi* (Grand Chamberlain), to the point that some researchers stated that "in the Eastern Empire especially, the real power lay in the hands not of the emperor nor of his aristocrats, but of his chief eunuch" [6, 8].

Despite being discouraged by Christianity, the phenomenon was still present in the Middle Ages in the Byzantium empire where slaves were castrated in childhood

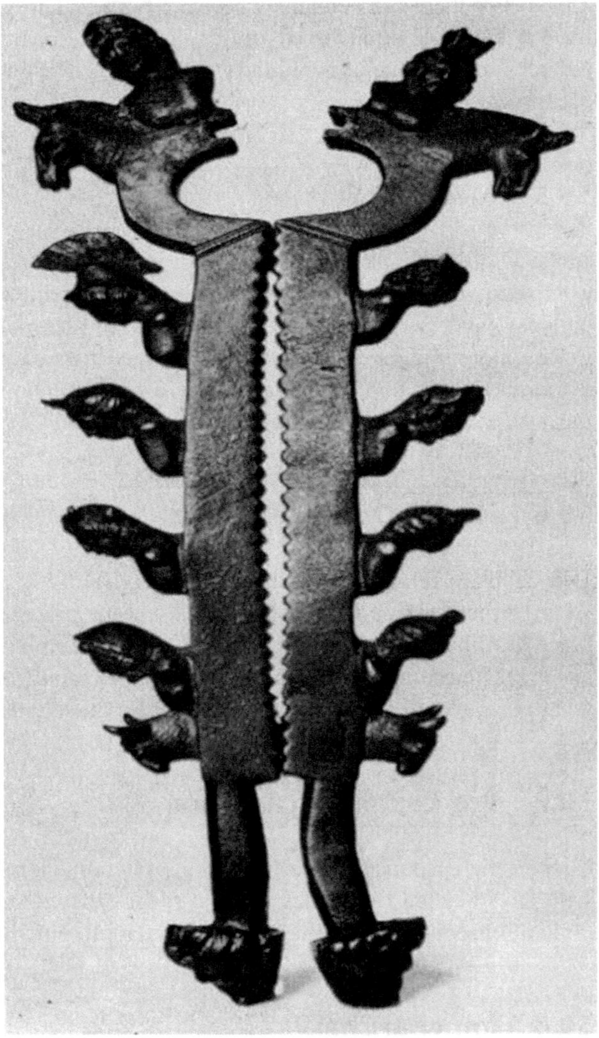

Fig. 50.1 Cult of Cybele castration clamp (Public Domain). Bronze Clamp from River Thames at London Bridge. Room of Roman Britain, Case D, British Museum. J scale

in a radical manner consisting of total removal of testes and penises. Such a radically castrated young boy was notoriously known as "**Carzimasium**". According to Grabowski, the Jewish origin of this name suggests that certain Jews were involved in the commerce of Eunuchs during that period [9]. However, it is important to remind our readers that castration is absolutely proscribed in the Hebraic religion, and Eunuchs are not accepted as priests. Indeed, this fact is unequivocally written in Deuteronomy 23:1 "No one who has been emasculated by crushing or cutting may enter the assembly of the Lord."

In Christianity also, the First Council of Nicaea in 325 has formally forbidden whoever has undergone a voluntary emasculation to enter the priesthood, but this did not discourage fanatics to continue a literal interpretation of Matthew Gospel,

19:12 "For there are eunuchs who were born that way, and there are eunuchs who have been made eunuchs by others, and there are those who choose to live like eunuchs for the sake of the kingdom of heaven. The one who can accept this should accept it" [1, 10].

50.5 Medieval Europe

In the Middle age, all of Europe was practicing castration either as a punishment or as preventive or curative treatment for various conditions such as leprosy, dementia, epilepsy, hydrocele, inguinal hernia, gout, and certain inflammatory diseases [1]. Furthermore, the interest to castrate younger boys between 7 and 12 years in order to preserve their soprano voice also grew with time, despite the poor anesthetics means and a mortality varying from 10% to 80% [1].

50.6 Islamic Ottoman Empire

Like Hebraic religion and Christianity, castration is also absolutely forbidden in Islam, either for free men or for slaves. Yet the presence of eunuchs was commonplace in Abbasside caliphates and the Ottoman Empire. From the sixteenth century, an increasing number of Eunuchs came to Istanbul from Africa, and by the nineteenth century, all eunuchs were slaves from outside the Empire [11].

50.7 Pre-Columbian America

Despite the existence of the transsexual phenomenon in ancient native Americans with the so-called Berdaches or "two-spirit," there is no robust evidence that these populations were performing self-emasculation to realize their will [12].

50.8 Imperial China

Castration and its corollary eunuch system are thought to have existed in Imperial China all over its 25 dynasties, covering an approximate period of 4000 years, only to disappear by the early twentieth century with the overthrowing of the last Emperor [13]. It is estimated that the total number of Eunuchs reached a 100,000 at the time of the establishment of the Qing dynasty in 1644, while the total empire population was 130 million people [14]. And this phenomenon has reached a so high magnitude that Historians and commentators referred to late Imperial China as a "**Castrated civilization**" [15]. In addition, many Chinese eunuchs were slaves being trusted in the royal court and utilized their position to gain political power. By the last period of the Ming dynasty (1368–1644 CE), they had established a nearly complete domination of the imperial court, and four infamous dictators in that period, namely Wang Zhen, Wang Zhi, Liu Jin, and Wei Zhongxian were all eunuchs [16, 17]. In China, castration involved the total removal of external genitalia (testes and penis) at the same time, and with increased experience, the mortality rate was lower (2%) than in other countries (25% or higher) [13].

Many families castrated their own children, and many young adults voluntarily underwent the same mutilation for socio-economical purposes, aiming at being employed as servants and getting protection in the Royal Palace (Fig. 50.2). Castrates were providing material advantages to their relatives; however, they were referred to as "Chujia" (leaving home) and their return home was considered too shameful for their families [18]. The last Imperial eunuch, Sun Yaoting, who died in December 1996 at the age of 94, was himself castrated at the age of 8 to save his father from bankruptcy [18].

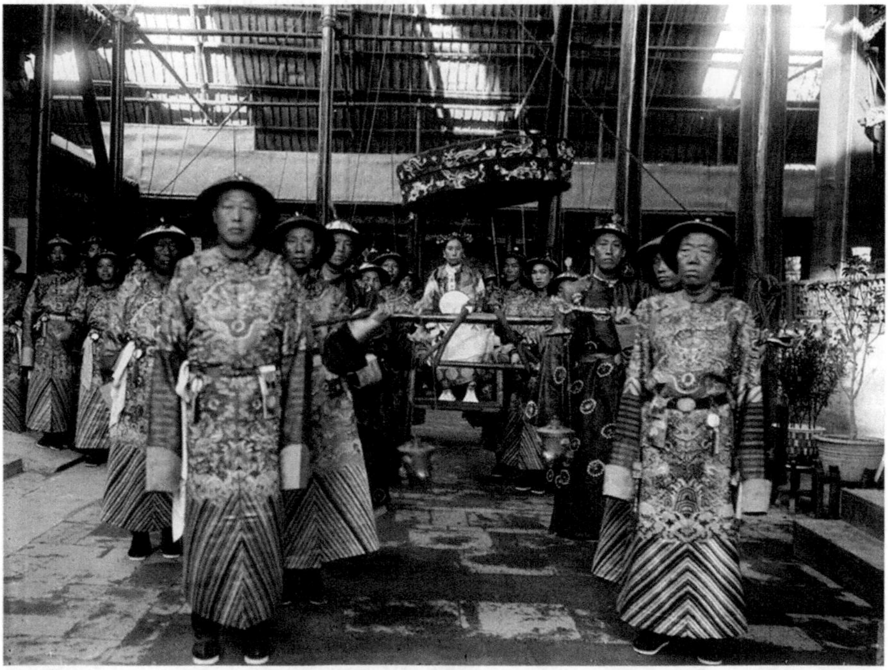

Fig. 50.2 The Empress Dowager Cixi (1835–1908) in sedan chair carried and surrounded by eunuchs in front of Renshoudian, Summer Palace, Beijing. (Photographer: Xunling, 1874–1943. (Public domain))

50.9 Early Modern England

There are many reports from the seventeenth and eighteenth centuries referring to self-castration and phallectomy in England, probably with religious delusions. This practice was however considered very shameful and humiliating by English society [19].

50.10 Russia

Founded by a fugitive peasant, Kondratii Selivanov, in around the 1760s, the **Skoptsy**, also called the **White Doves**, were a Christian sect in the Russian Empire that was encouraging genital self-amputations (orchidectomy with or without phallectomy for males, and mastectomy with clitoridectomy and excision of the labia majora for females) to attain purification. Male members of the sect had a choice between either the "**great seal**" (removal of the penis, the scrotum, and the testes) or the "**lesser seal**" (removal of the scrotum and testes, leaving the penis intact) (Fig. 50.3). They did so to atone for the so-called original sin committed by Adam

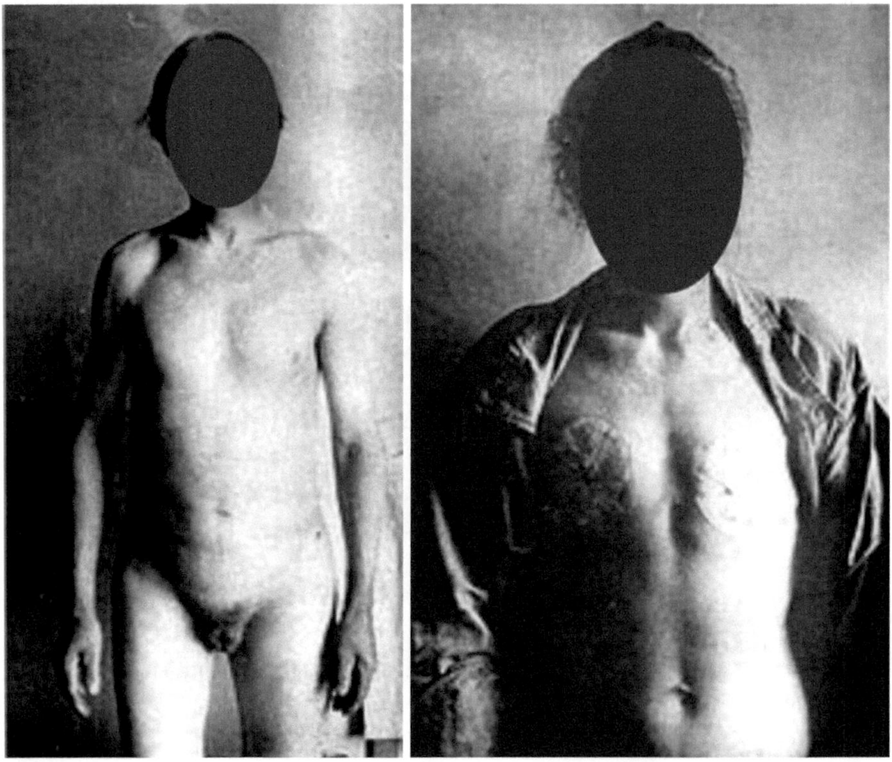

Fig. 50.3 Skoptsy man and woman with "greater seal". (Public domain)

and Eve through their genitals and were also referring to the early mentioned Mathew gospel 19:12. Obviously, adepts of this sect literally interpreted the last part of this verse not only as a spiritual purification but also as physical castration. The Skoptsy were severely persecuted by the Tsar governments and later by the Soviet authorities and started declining in the nineteenth and twentieth centuries. Today the sect is believed to have completely disappeared [20, 21].

50.11 India

The **hijra** (eunuch/transvestite) is a well-known institutionalized third gender in India. In 2014, a Supreme Court verdict ordered that Hijras should be recognized under a separate "third gender" category [22]. However, it is important to know that among Hijras, there is a minority born with ambiguous genitalia (Khusra), while the majority are unequivocally born males, then self-castrate (Khoja/Chhinni) through a process called "**Nirvan**" to attain purification for the cult of the Mother Goddess Bahuchara Mata. Besides these two categories, there are also cross-dressers or transvestites (Aqua), impotent male homosexuals or bisexuals (Zananay), or even biological true female with false Hijra identity (Chhibri) [22].

In view of the above facts, it became obvious to some researchers that many hijras are prostitutes, undermining the valued sacred role of their devotion [22–24]. By 2012, the estimated number of Hijras was five to six million in India but they are still a marginal community living in ghettos [22, 25].

50.12 Australia

Some aborigines traditionally perform urethrotomy by incising the undersurface of the penis. They do so in a stepwise manner starting at younger ages until adulthood to complete the incision which starts from the external meatus up to the base of the scrotum, resulting in a long ventral urethral slit. To date, the reason for this incision is still subject to debate. Speculations include hygiene reasons, contraceptive measures as the semen would flow too proximally to enter the vagina, enhancement of self-sexual stimulation for males with increased ventral sensation, or a desire to stimulate the females with a larger penile girth on erection, etc. [26–28].

Another proposed explanation is that aborigines' ancestors envied male kangaroos' penises which were believed to be anatomically bifurcated to adapt to the complex vaginal system of the female marsupials (two lateral vaginas for sperm carriage to the two uteruses, and one middle vagina for joey birth) [27]. However, modern studies disproved this fact and demonstrated that Kangaroos have unsplit penises [29], but many other marsupial species such as the Koala do effectively have bifurcated penises.

50.13 Famous Eunuchs in History

Although non-exhaustive, the following list portrays the fact that Eunuchs, either forced or voluntary, originated from various cultures, professions, and social positions, and embodied different personalities. This should always be borne in mind when facing a case of self-castration.

- **Pothinus (First century BC)**: **Pothinus** was the regent for the underaged Pharaoh Ptolemy XIII Theos Philopator, who co-ruled Egypt with his sister and wife Cleopatra VII after the death of their father Ptolemy XII.
- **Sporus (First century CE)**: He was one of the most known eunuchs in Roman history. This young man was favored, castrated, and officially married by Emperor Nero in the year 67 after the death of his wife Poppeae Sabina [30].
- **Cai Lun (First to Second century CE)**: He is traditionally regarded as the inventor of paper and the modern papermaking process. It is enough to realize that had Cai Lun not invented the paper, Johannes Gutenberg would not have invented his mechanical printing press at around 1440, mass communication would not have been possible at that time, and Renaissance would not have happened in Europe in the fifteenth Century.
- **Origen of Alexandria (185–254)**: Origen was considered the most brilliant Christian scholar and Theologian for centuries. As an ascetic, he reportedly self-castrated at a young age to freely work in instructing female catechumens. However, this version is not universally accepted [31].
- **Narses (Fifth to Sixthcentury CE)**: A Romanized Armenian, Narses was one of the Great Generals in the service of the Byzantine Emperor Justinian I.
- **Peter Abelard (1079–1142)**: Abelard was a famous French Philosopher, logician, and teacher who fell in love with his pupil Héloïse and had an affair and a son with her. Héloïse's uncle, Canon Fulbert then obliged Abelard to marry Héloïse in order to repair the dishonor and cover the shame. However soon after their marriage, Abelard, embarrassed and aiming at protecting his own reputation, sent his wife to a convent. This provoked Fulbert's furor, who felt betrayed and punished Abelard by getting him assaulted and castrated [32].
- **Zheng He (1371–1433)**: This Chinese mariner, explorer, Admiral, and Diplomat during the Ming Dynasty, was born in a Muslim family under the name "Ma He." He was captured and castrated at the age of 10 years soon after China reconquered Yunnan, the last territory held by Mongols [33].
- **Judar Pasha (1550–1606)**: This Spanish-born man was captured and castrated by Muslim Slave-raiders as a young boy. His original name was Diego de Guevara. He became a Moroccan military leader who notoriously conquered the Songhai Empire, with its historical cities Gao, Djenné, and Timbuktu (today located in the Republic of Mali).
- **Wei Zhongxian (1568–1627)**: Wei is considered as the most powerful and most notorious eunuch in Chinese history. He castrated himself at the age of 21 to enter the Royal court where he became progressively influential to the point that he took maximum advantage of the Tianqi Emperor's (Zhu Youjiao) weakness to

become the actual ruler by the end of his life along with the Emperor's wet nurse Madam Ke [34].

- **Thomas "Boston" Corbett (1832–1894)**: Corbett was a Union Army soldier who killed President Abraham Lincoln's assassin, John Wilkes. He was a fervent Christian, and in 1858, he was ogled by two prostitutes on his way back from a church meeting and got some sexual excitation. This encounter strongly disturbed him to the point that when he reached home, he deeply meditated about the Gospel of Mathew 19:12 (see above) and 5:29 'And if thy right eye offend thee, pluck it out, and cast it from thee: for it is profitable for thee that one of thy members should perish, and not that thy whole body should be cast into hell'. He immediately understood what he had to do and castrated himself with a pair of scissors as atonement [35]. After this act, he remained calm, continued praying, had dinner, then took a light stroll through the city before reporting to the hospital as the last, but also the least of his concerns.
- **Alessandro Moreschi (1858–1922)**: This famous Italian castrato singer of the late nineteenth century was also known as the "Angel of Rome" [36, 37].

References

1. Androutsos G, Marketos S. La castration à travers les âges. Andrologie. 1993;3(1):61–6.
2. Jonckheere F. L'Eunuque dans l'Égypte pharaonique. Revue d'Histoire des Sciences. 1954;7(2):139–55.
3. Hong CC, Ediger RD. Self-mutilation of the penis in C57BL/6N mice. Lab Anim. 1978;12:55–7.
4. Taylor G. Castration: an abbreviated history of western manhood. New York: Routledge; 2002. p. 285.
5. Photis Theodoropoulos. https://www.quora.com/What-was-the-role-of-eunuchs-in-Ancient-Greek-society.
6. Kontani Y. Castration under Roman Law: a study of the codification during the Reign of Justinian I (527–565). Ancient Soc. 2018;48:305–31. https://doi.org/10.2143/AS.48.0.3285205.
7. The Panarion of Epiphanius of Salamis: Sects 47–80, De Fide By Epiphanius, p 98–100. Epiphanius of Salamis. Panarion. p 4.38.1–4. Translated by Frank Williams in The Panarion of Epiphanius of Salamis. New York: E.J. Brill; 1987. https://people.well.com/user/aquarius/epiphanius-panarion-fide.htm.
8. Hopkins K. Eunuchs in politics in the later Roman Empire. Proc Camb Philol Soc. 1962;9:62–80.
9. Grabowski A. Eunuch between economy and philology. The case of *carzimasium*. In: Mélanges de l'École française de Rome—Moyen Âge [En ligne]; 2015. p. 127–31.
10. Caner DF. The practice and prohibition of self-castration in early Christianity. Vigiliae Christianae. 1997;51(4):396–415.
11. Toledano ER. The Imperial eunuchs of Istanbul: from Africa to the heart of Islam. Middle East Stud. 1984;20(3):379–90. Accessed 7 Apr 2021.
12. Boag P. Sexuality, gender, and identity in great plains history and myth. Great Plains Q. 1998;1998:1271.
13. Eng JT, Zhang Q, Zhu H. Skeletal effects of castration on two eunuchs of Ming China. Anthropol Sci. 2010;118:107–16. https://doi.org/10.1537/ase.090430.
14. Tsai S. The demand and supply of Ming eunuchs. J Asian Hist. 1991;25(2):121–46. http://www.jstor.org/stable/41930824. Accessed 7 Apr 2021.

15. Chiang H. How China became a "castrated civilization" and eunuchs a "third sex". In: Chiang H, editor. Transgender China. New York: Palgrave Macmillan; 2012. https://doi.org/10.1057/9781137082503_2.
16. Cartwright M. Eunuchs in Ancient China. World History Encyclopedia. 2017. Web 25 Jun 2021.
17. Crawford R. Eunuch power in the Ming dynasty. T'oung Pao. 1961;49(3, second series):115–48.
18. Chatterton J, Bultitude M. Castration; The eunuchs of Qing dynasty China; a medical and historical review. de Historia Urologie Europace. 2008;15:39–47.
19. Skuse A. 'One stroak of his razour': tales of self-gelding in early modern England. Soc Hist Med. 2020;33(2):377–93.
20. Engelstein L. From heresy to harm: self-castrators in the civic discourse of late tsarist Russia. In: Castration and the Heavenly Kingdom: a Russian folktale. Cornell University Press; 2003.
21. Tulpe IA, Torchinov EA. The Castrati ("Skoptsy") sect in Russia: history, teaching, and religious practice. Int J Transpers Stud. 2000;19(1):77–87.
22. Mal S. The hijras of India: a marginal community with paradox sexual identity. Indian J Soc Psychiatry. 2018;34:79–85.
23. Nanda S. The hijras of India: cultural and individual dimensions of an institutionalized third gender role. J Homosex. 1985;11(3–4):35–54. PMID: 4093603.
24. Lal V. Not this, not that: the hijras of India and the cultural politics of sexuality. Social Text. 1999;61:119–40.
25. Kalra G. Hijras: the unique transgender culture of India. Int J Cult Ment Health. 2012;5:121–6.
26. Cawte JE, Djagamara N, Barrett MG. The meaning of subincision of the urethra to aboriginal Australians. Br J Med Psychol. 1966;39:245–53. https://doi.org/10.1111/j.2044-8341.1966.tb01334.x.
27. Singer P, Desole D. The Australian subincision ceremony reconsidered: vaginal envy or kangaroo bifid penis envy. Am Anthropol. 1967;69(3/4, new series):355–8. http://www.jstor.org/stable/669931. Accessed 5 Apr 2021.
28. Pounder DJ. Ritual mutilation. Subincision of the penis among Australian Aborigines. Am J Forensic Med Pathol. 1983;4(3):227–9.
29. Warburton NM, Bateman PW, Fleming PA. Anatomy of the cavernous muscles of the kangaroo penis highlights marsupial-placental dichotomy. J Anat. 2019;234(3):306–15. https://doi.org/10.1111/joa.12930. Epub 2019 Jan 6. PMID: 30613968; PMCID: PMC6365618.
30. Woods D. Nero and Sporus. Latomus Revue d'etudes Latines. 2009;68(1):73–82.
31. Chadwick H. Origen. Encyclopedia Britannica. 2020. https://www.britannica.com/biography/Origen. Accessed 8 Apr 2021.
32. Guillaumard F. Le travail de l'écriture d'Héloïse dans ses lettres à Abélard. Analyse Freudienne Presse. 2005;2(2):153–66. https://doi.org/10.3917/afp.012.0153.
33. Lo J-p. Zheng He. Encyclopedia Britannica. 2021; https://www.britannica.com/biography/Zheng-He. Accessed 9 Apr 2021
34. Britannica, The Editors of Encyclopaedia. Wei Zhongxian. Encyclopedia Britannica. 2021. https://www.britannica.com/biography/Wei-Zhongxian. Accessed 8 Apr 2021.
35. Jensen B. The insane story of the guy who killed the guy who killed Lincoln. Meet Boston Corbett, the self-castrated hatmaker who was John Wilkes Booth's Jack Ruby. Published online in April 2015. https://www.washingtonian.com/2015/04/12/the-man-who-killed-john-wilkes-booth/.
36. Clapton N. Moreschi and the voice of the castrato. London: Haus; 2008. p. 60–2.
37. Koutsiaris EA, Alamanis C, Eftychiadis A, Zervas A. Castrati singers: surgery for religion and art. Ital J Anat Embryol. 2014;119(2):106–10. PMID: 25665280

Male Genital Self-Mutilation in the Modern Medical Literature

51

Many authors refer to the phenomenon of male genital self-mutilation as "**Klingsor Syndrome**" or "**Eshmum Complex**." The first eponym comes from a fictitious character in the Wagner's opera "Parsifal" where Klingsor was a magician who castrated himself in an unsuccessful attempt to gain acceptance from the Knights of the Grail [1]. The second one comes from the legendary beautiful young man mentioned above in the Phoenician mythology (see Chap. 49).

While exclusively concentrating on the male aspect of this malady in the present work, it should be borne in mind that the female counterpart of this phenomenon has also been reported in the modern medical literature, but articles are extremely scanty [2, 3]. Furthermore, a psychiatric pathological entity consisting of female genital self-mutilations, dysorexia, and a hysterical personality has been proposed as **Caenis Syndrome**. This eponym refers to Caenis, who was the loveliest of all girls in Thessaly but refused to marry anyone and was abducted and raped by Poseidon (or Neptune), the God of the Sea. Poseidon then offered her one wish, and she demanded to be changed into a man so that she might never be wronged again [4].

It is generally assumed that the first case of GSM in the modern literature was reported by Daniel Stroch in 1901 [5]. However, there is an older report authored by MacDonald in 1884 [6] about a 50-year-old Indian cultivator who auto-inflicted a bilateral orchidectomy and presented after 36 h. After local treatment according to available antiseptic means in that pre-antibiotic era, the patient's condition needed almost 40 days to improve, only to allow him to be sentenced by a court to 7 days' imprisonment for this self-inflicting injury.

Many cases were soon reported in the twentieth century, lifting the veil on this phenomenon, and enriching the modern medical literature, with an increasing trend that continues to date (Fig. 51.1). By the time this review was concluded, there were not less than 246 articles written, for a total of 337 cases arising from all 6 inhabited continents, comprising individual case reports and monocentric series.

S. A. AL-Mamari, *Urogenital Trauma: A Practical Guide*,
https://doi.org/10.1007/978-981-99-6171-9_51

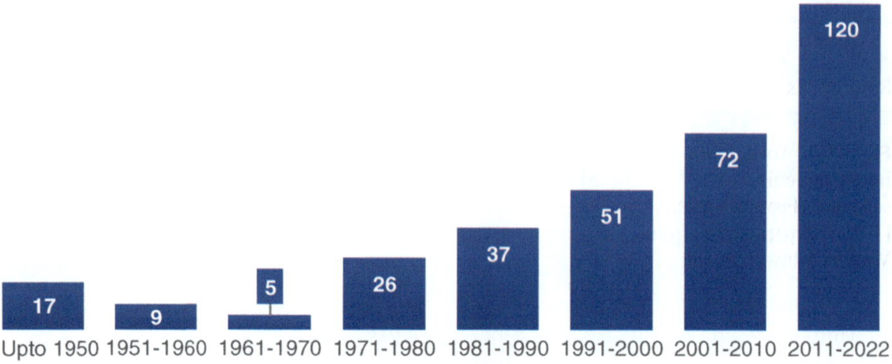

Fig. 51.1 Number of GSM cases per decade (total 337)

Not strictly considered as amputations, cases of urethral foreign bodies insertion should not be considered as GSM as well as those of self-insertion of plastic spherules in the penile skin reported in Japanese racketeers known as "**Yakuza**" [7].

Overall, apart from the Hijras in India, male GSM remains sporadic. However, a series study in a single tertiary hospital in the USA over a 5-year period revealed a total of 118 cases with male genital trauma, of whom 39% (46 patients) had a penetrating injury and 61% had a blunt trauma. Among the penetrating injury, the most common mechanism was external violence (48%) and self-inflicted injury (40%). Hence, 18 cases of GSM were recorded in that period, giving an average of more than 3 patients per year [8].

In addition to hundreds of sporadic case reports here and there, there is a handful of review articles treating this phenomenon, the latest three being written in 1979, 1996, and 2017, and inventorying 53, 98 cases, and 173 cases, respectively [9–11].

There have been also a dozen series treating this phenomenon. The oldest was written by Bigot in 1938 (cited from Hemphill 1951) about ten Indochina Buddhists, aged from 20 to 70 years, who self-amputated their penises to prevent incestuous or immoral acts or from indulging in sexual thoughts [12]. One by one, more series continued to be reported with slowly increasing sizes [13–16]. Review articles have also been published addressing the psychiatric aspect of major self-mutilations in general [17, 18] or the GSM aspect in particular [19, 20].

There have also been many online surveys addressing the motivations behind castration [21–25], while others were specific to men who performed voluntary penectomy with testicular preservation [26] or to responses to orchidectomy [27]. Authors also published reviews and meta-analysis about the penile replantation outcome [28], and the cosmetic and functional results [29].

Reports came from all the continents, especially North America, Europe, and Asia (India, Japan). Christian and Asian Polytheist worlds have shown the highest incidence of GSM. Arabic countries did also report dozens of cases, especially Morocco which has published the highest number of male GSM in the Islamic world [30–33], in addition to two monocentric review articles consisting of 14 and 8 cases, respectively [16, 34], followed by Turkey [35, 36] (Fig. 51.2).

Other countries include:

- Russia, Israel, Spain: four cases each.
- Italy, Sweden, Ireland, Gabon, Hungary, Ghana, Poland, Taiwan, China, and Malaysia: three cases each.
- Brazil, Serbia, and Kenya: two cases each.
- Oman, UAE, KSA, Columbia, Belgium, South Korea, Trinidad, Iran, Switzerland, Yugoslavia, Denmark, Netherlands, Georgia, Chad, Slovenia, Hong-Kong, Tunisia, Cameroun, Bangladesh, Indonesia, South-Africa, Thailand: one case each.

In contrast, extremely rare cases were reported elsewhere in the Arab world, including one case in each of the following countries: Tunisia, the United Arab Emirates, the Kingdom of Saudi Arabia, and the Sultanate of Oman [37–40]. Surprisingly, no article came from Egypt. Although there is no report on religious delusion in relation to GSM in the Islamic world, other types of hallucination can still play a role here like in other regions of the world. Underreporting plays a possible role in the rarity of cases of male GSM in Arab-Islamic countries. Indeed, only one case has been published from Oman just a few months before concluding this review. It consisted of bilateral orchidectomy and partial penectomy in a married Omani citizen [40], while cases of self-orchidectomy by a young boy and self-penectomy by an expatriate working in the countryside have been recorded in this

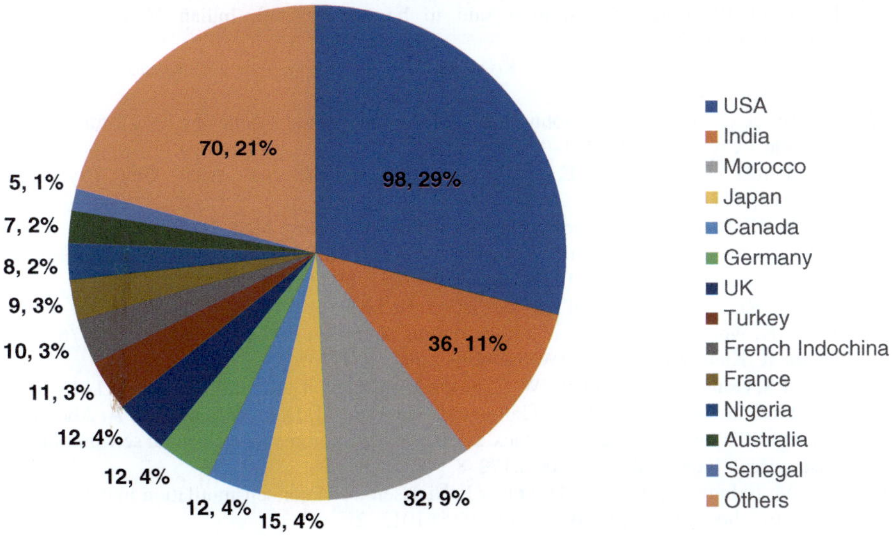

Fig. 51.2 Number and percentage of GSM cases per country (total 337)

country. Unfortunately, the last two cases remained unreported in the medical literature.

Anumonye was the first author to report cases of auto-penectomy (two) in Sub-Saharan Africa in 1973 [41], and to date, cases arose mainly from the West-Africa (Nigeria, Senegal, Côte d'Ivoire) [42–48], and even a review article in GSM, as well as a series on traumatic penile injuries in general, were produced from this region substantiating the local interest in research and publications about this pathology [49, 50]. More scanty articles arose from other African regions such as Central Africa (Gabon) and East Africa (Kenya) [51, 52]. Only one case report was found from the Southern African Subcontinent [53]. However, efforts to discover publications from other great African countries (Ethiopia, DR Congo, Tanzania, etc.) remained fruitless.

Similarly, few cases were reported from Australia, and paradoxically even more scanty articles were published from more populated countries such as China, Russia, and Brazil.

References

1. Bhattacharyya R, Sanyal D, Roy K. A case of Klingsor Syndrome: when there is no longer psychosis. Isr J Psychiatry Relat Sci. 2011;48(1):30–3. PMID: 21572240.
2. Simpson MA, Anstee BH. Female genital self-mutilation as a cause of vaginal bleeding. Postgrad Med J. 1974;50(583):308–9.
3. Wise TN, Dietrich AM, Segall E. Female genital self-mutilation: case reports and literature review. J Sex Marital Ther. 1989;15(4):269–74.
4. Goldney RD, Simpson IG. Female genital self-mutilation, dysorexia and the hysterical personality: the Caenis Syndrome. Can Psychiatr Assoc J. 1975;20(6):435–41.
5. Stroch D. Self-castration. Letter to the editor. JAMA. 1901;36:220.
6. Macdonald JR. Case of castration said to be self-inflicted. Indian Medical Gazette. 1884;19(11):326–7.
7. Tsunenari S, Idaka T, Kanda M, Koga Y. Self-mutilation. Am J Forensic Med Pathol. 1981;2(3):203–8.
8. McCormick CS, Dumais MG, Johnsen NV, et al. Male genital trauma at a level 1 trauma center. World J Urol. 2020;38:3283–9.
9. Greilsheimer H, Groves JE. Male genital self-mutilation. Arch Gen Psychiatry. 1979;36(4):441–6.
10. Romilly CS, Isaac MT. Male genital self-mutilation. Br J Hosp Med. 1996;55(7):427–31.
11. Veeder TA, Leo RJ. Male genital self-mutilation: a systematic review of psychiatric disorders and psychosocial factors. Gen Hosp Psychiatry. 2017;44:43–50.
12. Hemphill RE. A case of genital self-mutilation. Br J Med Psychol. 1951;24(4):291–5.
13. Blacker K, Wong N. Four cases of autocastration. Arch Gen Psychiatry. 1963;8:169–76.
14. Mendez R, Kiely WF, Morrow JW. Self-emasculation. J Urol. 1972;107(6):981–5.
15. Aboseif S, Gomez R, McAninch JW. Genital self-mutilation. J Urol. 1993;150(4):1143–6.
16. Mawuko-Gadosseh Y, Mayele M, Gallouo M, Graiouid M, Dakir M, Debbagh A, Aboutaieb R. Automutilation des organes génitaux externes chez l'homme [Male genital self-mutilation: a case series]. Prog Urol. 2020;30(3):172–8.
17. Large M, Babidge N, Andrews D, Storey P, Nielssen O. Major self-mutilation in the first episode of psychosis. Schizophr Bull. 2009;35(5):1012–21.

18. Gahr M, Plener PL, Kölle MA, Freudenmann RW, Schönfeldt-Lecuona C. Self-mutilation induced by psychotropic substances: a systematic review. Psychiatry Res. 2012;200(2–3):977–83.
19. Bourgeois M, Daubech JF, Benezech M, Lemerle AM. Enquête sur l'automutilation chez l'adulte en milieu psychiatrique (a propos de 90 cas) [Survey on self-mutilation in adults in psychiatric milieu (a propos of 90 cases)]. Ann Med Psychol (Paris). 1984;142(10):1287–95.
20. Martin T, Gattaz WF. Psychiatric aspects of male genital self-mutilation. Psychopathology. 1991;24(3):170–8.
21. Vale K, Siemens I, Johnson TW, Wassersug RJ. Religiosity, childhood abuse, and other risk factors associated with voluntary genital ablation. Can J Behav Sci. 2013;45:230–7.
22. Jackowich RA, Vale R, Vale K, Wassersug RJ, Johnson TW. Voluntary genital ablations: contrasting the cutters and their clients. Sex Med. 2014;2:121–32.
23. Roberts LF, Brett MA, Johnson TW, Wassersug RJ. A passion for castration: characterizing men who are fascinated with castration, but have not been castrated. J Sex Med. 2008;5:1669–80.
24. Johnson TW, Brett MA, Roberts LF, Wassersug RJ. Eunuchs in contemporary society: characterizing men who are voluntarily castrated (Part I). J Sex Med. 2007;4(4 Pt 1):930–45.
25. Wong STS, Wassersug RJ, Johnson TW, et al. Differences in the psychological, sexual, and childhood experiences among men with extreme interests in voluntary castration. Arch Sex Behav. 2021;50:1167–82. https://doi.org/10.1007/s10508-020-01808-6.
26. Wibowo E, Wong STS, Wassersug RJ, Johnson TW. Characteristics of males who obtained a voluntary penectomy. Arch Sex Behav. 2020;49(2):793–803.
27. Brett MA, Roberts LF, Johnson TW, Wassersug RJ. Eunuchs in contemporary society: expectations, consequences, and adjustments to castration (Part II). J Sex Med. 2007;4(4 Pt 1):946–55.
28. Li GZ, Man LB, He F, Huang GL. Replantation of amputated penis in Chinese men: a meta-analysis. Zhonghua Nan Ke Xue. 2013;19(8):722–6.
29. Virasoro R, Tonkin JB, McCammon KA, Jordan GH. Penile amputation: cosmetic and functional results. Sex Med Rev. 2015;3(3):214–22.
30. Outarahout M, Sekkat FZ. Automutilation de la verge ou le suicide de genre. Trois cas de schizophrènes. L'Information Psychiatrique. 2014;90:207–11. https://doi.org/10.1684/ipe.2014.1177.
31. Kharbach Y, Amiroune D, Ahsaini M, et al. Penile self-mutilation preceded by bizarre delusions: two case reports. J Med Case Rep. 2014;8:246.
32. Aalouane R, Rammouz I, Hafidi H, Boujraf S. Genital self-mutilation in an attempt of suicide by a patient with a borderline personality. J Neurosci Rural Pract. 2013;4:199–203. https://doi.org/10.4103/0976-3147.112769.
33. Riyach O, El Majdoub A, Tazi MF, El Ammari JE, El Fassi MJ, Khallouk A, Farih MH. Successful replantation of an amputated penis: a case report and review of the literature. J Med Case Rep. 2014;8:125. https://doi.org/10.1186/1752-1947-8-125.
34. Ziba OJ, Mzyiene M, Ahsaini M, Soufiane M, Tazi M, El Ammari J, Mohammed J, Farih F. Characteristics and management of male genital self-mutilation: a series of 08 cases. Int J Innov Res Sci Eng Technol. 2021;6(10):128–34.
35. Erkol Z, Sirin G, Erkol H, Yilmaz R, Ince H, Konuk N. Subtotal self-amputation of the penis and bilateral self-orchiectomy followed by suicide by hanging: case report. Turkiye Klinikleri J Med Sci. 2012;32:869–73.
36. Lok U, Gulacti U, Benlioglu C, Buyukaslan H, Aktas N. Self-mutilation of genitalia-using teeth. J Clin Diagn Res. 2014;8(2):179–80. https://doi.org/10.7860/JCDR/2014/7552.4052.
37. Kamoun-Siala M, Fellaj-Lachtar DM, Amami O, Jarraya A. De la dysérection à l'automutilation génitale (à propos d'un cas). Annales Médico-Psychologiques Revue Psychiatrique. 2005;163:588–94.
38. Shirodkar SS, Hammad FT, Qureshi NA. Male genital self-amputation in the Middle East. A simple repair by anterior urethrostomy. Saudi Med J. 2007;28(5):791–3.
39. Qureshi NA. Male genital self-mutilation with special emphasis on the sociocultural meanings. Neurosciences (Riyadh). 2009;14(2):178–81.

40. Al-Fahdi A, Al-Mahrouqi T, Al-Zain I, et al. Self-inflicted total amputation of the external genitalia as a psychological repercussion of the COVID-19 pandemic: a case report. Cureus. 2022;14(12):e32725. https://doi.org/10.7759/cureus.32725.
41. Anumonye A. Case report. Self-inflicted amputation of the penis in two Nigerian males. Niger Med J. 1973;3(1):51–2.
42. Tabowei BI, Kombo BB. Genital self-mutilation. Niger Del Med J. 2015;1(2):40–4.
43. Ajape AA, Issa BA, Buhari OI, Adeoye PO, Babata AL, Abiola OO. Genital self-mutilation. Ann Afr Med. 2010;9(1):31–4.
44. Yusuf AJ, Bello A, Abubakar ML, et al. Genital self-mutilation in schizophrenic patients. A report of two cases. Afr J Urol. 2009;15:189–91.
45. Jalloh M, Ndoye M, Niang L et al. Automutilation avec amputation de la verge chez des patients schizophrènes: à propos de 2 cas. Revue Africaine de Chirurgie et Spécialités. 2013;7(1).
46. Sarr Adiouma S, Sow Y, Ndiaye B, et al. Automutilation génitale masculine: à propos de 2 observations. Theol Sex. 2015;24:65–8. https://doi.org/10.1016/j.sexol.2014.06.002.
47. Kabore FA, Fall PA, Diao B, et al. Auto-amputation récidivante du pénis sur terrain schizophrène: à propos d'un cas. Andrologie. 2008;18:224–6.
48. Dékou A, Vé D, Koffi A, et al. L'automutilation génitale: intérêt d'un avis psychiatrique dans la prise en charge urologique. Afr J Urol. 2009;15:227–32.
49. Eke N. Genital self-mutilation: there is no method in this madness. BJU Int. 2000;85(3):295–8.
50. Oranusi CK, Nwofor A. Traumatic penile injuries: mechanisms and problems of treatment in a tertiary institution in Nigeria. Niger J Clin Pract. 2014;17(6):763–6.
51. Massande Mouyendi J, Ndang Ngou Milama S, Mougougou A, Nguema Asseko B, Bayonne Manou S. Automutilation penienne sur terrain psychotique: a propos de 4 cas. Bull Med Owendo. 2017;15(43):58–62.
52. Muluka EAP, Dhaphale M. Severe self-mutilation among Kenyan psychotics. Br J Psychiatry. 1986;149:778–80.
53. Lebelo LT, Grobler GP. Case study: a patient with severe delusions who self-mutilates. S Afr J Psychiatry. 2020;26:1403. https://doi.org/10.4102/sajpsychiatry.v26i0.1403.

Etiology of Male Genital Self-Mutilation 52

GSM can be understood as a special part of **apotemnophilia** (from Greek words "apo" = away from, "temno" = piece cut off, and "philia" = love) which is simply defined as an overwhelming or obsessive desire to have a healthy limb or organ amputated. **Dermatillomania** is a very minor stage of apotemnophilia consisting of skin-picking, scratching, and **excoriation** [1]. Importantly, genital dermatillomania was reported to cause recurrent penile ulcers that prompted multiple reconstructive surgeries ending in penis loss in one patient [2]. The tendency for repetitive self-mutilation is also referred to as "**Van Gogh syndrome**" after the famous Dutch painter who cut off the lower half of his left ear and gave it to a prostitute [3].

In addition to sharing the same psychiatric background with apotemnophilia in general, GSM has two frequent additional causes: **religious delusions and transsexualism or gender dysphoria**. There is an overlap between the etiological factors of GSM and categorizing them as equals navigating through a labyrinth. To unravel this conundrum, male GSM can be roughly ranged into two categories: **Psychiatric imbalances and transsexualism**. Yet in many cases of transsexualism, some degree of psychopathy can be present. Also, religious delusions are sometimes evoked as a distinct group despite being obviously driven by psychosis. Studies have shown a total rate of psychiatric cause of 80 to 90% including schizophrenia (49–51%), organic psychosis (substance abuse, epilepsy, brain damage…) (17–19%), and neuroses (16–19%). In addition, there were gender dysphoria and normal subjects rates of 6-15% and 7%, respectively [4–7].

52.1 Psychiatric Imbalances

In a recent psychiatric review of major self-mutilations (MSM) including orchidectomy, penectomy, eye enucleation, or removal of a portion of the limbs, Large et al. studied the proportion of patients who were in their first episode of psychosis. They

S. A. AL-Mamari, *Urogenital Trauma: A Practical Guide*, https://doi.org/10.1007/978-981-99-6171-9_52

documented a psychotic illness in 143 of 189 cases (75.6%) of MSM, and 119 of the 143 psychotic patients (83.2%) were schizophrenic [8].

Underlying causes of psychosis in relation to GSM:

(a) **Religious delusions**: already discussed above.
(b) **Drug abuse**: A review article found **Cannabis** (33.3–51.5%), **alcohol** (16.7–44.3%), and **tobacco/nicotine** (16–34.4%) to be the most used substances in association with secondary psychosis [9]. Others are Opioids, sedatives, cocaine, stimulants, hallucinogens, solvents, amphetamine, barbiturates, hypnotics, Ecstasy, and Phencyclidine.

    Limiting the study to drug-induced self-mutilation alone, Gahr et al. found in their review that the majority of patients were male (85%) with a mean age of 30 years and that 73% of patients self-mutilated subsequently to the use of one substance, while 27% self-mutilated after the use of more than one [6]. Here, among the psychotic substances, **alcohol** (25%), **hallucinogens** (25%), and **amphetamines** (22%) were the most frequently found and major psychotic impairment was present in 80% of patients.
(c) **Prison-induced psychosis**: This is a recognized psychiatric entity since the nineteenth century [10]. Indeed, the current review revealed many cases of self-castrations and emasculations in penitentiary environments [11, 12].
(d) "**Folie à deux ou à plusieurs**": Some curiosities have been documented during this research including two cases of male GSM occurring in the same family ("folie à deux") [13], or contagious self-inflicted genital injury in a hospital ("folie à plusieurs") [14].

GSMs have no limit and can even occur in public, like what was commonplace in Hierapolis, Syria, during the cult of the Goddess Astarte (see Chap. 49) [15]. This case illustrates the fact that patients in a schizophrenia crisis are disconnected from reality and do not care about being observed while under the influence of their delusions. In modern times, some Christians show special attraction to Jerusalem as the central place to express their devotion. And for those who have pre-existing or latent psychotic disturbances, this holy city is the ideal place to act out their delusion, including self-mutilating the genital organs under extreme religious excitement. This phenomenon has been coined '**The Jerusalem Syndrome**' [16, 17].

52.2 Transsexualism

Transsexualism is the second most important cause of GSM after schizophrenia. Voluntary eunuchs (also referred to as "**eunuch wannabes**" in certain publications) account for the greatest percentage in this group: These are individuals who desire or are planning to undergo castration. They generally do not consult medical professionals regarding their desire and therefore resort to self-castration, castration by non-medical professionals, or self-inflicted intratesticular injections of toxic substances aiming at obliging the Urologists to remove the damaged testicles [18].

A survey revealed two big categories of voluntary eunuch [19]: a large proportion (40%) of them merely showed a fetishistic interest and appeared to be at relatively low risk of irreversible genital mutilation. The other category (20%) appeared to be at great risk of genital mutilation, showing a greater desire to reduce libido, change their male genital appearance, and prevent sexually offensive behavior. Between these two categories are individuals who were just interested in castration but not seeking it.

This survey showed that 19% of all voluntary eunuchs have attempted self-castration, but only 10% have sought medical assistance. Interestingly, this study shed the light on the fact that gender identity disorder in voluntary eunuchs may be other than the traditional male-to-female (MtF) transsexual and launched the concept of **male-to-eunuch transsexuality**, i.e., many eunuchs just want to lose their male attributes without necessarily adopting the female ones [19, 20]. It was also shown that the act of castration is largely premeditated with an 18-year elapsed time from the onset of an individual's desire to be a eunuch to the time of his actual castration, and **four etiological factors** were identified: **abuse during childhood, homosexuality, exposure to animal castration at a younger age, and religious condemnation of sexuality** [20].

Interestingly another survey addressing the personality of cutters who performed castration in voluntary eunuchs showed that they shared many of the above-mentioned etiological factors with their clients, many of them being themselves castrated [21].

A recent survey of 11 voluntarily penectomized subjects who did not desire testicular ablation showed a rather homosexual attraction with aesthetic and eroticist motivations. The study group was less likely to identify as male, was more likely to have attempted self-injury to their penis in the past, showed attraction to males without penises, and felt that they were more physically attractive without a penis than the controls [22].

Yet again, even in transexuals, there is no limit to the odd: What to say about this married patient who performed self-bilateral orchidectomy to fulfill his transsexual fantasy but had to take a low dose of exogenous androgen to maintain sexual marital activity due to an extraordinarily strong pair-bonding with his wife? [23].

52.3 "Normal Patients"

One might logically wonder how a reportedly normal person can self-mutilate his genitalia, or whether a person with no psychiatric background can still be considered normal after self-amputating his genitalia or any other important part of his body. These questions, though very pertinent, are better left to psychiatric expertise and will not be addressed in this discussion which will be limited to the precipitating causes of GSM in these so-called normal persons.

Thus, we have found various reasons such as conflict and frustration (increased stress) either within the family or in the professional environment [24–27], low self-esteem, and insecure personality structure with or without suicidal intention [28–32], bizarre sexual arousal [33], hypogonadism and sexual impotence ("Why to keep it if it is useless?") [34], heavily indebted man after spoiling all his resources [35], and a married man who attempted suicide because of the inability to cope with loneliness in quarantine and the fear of COVID-19 [36]. There is also a reported case of self-castration as a treatment for alopecia [37]. It is not known whether this man has made his dream come true after this sacrifice.

References

1. Lochner C, Roos A, Stein DJ. Excoriation (skin-picking) disorder: a systematic review of treatment options. Neuropsychiatr Dis Treat. 2017;13:1867–72. https://doi.org/10.2147/NDT.S121138. PMID: 28761349; PMCID: PMC5522672.
2. Alexandrov P, Tan WP, Elterman L. Genital dermatillomania. Curr Urol. 2017;11(1):54–6.
3. Runyan WM. Why did Van Gogh cut off his ear? The problem of alternative explanations in psychobiography. J Pers Soc Psychol. 1981;40(6):1070–7.
4. Greilsheimer H, Groves JE. Male genital self-mutilation. Arch Gen Psychiatry. 1979;36(4):441–6.
5. Veeder TA, Leo RJ. Male genital self-mutilation: a systematic review of psychiatric disorders and psychosocial factors. Gen Hosp Psychiatry. 2017;44:43–50.
6. Gahr M, Plener PL, Kölle MA, Freudenmann RW, Schönfeldt-Lecuona C. Self-mutilation induced by psychotropic substances: a systematic review. Psychiatry Res. 2012;200(2–3):977–83.
7. Boyer ER, Tucker P. Genital self-mutilation: a cutting conundrum. Psychiatric Times. 2020;37(7).
8. Large M, Babidge N, Andrews D, Storey P, Nielssen O. Major self-mutilation in the first episode of psychosis. Schizophr Bull. 2009;35(5):1012–21.
9. Addington J, Case N, Saleem MM, Auther AM, Cornblatt BA, Cadenhead KS. Substance use in clinical high risk for psychosis: a review of the literature. Early Interv Psychiatry. 2014;8(2):104–12. https://doi.org/10.1111/eip.12100.
10. Al Chaabani S, Bataille M. Troubles psychotiques et dissociatifs en milieu carcéral [Prison psychosis and dissociative disorders]. Rev Med Liege. 2002;57(12):793–8.
11. Conacher GN, Westwood GH. Autocastration in Ontario Federal Penitentiary. Br J Psychiatry. 1987;150:565–6.
12. Brown GR. Autocastration and autopenectomy as surgical self-treatment in incarcerated persons with gender identity disorder. Int J Transgenderism. 2010;12(1):31–9. https://doi.org/10.1080/15532731003688970.
13. Ristić DI, Petrović D, Cirić Z. Penile self-mutilation—two cases in one family. Psychiatr Danub. 2008;20(3):332–6.
14. Rada RT, James W. Urethral insertion of foreign bodies. A report of contagious self-mutilation in a maximum-security hospital. Arch Gen Psychiatry. 1982;39(4):423–9.
15. Wilcox Vanden Berg RN, Gaffney CD, Paduch DA. Presentation and resolution of gender dysphoria as a positive symptom in a young schizophrenic man who presented with self-emasculation: frontiers of bioethics, psychiatry, and microsurgical genital reconstruction. Clin Case Rep. 2020;8(9):1735–40.
16. Zislin J, Katz G, Raskin S, Strauss Z, Teitelbaum A, Durst R. Male genital self-mutilation in the context of religious belief: the Jerusalem syndrome. Transcult Psychiatry. 2002;39(2):257–64. https://doi.org/10.1177/136346150203900208.
17. Bar-el Y, Durst R, Katz G, Zislin J, Strauss Z, Knobler HY. Jerusalem syndrome. Br J Psychiatry. 2000;176:86–90. https://doi.org/10.1192/bjp.176.1.86. PMID: 10789334.
18. Johnson TW, Irwig MS. The hidden world of self-castration and testicular self-injury. Nat Rev Urol. 2014;11(5):297–300. https://doi.org/10.1038/nrurol.2014.84.
19. Roberts LF, Brett MA, Johnson TW, Wassersug RJ. A passion for castration: characterizing men who are fascinated with castration, but have not been castrated. J Sex Med. 2008;5:1669–80.
20. Johnson TW, Brett MA, Roberts LF, Wassersug RJ. Eunuchs in contemporary society: characterizing men who are voluntarily castrated (Part I). J Sex Med. 2007;4(4 Pt 1):930–45.

21. Jackowich RA, Vale R, Vale K, Wassersug RJ, Johnson TW. Voluntary genital ablations: contrasting the cutters and their clients. Sex Med. 2014;2:121–32.
22. Wibowo E, Wong STS, Wassersug RJ, Johnson TW. Characteristics of males who obtained a voluntary penectomy. Arch Sex Behav. 2020;49(2):793–803.
23. van Kammen DP, Money J. Erotic imagery and self-castration in transvestism/transsexualism: a case report. J Homosex. 1977;2(4):359–6.
24. Mago V. Male genital self-mutilation. Indian J Psychiatry. 2011;53:168–9.
25. Nerli RB, Ravish IR, Amarkhed SS, Manoranjan UD, Prabha V, Koura A. Genital self-mutilation in nonpsychotic heterosexual males: case report of two cases. Indian J Psychiatry. 2008;50(4):285–7. https://doi.org/10.4103/0019-5545.44753.
26. Shimizu A, Mizuta I. Male genital self-mutilation: a case report. Br J Med Psychol. 1995;68:187–9.
27. Terayama T, Sakamoto T, Ikeuchi H, Tanaka Y. Self-penile glans amputation: a report of two cases. Acute Med Surg. 2016;4(1):101–4. Published 2016 May 27. https://doi.org/10.1002/ams2.199.
28. Wong STS, Wassersug RJ, Johnson TW, et al. Differences in the psychological, sexual, and childhood experiences among men with extreme interests in voluntary castration. Arch Sex Behav. 2021;50:1167–82. https://doi.org/10.1007/s10508-020-01808-6.
29. Nerli RB, Srikanth P, Kumar GA, Abhijith SM. Genital self-mutilation: two case reports. J Case Rep. 2015;5:100–2.
30. Rudhran V, Thippeswamy H, Chaturvedi SK. Phallicide: a case of auto penile amputation as a mode of suicide. Aust N Z J Psychiatry. 2013;47(5):491–2.
31. Tharoor H. A case of genital self-mutilation in an elderly man. Prim Care Companion J Clin Psychiatry. 2007;9(5):396–7. https://doi.org/10.4088/pcc.v09n0511e. PMID: 17998964; PMCID: PMC2040280.
32. Yang JG, Bullard MJ. Failed suicide or successful male genital self-amputation? Am J Psychiatry. 1993;150(2):350–1.
33. Ilgi M, Kutsal C, Abdullayev E, Aykanlı E, Kirecci SL. Genital self-mutilation case in high-level educated person. Urol Case Rep. 2016;10:19–22.
34. Sudarshan CY, Rao KN, Santosh SV. Genital self-mutilation in erectile disorder. Indian J Psychiatry. 2006;48(1):64–5. https://doi.org/10.4103/0019-5545.31623.
35. Tabowei BI, Kombo BB. Genital self mutilation. Nig Del Med J. 2015;1(2):40–4.
36. Al-Fahdi A, Al-Mahrouqi T, Al-Zain I, et al. Self-inflicted total amputation of the external genitalia as a psychological repercussion of the COVID-19 pandemic: a case report. Cureus. 2022;14(12):e32725. https://doi.org/10.7759/cureus.32725.
37. Gleeson MJ, Connolly J, Grainger R. Self-castration as treatment for alopecia. Br J Urol. 1993;71(5):614–5.

53 Used Instruments, Organ Disposal, and Anatomopathology of Male Genital Self-Mutilation

A broad variety of instruments are used for GSM including cutting tools (knives, razors, scissors, sickle, broken glass, chisel with hammer, box cutter, electrical chain saw, pruning shears) and constricting materials (bottleneck, metallic ring, metallic wire, rubber band, thread tie, buckle). Other means include masturbation machine, teeth, fingernails, radiofrequency ablation, vegetable mill, and injectable chemical agents (Buprenorphine, paraffin, alcohol, printer ink).

The removed organs may be kept, thrown away, or into the toilet [1]. Cases of autophagia have been reported where patients ate the amputated genitals (penis, testes, scrotum) as well as other organs (ears, distal phalanx of fifth fingers) [2, 3].

With data collected from 173 cases, Veeder et al. found that phallectomy alone is the predominant anatomopathological injury in GSM, (35.8%), followed by orchidectomy (32.4%), combined phallectomy and orchidectomy (19.7%), and genital lacerations (12.1%) [4]. A Japanese publication provided a detailed study on the site of penectomy showing the following distribution: peri-pubic area in 7.4%, proximal penile part in 88.9%, and glans in 3.7% [5]. There is one case from Spain with multiple penile cuts and penectomy [6]. There are also cases of metachronous orchidectomy and penectomy where the patients started first with bilateral orchidectomy before penectomy with variable intervals [7, 8]. Extragenital injuries associated with GSM, include wrist incisions, tongue, nipples, ear excision, anterior abdominal stabbing with viscera perforations, chest stabbing, attempt to enucleate the eyes [9]. The most appalling cases are perhaps two young men who self-inflicted penectomy and cut throat in the same country (Ghana) with a 5-year-interval; both patients were rapidly managed with tracheostomy and penile stump refashioning and survived [10, 11]. Noteworthy is also the case of a heterosexual patient who performed bilateral self-orchidectomy in order to prevent sexual aggressiveness and soften his approach to women, and later embarked on a self-laparotomy in an attempt to "denervate his adrenal glands". His aim was to stop catecholamines secretion that he incriminated as the cause of his undue nervousness. After thorough documentation in libraries, he wore gloves and a mask, lay supine, positioned multiple mirrors

S. A. AL-Mamari, *Urogenital Trauma: A Practical Guide*,
https://doi.org/10.1007/978-981-99-6171-9_53

at different angles to optimize his views, and used antiseptics and local anesthetics. He performed a 14-cm incision from the xiphoid process to the umbilicus, ligated the abdominal wall vessels, entered the peritoneal cavity, and only stopped when he experienced severe pain upon liver retraction [12].

References

1. Yeniyol CÖ, Yener H, Keçeci Y, Ayder AR. Microvascular replantation of a self amputated penis. Int Urol Nephrol. 2002;33(1):117–9. https://doi.org/10.1023/a:1014437927083.
2. Mendez R, Kiely WF, Morrow JW. Self-emasculation. J Urol. 1972;107(6):981–5.
3. Koops E, Püschel K. Selbstverstümmelung und Autophagie [Self-mutilation and autophagia]. Arch Kriminol. 1990;186(1–2):29–36.
4. Veeder TA, Leo RJ. Male genital self-mutilation: a systematic review of psychiatric disorders and psychosocial factors. Gen Hosp Psychiatry. 2017;44:43–50.
5. Terayama T, Sakamoto T, Ikeuchi H, Tanaka Y. Self-penile glans amputation: a report of two cases. Acute Med Surg. 2016;4(1):101–4. Published 2016 May 27. https://doi.org/10.1002/ams2.199.
6. Toribio-Vázquez C, Yebes Á, Quesada-Olarte J, Rodriguez A, Alonso-Bartolomé M, Ayllon H, Martinez-Piñeiro L. Genital mutilation in males. Curr Urol Rep. 2022;24:121. https://doi.org/10.1007/s11934-022-01129-2. Epub ahead of print. PMID: 36401111.
7. Boualaoui I, El Bote H, Bellouki O, Ibrahimi A, El Sayegh H, Nouini Y. Rudy and Borden technique for penile self-mutilation in Klingsor syndrome: a case report. Pan Afr Med J. 2021;38:334. https://doi.org/10.11604/pamj.2021.38.334.28897. PMID: 34285757; PMCID: PMC8265253.
8. Ravichandran S, Smith PM, Tang V. Genital self-amputation—its psychological urge. J Surg Case Rep. 2022;2022(12):rjac569. https://doi.org/10.1093/jscr/rjac569. PMID: 36518649; PMCID: PMC9741515.
9. Tsanakalis F, Almadhyan A, Flondell-Sité D. A rare case of complete male genital self-amputation posing challenges in the psychiatric diagnosis and management. Heliyon. 2021;7(6):e07349. https://doi.org/10.1016/j.heliyon.2021.e07349. PMID: 34195445; PMCID: PMC8239729.
10. Gudugbe S, Asiedu IO, Lamptey J, Kyei M, Baidoo K. Self-genital mutilation and attempted suicide by cut throat in the same patient at presentation: a rare event. Open J Psychiatry. 2015;05:330–3.
11. Thompson PA, Obeng K, Maison P, Quansah K, Nortey M. A case of cut throat and penis. J Adv Med Medical Res. 2020;32(12):87–91.
12. Kalin NH. Genital and abdominal self-surgery. JAMA. 1979;241(20):2188.

Management of Male Genital Self-Mutilation

54

Principles to be observed once a patient arrives in the hospital after self-inflicted genital mutilation include rapidly taking the history from him if he has a lucid speech or from the accompanying persons. However, no time should be lost before requesting routine blood tests as well as blood cross-matching as the patient might develop hypovolemic shock requiring urgent transfusion. If the patient is not psychiatrically stable, he should be sedated, his vitals monitored, and the opinion and intervention of the psychiatrist are urgently requested.

The wound must be cleaned and packed for provisional hemostasis, broad-spectrum antibiotics, IV fluid, and analgesics should be initiated without delay, and an antitetanic vaccine should also be given.

If the amputated distal penile part is not available or not viable, efforts will consist of cleaning the wound, ensuring the hemostasis, and either refashioning the penile stump if it has enough length to allow urination in standing position [1], or closing the stump if it is too short and creating a urethro-perineal fistula. If the part is available and has an apparently good shape, i.e., non-crushed penis or testis, it should be thoroughly washed with 0.9% saline and kept in a pressurized container at 4 °C by wrapping it in moist gauze inside a plastic bag sealed within a second plastic bag containing ices, then placed in an ice container. Before the anastomosis, the amputated part should be sterilized with 1% chlorhexidine solution and immersed in a 1% sodium heparin-saline solution, then irrigated with normal saline and antibiotics [2].

Except for cases of self-testicular contusion of torsion, imaging investigations (ultrasonography, etc.) are superfluous in the majority of GSM who present with an overt injury and no time should be lost before taking them in the operating theater.

An adult and well-oriented patient should be rapidly posted for and consented to surgery; otherwise, consent should be taken from an adult relative. The anesthetist clearance should be obtained in the accident and emergencies department, and the patient be shifted as soon as possible to the OT. When the patient is in an acute psychotic phase and refuses replantation and family members are absent, **it is worth**

S. A. AL-Mamari, *Urogenital Trauma: A Practical Guide*,
https://doi.org/10.1007/978-981-99-6171-9_54

considering that his mental status makes him unfit to take a lucid decision, and therefore the team (Urologist, Psychiatrist, Plastic Surgeon, Anesthetist, the Hospital Public Relations Officer) **should decide for the best to the patient including taking him for an urgent reimplantation procedure despite the lack of his consent** [3].

Obviously, the surgical approach depends on the time to presentation and whether the amputated parts have been well preserved. In a Moroccan series, the average time to presentation was 6 h after the removal of one case with extreme delay (2 months) [4].

If the patient presents early and organs are transected sharply, i.e., non-crushed, every effort should be made for their re-anastomosis. The clinical experience with testicular torsion has allowed defining the limit for testicular survival in warm ischemia at 4–6 h. However, **the limit for penile survival is not clearly known**, and there are encouraging reports of successful microscopic penile replantation after a 9.5-h-warm ischemia time and a 14-h-total ischemia time [5].

Presently, it is out of the question to propose to these patients any plan for penile transplantation. Since its first reported case in China in 2006 [6], this procedure is still in its infancy and only a few cases have been performed so far in the world, especially in South Africa [7] and in the USA [8], being **exclusively reserved to accidentally injured or well-cooperative cancer survivors** [9]. Research is being made for the bioengineering of various organs including penises [10], but its clinical application will need many more years or decades to appear on the horizon.

54.1 Surgical Management

54.1.1 Unilateral or Bilateral Orchidectomy

The operation consists of a **re-anastomosis of the spermatic artery and vein as well as the vas deferens**. Unfortunately, reports of successful re-anastomosis of testes are exceedingly rare. This might be explained by the fact that testicles are seldom brought by the patients after castration. Another explanation is the paired nature of these organs that affects surgeons' motivation to perform a tedious re-anastomosis of one testis if the other one is intact. But this argument stands valid only for a minority of cases because bilateral orchidectomy appears to be statistically more frequent than unilateral.

The first attempt at testicular salvage was reported by Evins et al. in 1977 but was unsuccessful [11]. It did not take long before Rodriguez Costa et al. performed the first successful testicular re-anastomosis in a 3-year-old boy [12], and in the following decade, Lin et al. published a report on two cases of successful testicular re-anastomoses [13].

Other publications contributed to this experience with a total testicular ischemia time of 4–6 h including a 3-h warm ischemia, showing excellent ultrasonographic (homogeneous parenchymal echo pattern and normal blood flow), hormonal (testosterone level) and histopathological outcomes (presence germ cells and Leydig cells on biopsy), and a good vasography after a 4- to 6-month follow-up [14–16].

Cooling the testis before re-anastomosis is essential to prevent warm ischemia damage. Obviously, the great challenge in testicular salvage after amputation is the exceedingly small size of the spermatic artery which measures only 1 mm diameter on average. Under a surgical microscope, the plastic surgeon will first perform the arterial anastomosis using an atraumatic needle and 10/0 Ethilon or Prolene suture, then the venous anastomosis (two veins are generally present and are at least twice larger than the artery with a 2–3 mm diameter), and finally the vasovasostomy with a 7/0 suture [13].

Further successful experiences of testicular salvage were published in the twenty-first century including ingenious innovations such as a permanent ectopic testicular replantation in the forearm or a temporary replantation in the forearm allowing refabrication of a long pedicle before orthotopic transfer to the perineum [17].

Unfortunately, efforts to reimplant the testes are not always rewarding, as shown by a review of 17 patients with autocastration with a testicular salvage rate of 24% only [18].

54.1.2 Penectomy

The first case of penile replantation was reported by Ehrich in 1929 [19]. It was a **macroscopic procedure** roughly performed by just fixing the distal penis to the stump with urethral and tunica albuginea anastomosis covered with skin sutures. No neurovascular re-anastomosis is made in the macroscopic approach, and the graft survival depends on corporal sinusoidal blood flow. The operation harbors many complications (necrosis) and a high failure rate. It took almost half a century before Tamai and Cohen separately described a **microsurgical repair** of the penis with satisfactory results in 1977 [20, 21]. A Chinese metanalysis found significant differences in erectile dysfunction, urethral stricture, and urinary fistula between the two techniques and suggested that early microscopic anastomosis of the most possible penile dorsal veins, arteries, and dorsal nerves is essential for the survival of the replanted penis and reduction of complications [22].

Today there is a consensus that microsurgical penile re-anastomosis is the best treatment for penile amputation [23–27]. The following surgical steps are advocated by many authors [2, 25, 27–29] and can be divided into three phases:

Phase 1: Steps performed by the urologist.

- Cystourethroscopy into the posterior urethra to assess the normality of the proximal urethra and the bladder.
- Suprapubic catheter placement.
- Debridement of nonviable tissue to allow identification of the veins, nerves, and arteries.
- Spatulation of the urethral stump and anastomosis including the underlying corpus spongiosum with interrupted 4/0 Vicryl or 5/0 to 6/0 Monocryl sutures.

When half of the anastomosis is done, a 16- or 18-Fr silastic catheter is inserted and the anastomosis is completed in a tension-free technique.
- Tunica albuginea closure with 3/0 Polydioxanone (PDS) sutures.
- Repair of both corpora cavernosa with interrupted 3/0 or 4/0 Monocryl or 5/0 Vicryl sutures.

Phase 2: Steps performed by the plastic surgeon (with the use of a surgical microscope).

- Anastomosis of the dorsal artery and dorsal vein as well as the dorsal sensory nerves.
- Anastomosis of the dorsal superficial vein and nerve using a microsurgical technique with 9/0 or 10/0 Ethilon or Prolene.
- Anastomosis of the dorsal deep vein and the deep arteries with 10/0 Ethilon or Prolene.

Phase 3: Closure.

- Placement of two drains and skin closure with interrupted 4/0 Vicryl or Monocryl.
- Dressing of the wound with Jelonet paraffin gauze.
- Immobilization and protection of the penis by bulky dressing or padding in a special ventral foam splint to avoid kinking and compromising vascularization of the distal part.

To prevent skin necrosis, one can proceed to debridement of the penile skin with the subsequent burying of the penis in the scrotum, and the creation of a subcutaneous tunnel in the suprapubic area has also been suggested. Repair of the **external pudendal system** was also suggested as an option to prevent skin necrosis problems in the presence of pubic-level amputations (present in 7.4% of cases in a Japanese study [30]), since the penoscrotal skin is perfused from the external pudendal artery system [31]. In cases where proximal penile vessels are damaged, the **deep inferior epigastric vessels** have been utilized for microvascular penile replantation [29].

Post-operative care:

- Direct inspection and Doppler ultrasound every 30 min [25].
- Low-molecular weight heparin.
- Continue broad-spectrum antibiotics.
- Hyperbaric oxygen can be useful.

Leech therapy can be used to prevent congestion when restoration of venous return is suboptimal [32].

When there is a lack of expertise in microsurgery, it is advised to attempt a non-microsurgical repair where no dorsal vein, artery, or nerve anastomosis is performed [33]. Here the whole procedure is performed by the urologist and includes the following steps:

- Placement of a suprapubic catheter.
- Insertion of a 16- to 18-Fr catheter through the urethra of the dissevered part, then through the proximal urethra into the bladder.
- End-to-end urethral anastomosis made with a two-layer closure using a 5/0 polyglycolic acid (PGA) suture.
- Connection of the cavernous bodies of the penis with 3/0 polyglycolic acid continuous suture.
- Reapproximation of the Buck's and dartos fascia.
- Closure of the skin.

In cases of **glansectomy**, some authors have suggested merely performing a **stump plasty** as an easy technique for the preservation of sexual activity despite the resulting shorter penis [30]. A **sensate radial forearm free flap** can also be used, not necessarily to reconstruct the whole penis, but only an amputated glans, further widening the human ingenuity horizon. This was successfully performed on a 28-year-old psychotic man who presented 3 years after a self-amputation [34].

54.2 Psychiatric Management

Psychiatric expertise and management are essential in GSMs in acute as well as in the post-crisis phase for all patients, including those with no known psychiatric troubles. A patient who has self-injured should be closely followed up by a psychiatrist to avoid recurrence which can occur any time within hours, days, weeks, months, or even after years or decades. Details of psychiatric management are beyond the scope of this study. However, its importance can be apprehended through the following few scenarios which are self-explanatory.

- Patients have self-amputated their penises twice in up to a 10-year interval, and surgeons had to repeat microsurgical penile replantation on them [35, 36].
- What to do in response to the unlimited madness if not by showing unlimited patience and effort? This was experienced by some urologists who performed penile replantation on a psychotic patient. The patient re-amputated his penis 2 days later. This did not discourage the surgeons but prompted them to reimplant the organ for a second time! However, when the patient violently pulled out his urinary catheter 2 weeks later, the subsequent penile necrosis caused by the traction left no other solution than a penectomy and perineal urethrostomy [37]. This case amply demonstrates that however great the surgeons' achievements are, their launch window and ammunition are unfortunately limited, and their success largely depends on the effectiveness of the psychiatric management.
- More troubling is the possibility of a patient to self-inflict genital mutilation, even in an apparently symptom-free phase of his illness [38].
- Patients in a schizophrenia crisis are disconnected from reality and do not care about being observed while under the influence of their delusions. GSMs have no

limit and can even occur in public, like what was commonplace in Hierapolis during the cult of the Goddess Astarte (see above) [3].

- Finally, how dejected would you feel after successful penile reimplantation achieved at the cost of hours of meticulous effort and concentration in a psychotic patient, only to hear that he committed suicide 4 days after leaving the hospital [39]?

References

1. Boualaoui I, et al. Rudy and Borden technique for penile self-mutilation in Klingsor syndrome: a case report. Pan Afr Med J. 2021;38:334. https://doi.org/10.11604/pamj.2021.38.334.28897.
2. Babaei AR, Safarinejad MR. Penile replantation, science or myth? A systematic review. Urol J. 2009;4(2):62–5.
3. Wilcox Vanden Berg RN, Gaffney CD, Paduch DA. Presentation and resolution of gender dysphoria as a positive symptom in a young schizophrenic man who presented with self-emasculation: frontiers of bioethics, psychiatry, and microsurgical genital reconstruction. Clin Case Rep. 2020;8(9):1735–40.
4. Mawuko-Gadosseh Y, Mayele M, Gallouo M, Graiouid M, Dakir M, Debbagh A, Aboutaieb R. Automutilation des organes génitaux externes chez l'homme [Male genital self-mutilation: a case series]. Prog Urol. 2020;30(3):172–8.
5. Mosahebi A, Butterworth M, Knight R, Berger L, Kaisary A, Butler PEM. Delayed penile replantation after prolonged warm ischemia. Microsurgery. 2001;21(2):52–4.
6. Hu W, Lu J, Zhang L, Wu W, Nie H, Zhu Y, Deng Z, Zhao Y, Sheng W, Chao Q, Qiu X, Yang J, Bai Y. A preliminary report of penile transplantation. Eur Urol. 2006;50(4):851–3.
7. van der Merwe A, Graewe F, Zühlke A, et al. Penile allotransplantation for penis amputation following ritual circumcision: a case report with 24 months of follow-up. Lancet. 2017;390:1038–47.
8. Cetrulo CL Jr, Li K, Salinas HM, et al. Penis transplantation: first US experience. Ann Surg. 2018;267(5):983–8.
9. Szafran AA, Redett R, Burnett AL. Penile transplantation: the US experience and institutional program set-up. Transl Androl Urol. 2018;7(4):639–45. https://doi.org/10.21037/tau.2018.03.14.
10. Mohammadi D. The lab-grown penis: approaching a medical milestone. The Observer. 2014; https://www.theguardian.com/education/2014/oct/04/penis-transplants-anthony-atala-interview. Accessed 16 Mar 2015.
11. Evins SC, Whittle T, Rous SN. Self-emasculation: review of the literature, report of a case and outline of the objectives of management. J Urol. 1977;118(5):775–6.
12. Rodríguez Costa A, Romeo C, De Viedma LG, Agra Cadarso B. Amputación testicular traumática. Reimplantación con éxito mediante microcirugía [Traumatic amputation of the testicle. Successful reimplantation using microsurgery (author's transl)]. An Esp Pediatr. 1978;11(12):865–7.
13. Lin SD, Lai CS, Su PY. Replantation of the testis by microsurgical technique. Plast Reconstr Surg. 1985;76(4):620–5.
14. Xu YM, Wu P, Cai PC, Cheng ZC. Replantation of the testis: report of a case. J Urol. 1988;139(3):596–8.
15. Altarac S. A case of testicle replantation. J Urol. 1993;150(5 Pt 1):1507–8.
16. Shioshvili TI. A case of successful replantation of testis after autohemicastration. Eur Urol. 1987;13(4):285–6.

17. Ramdas S, Thomas A, Arun Kumar S. Temporary ectopic testicular replantation, refabrication and orthotopic transfer. J Plast Reconstr Aesthet Surg. 2007;60(7):700–3.
18. Phonsombat S, Master VA, McAninch JW. Penetrating external genital trauma: a 30-year single institution experience. J Urol. 2008;180(1):192–5; discussion 195–6.
19. Ehrich WS. Two unusual penile injuries. J Urol. 1929;21:239–41.
20. Cohen BE, May JW Jr, Daly JS, Young HH. Successful clinical replantation of an amputated penis by microneurovascular repair. Case report. Plast Reconstr Surg. 1977;59:276–80.
21. Tamai S, Nakamura Y, Motomiya Y. Microsurgical replantation of a completely amputated penis and scrotum: case report. Plast Reconstr Surg. 1977;60(2):287–91.
22. Li GZ, Man LB, He F, Huang GL. Replantation of amputated penis in Chinese men: a meta-analysis. Zhonghua Nan Ke Xue. 2013;19(8):722–6.
23. McCormick C, Dumais MG, Johnsen NV, et al. Male genital trauma at a level 1 trauma center. World J Urol. 2020;38:3283–9.
24. Biswas G. Technical considerations and outcomes in penile replantation. Semin Plast Surg. 2013;27(4):205–10.
25. Roche NA, Vermeulen BT, Blondeel PN, Stillaert FB. Technical recommendations for penile replantation based on lessons learned from penile reconstruction. J Reconstr Microsurg. 2012;28(4):247–50.
26. Becker M, Höfner K, Lassner F, Pallua N, Berger A. Replantation of the complete external genitals. Plast Reconstr Surg. 1997;99(4):1165–8.
27. Caygill PL, Floyd MS Jr, New FJ, Davies MC. A successful microsurgical approach to treating penile amputation following genital self mutilation. J Surg Case Rep. 2018;2018(10):rjy271.
28. Raheem OA, Mirheydar HS, Patel ND, Patel SH, Suliman A, Buckley JC. Surgical management of traumatic penile amputation: a case report and review of the world literature. Sex Med. 2015;3(1):49–53. https://doi.org/10.1002/sm2.54.
29. Leyngold MM, Rivera-Serrano CM. Microvascular penile replantation utilizing the deep inferior epigastric vessels. J Reconstr Microsurg. 2014;30:581–4.
30. Terayama T, Sakamoto T, Ikeuchi H, Tanaka Y. Self-penile glans amputation: a report of two cases. Acute Med Surg. 2016;4(1):101–4. Published 2016 May 27. https://doi.org/10.1002/ams2.199.
31. Manav S, Erdal AI, Genç İG, et al. Klingsor syndrome—microvascular replantation of penis after self-mutilation in schizophrenia. Indian J Surg. 2021;84:379.
32. Mineo M, Jolley T, Rodriguez G. Leech therapy in penile replantation: a case of recurrent penile self-amputation. Urology. 2004;63:981–3.
33. El Harrech Y, Abaka N, Ghoundale O, Touiti D. Genital self-amputation or the Klingsor syndrome: successful non-microsurgical penile replantation. Urol Ann. 2013;5(4):305–8.
34. Hage JJ. A unique case of secondary microvascular glansplasty: the last genitoreconstructive frontier? Ann Plast Surg. 2000;45(4):422–6.
35. Volkmer B, Maier S. Successful penile replantation following autoamputation: twice! Int J Impot Res. 2002;14:197–8.
36. Sanger JR, Matloub HS, Yousif NJ, Begun FP. Penile replantation after self-inflicted amputation. Ann Plast Surg. 1992;29(6):579–84.
37. Kabore FA, Fall PA, Diao B, et al. Auto-amputation récidivante du pénis sur terrain schizophrène: à propos d'un cas. Andrologie. 2008;18:224–6.
38. Sharma V, Sharma A. Autoamputation of genitalia in bipolar patient. Case Rep Psychiatry. 2017;2017:1–3.
39. Jandou I, Ettanji A, Kbirou A, Rkik M, Moataz A, Mohammed D, Debbagh A, Aboutaieb R. Penile strangulation and amputation in schizophrenic patients: a reports of two cases. Ann Med Surg (Lond). 2020;60:263–5.

Prognosis of Male Genital Self-Mutilation

55

Immediate consequences of GSM are bleeding whose severity depends on the anatomopathological level of injury. For obvious vascular reasons, penectomies provoke more severe bleeding than orchidectomy and may cause hypovolemic shock and even lead to death if unattended. Our review revealed not less than six deaths caused by GSM. One of them was a patient with self-penectomy and extragenital mutilations and autophagia who bled to death [1]. Other consequences are local infections and sepsis. Maggots and secondary myiasis of the penile stump were also described in a case with a late presentation [2]. In the great majority of the patients who survived a GSM, the prognosis can be studied in two separate subgroups: voluntary eunuchs and patients undergoing penile replantation.

55.1 Voluntary Eunuchs

Young age castrates were historically known to have gynecomastia, female muscular development, female fat distribution, taller height, absence, or smaller Adam's apple, and reduced pilosity compared to normal subjects. Bilateral orchidectomy provokes the so-called **impotentia generandi** (incapacity to procreate) but not **impotentia coeundi** (coital incapacity) [3, 4], hence castrates might still have an erection and perform sexual intercourses. This is the reason why captives were subjected to orchidectomies and phallectomy.

Through scientific studies on Skoptzy, Chinese, and Ottoman court eunuchs, Wilson and Roehrborn reported evidence of osteoporosis and consequent kyphosis, failure of closure of the epiphyses, reactive pituitary hyperplasia, shrinkage of the prostate, and development of gynecomastia [5]. In a survey of 92 voluntarily orchiectomized eunuchs, Brett et al. found that 52% of them appreciated the sense of control over sexual urges and appetite. There was a loss of libido in 66%, hot flashes in 63%, and genital shrinkage in 55%. Twenty-two percent reported a change in sexual orientation, and 60% had to take supplemental hormone treatments to

S. A. AL-Mamari, *Urogenital Trauma: A Practical Guide*,
https://doi.org/10.1007/978-981-99-6171-9_55

counteract the side effects of castration. The survey also showed that 53% of the castrations were not performed by medical professionals [6].

55.2 Post-penile Replantation

The following discussion must be considered only in situations where effective psychiatric management is achieved, and full collaboration is gained from the patients.

Two metanalyses recruiting a total of 217 patients have shown an overall complication rate of 73% with the most frequent being skin necrosis (54.8–58%), followed by skin sensory abnormality (27.9–31.6%), venous congestion (20.2%), erectile dysfunction (12.6–22.5%), urethral stricture (11–14.4%), and fistula (6.6–7.2%). Nonetheless **91.6% of patients reported overall satisfaction** [7, 8]. Babaei and Safarinejad reported on 27 successful microsurgical reimplantations out of 30 in a review that clearly demonstrated that the macrosurgical technique which was performed in 50 cases exposed to higher rates of fistula formation, urethral stenosis, skin necrosis, loss of sensation, and erectile dysfunction. Nonetheless, they found that microsurgical replantation is not a panacea since spontaneous erections and penetration ability with a full sensation of the glans are rare [9].

References

1. Koops E, Püschel K. Selbstverstümmelung und Autophagie [Self-mutilation and autophagia]. Arch Kriminol. 1990;186(1–2):29–36.
2. Tomita M, Uchijima Y, Okada K, Yamaguchi N. A report of self-amputation of the penis with subsequent complication of myiasis. Hinyokika Kiyo. 1984;30(9):1293–6.
3. Androutsos G, Marketos S. La castration à travers les âges. Andrologie. 1993;3(1):61–6.
4. Aucoin MW, Wassersug RJ. The sexuality and social performance of androgen-deprived (castrated) men throughout history: implications for modern day cancer patients. Soc Sci Med. 2006;63(12):3162–73.
5. Wilson JD, Roehrborn C. Long-term consequences of castration in men: lessons from the Skoptzy and the eunuchs of the Chinese and Ottoman courts. J Clin Endocrinol Metab. 1999;84(12):4324–31.
6. Brett MA, Roberts LF, Johnson TW, Wassersug RJ. Eunuchs in contemporary society: expectations, consequences, and adjustments to castration (Part II). J Sex Med. 2007;4(4 Pt 1):946–55.
7. Li GZ, Man LB, He F, Huang GL. Replantation of amputated penis in Chinese men: a meta-analysis. Zhonghua Nan Ke Xue. 2013;19(8):722–6.
8. Morrison SD, Shakir A, Vyas KS, Remington AC, Mogni B, Wilson SC, Grant DW, Cho DY, Rahnemai-Azar AA, Lee GK, Friedrich JB, Mardini S. Penile replantation: a retrospective analysis of outcomes and complications. J Reconstr Microsurg. 2017;33(4):227–32.
9. Babaei AR, Safarinejad MR. Penile replantation, science or myth? A systematic review. Urol J. 2009;4(2):62–5.

Summary of Male Genital Self-Mutilations (GSM)

56

Male genital self-mutilation is an old phenomenon accompanying humanity since the dawn of time.

Having no racial, religious, social, or geographical barriers, this multifactorial malady is mostly governed by either acute or chronic impaired mental statuses of various degrees, where schizophrenia plays an important role with the contribution of many imbricated direct or indirect causes.

Besides schizophrenia, another important subgroup is made of voluntary eunuchs. However, even the motivations of the latter are multiple and sometimes unclear, adding to the complexity of this maze.

Except for a minority of subjects who disclose their intentions or who have already attempted self-inflicted injuries, preventive management is not applicable to the great majority of the patients.

Nowadays, apart from the Hijras in India, GSMs are sporadic. Nonetheless, they can be assumed to occur all over the world, although the interest of local researchers varies from one region to another.

In more than one-third of the cases, male GSM involves the removal of the penis alone. Bilateral orchidectomy is second in occurrence followed by combined bilateral orchidectomy with penectomy, while unilateral orchidectomy and other minor mutilations or lacerations are found in a small percentage only.

Provided early and effective psychiatric management is initiated peri-operatively and maintained well beyond, modern surgical refinement with the introduction of microvascular technique allows better cosmetic and functional results in penile replantation which should always be considered whenever possible. Yet macrovascular replantation remains an option when a microvascular technique cannot be performed either due to the absence of equipment or lack of expertise.

Although GSM cannot be fully comprehended and anticipated in the great majority of cases, learning the fundamentals of the surgical management of these injuries is of paramount importance for any urologist who wishes to prepare himself/herself for an encounter with a GSM case in his/her daily practice, and early management

S. A. AL-Mamari, *Urogenital Trauma: A Practical Guide*,
https://doi.org/10.1007/978-981-99-6171-9_56

and continuous surveillance by the psychiatrist are a sine qua non for the success of the intervention in short and long term.

Correction to: Grading of Renal Trauma

Correction to:
Chapter 5 in: S. A. AL-Mamari, *Urogenital Trauma: A Practical Guide*, https://doi.org/10.1007/978-981-99-6171-9_5

Figure 5.2 has been removed for copyright reasons.

The updated version of this chapter can be found at
https://doi.org/10.1007/978-981-99-6171-9_5

S. A. AL-Mamari, *Urogenital Trauma: A Practical Guide*,
https://doi.org/10.1007/978-981-99-6171-9_57

Index

S. A. AL-Mamari, *Urogenital Trauma: A Practical Guide*,
https://doi.org/10.1007/978-981-99-6171-9

U

V

W

Y

GPSR Compliance

The European Union's (EU) General Product Safety Regulation (GPSR) is a set of rules that requires consumer products to be safe and our obligations to ensure this.

If you have any concerns about our products, you can contact us on ProductSafety@springernature.com

In case Publisher is established outside the EU, the EU authorized representative is:

Springer Nature Customer Service Center GmbH
Europaplatz 3
69115 Heidelberg, Germany

Batch number: 10726058

Printed by Printforce, the Netherlands